AAS
Agents and Actions Supplements
Vol. 38/I

Series Editors
K. Brune, Erlangen
M. J. Parnham, Bonn

Birkhäuser Verlag
Basel · Boston · Berlin

Recent Progress on Kinins

Biochemistry and Molecular Biology
of the Kallikrein-Kinin System

Proceedings of the International Conference "Kinin 91 Munich",
held in Munich, September 8–14, 1991

Edited by

H. Fritz
W. Müller-Esterl
M. Jochum
A. Roscher
K. Luppertz
(Technical Editor)

Birkhäuser Verlag
Basel · Boston · Berlin

Volume Editors' Addresses:

Editors:

Prof. Dr. Hans Fritz
Abteilung für Klinische Chemie
und Klinische Biochemie in der
Chirurgischen Klinik Innenstadt
der Universität München
Nussbaumstrasse 20
D–8000 München 2

Prof. Dr. Marianne Jochum
Abteilung für Klinische Chemie
und Klinische Biochemie in der
Chirurgischen Klinik Innenstadt
der Universität München
Nussbaumstrasse 20
D–8000 München 2

Technical Editor:

Dr. Karin Luppertz
Abteilung für Klinische Chemie
und Klinische Biochemie in der
Chirurgischen Klinik Innenstadt
der Universität München
Nussbaumstrasse 20
D–8000 München 2

Prof. Dr. Werner Müller-Esterl
Institut für Physiol. Chemie
Johannes-Gutenberg-Universität
Duesbergweg 6
D–6500 Mainz 1

Prof. Dr. Adelbert Roscher
Dr. von Haunersches Kinderspital
der Universität München
Lindwurmstrasse 4
D–8000 München 40

A CIP catalogue record for this book is available from the Library of Congress,
Washington D.C., USA

Deutsche Bibliothek Cataloging-in-Publication Data

Recent progress on kinins. – Basel ; Boston ; Berlin : Birkhäuser.
  (Agents and actions : Supplements ; Vol. 38)
  ISBN-13: 978-3-0348-7323-9
NE: International Conference Kinin <1991, München>; Agents and actions / Supplements
1. Biochemistry and molecular biology of the kallikrein kinin system. – 1992

**Biochemistry and molecular biology of the kallikrein kinin
system** : proceedings of the International Conference "Kinin 91
Munich", held in Munich, September 8–14, 1991 / ed. by
H. Fritz ... – Basel ; Boston ; Berlin : Birkhäuser, 1992
  (Recent progress on kinins ; 1)
  (Agents and actions : Supplements ; Vol. 38)
  ISBN-13: 978-3-0348-7323-9
NE: Fritz, Hans [Hrsg.]

© 1992 Birkhäuser Verlag
Softcover reprint of the hardcover 1st edition 1992
  P.O. Box 133
  4010 Basel/Switzerland

ISBN-13: 978-3-0348-7323-9   e-ISBN-13: 978-3-0348-7321-5
DOI: 10.1007/978-3-0348-7321-5

CONTENTS

Kallikreins and Kallikrein Inhibitors

Kininogens and Cysteine Proteinase Inhibitors

Kininases and Kininase Inhibitors

Kinin Receptors and Kinin Antagonists

Localization of Kallikreins and Kininogens

Opening Address

Hans FRITZ

Department of Clinical Chemistry and Clinical Biochemistry, Surgical Clinic City,
University of Munich, Nussbaumstr. 20, D-8000 Munich 2, F.R.G.

Dear colleagues, dear friends, ladies and gentlemen:

Welcome to KININ '91 MUNICH nearly exactly 10 years after KININ '81 MUNICH!

The International KININ Conferences and KININ '91 MUNICH

The International KININ Conferences are meetings with tradition. I had the pleasure to participate in seven of them, starting with ROCHA E SILVA's meeting in Rio de Janeiro in 1967, which was followed by the Conferences in Reston (1974), Tokyo (1978), Munich (1981), Savannah (1984), and again in Tokyo (1987).

It is my great regret that the president of the last KININ Conference, Prof. Hiroshi MORIYA from the Science University of Tokyo, passed away on June 27th of this year.

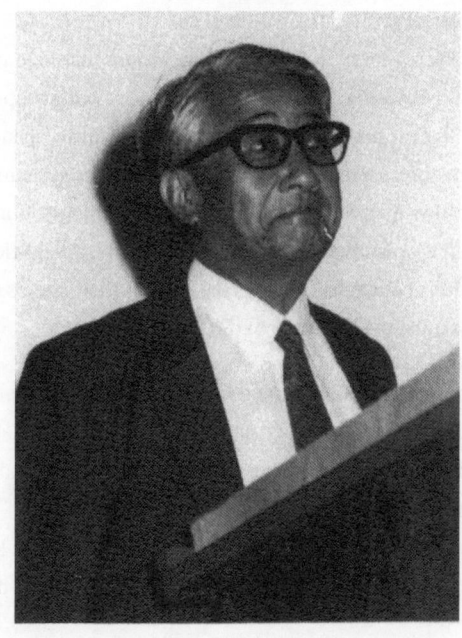

With the death of Hiroshi MORIYA the KININ family has lost a great scientist with a warm personality, and many of us a good friend. His major scientific achievements were his early studies on porcine pancreatic kallikrein in the late fifties and his subsequent studies on (1) the microheterogeneity of tissue kallikreins, (2) the carbohydrate structures of porcine and human urinary kallikrein, (3) the structure and activation mechanism of prokallikrein, (4) the characteristics of kinin-inactivating enzymes from mushrooms, (5) the resorption of kallikrein and its effect on the absorption of amino acids and glucose from small intestine, and (6) very recently, the localization of kallikrein in prolactin-producing cells in the rat anterior pituitary and pineal glands together with KIZUKI and KITAGAWA.

Next Thursday afternoon the International Advisory Board will recommend or probably decide where the next KININ Conference will take place. The major problem for each organizer is the financing: 10 years ago in 1981 we had total costs of approx. 350 000 DM (which equals 200 000 US $); this year we will approach 900 000 DM or 500 000 $. This is a 2.5 fold increase in 10 years, and only approx. 30% is income from participants.

This situation caused a special problem in view of the participation of junior scientists and of scientists coming from countries with weak currency. They comprise approx. 20% of the audience of this Conference. Their participation on a low or even zero cost level was made possible by the generous financial support provided by the institutions, companies and individuals listed in the program. The organizers and the participants would like to express their sincere thanks to all of them. *We are especially greatful to the E.K. Frey-E. Werle Foundation of the Henning L. Voigt Family for taking over the auspieces and providing the financial basis for KININ '91 MUNICH.*

I will point out some peculiarities of this KININ Conference.
First the program: Despite the fact that no scientist presents more than one talk, the program contains 132 oral contributions and over 190 posters in the various symposia, workshops, poster sessions and special lectures. In addition, approx. 30 oral presentations are anticipated in the panel discussions. The scientific program covers also important topics related to the kallikrein-kinin systems such as pathophysiology of inflammation, proteinase inhibition as a therapeutic tool, coagulation and fibrinolysis as well as kinins and nitric oxide or ion channels. The planning of this comprehensive scientific program was possible only because of the efforts of numerous colleagues all over the world - their names are given in the program - and especially the concentrated work and the expertise of the local organizers.

For those participants joining for the first time an International KININ Conference, I would like to introduce the local organizers:
GERD BÖNNER, Cologne: The expert in physiological, pharmacological and medical aspects of the kallikrein-kinin systems and their components.
GÜNTHER DIETZE, Bühl: Internal medicine is his hobby and profession, kinin-mediated effects are his scientific interest since he met E.K. FREY in Munich and became his personal doctor.

MARIANNE JOCHUM, Munich: She is an expert in pathophysiology of inflammation and proteinase inhibition therapies. She will become professor of pathobiochemistry in a few days.

KRISTIAN RETT, Munich: Scholar of Günther Dietze with the same profession and scientific interest.

ADALBERT ROSCHER, Munich: A clinical biochemist; his scientific work is focussed on the pharmacology of kinin receptors.

BERNWARD SCHÖLKENS, Frankfurt: Expert for kinin receptor antagonists, their design, synthesis and pharmacological or clinical effectiveness.

THOMAS UNGER, Heidelberg: A professional pharmacologist for kininases, ACE inhibitors and kinin receptor antagonists.

WERNER MÜLLER-ESTERL, Mainz: A biochemist; his scientific hobby are the kininogens as well as the kinin receptors and everything which is somehow related to these multifunctional proteins.

On behalf of the local organizing committee and myself I want to thank everyone in the audience who contributed to making the program comprehensive, exciting and up-dated, and especially the following collegues: T. BERG, Oslo, K. BHOOLA, Bristol, A. CUTHBERT, Cambridge, C. KLUFT, Leiden, R. MAC-DONALD, Dallas, M. SCHACHTER, London, E. FINK, Munich, M. KATORI, Kanagawa, W. HELLER, Tübingen, M. GALLIMORE, Tübingen, R. BURCH, Baltimore, R.J. MILLER, Chicago, J. STEWART, Denver, E. WHALLEY, Denver, D. PROUD, Baltimore, and A. SCHMAIER, Ann Arbor.

The second event I would like to mention with great satisfaction is the participation - for the first time - of scientists and colleagues from East Germany, the former GFR, and East Europe including the Soviet Union or Russia (now GUS). We should congratulate them and the entire world on the political developments of these days which were incredible to us at the last KININ Conference in Tokyo.

My personal request to the scientists of the KININ family in USA, Japan and Brazil is: Please, invite our colleagues from these countries to visit your laboratories so that they can see the progress there from first hand and, please, visit their labs in order to transfer thereby as much knowledge as possible to a generation of scientists, which did not give up contact with KININS despite the long, frustating period they had to experience without what we feel is most necessary to enjoy life: Liberty and - from their point of view - nearly unbelievable good priviledges. Collaboration on a worldwide basis is the best guarantee for a peaceful future for all of us.

The third event which is new here, is the award of the *FREY-WERLE Commemorative Medal* and the *FREY-WERLE Promotion Prize* (5000,- US $), donated by the *E.K. Frey-E. Werle Foundation of the Henning L. Voigt Family*, for outstanding scientific contributions in the field of the kallikrein-kinin systems. All participants of KININ '91 MUNICH are cordially invited to join this academic event which will take place Friday evening in the Auditorium Maximum of the University of Munich; on this occasion a famous string quartett will play Mozart and Beethoven. The Rektor of the University and the Foundation with its promotor Henning L. VOIGT would be pleased to welcome you at the final reception.

Such an academic event could become tradition in forthcoming KININ Conferences. We believe that the public appreciation of outstanding scientific contributions in the field would be also a great stimulus for scientists all over the world to the benefit of the scientific progress and patients as well.

The Scientific Program of KININ '91 MUNICH

Originally I intended to finish now my introduction by wishing you an exciting and motivating stay in the Bavarian Capital, Munich. We had agreed that Werner MÜLLER-ESTERL - he has a chair at Institute for Pathobiochemistry in Mainz - should, as second speaker, reflect on the highlights of the scientific program and the historical development in the area during the last decade. He is especially qualified for such a task because of the broad experience he gained in the kallikrein-kinin field during his long stay in our Department, which came out of Eugen WERLE's chair and Institute for Clinical Chemistry and Clinical Biochemistry at the University of Munich. However, a severe accident at home has made it impossible for Werner to join us this week. He sends all participants of KININ '91 MUNICH and especially his numerous friends in the audience his kindest regards. He has promised me to train hard to achieve an early recovery, that means, his physical comeback. As far as his scientific input is concerned, Werner is on the top as ever; this can be easily appreciated from *his ideas and words in the following text* he faxed to me some days ago.

The motto of this Conference was deliberately chosen: "Towards a better understanding of the molecular basis of kinin action"; it reflects the status quo of the field and outlines one of the major goals, i.e. the precise comprehension of the molecular mechanisms underlying the pleiotropic effects of the pluripotent kinin peptides.

Looking back: Since the days of the last KININ meeting in Munich we have witnessed a tremendous development of our field. Profiting from the then newly developed techniques of molecular biology an unanticipated progress has been made including the following hallmarks:

1. Molecular cloning and structural definition of the large *kallikrein gene family* as well as elucidation of the subtle structural differences determining the spectrum of specificities of otherwise closely related enzymes.
2. Molecular cloning and primary structure analysis of the various types of *mammalian kininogens*; they are now known as paradigms of multifunctional proteins; they have taught us a lesson in the evolution of multidomain proteins. We have witnessed the merger of the research areas of kininogens and plasma cysteine proteinase inhibitors and the major acute phase protein.
3. Molecular cloning of the kininases, above all the angiotensin-converting enzyme, revealing the key structural features of that particular exopeptidase. We have witnessed an unforeseen success of specific ACE inhibitors in the therapy of essential hypertension, a convincing example for the benefitial application of *proteinase inhibition therapy*.
4. The very recent molecular cloning of the kinin B2 receptor indicating the kinins' actions are mediated by the heptahelical rhodopsin-like receptor type. This salient feature has become the *self-explanatory logo of the Conference.*

5. Last but not least the *development of specific kinin receptor antagonists* of the first and the second gene-
    ration which aid in exploring and differentiating the multiple physiological effects of the kinins.

This only highlights some of the major achievements of the KININ community in the past ten years or so; of
course, considerable progress has been made in related areas such as the physiology and pathophysiology of
the kallikrein-kinin systems. These achievements reflect a concerted effort of a truly international endeavour
involving groups from all over the world. In this respect it is a pleasure to point out that the kallikrein-kinin
research area is among the few biochemical fields that has entertained an active community in the eastern
countries, especially in the Soviet Union (GUS).

Looking ahead - the prospects are bright. With the available tools we are in the position to pinpoint every
single component of the kallikrein-kinin systems (KKS) in any given tissue both on the gene and the protein
level. This should allow us to learn about the tissue distribution of kinin receptors, and the potential role of
kinins as candidate neurotransmitters in the brain. The *kinin antagonists* will proof indispensable work
horses to discriminate between the various physiological, pharmacological, and pathological effects of the
kinins. In addition, they will become valuable drugs to treat various diseases. Moreover, we will learn about
the evolution of the KKS as a prototypic peptidergic system fulfilling complex biological roles.

To illustrate this evolutionary issue: Finding that the kinin and the angiotensin receptors share an unexpected degree of sequence coincidence points to the fact that the two underlying systems share more than
just one cross-road, i.e. the converting enzyme. Rather this finding might be indicative of a common ancestor
of the two counteracting systems suggesting that they evolved from a much more primitive precursor system
driving blood pressure in an undirectional way. So this is why investigation into more esoteric species such
as insects or primitive chordates is considered to be meaningful because it might reveal predicted precursor
systems or - equally interesting - uncover an unique case of convergent evolution. So let's go Drosophila...!

Furthermore, getting a clearer picture of the structures of the various constituents of the KKS, their molecular interplay and mechanisms should, in turn, aid in the rational design of drugs that either inhibit or augment
the inherent activities of the system depending on what is needed to treat conditions such as hypertension,
inflammation, or contact-mediated hyperçoagulability.

Two requests: *First*, our achievements should release the brakes imposed on our research effort - intellec-
tually, financially, personally, institutionally - and guide us to the long-searched "true" physiological roles of
the kinins. *Second*, we strongly vote for a (often practiced) free exchange of reagents that have been developed in our community, without any constraints, for the benefit of our scientific enterprise, and in the spirit
of an international community with far-reaching and ambitious goals in perspective.

In this way we will collect the missing Rosetta stones which will allow us to decipher the remaining myste-
ries of the kallikrein-kinin system.

The E.K. Frey-E. Werle Foundation
of the Henning L. Voigt Family

In September 1988 the businessman and publisher *Henning Leonard Voigt* gave one million DM to establish an incorporated public foundation according to civil law with its seat in Munich. The purpose of this foundation, the *E.K. Frey-E. Werle Foundation of the Henning L. Voigt Family*, is the promotion of science and research in the field of cardiology, haemostasiology and metabolism in particular to explain the significance of the kallikrein-kinin system and systems communicating with it. The Foundation pursues exclusively and directly nonprofit-making purposes and is selflessly active. Its basic assets are currently in excess of one million DM. *Organs of the Foundation* are the Foundation Executives and the Board of Trustees, which has 8 to 10 members in accordance with the articles. The Board of Trustees currently includes Dr. J. Burkhardt (*Judicial Officer*), Prof. Dr. G. Dietze (Head of Max-Grundig-Klinik, Bühl), F. Friedberger (LMU Honorary Senator, former LMU Chancellor), Prof. Dr. H. Fritz (*2nd Chairman*), Prof. Dr. K. Peter (*1st Chairman*, Dean of the LMU Medical Faculty), Prof. Dr. F.W. Schildberg (Head of LMU Surgical Clinic Großhadern), Prof. Dr. W. Steinmann (Rektor of LMU), Prof. Dr. L. Schweiberer (Head of LMU Surgical Clinic City), Prof. Dr. N. Zöllner (*Vice-chairman*, Head of LMU Medical Policlinic City), Mr. Henning L. Voigt (Promoter of the Foundation, LMU Honorary Senator).

On the occasion of the "E.K. Frey Week" (symposia in memoriam to E.K. Frey's 100th birthday) the Foundation awarded in 1988 (Sept. 14) during an academic celebration in the Auditorium Maximum of the Ludwig-Maximilians-Universität München (LMU Munich) for the first time the

> *E.K. Frey - E. Werle Promotion Prize* and the
> *E.K. Frey - E. Werle Commemorative Medal*

by the President of the LMU Munich, the *Prize to G. Bönner* (Cologne/Germany) and *W. Jauch* (Munich/Germany) and the *Medal to E.G. Erdös* (Chicago/USA). On the occasion of an academic celebration of the "Sonderforschungsbereich 207 der Ludwig-Maximilians-Universität München" in 1989 (April 28) at the same place, the President of the LMU Munich awarded the Promotion Prize and Commemorative Medal of the Foundation the second time, the *Prize to W. Bode* (Munich/Germany) and the *Medal to R. Huber* (Munich/Germany).

On the occasion of KININ '91 MUNICH the Promotion Prize and Commemorative Medal of the Foundation have been awarded the third time, again at the same place, by the Rektor of the LMU Munich, Professor Dr. W. Steinmann, to three scientists from abroad,

> the *Medal* to   *J. Stewart* (Denver/USA) and
> the *Prize* to   *C.D. Figueroa* (Valdivia/Chile) and
>   *A. Schmaier* (Ann Harbor/USA).

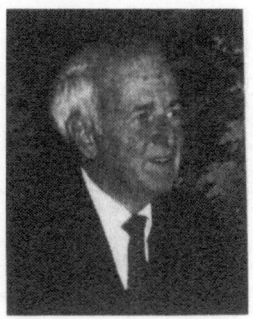

Henning L. Voigt
Promotor of the Foundation
Honorary Senator of
the LMU Munich

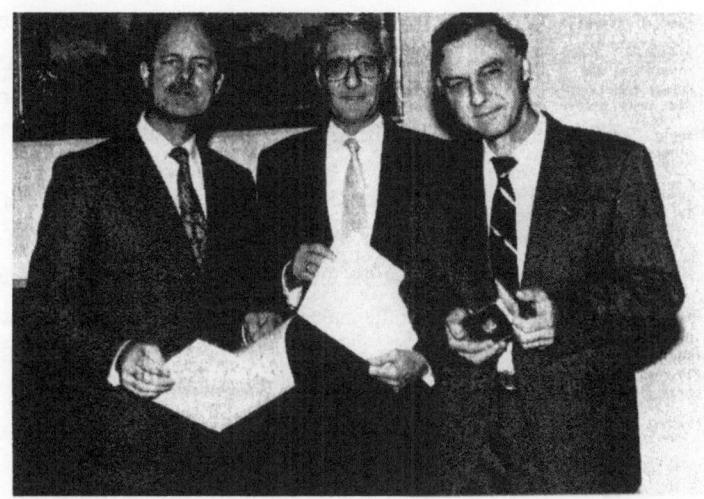

W. Bode	**W. Steinmann**	**R. Huber**
Prize	President of the	Medal
1989	LMU Munich	1989

Prize and Medal 1988
See "The Kallikrein-Kinin System in Health and Disease". International Symposium,
Munich, September 12-17, 1988. H. Fritz, I. Schmidt and G. Dietze (Eds.), Limbach-
Verlag Braunschweig, pp. 35-45, 1989.

AAS 38/I
Recent Progress on Kinins
© 1992 Birkhäuser Verlag Basel

The E.K. FREY - E. WERLE FOUNDATION
of the HENNING L. VOIGT FAMILY

Academic Celebration on Friday, September 13, 1991

Prof. Dr. Wulf Steinmann

Rektor of the Ludwig-Maximilians-University Munich

The KININs: A "Münchner Kindl"

In 1925 the surgeon E.K. FREY, a scholar of Sauerbruch, injected human urine into dogs while searching for the substance inducing anuria in newly operated patients. At that time he could not imagine the significance of the hypotension he observed and what this observation would lead to. His experiment, the first of a series of studies performed together with the physiologist H. KRAUT in the basement of the Surgical Department of the University at the Nußbaumstraße, was the birth of the KININs.

How KININs "appear and disappear" was unravelled later by the chemist E. WERLE, the third of the German pioneers in the field of the KININs. Later, WERLE was first to become head of a Department of Clinical Chemistry in Germany, again located at the Surgical Department at the Nußbaumstraße. FREY, KRAUT, and WERLE observed and documented the majority of the biologic effects of the KININs, until - starting in the 50'ies - the KININs were recognized world-wide. From about 1939, the Brazilian scientist ROCHA E SYLVA contributed significantly to the understanding of the KININs.

The KININs and the Kallikrein-KININ System

KININs can be imagined as a chain of 9-11 pearls (i.e. amino acids). This chain of pearls is cut from larger chains consisting of several hundreds of amino acids, the *kininogens*, high molecular weight proteins ubiquitous in the organism. The two cuts are made by highly specialized scissors (i.e. proteolytic enzymes or proteinases), the *kallikreins*. The KININs are much too potent to be left in the organism without causing harm - within seconds they are broken apart by other specialized proteases, the *kininases*.

In a healthy organism the cooperation of all components of this kallikrein-kinin system is well organized. Thus, KININs are liberated only on demand and are subsequently inactivated rapidly and metabolized. Already in minute amounts (1/1,000,000,000,000 of a gram) they are biologically active, causing diverse effects such as contraction of smooth muscle cells (thus regulating the tension of the capillary vascular bed and the blood pressure) and transport of salts and water through membranes (thus regulating kidney function and urine production).

An excessive liberation of KININs caused either by an abnormal stimulation of the kallikrein-kinin system or by a defective or missing component of this system potentially may lead to diseases - I will go into detail later.

Recognition of Superb Scientific Achievements

320 scientific reports presented and discussed during the 6 days of the international congress KININ '91 MUNICH indicate the central role played by KININs and the kallkrein-kinin system today. However, despite being well recognized by specialists, the outstanding achievements in this field are little known to the general public. Therefore, it is particularly meritorious that the businessman and publicist Henning L. VOIGT - he has recently been appointed honorary senator of the Ludwig-Maximilians-University - supported with generous donations the establishment of a foundation dedicated to honour outstanding scientific contributions in this complex field and to relate them to the public.

In the name of the *E.K. Frey - E. Werle Foundation and the Henning L. Voigt Family* I twice had the honour and the pleasure to award distinguished scientists with the *E.K. Frey - E. Werle Commemorative Medal* and the *E.K. Frey - E. Werle Prize*.

In 1988 the medal was awarded for the first time to Ervin ERDÖS (Chicago) for his fundamental work on the structure, properties and function of kininases. This work led to the development of synthetic inhibitors of kininase II, also called "angiotensin converting enzyme" or ACE. Inhibition of this enzyme has been proven useful for the therapy of essential hypertension and is now used world-wide. On the same occasion the prize was given to Gerd BÖNNER (Cologne) for his investigations concerning the role of the renal kallikrein-kinin system in the pathogenesis of arterial hypertension and the fate of ACE inhibitors in the human organism, and to Karl-Walter JAUCH (Munich) for the first application of KININs and ACE inhibitors as therapeutic drugs in severely ill intensive care patients.

In 1989, medal and prize were awarded to the Nobel laureate Robert HUBER and to Wolfram BODE, his long time colleague at the Max-Planck-Institute for Biochemistry in Martinsried. Together they revealed many three dimensional structures of proteases, inhibitors and protease-inhibitor complexes. Their results made it possible to understand the interaction of inhibitors and proteases in detail on a molecular basis. Currently, their results are utilized for the "computer-aided" construction of inhibitors targeted at specific enzymes, potential drugs in the therapy of protease-related diseases.

Today, the *Prize* will be awarded for the third time to two scientists with outstanding contributions in the field of the kallikrein-kinin system. Both scientists share a mutual interest in aspects of the cell biology of the kallikrein-kinin system. Due to the limited time during this celebration it is obvious that I can address only some highlights of their work.

First to the recipients, Carlos FIGUEROA from Valdivia/Chile and Alvin SCHMAIER from Ann Arbor/USA.

Neutrophil granulocytes are among the most important, rapidly reacting defense cells, constituting an emergency system guarding the organism against invaders such as bacteria, fungi and viruses, and initiating wound healing after injuries. Until recently the link between the tissue kallikrein-kinin system and the reaction of these cells during the inflammatory response of the organism was not recognized. Carlos FIGUEROA in the group of Kanti BHOOLA (Bristol/England) was the first to detect *tissue kallikrein in lysosomal granules of neutrophil leukocytes*, thus presenting the first clear cut evidence for the involvement of tissue kallikrein and KININs in this important cellular defense mechanism. In addition, the same group demonstrated that kininogens, the parent substance of KININs, are present on the outer membrane of these cells. Together, both observations were the basis of a new and exciting working hypothesis: During the activation of defense cells tissue kallikrein is released which in turn liberates KININs from membrane-bound kininogens. KININs were already known to open the intercellular junctions between the endothelial cells of the inner surface of the blood vessels; thus, the liberation of KININs near defense cells may facilitate their passage through endothelial layers and thus their entrance into the surrounding tissue, accelerating their arrival at injured, inflamed, or infected areas. Although further cell biologic studies are required to verify this hypothesis, the results of Carlos FIGUEROA and his colleagues clearly indicate a role of the kallikrein-kinin system in the defense function of neutrophil leukocytes. In addition, their work has a major impact on the medical research in the area of the inflammatory response, particularly on the development of novel anti-inflammatory drugs.

Platelets constitute another important cell population of the organism. These cells carry multiple functions involved in the healing of wounds and essential for the rapid occlusion of vessels after injuries. Platelets are rapidly activated by the clotting protease thrombin which induces their aggregation, leading to a primary occlusion of the injured vessel. Subsequently, plasmatic clotting processes are initiated on the surface of platelets, causing the formation of a fibrin clot and a stable occlusion of the vessel. However, initiation of these processes in the wrong place, e.g. at stenoses or at vessel endothelium injured by smoking, may also lead to vessel occlusion and thus to diseases such as thrombosis or cardiac infarction. Our current knowledge of the *role of kininogens in the cellular reaction of platelets* stems predominantly from the work of Alvin SCHMAIER who performed most of these studies together with Robert COLEMAN in Philadelphia/USA. He demonstrated that kininogens bear special binding regions for their attachment to the outer membrane of platelets, and that platelets themselves are capable to synthesize kininogens which may in turn bind to platelets after being released during platelet activation. After being bound, kininogens may act in opposite ways: high molecular kininogen may support clotting whereas both high and low molecular weight kininogen (the latter species is normally present in much higher amounts) may inhibit activation of platelets by thrombin. Alvin SCHMAIER's demonstration of this dual function of kininogens, which may induce or block coagulation, depending on demand, is rather exciting. From a medical point of view the binding regions for platelets located in the heavy chains of both kininogens are of particular interest: They may be identified and partial, homologue structures may be produced using chemical synthesis or genetic engineering with the aim to develop "natural" inhibitors of coagulation as drugs for the prophylaxis of thrombosis.

In the last part of my talk I will come to the KININs and thus to the reason to award the *E.K. Frey - E. Werle Commemorative Medal* to John STEWART (Denver/USA). As the scientists among us know, already minute amounts of KININs activate many cells, inducing various biologic effects mandatory for diverse physiological functions of the organism. However, in excessive amounts KININs may act as inflammatory mediators, causing major harm to the organism, e.g. by inducing

- edema leading to dysfunction of organs and possibly death,
- contraction of bronchial muscles, thus initiating asthma attacks,
- a massive drop of blood pressure leading to the severe shock,
- severe pain.

Pathological effects of KININs are also mediated by cells, i.e. they are caused by excessive activation of specific cell types. The first and most important step involved is the binding of KININs to special KININ receptors on the surface of cells. The binding of KININs to these receptors causes the activation of the cell, inducing a response specific for each cell type, e.g. contraction of smooth muscle cells.

John STEWART concentrated early on KININ receptors as an approach to block the KININ-induced activation of cells and thus their pathological effects. After 22 years of laborious work he succeeded in synthesizing the first compounds active as antagonists of KININs. Similar to KININs themselves, these antagonists bind to KININ receptors, however, without activating cells. Although the principles involved appear elementary, the construction of compounds with high specificity and activity and thus with a high therapeutic impact was very difficult. With his pioneering work John STEWART provided the guidance for the continuing effort of many scientists.

Currently, the production of KININ antagonists for therapeutic use has a high priority in many pharmaceutical companies. The usefulness of KININ antagonists as therapeutic drugs for inflammatory and allergic diseases as well as a tool in the research on the physiological and pathophysiological action of KININs is a priority topic of the International KININ Congress held this week in Munich, demonstrating the accelerating development in the area of KININ receptors and their antagonists.

Finally, in the name of the *E.K. Frey - E. Werle Foundation of the Henning L. Voigt Family* I like to express my satisfaction that we may demonstrate these rapid developments to you and the public during this celebration.

(Translated from the German version by Dr. Christian Sommerhoff, Munich)

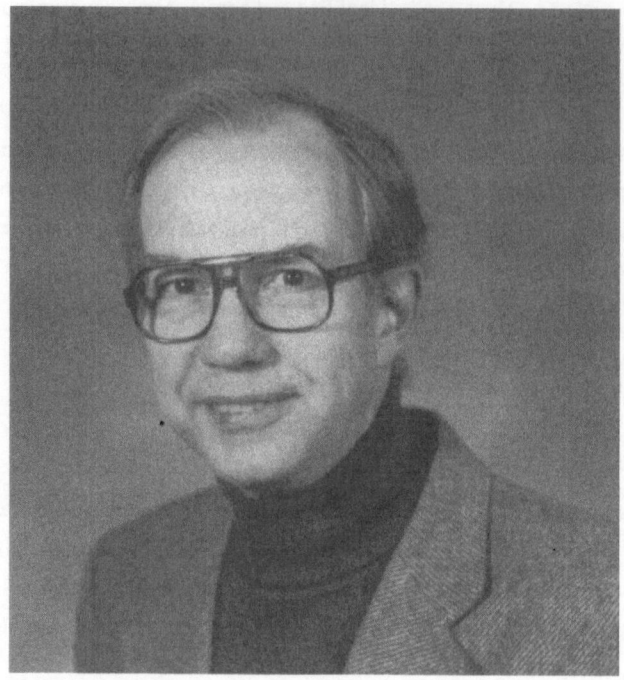

The

E.K. FREY - E. WERLE FOUNDATION

of the HENNING L. VOIGT FAMILY

awarded during an
academic celebration
on the occasion of
the International Conference
KININ '91 MUNICH
in Munich on September 13, 1991

**Professor Dr.
John M. STEWART**

Professor of Biochemistry
at the University of Colorado
School of Medicine,
in Denver, Colorado/USA

The

E.K. FREY - E. WERLE

COMMEMORATIVE MEDAL

in recognition
of his outstanding investigations
on
chemistry and pharmacology of

PEPTIDE HORMONES

and especially on
the design and synthesis of potent

KININ AGONISTS and ANTAGONISTS

.

E.K. FREY - E. WERLE
FOUNDATION of the
HENNING L. VOIGT FAMILY

H.L. Voigt   G. Dietze   H. Fritz
The promoter   *The Foundation Executives*

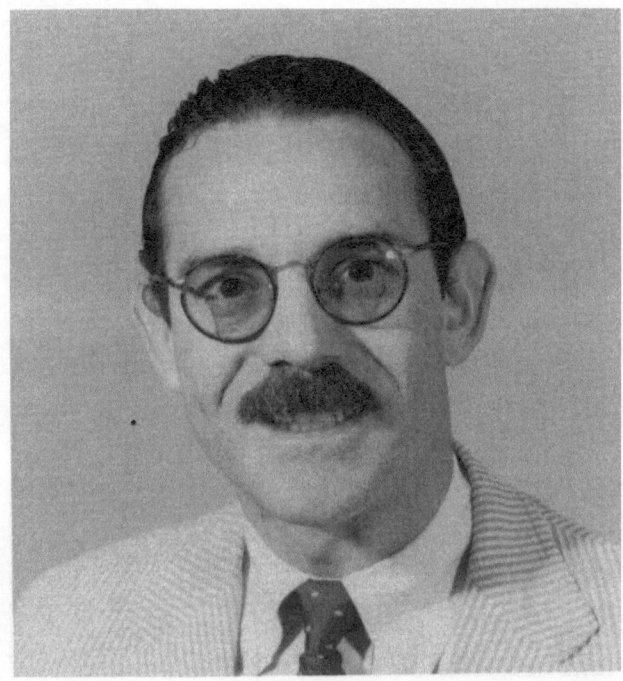

<table>
<tr><td>

The

E.K. FREY - E. WERLE FOUNDATION

of the HENNING L. VOIGT FAMILY

awarded during an
academic celebration
on the occasion of the
International Conference
KININ '91 MUNICH
in Munich on September 13, 1991

Professor Dr.
Alvin H. SCHMAIER

Professor of Internal Medicine
at the
Temple University School of Medicine
in Philadelphia,
Pennsylvania/USA

</td><td>

The

E.K. FREY - E. WERLE

PROMOTION PRIZE

in recognition
of his outstanding investigations
on
the effects, mechanisms of action,
and functional roles of

KININOGENS

and their interactions with cells
mediating blood coagulation and inflammation

E.K. FREY - E. WERLE
FOUNDATION of the
HENNING L. VOIGT FAMILY

H.L. Voigt   G. Dietze   H. Fritz
The promoter   *The Foundation Executives*

</td></tr>
</table>

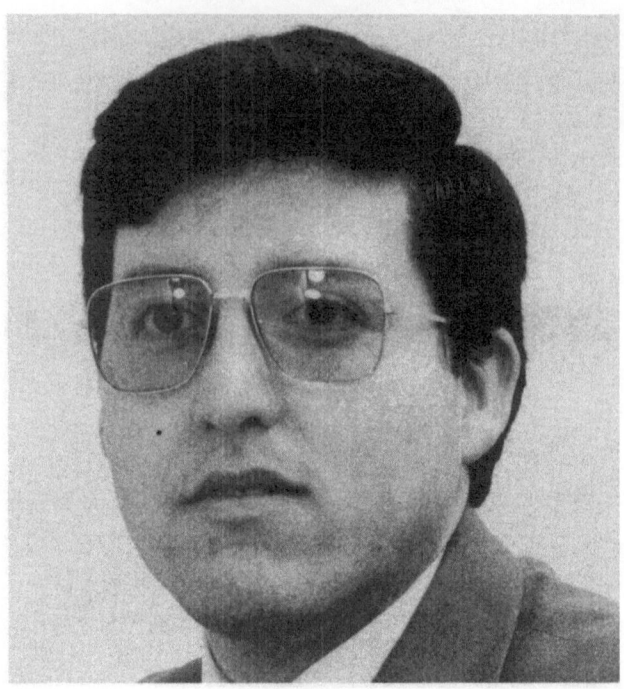

The	The
E.K. FREY - E. WERLE FOUNDATION	E.K. FREY - E. WERLE
of the HENNING L. VOIGT FAMILY	PROMOTION PRIZE

The

E.K. FREY - E. WERLE FOUNDATION

of the HENNING L. VOIGT FAMILY

awarded during
an academic celebration
on the occasion of the
International Conference
KININ '91 MUNICH
in Munich on September 13, 1991

Dr. Carlos D. FIGUEROA

Lecturer in Pathology
at the Austral University
in Valdivia, Chile

The

E.K. FREY - E. WERLE

PROMOTION PRIZE

in recognition of his outstanding
investigations on the cellular
and subcellular localization of

TISSUE KALLIKREIN and KININOGENS

in various organ tissues and cells
and in neutrophils implying new functional
roles of the kallikrein-kinin systems
in the inflammatory response

E.K. FREY - E. WERLE
FOUNDATION of the
HENNING L. VOIGT FAMILY

H.L. Voigt   G. Dietze   H. Fritz
The promoter   *The Foundation Executives*

© 1992 Birkhäuser Verlag Basel

Acceptance of the Frey-Werle Medal

John M. STEWART

Professor STEINMANN, Senator VOIGT, Members of the E.K. FREY-E. WERLE Foundation of the Henning L. VOIGT Family, Ladies and Gentlemen:

It is a great honor for me to receive the E.K. Frey-E. Werle Memorial Medal as the third recipient, following Ervin ERDÖS and Robert HUBER. I am happy to accept this medal, not only for myself, but also on behalf of all those persons who have worked on the bradykinin project in my laboratory. I wish to acknowledge especially the work of Dr. Raymond VAVREK in development and synthesis of bradykinin antagonists.

It is now 65 years since Professor FREY published his initial studies on the kallikrein system, and 30 years since announcement of the amino acid sequence of bradykinin by ELLIOTT and synthesis by BOISSONNAS. I began the search for a bradykinin antagonist two years later, in 1962, at Rockefeller University, with the encouragement of Professor D.W. WOOLLEY. That search eventually led to discovery of practical bradykinin antagonists in 1984.

I first had the opportunity to meet Professor WERLE in 1965 at the KININ symposium in Florence, Italy. Then and ever since I have greatly admired him for his pioneering, careful work with Professor FREY in the kallikrein-kinin field.

The long time between knowledge of the structure of bradykinin and discovery of useful antagonists is a reflection of the uncharted paths to be followed and the lack of guidelines to show the way. The problem was to design an analog of bradykinin modified in such a way that it still retained high affinity for bradykinin receptors on cells, but lacked any efficacy; it could not "turn on" the cells to perform the functions normally evoked by bradykinin. Even today, with our knowledge of the primary structures of receptors for bradykinin and other peptide hormones, the search is still largely one of trial and error. Our eventual discovery of the antagonists came after many unsuccessful trials. But in these unsuccessful attempts we learned many things that eventually proved useful after we had discovered the critical structure modification that yielded the first antagonists.

Work by many scientists during many years has shown that bradykinin and related kinins are directly involved in the regulation of every physiological system in the body, and that many illnesses arise from pathological over-production of these kinins. Such conditions as asthma, the common cold, arthritis and septic shock can be mentioned. Drugs available now for treatment of these, and other, kinin-mediated diseases are far from beeing completely sucessful. Bradykinin antagonists now offer the hope of much better drugs for these diseases.

Since our demonstration of successful bradykinin antagonists, many others have entered the search for improved antagonists. At this time probably fifteen pharmaceutical companies have bradykinin antagonist programs. At this congress we have heard announcements of remarkable progress in this direction. It is a source of great personal pleasure to me to have been instrumental in helping to make such progress possible. I look forward eagerly to the future years, for I am sure we shall see many exciting new developments in the bradykinin antagonist field.

Again, I wish to express my great thanks to the FREY-WERLE Foundation for this honor, and to the Henning L. VOIGT FAMILY for their generosity.

Thank you.

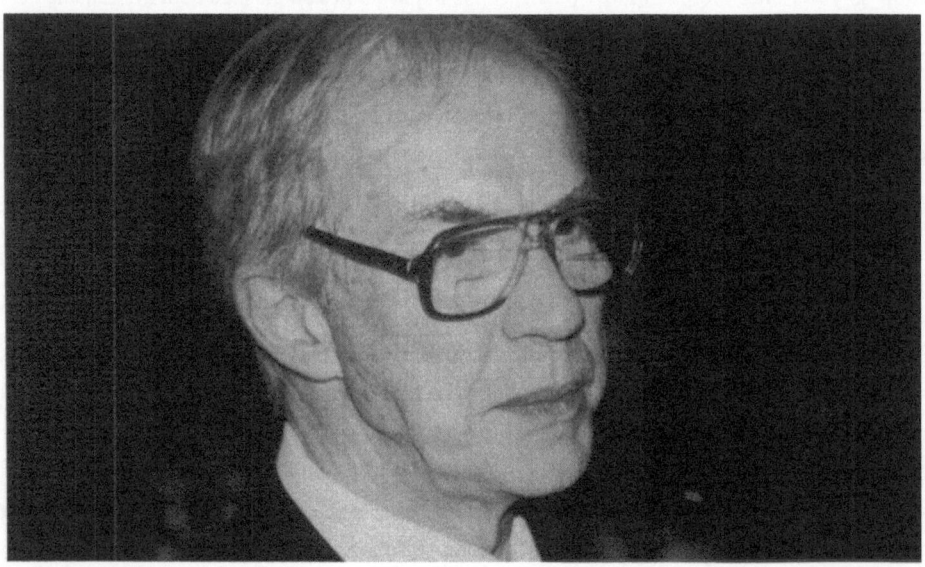

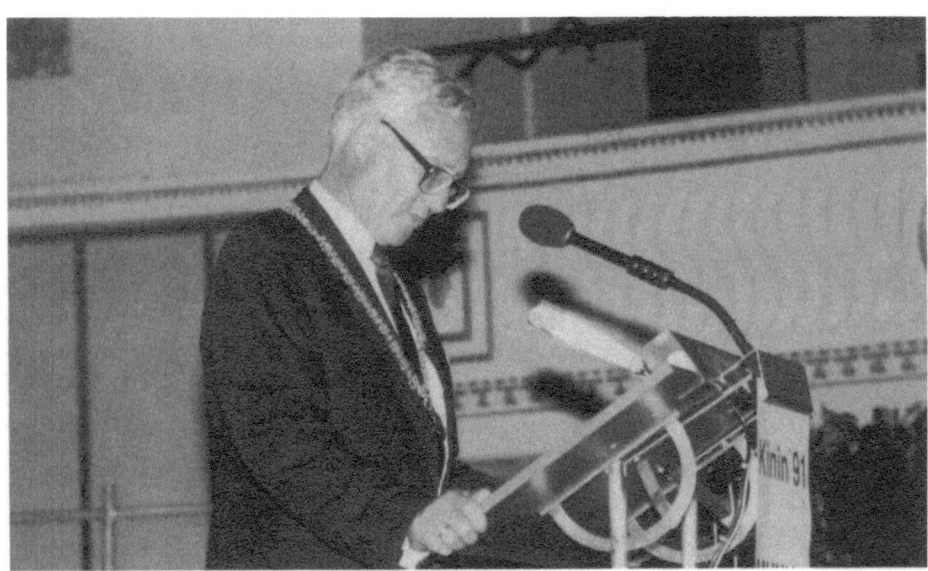

Prof. Dr. Wulf Steinmann,
Rektor of the Ludwig-Maximilians University Munich,
during his eulogy at the Academic Celebration

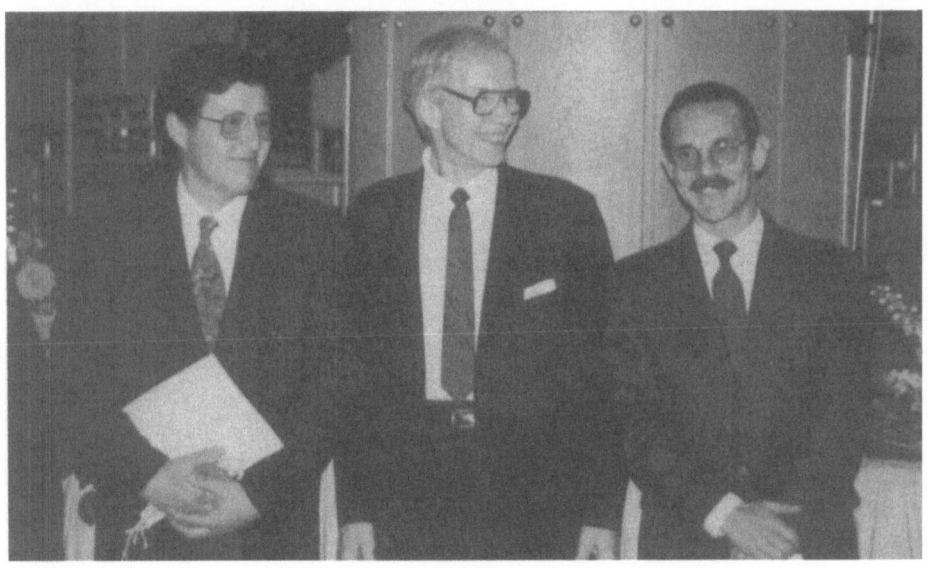

The honoured scientists
Carlos D. Figueroa, John M. Stewart, and Alvin H. Schmaier

Kallikreins and Kallikrein Inhibitors

A COMMON NOMENCLATURE FOR MEMBERS OF THE TISSUE (GLANDULAR) KALLIKREIN GENE FAMILIES

T. Berg[1], R. A. Bradshaw[2], O. A. Carretero[3], J. Chao[4], L. Chao[4], J. A. Clements[5], M. Fahnestock[6], H. Fritz[7], F. Gauthier[8], R. J. MacDonald[9], H. S. Margolius[10], B. J. Morris[11], R. I. Richards[12], A. G. Scicli[3].

[1]Institute of Physiology, University of Oslo, 0317 Oslo 3, Norway;

[2]Department of Biological Chemistry, California College of Medicine, University of California, Irvine, CA 92717;

[3]Hypertension and Vascular Research Division, Henry Ford Hospital, Detroit, MI 48202;

[4]Department of Biochemistry and Molecular Biology, Medical University of South Carolina, Charleston, SC 29425;

[5]Prince Henry's Institute of Medical Research, Clayton, Vic 3168 Australia;

[6]Department of Biomedical Sciences, McMaster University, Hamilton, Ontario, L8N 3Z5, Canada;

[7]Abteilung fur Klinische Chemie und Biochemie, Universitat Munchen, 8000 Munchen 2, Germany;

[8]University Francois Rabelais, CNRS URA1334, F-37032 Tours Cedex, France;

[9]Department of Biochemistry, UT Southwestern, Dallas, TX 75235-9038;

[10]Department of Pharmacology, Medical University of South Carolina, Charleston, SC 29425;

[11]Department of Physiology, University of Sydney, Sydney, N.S.W. 2006, Australia;

[12]Department of Cytogenetics and Molecular Genetics, Adelaide Children's Hospital, North Adelaide S.A. 5006, Australia.

During the KININ '91 MUNICH Symposium a workshop met to formulate a common nomenclature for tissue kallikreins that would codify family member designations, correct redundancies and clarify ambiguities. A common designation, based on the stem KLK, was proposed for the kallikrein gene families (Table I). KLK is the designation assigned to human kallikrein gene family members by the Human Genome Mapping Nomenclature Committee (HGMNC) and has recently been accepted by the International Committee on Standardized Genetic Nomenclature for Mice.

To conform with the conventions for genetic loci, the designation for all species but mouse will be italicized upper case letters (*KLK*); the designation for mouse is *Klk* (also italicized). Individual genes of the family for each species will have assigned Arabic numerals. A hyphen precedes the numeral for the mouse gene designations only. For currently known family

Table I. Recommended Nomenclature for Tissue Kallikrein Gene Families.

Species	HGMNC approved gene designation	abbreviated designations Genes/mRNAs	Proteins
mouse	*MMU Klk-1*, etc.	*mKlk-1*, etc.	mK1, etc.
human	*HSA KLK1*, etc.	*hKLK1*, etc.	hK1, etc.
rat	*RNO KLK1*, etc.	*rKLK1*, etc.	rK1, etc.

members the assigned identifying numbers will coincide as much as possible with currently used numbering (see Tables II through V). Newly discovered members will be assigned higher numbers in the order of their publication or submission for publication. The use of the same numerical designation for kallikrein genes in different species is not meant to indicate genes whose encoded proteins have homologous functions, except for the tissue (renal) kallikreins for human, mouse, rat and possibly pig, all of which now have the numerical designation 1 (one).

The species designation approved by the HGMNC is a three-letter upper case abbreviation (italicized) comprising the first letter of the genus and the first two letters of the species [Table I and *SSC* for *Sus scrofa* (pig); *CCO* for *Cavia cobaya* (guinea pig); *CFA* for *Canus familiaris* (dog)]. The workshop recommended that for convenience an abbreviated designation may be used, if desired, that includes a single (or when necessary a double) lower case letter designation for the species (e.g., *mKlk* for the mouse, *gpKLK* for the guinea pig, etc.; see Tables II through V). If the abbreviated designation is used, the family members should always be identified in a manuscript first by their formal designations as defined above. An mRNA will be designated according to the gene that encodes it (e.g., *RNO KLK1* mRNA or *rKLK1* mRNA; see Table I).

The workshop also recommended a modified designation that would distinguish the protein form of family members. This designation will be an upper case K, preceded by the lower case species designation and followed by the family member identification number (see Table I). Proteins with generic names already in use would retain that name (e.g., tissue kallikrein or renal kallikrein for the products of *hKLK1, mKlk-1* and *rKLK1*), but could also (or simultaneously) be designated as hK1, mK1 and rK1, respectively. For discussions of protein structure, it was recommended strongly that amino acid sequence numbering follow the chymotrypsin convention.

The workshop established a nomenclature group to assign identification numbers to newly discovered family members. New members of a family for each species would be added sequentially regardless of whether the gene, mRNA or protein was described first. However, to attain a designation with a number, sufficient amino acid or nucleotide sequence information must be available to uniquely identify a new member and to distinguish it from the others. Numbers will be assigned only for manuscripts published or in press to prevent reserving numbers for unsubstantiated members. Researchers who identify new kallikrein genes are requested to contact a member of the nomenclature group prior to submission for publication. The nomenclature group is Ray MacDonald [(214) 688-3477; FAX (214) 688-8856], Lee Chao [(803) 792-4321; FAX (803) 792-4322], Margaret Fahnestock [(416) 525-9140, Ext. 3344; FAX (416) 521-0048] and Francis Gauthier [(33) 47 36 60 45; FAX (33) 47 36 60 46].

Tables II through IV contain a compilation of known members for the human, mouse and rat families; Table V lists tissue kallikreins from other species. The tables include the new designation (abbreviated form), previous designations and synonyms for each family member. Only those proteins with sufficient amino acid sequence information to identify a corresponding gene are included in the listings.

Table II. The Human Tissue Kallikrein Gene Family (approved species designation: HSA)

New Designation	Previous Designations	mRNA/cDNA	Protein	New Protein Designation
hKLK1	KLK1[1,2], hRKALL[3]	λHK1[4] & phKK25[5] cDNAs	tissue kallikrein[6,14] (renal/pancreas/salivary)	hK1
hKLK2	KLK2[7], hGK-1[8], hKK-3[5]			hK2
hKLK3	PSA[9], PA[10], APS[1,2]	λHPSA-1[11] & PSA[12] cDNAs	PSA[13] (prostate -specific antigen)	hK3

1. Sutherland, G.R., Baker, E., Hyland, V.J., Callen, D.F., Close, J.A., Tregear, G.W., Evans, B.A., and Richards, R.I. (1988). Cytogenet. Cell Genet. 48:205-207.
2. Le Beau, M.M., Ryan, D., and Pericak-Vance, M.A. (1989). Cytogenet. Cell Genet. (Human Gene Mapping 10) 51:338-357.
3. Evans, B.A., Yun, Z.X., Close, J.A., Tregear, G.W., Kitamura, N., Nakanishi, S., Callen, D.F., Baker, E., Hyland, V.J., Sutherland, G.R., and Richards, R.I. (1988). Biochemistry 27:3124-3129.
4. Baker, A.R., and Shine, J. (1985). DNA 4:445-450.
5. Fukushima, D., Kitamura, N. and Nakanishi, S. (1985). Biochemistry 24:8037-8043.
6. Lottspeich, F., Geiger, R., Henschen, A., and Kutzbach, C. (1979). Hoppe-Seyler's Z. Physiol. Chem. 360:1947-1950.
7. Ropers, H.H., and Pericak-Vance, M.A. (1990). Cytogenet. Cell Genet. (Human Gene Mapping 10.5) 55:218-228.
8. Schedlich, L.J., Bennetts, B.H., and Morris, B.J. (1987). DNA 6:429-437.
9. Digby, M., Zhang, X-Y., and Richards, R.I. (1989). Nuc. Acids Res. 17:2137.
10. Riegman, P.H.J., Vlietstra, R.J., van der Korput, J.A.G.M., Romijn, J.C., and Trapman, J. (1989). Biochem. Biophys. Res. Commun. 159:95-102.
11. Lundwall, A., and Lilja, H. (1987). FEBS Lett. 214:317-322.
12. Schulz, P., Stucka, R., Feldmann, H., Combriato, G., Klobeck, H.-G., and Fittler, F. (1988). Nuc. Acids Res. 16:6226.
13. Watt, K.W.K., Lee, P-J., M'Timkulu, T., Chan, W-P., and Loor, R. (1986). Proc. Natl. Acat. Sci. USA 83:3166-3170.
14. Lu, H.S., Lin, F-K., Chao, L., and Chao, J. (1989). Int. J. Peptide Protein Res. 33:237-249.

Table III. The Mouse Tissue Kallikrein Gene Family (approved species designation: MMU)

New Designation	Previous Designations	mRNA/cDNA	Protein	New Protein Designation
mKlk-1	mGK-6[2,11]	pMAK3[24]	tissue/renal kallikrein	mK1
mKlk-2	mGK-2[1,2]	pseudogene		
mKlk-3	mGK-3[2,3]	pmγN[4] & pSM676[6] cDNAs	γNGF[5]	mK3
mKlk-4	mGK-4[2,3]	2A4 cDNA[7]	αNGF[8,9]	mK4
mKlk-5	mGK-5[2,10]			mK5
mKlk-6	mGK-1[1]			mK6
mKlk-7	mGK-7[2]	pseudogene		
mKlk-8	mGK-8[2]	pMF-2 cDNA[12]		mK8
mKlk-9	mGK-9[2,13]	MB1-73 cDNA[14]	EGF-BP C[15]	mK9
mKlk-10	mGK-10[2]	pseudogene		
mKlk-11	mGK-11[2,16]			mK11
mKlk-12	mGK-12[2]	pseudogene		
mKlk-13	mGK-13[2,13]	pPRECE cDNA[22]	EGF-BP B[18], PRECE[22]	mK13
mKlk-14	mGK-14[2]			mK14
mKlk-15	mGK-15[2]	pseudogene		
mKlk-16	mGK-16[2,19]		γ–renin[20]	mK16
mKlk-17	mGK-17[2]	pseudogene		
mKlk-18	mGK-18[2]	pseudogene		
mKlk-19	mGK-19[2]	pseudogene		
mKlk-21	mGK-21[2]			mK21
mKlk-22	mGK-22[2,13]		βNGF-endopeptidase[21], EGF-BP A[18], enzyme A[25]	mK22
mKlk-23	mGK-23[2]	pseudogene		
mKlk-24	mGK-24[2]			mK24
mKlk-25	mGK-25[2]	pseudogene		
mKlk-26		pSGP-2[17] & pPRECE-2[23] cDNAs	PRECE-2[23]	mK26

1. Mason, A.J., Evans, B.A., Cox, D.R., Shine, J., and Richards, R.I. (1983). Nature 303:300-307.
2. Evans, B.A., Drinkwater, C.C., and Richards, R.K. (1987). J. Biol. Chem. 262:8027-8034.
3. Evans, B.A., and Richards, R.I. (1985). EMBO J. 4:133-138.
4. Ullrich, A., Gray, A., Wood, W.I., Hayflick, J. and Seeburg, P.H. (1984). DNA 3:387-392.
5. Thomas, K.A., Baglan, N.C., and Bradshaw, R.A. (1981). J. Biol. Chem. 256:9156-9166.
6. Howles, P.N., Dickinson, D.P., DiCaprio L.L. , Woodworth-Gutai, M., and Gross, K.W. (1984). Nuc. Acids Res. 12:2791-2805.
7. Isackson, P.J., Ullrich, A., and Bradshaw, R.A. (1984). Biochemistry 23:5997-6002.
8. Ronne, H., Anundi, H., Rask, L., and Peterson, P.A. (1984). Biochemistry 23:1229-1234
9. Isackson, P.J., and Bradshaw, R.A. (1984). J. Biol. Chem. 259:5380-5383.
10. Drinkwater, C.C., and Richards, R.I. (1987). Nuc. Acids Res. 15:10052.
11. van Leeuwen, B.H., Evans, B.A., Tregear, G., and Richards, R.I. (1986). J. Biol. Chem. 261:5529-5535.
12. Fahnestock, M., Brundage, S., and Shooter, E.M. (1986). Nuc. Acids Res. 14:4823-4835.
13. Drinkwater, C.C., Evans, B.A., and Richards, R.K. (1987). Biochemistry 26:6750-6756.
14. Blaber, M., Isackson, P.J., and Bradshaw, R.A. (1987). Biochemistry 26:6742-6749.

15. Isackson, P.J., Silverman, R.E., Blaber, M., Server, A.C., Nichols, R.A., Shooter, E.M., and Bradshaw, R.A. (1987). Biochemistry 26:2082-2085.
16. Drinkwater, C.C., and Richards, R.I. (1988). Nuc. Acids Res. 16:10918.
17. Lundgren, S., Ronne, H., Rask, L., and Peterson, P.A. (1984). J. Biol. Chem. 259:7780-7784.
18. Anundi, H., Ronne, H., Peterson, P.A., and Rask, L. (1982). Eur. J. Biochem. 129:365-371.
19. Drinkwater, C.C., Evans, B.A., and Richards, R.I. (1988). J. Biol. Chem. 263:8565-8568.
20. Poe, M., Wu, J.K., Florance, J.R., Rodkey, J.A., Bennett, C.D., and Hoogsteen, K. (1983). J. Biol. Chem. 258:2209-2216.
21. Fahnestock, M., Woo, J.E., Lopez, G.A., Snow, J., Walz, D.A., Arici, M.J., and Mobley, W.C. (1991). Biochemistry 30:3443-3450.
22. Kim, W-S., Kazuhisa, N., Nakagawa, T., Kawamura, Y., Haraguchi, K., and Murakami, K. (1991). J. Biol. Chem. 266:19283-19287.
23. Kim, W-S., Nakayama, K., and Murakami, K. (1991). FEBS Lett. 293:142-144.
24. Douglass, J., Ranney, K., Uhler, M., Little, G., and Herbert, E. (1984). In *Molecular Biology of Development*. (Alan R. Liss) pp. 573-588.
25. Schenkein, I., Franklin, E.C., and Frangione, B. (1981). Arch. Biochem. Biophys. 209:57-62.

Table IV. The Rat Tissue Kallikrein Gene Family (approved species designation: RNO)

New Designation	Previous Designations	mRNA/cDNA	Protein	New Protein Designation
rKLK1	rGK-1[1] true tiss. kall.[19]	PS[2] RSK1105 cDNA[18]	tissue kallikrein[3], renal kallikrein	rK1
rKLK2	rGK-2[1] RSKG-5[5]	S2[2]	tonin[4]	rK2[20]
rKLK3	rGK-3[1,6] RSKG-50[5]	S1[2]		rK3
rKLK4	rGK-4[1,6]			rK4
rKLK5	rGK-5[1]	pseudogene?		
rKLK6	rGK-6[1,6]			rK6
rKLK7	RSKG-7[7]	K1[8]	k7[9], esterase B[10], proteinase A[11]	rK7
rKLK8	rGK-8[1]	P1[12]	k8[9]	rK8
rKLK9		S3[2]	SEV[13], KLP-S3[14], prostate K[21]	rK9[20]
rKLK10		rKLK10 mRNA[22]	endopeptidase k[15], antigen gamma[16], proteinase B[11] & T-kininogenase[17]	rK10[15]
rKLK11	rGK-7[1]	pseudogene?		
rKLK12	RSKG-3[7]			rK12
rKLK13	RSKG-9[18]	pseudogene		

1. Wines, D.R., Brady, J.M., Pritchett, D.B., Roberts, J.L., and MacDonald, R.J. (1989). J. Biol. Chem. 264:7653-7662.
2. Ashley, P.L., and MacDonald, R.J. (1984). Biochemistry 24:4512-4520.

3. Lazure, C., Seidah, N.G., Thibault, G., Genest, J. and Chretien, M. (1981). In *Peptides: Synthesis, Structure and Function. Proceedings of the VIIth American Peptide Symposium*, eds. D.H. Rich and M.R. Gross. (Pierce Chemical, Rockford, IL), pp. 517-520.
4. Boucher, R., Asselin, J., and Genest, J. (1974). Circ. Res. 34(Suppl. 1):203-209.
5. Shai, S-Y., Woodley-Miller, C., Chao, J., and Chao, L. (1989). Biochemistry 28:5334-5343.
6. Wines, D.R., Brady, J.M., Southard, E.M., and MacDonald, R.J. (1991). J. Mol. Evol. 32: 476-492.
7. Chen, Y-P., Chao, J., and Chao, L. (1988). Biochemistry 27:7189-7196.
8. Brady, J.M., and MacDonald, R.J. (1990). Arch. Biochem. Biophys. 278:342-349.
9. Elmoujahed, A., Gutman, N., Brillard, M., and Gauthier, F. (1990). FEBS Lett. 265:137-140.
10. Berg, T., Wassdal, I., and Sletten, K. (1992). J. Histochem. Cytochem. 40:83-92.
11. Kato, H., Nakanishi, E., Enjyoji, K., Hayashi, I., Oh-Ishi, S. and Iwanaga, S. (1987). J. Biochem. (Tokyo) 102:1389-1404.
12. Brady, J.M., Wines, D.R., and MacDonald, R.J. (1989). Biochemistry 28:5203-5210.
13. Yamaguchi, Y.T., Carretero, O.A., and Scicli, A.G. (1991). J. Biol. Chem. 266:5011-5017.
14. Berg, T., Schoyen, H., Wassdal, I., Hull, R., Gerskowitch, V.P., and Toft, K. (1992). Biochem. J., 281:819-828.
15. Gutman, N., Moreau, T., Alhenc-gelas, F., Baussant, T., Elmoujahed, A., Akpona, S., and Gauthier, F. (1988). Eur. J. Biochem. 171:577-582.
16. Berg, T., Wassdal, I., Mindroiu, T., Sletten, K., Scicli, G., Carretero, O.A., and Scicli, A.G. (1991). Biochem. J. 280:19-25.
17. Xiong, W., Chen, L.M., and Chao, J. (1990). J. Biol. Chem. 265:2822-2827.
18. Gerald, W.L., Chao, J., and Chao, L. (1986). Biochim. Biophys. Acta 866:1-14.
19. Inoue, H., Fukui, K., and Miyake, Y. (1989). J. Biochem. (Tokyo) 105:834-840.
20. Moreau, T., Brillard-Bourdet, M., Bouhnik, J., and Gauthier, F. (1992). J. Biol. Chem., in press.
21. Wang, C., Tang, C.Q., Zhou, G.X., Chao, L., and Chao, J. (1992). Biochem. Biophys. Acta, in press.
22. Ma, J.X., J. Chao, L. Chao, personal communication.

Table V. Tissue Kallikrein Genes of Other Species

New Designation	Previous Designations	Protein	New Protein Designation
PIG (approved species designation: *SSC*)			
pKLK1		pancreatic kallikrein[1,2,3,4]	pK1
GUINEA PIG (approved species designation: *CCO*)			
gpKLK1		tissue kallikrein I[5,6] (submaxillary)	gpK1
gpKLK2		tissue kallikrein II[5,6] (prostate), gpPK[7]	gpK2
DOG (approved species designation: *CFA*)			
dKLK1	DAgE1[8] cDNA	androgen-dependent arginine esterase[9]	dK1

1. Tschesche, H., Mair, G., Godec, G., Fiedler, F., Ehret, W., Hirschauer, C., Lemon, M., and Fritz, H. (1979) *Adv. Exp. Med. Biol. (Kinins II: Biochemistry, Pathophysiology and Clinical Aspects)* Vol. 120, Part A, pp. 245-260.
2. Fiedler, F., Fink, E., Tschesche, H., and Fritz, H. (1981). Methods Enzymol. 80:493-532.
3. Kamada, M., Ikekita, M., Kurahashi, T., Aoki, K., Kizuki, K., Moriya, H., Sweeley, C.C., Kamo, M., and Tsugita, A. (1990). Chem. Pharm. Bull. 38:1053-1057.

4. Bode, W., Chen, Z., Bartels, K., Kutzbach, C., Schmidt-Kastner, G., and Bartunik, H. (1983). J. Mol. Biol. 164:237-282.
5. Fiedler, F., Lemon, M.J.C., Hirschauer, C., Leysath, G. Lottspeich, F., Henschen, A., Gau, W., and Bhoola, K.D. (1983). Biochem J. 209:125-134.
6. Mayer, G., Bhoola, K.D., and Fiedler, F. (1989). *Adv. Exp. Med. Biol. (Kinins V)* 247:201-206.
7. Dunbar, J.C., and Bradshaw, R.A. (1987). Biochemistry 26:3471-3478.
8. Chapdelaine, P., Gauthier, E., Ho-Kim, M.A., Bissonnette, L., Tremblay, R.R., and Dube, J.Y. (1991). DNA and Cell Biol. 10:49-59.
9. Lazure, C., Leduc, R., Seidah, N.G., Chretien, M., Dube, J.Y., Chapdelaine, P., Frenette, G., Paquin, R., Tremblay, R.R. (1984). FEBS Lett. 175:1-7.

Note Added in Proof: According to international nomenclature conventions gene symbols do not include a designation for the species of origin, i.e. gene symbols are *Klk-1* (mouse), *KLK1* (all other species); *Klk-2, KLK2*; etc.

AAS 38/I
Recent Progress on Kinins
© 1992 Birkhäuser Verlag Basel

EVOLUTION OF THE KALLIKREIN GENE FAMILY

Stephen R. Murray, Julie Chao and Lee Chao

Department of Biochemistry and Molecular Biology
Medical University of South Carolina, Charleston, S.C., 29425, USA

SUMMARY: All kallikrein-like genes that have been studied to date are composed of 5 exons and the tertiary structures of the encoded enzymes are remarkably similar. In the mouse and rat, these genes are highly conserved, tightly linked and tandemly arranged. In other species, such as the human, the family is less well defined and seems to be much smaller than that of the mouse and rat. Although extensively studied, the exact physiologic significance is not known for many kallikrein gene family members, however, they are thought to play important roles in processing biologically important peptide precursors. Given the potential importance of these mammalian enzymes as a group of highly selective peptide processing enzymes, it would be helpful to know more about the ways in which this family varies from species to species, especially with respect to the size of the family in each species. The evolutionary mechanisms which have shaped this family of genes are largely unknown, however, enough data has been generated to begin understanding the pathway by which this gene family has evolved.

INTRODUCTION

The serine proteases are a large group of well-studied enzymes which have both general proteolytic and specific protein processing functions. Tissue kallikrein and related enzymes share extensive structural similarity with chymotrypsin and the other mammalian serine proteases. These enzymes have a common gene structure, their nucleic acid and amino acid sequences have a high degree of identity, and the tertiary structure of the proteins is very similar. The major structural changes that have occurred during evolution represent modifications of the same basic plan, mostly in the form of additions. Some proteases, such as blood coagulation factors, have added new domains to include Ca^{++}-binding activity and EGF-like regions while others have added the ability to bind to fibrin via the "kringle" domain (1). However, the kallikreins and their closest relatives, trypsin and chymotrypsin, have retained only the protease function.

Mice and rats have been shown to have large families of highly conserved tissue kallikrein-like genes encoding homologous enzymes which differ in their substrate specificities and tissue expression patterns (2). In the mouse, these genes number approximately 24 and are all tandemly arranged on chromosome 7 (3). The rat has between 10 and 17 kallikrein-like genes and they may be as closely linked as those in the mouse (4,5,6).

Curiously, other mammalian species do not seem to have such large families of kallikrein-like enzymes, and humans may have as few as 3-5 kallikrein-like genes (7,8), and to date only four human kallikrein-like genes or gene products have been described (reviewed in 9). These are tissue kallikrein (7,8,10), prostate-specific antigen (11,12), hKG-1, a kallikrein-like gene (13), and a fourth, partially characterized, gene (10). It is interesting to note however that two of the four known human kallikrein genes are tandemly arranged, and therefore at least two members of the human kallikrein gene family are as closely linked as those of the rodents (14). Previously we have used Southern blotting to show that the size of the kallikrein family seems to vary among the mammals (9). Within the rat and mouse families, the members are all tandemly linked and highly homologous (3,6), and the three well-characterized human genes are 60-70% identical to one another in both amino acid and nucleic acid sequences. All of the kallikrein genes described to date are 5-7kb long and consist of 5 exons. Furthermore, the exon-exon splice sites are conserved and the genes share a high degree of nucleotide sequence identity, both within and between species.

Kallikreins, and all members of the mammalian serine protease family, are thought to have arisen from a single common ancestral gene through gene duplications, exon shuffling and subsequent divergence (1,15). Wines et al (16) pointed out the importance of sequence exchanges and gene conversion in the concerted evolution of the members of the rat kallikrein family. However, we have looked at numerous mammalian species using genomic DNA Southern blotting and found that tissue kallikrein genes are conserved throughout the mammals (9). In this paper, we examine the primate kallikrein gene family in greater detail, and propose a model for the evolution of this family that includes separation events and divergent evolution to account for the differences found between the human and rodent gene families.

MATERIALS AND METHODS

Genomic DNA Preparation. DNA was prepared as follows. Three grams of animal tissue (usually liver) were pulverized in liquid nitrogen and the resulting powder was slowly added to 30 ml of 0.1M Na_2EDTA, pH 8.0, 4% Sarkosyl NL30, and mixed until dissolved. Cesium chloride was then added to a concentration of 1 g/ml and the resulting solution centrifuged at 17,000 x g for 30 min in a Beckman J21B centrifuge at 20°C. The protein layer was removed from the top of the solution and the underlying supernatant was layered over a 1.5 ml, 5.7 M CsCl cushion and spun at 150,000 x g at 20°C for 20 hr. The banded DNA was collected using a wide-bore Pasteur pipet, dialyzed against 100 mM Na_2EDTA, pH 8.0, treated with 20 µg/ml RNase A and 5 units/ml T_1RNase at 55°C for 1.5 hr., digested with 100 µg/ml proteinase K at 55°C for 1 hr., and extracted 3 times with phenol:choloroform:isoamyl alcohol (25:24:1) and 2 times with chloroform:isoamyl alcohol (24:1). Finally the DNA was dialyzed against 3 changes, 4 L each, of NATE (10 mM Tris-HCl, pH 8.0, 10 mM NaCl, 1 mM Na$_2$EDTA).

Southern Blotting.   Southern blots were performed essentially according to Southern (17). Ten µg of genomic DNA were digested with 50 units of restriction endonuclease for 18 hr.   The resulting DNA fragments were separated by electrophoresis through a 0.8% agarose gel and transferred to either nitrocellulose filters or Immobilon-N membranes (Millipore, Bedford, MA) via capillary action according to the method of Maniatis et al (18). Following baking, the filters were prehybridized and then hybridized with a ^{32}P nick-translated (1 X 10^8 CPM/µg) monkey tissue kallikrein cDNA probe (Lin et al, unpublished data).   After overnight hybridization, the filters were washed, dried and exposed to Kodak AR film at -80°C.

Sequence Comparisons.   The sequences of 10 kallikrein-like enzymes were aligned allowing for insertions and deletions according to their best fit. This process was aided by taking into account conserved features such as the aspartate-histidine-serine charge relay system and the position of cystine residues known to participate in disulfide bonds. The degree of identity was calculated according to the following formula:

$$\% \text{ Identity} = \frac{\text{Total residues - (\#mismatches + \#insertions +\#deletions)}}{\text{Total residues}}$$

This procedure was performed for both cDNA and amino acid sequence data.

Model Drawing. A model of the three dimensional structure of kallikrein-like enzymes was drawn based on the x-ray crystallographic findings for mammalian serine proteases. The numbering scheme follows the convention for chymotrypsin with the charge relay system members designated his-57, asp-102 and ser-195. The drawing represents a generalized structure for this class of related serine proteases and is shaded according to the sequence comparison findings (see above). Those areas of high conservation are darker than those of low conservation. The shading reflects general trends, and not the degree of identity of specific residues.

RESULTS

Anthropoidea Species Genomic DNA Southern Blot. Genomic DNA from all 5 hominoid primates (*Homo, Pan, Gorilla, Pongo* and *Hylobates*) as well as one old world monkey (*Papio*) and one new world monkey (*Saimiri*) was digested with Eco RI, blotted, and hybridized to a monkey (*Saimiri*) kallikrein cDNA probe according to the procedure in Materials and Methods (Figure 1). There are between 2 and 5 bands present in each species, and the overall pattern is similar between all 7 species demonstrating the conserved nature of the kallikrein gene family among the primates. A similar conservation of patterns is observed when other restriction enzymes are used (data not shown).

Human Genomic Blot. Human genomic DNA was digested with 8 different restriction

Human Genomic Blot. Human genomic DNA was digested with 8 different restriction endonucleases, fractionated on an agarose gel, and subsequently blotted and hybridized with a monkey tissue kallikrein cDNA probe. The resulting autoradiogram is shown in Figure 2. Most enzymes produced 3 or 4 bands of varying intensity. Comparison with the restriction patterns of the known human kallikrein genes reveals that not all of the bands can be accounted for by the known human kallikrein-like genes and each lane contains several weakly-hybridizing bands, suggesting the existence of several less-well conserved kallikrein-like genes.

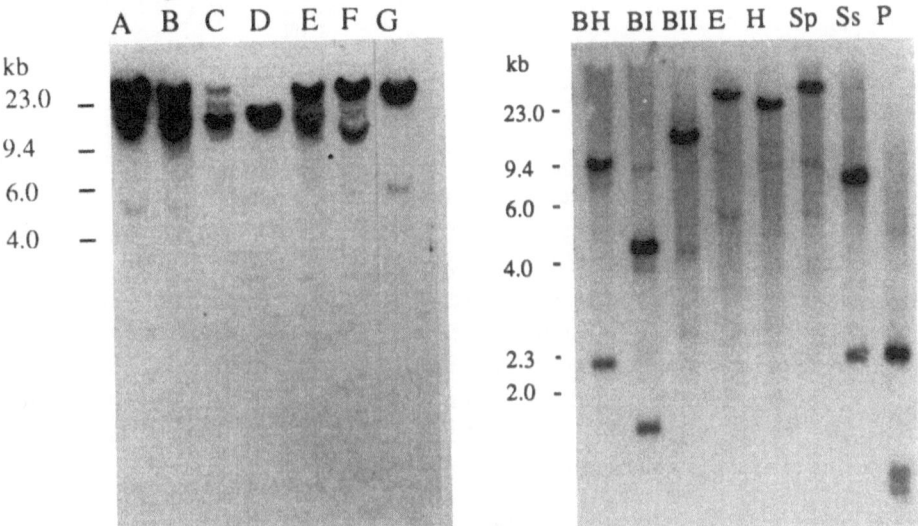

Figure 1 (left). Anthropoidea Species Genomic DNA Southern Blot. Samples are from (A) human (B) chimpanzee (C) gorilla (D) orangutan (E) gibbon (F) baboon and (G) monkey. Eco RI digested DNA was hybridized to a monkey kallikrein cDNA probe.

Figure 2 (right). Human Genomic Southern Blot. Human DNA was digested with: BamHI (BH), Bgl I (BI), Bgl II (BII), Eco RI (E), Hind III (H), Sph I (Sp), Sst I (Ss), and Pst I (P), and hyridized to a monkey kallikrein cDNA probe.

Sequence Comparisons. The cDNA and protein sequences for 10 kallikrein-like enzymes including 3 human kallikrein gene family members, 1 monkey kallikrein, 5 rat kallikreins, and 2 mouse kallikreins were aligned and the percent identity calculated as described in Materials and Methods. The calculated percent identities are tabulated in Table I. The identity varies from a high of 94% for the nucleic acid sequences and 91% for protein, between human and monkey kallikrein, to a low of 61% for nucleic acid sequences between RSKG-50 and human prostate-specific antigen, and 51% for protein, between rat tissue (pancreatic) kallikrein and human prostate-specific antigen. Note that the degree of identity follows the general phylogenetic relationship between the various species in that those that are more closely related have a higher degree of identity than those that are relatively more distant.

Table I: Degree of Identity Between Human Kallikrein and Other Kallikrein-Like Enzymes

Sequence	cDNA	Protein
Human Kallikrein (7,8)	100%	100%
Human Prostate-Specific Antigen (12)	73%	60%
hKG-1 (13)	74%	66%
Monkey Kallikrein (unpub. data)	97%	91%
Rat Pancreatic Kallikrein (19)	73%	59%
Tonin (4,20)	67%	53%
RSKG-50 (20)	68%	60%
RSKG-7 (21)	70%	60%
Mouse mGK-1 (22)	70%	61%
Mouse EBP (23)	69%	59%

Structural Comparisons. A generalized model for the 3-dimensional structure of kallikrein, as drawn from the x-ray crystallographic data for 5 mammalian serine proteases, is shown in Figure 3. The C-terminal helical region and the 12 b-sheets are represented by ribbons, and the connecting turns by bold lines. The numbering scheme follows the convention for chymotrypsin, with the charge relay system being numbered his-57, asp-102 and ser-195. The figure is shaded to reflect regional trends in the conservation of amino acid residues between the sequences compared above, with darker shading reflecting a higher degree of identity. Note that the most highly conserved residues are found on the interior of the molecule, while the external loop structures are more variable.

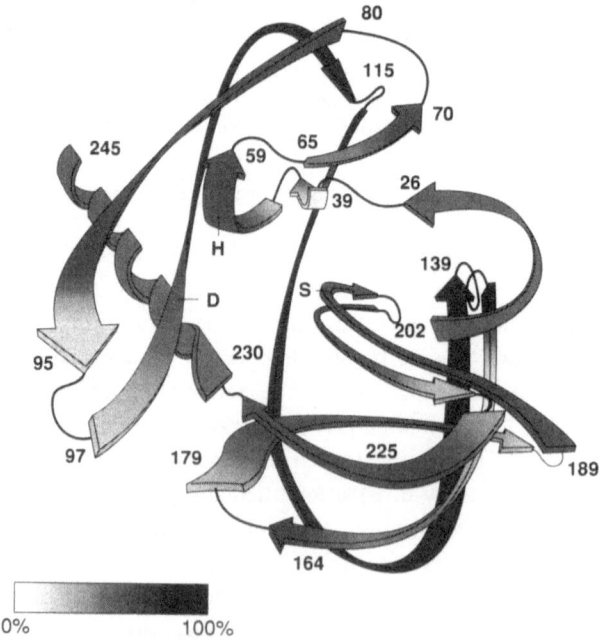

Figure 3. Regional conservation patterns of kallirein-like enzymes. The intensity of the shading reflects the degree of identity (0%-100%) of the various regions. Region 95-97 contains a 10 amino acid insertion called the kallikrein loop which is not present in other mammalian serine proteases.

DISCUSSION

The mammalian serine proteases are among the most thoroughly studied enzymes, and many members of this superfamily have been sequenced at either the protein or nucleic acid level. Despite a great diversity of activities, from the highly regulated and specific proteases of the blood coagulation cascade to the general digestive enzymes, all of the mammalian serine proteases have a great number of structural details in common.

Our Southern blots (Figures 1 and 2) demonstrate that tissue kallikreins are conserved throughout the primates. All species show 2 or 3 bands of similar size (Figure 1). Our previous studies of other mammals revealed a large variation in banding patterns that makes it difficult to determine the number of genes in the kallikrein family for a specific species without isolating and characterizing all the kallikrein-like genes in that species. However, despite these differences, all the mammals studied cross-hybridized with a monkey kallikrein nucleic acid probe, demonstrating the highly conserved nature of these enzymes (9).

Although the size of the mammalian kallikrein gene family is uncertain, enough sequence data is available to begin to study the relationships between the serine protease superfamily members. Based on x-ray crystallographic data, the tertiary structures of all mammalian serine proteases are remarkably similar. Figure 3 represents a general model of the mammalian serine proteases based on such data. By comparing the protein sequences for 10 kallikrein-like enzymes, we have shown that the most conserved regions line the substrate-binding pocket while the variable regions tend to lie on the exterior of the molecule. Kallikrein varies most from chymotrypsin in loop regions which surround the active-site cleft, thereby accounting for the reduced substrate specificity of kallikrein as opposed to trypsin. It is possible that the variation seen in the loop structures that lie on the exterior of the different kallikrein-like enzymes reflects their different substrate specificities (24).

The apparent small size of the human kallikrein gene family vis-a-vis the rodent family poses a problem with respect to the numerous proposed functions of the kallikrein family of enzymes. Given the importance of several of the mouse and rat enzymes, for example the mouse growth factor processing enzymes, it is probable that all mammals contain homologues of these enzymes. We have identified 19 unique human genomic clones which may represent the human homologues of some of the rodent enzymes which currently have no known counterpart in humans (9). We feel that all of the tissue kallikrein-like genes probably arose from a single ancestral gene via duplications. This probably happened early in mammalian evolution and all mammals may have large kallikrein gene families. We have proposed that the human kallikrein gene family contains two groups of kallikrein-like enzymes, those which are closely linked and have remained homologous, i.e. tissue kallikrein, human prostate-specific antigen and hKG-1, and those which have become dispersed throughout the genome and therefore have diverged. In some species, the rat and mouse for example, all of the kallikrein gene family members have remained closely linked and homologous, while in other species they have become separated. Such separated members of multigene families, or orphons, are widespread among animal species (25).

The possibility that the kallikrein family represents a battery of processing enzymes tailored to process or degrade a large number of peptide substrates depends on the existence of a large number of such enzymes, and indeed in the mouse and rat, such a family has been found (3,5,6). The same may be true of other mammals, but the degree of homology among the family members that are separated from the rest of the family, i.e. orphons, may be sufficiently low that they are no longer readily identifiable on Southern blotting. Our continuing work on the human kallikrein genes may help to clarify these issues, and further define the physiologic significance of these enzymes as well as provide insight into some of the molecular mechanisms which guide the evolution of gene families.

ACKNOWLEDGEMENT

We are grateful to Brent Swenson of the Yerkes Regional Primate Research Center at Emory University and Raoul Benveniste of the Laboratory of Viral Carcinogenesis at the National Institute of Cancer for their help in securing primate blood and DNA samples. Also, we thank Tim Sisco of the Department of Audiovisual Resources at MUSC for helping us with the artwork. This work is supported by NIH grants HL29397 and DE09731.

REFERENCES

1.   Rogers, J. 1985. Exon shuffling and intron insertion in serine protease genes. Nature 315:460-461.

2.   MacDonald, RJ, Margolius, HS, Erdos, EG. 1988. Molecular biology of tissue kallikrein. Biochem J 253:313-321.

3.   Evans, BA, Drinkwater, CC, Richards, RI. 1987. Mouse glandular kallikrein genes. Structure and partial sequence analysis of the kallikrein gene locus. J Biol Chem 262:8027-8034.

4.   Ashley, PL, MacDonald, RJ. 1985. Kallikrein-related mRNAs of the rat submaxillary gland: Nucleotide sequences of four distinct types including tonin. Biochemistry 24:4512-4520.

5.   Gerald, WL, Chao, J, Chao,L. 1989. Immunological identification of rat tissue kallikrein cDNA and characterization of the kallikrein gene family. Biochem Biophys Acta 866:1-14.

6.   Wines, DR, Brady, JM, Pritchett, DB, Roberts, JL, and MacDonald, RJ. 1989. Organization and expression of the rat kallikrein gene family. J Biol Chem 264(13):7653-7662.

7.   Fukushima, D, Kitamura, N, Nakanishi, S. 1985. Nucleotide sequence of cloned cDNA for human pancreatic kallikrein. Biochemistry 24:8037-43.

8.   Baker, AR, Shine, J. 1985. Human kidney kallikrein: cDNA cloning and sequence analysis. DNA 4:445-450.

9.   Murray, SR, Chao, J, Lin, F-K, Chao, L. 1990. Kallikrein multigene families and the regulation of their expression. J Cardiovas Pharm 15(Suppl 6):S7-S16.

10. Evans, BA, Yun, ZX, Close, JA, Tregear, GW, Kitamura, N, Nakanishi, S, Calen, DF, Baker, E, Sutherland, GE, Richards, R. 1988. Structure and chromosomal localization of the human renal kallikrein gene. Biochemistry 27:3124-29.

11. Watt, KWK, Lee, P-J, M'Timkulu, T, Chan, W-P, Loor, R. 1986.Human prostate-specific antigen: Structural and function similarity with serine proteases. Proc Natl Acad Sci USA 83:3166-3170.

12. Lundwall, A, Lilja, H. 1987. Molecular cloning of human prostate- specific antigen cDNA. FEBS Lett 214:317-322.

13. Schedlich, LJ, Bennetts, BH, Morris, BJ. 1987. Primary structure of a human glandular kallikrein gene. DNA 6:429-437.

14. Riegman, PHS, Vlietstra, RJ, Kaassen, P van der Korput, JAGM, Gearts Van Kessel, A, Romijn, JL, Trapman, J. 1989. The prostate-specific antigen and the human glandular kallikrein-1 gene are tandemly located on chromosome 19. FEBS Lett 247: 123-126.

15. Neurath, H. 1989. The diversity of proteolytic enzymes, pp 1-13. In Proteolytic enzymes: a practical approach. RJ Beynon and JS Bond, eds. IRL Press, New York.

16. Wines, DR, Brady, JM, Southard, M, MacDonald, RJ. 1991. Evolution of the rat kallikrein gene family: gene conversion leads to functional diversity. J Mol Evol 32:476-492.

17. Southern, EM. 1975. Detection of specific sequences among DNA fragments separated by gel electrophoresis. J Mol Biol 98: 503-517.

18. Maniatis, T, Fritsch, E, Sambrook, J. 1982. Molecular Cloning. A Laboratory Manual. Cold Spring Harbor Laboratory, New York.

19. Swift, GH, Dagorn, J-C, Ashely, PL, Cummings, SW, MacDonald, RJ. 1982. Rat pancreatic kallikrein mRNA: nucleotide sequence and amino acid sequence of the encoded preproenzyme. Proc Natl Acad Sci USA 79:7263-7267.

20. Shai, S-Y, Woodley-Miller, C, Chao, J, Chao, L. 1989. Characterization of genes encoding rat tonin and a kallikrein-like serine protease. Biochemistry 28(13):5334-5343.

21. Chen, YP, Chao, J, Chao, L. 1988. Molecular cloning and characterization of two rat renal kallikrein genes. Biochemistry 27:7189-7196.

22. Mason, AJ, Evans, BA, Cox, DR, Shine, J, Richards, RI. 1983. Structure of mouse kallikrein gene family suggests a role in specific processing of biologically active peptides. Nature 303:300-307.

23. Drinkwater, CC, Evans BA, Richards, RI. 1987. Mouse glandular kallikrein genes: identification and characterization of the genes encoding the epidermal growth factor binding proteins. Biochemistry 26:6750-6756.

24. Bode, W, Ghen, Z, Bartels, K. 1983. Refined 2 Å X-ray crystal structure of porcine pancreatic kallikrein A, a specific trypsin-like serine proteinase. J Mol Biol 164:237-282.

25. Childs, G, Maxson, R, Cohn, RH, Kedes, L. 1981. Orphons: dispersed genetic elements derived from tandem repetitive genes of eukaryotes. Cell 23:651-663.

AAS 38/I
Recent Progress on Kinins
© 1992 Birkhäuser Verlag Basel

A RE–EVALUATION OF THE TISSUE–SPECIFIC PATTERN OF EXPRESSION OF THE RAT KALLIKREIN GENE FAMILY

Judith Clements, Annie Mukhtar, Allison Ehrlich and Peter Fuller

Prince Henry's Institute of Medical Research, PO Box 152, Clayton, Victoria, Australia, 3168

SUMMARY

We have used reverse transcriptase–polymerase chain reaction (RT–PCR) analysis and insitu hybridization to further define the tissue and cell–specific pattern of expression of the rat kallikrein gene family. rKlk1 gene expression has been unequivocally demonstrated in the rat heart, ovary and testis. Similarly, rKlk3, 4 and 9 gene expression has been demonstrated in the testis/ovary, heart and testis respectively. Insitu hybridization has identified the expression of kallikrein gene family members to specific cell–types in the rat ovary (granulosa cell) and testis (germ cell).

INTRODUCTION

The glandular or tissue kallikreins are a family of serine proteases known for their high degree of sequence conservation but yet diverse range of enzymatic functions (reviewed in 1,2). The precise physiological role(s) played by members of this large family of enzymes in many tissues is, however, still not clear.

The tissue kallikreins are encoded by a multigene family in several species (1,2). From Southern blot analysis, the rat kallikrein gene family would appear to include up to 20 members although only 12 gene family members [rKlk1–12(new nomenclature, see these proceedings); rGK1–8, S3, RSKG3, RSKG7, RSKG9 (old nomenclature)] have been fully characterized (reviewed in 1,2). On Northern blot analysis with gene–specific oligonucleotide probes some of these genes are known to be expressed in a variety of tissues (see Table 1). Other biochemical and physiological evidence, however, suggests that kallikrein gene family members may be expressed in many other tissues. Kallikrein (–like) immunoreactivity and enzyme activity has been demonstrated in the rat heart (3,4) although expression of a definitive family member has yet to be shown. Similarly, kininogenase activity has been detected in the female reproductive tract (5) but gene expression has not yet been established in this tissue. A kallikrein–like (rKlk8/P1–like) mRNA has also been identified in the rat testis (6,7) but is yet to be fully characterized.

TABLE 1. TISSUE - SPECIFIC EXPRESSION OF RAT KALLIKREIN GENE FAMILY MEMBERS

GENE mRNA	rKlk1 rGK1 PS	2 rGK2 S2	3 rGK3 S1	4 rGK4 -	6 rGK6 -	7 RSKG7 K1	8 rGK8 P1	9 - S3	12 RSKG3 -
TISSUE									
SMG	+	+	+	+		+	+	+	+
Kidney	+	-	-	+		+	-	-	-
Pancreas	+	-	-			-	-	-	-
Stomach	+	-	-			-	-	-	-
Intestine	+	-	-			-	-	-	-
Liver	-	-	-			-	-	-	-
Blood vessels	+								
Pituitary	+	-	-			-	-	-	-
Brain	?								
Prostate	-	-	-			-	+	+	-
Spleen	?	-	-			-	-	-	-
Heart	-/+			/+					
Ovary	-/+	-	-/+			?	-	-	
Testis	-/+	-	-/+			-	?	-/+	?

Positive and negative demonstration of gene expression from Northern blot analysis with gene–specific olignucleotide probes (taken from ref.1) is indicated by + or −. The demonstration of gene expression by RT–PCR analysis (this study) is indicated by /+. Those tissues where expression of a kallikrein–like gene have been described but the mRNA is yet to be fully characterized are indicated by ?. Tissue/genes not yet tested are left blank.

In order to help elucidate the physiological role(s) played by the various members of this large gene family in these and other tissues, we have sought to determine the definitive kallikrein gene family member(s) expressed in these tissues. In the current study, we have used the more sensitive assay of mRNA detection, the reverse transcriptase–polymerase chain reaction (RT–PCR) to determine which kallikrein gene family member is expressed in the rat heart and ovary and to more fully characterise the novel kallikrein–like mRNA previously described in the rat testis. In addition, in the testis and ovary, we have used insitu hybridization with gene–specific oligonucleotide probes to explore the particular cell–type expressing kallikrein gene family member(s) in these tissues.

MATERIALS AND METHODS
PCR Strategy

Universal kallikrein gene PCR primers were derived from two highly conserved regions in the kallikrein mRNA sequence derived from exon 2 (5' primer; codons 10–17) and exon 4 (3' primer; codons 145–151) of the kallikrein genes to generate a PCR product of 426bp (Fig 1A). Gene–specific oligonucleotide probes (see asterisked arrows Fig 1A) derived from less homologous sequences, internal to these PCR primers, in exons 2 (codons 20–25), 3(codons 77–83) and overlapping exons 3 and 4 (codons 136–142) were used to discriminate between the different genes on Southern blot analysis of the PCR products. To confirm the expression of a particular kallikrein gene family member detected using the above strategy, RT–PCR was repeated using primers derived from the above–mentioned gene–specific regions in exon 2 and the overlapping exon 3/4 region to generate a PCR product of 366bp (Fig 1B). In this instance, the generation of a specific product was confirmed by Southern blot analysis of the PCR products with the oligonucleotide probe derived from the remaining gene–specific region, internal to the PCR primers, in exon 3 (asterisked arrow, Fig 1B).

PCR STRATEGIES

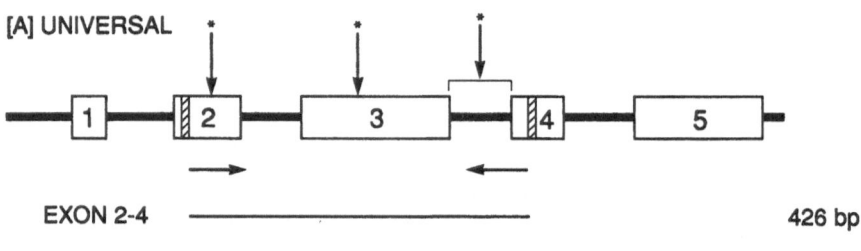

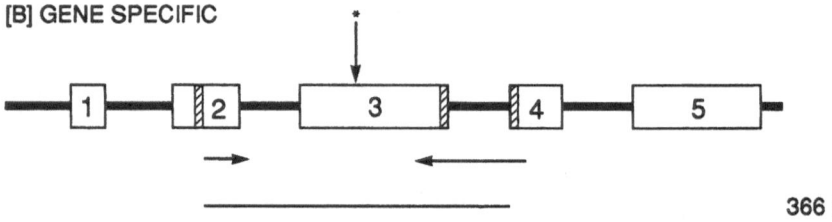

Figure 1. Schematic representation of universal (A) and gene–specific (B) PCR strategies. Exons are boxed and numbered. Regions from which the PCR primers were designed are indicated by horizontal arrows and hatched areas in the respective exons. Asterisked vertical arrows indicate the gene–specific regions from which the oligonucleotide probes for Southern blot analysis were designed. The length and size (bp) of the PCR product are indicated below.

RT–PCR Analysis

Total RNA was extracted from male or female rat Sprague–Dawley tissues (ovary, testis and heart; salivary gland and prostate – controls) as previously reported (6). RT–PCR was performed essentially as described previously (8). Briefly kallikrein cDNA was synthesized from the total RNA in a synthesis reaction primed with either the universal or gene–specific 3' PCR primers. Following cDNA synthesis, 5' PCR primers and Taq polymerase (Boehringer Mannheim) were added and amplification was performed for 30 cycles with an annealing temperature of 55°C. Southern blots of the RT–PCR products were hybridized with a rKlk1 (rGK1/PS) cRNA probe at 42°C (under non–stringent conditions) or with the appropriate gene specific oligonucleotide probe (18–21 mers) internal to the PCR primers as previously described (6,9). For sequence analysis RT–PCR products were subcloned into pGEM vectors (Promega) and dideoxysequencing performed using T7 or SP6 primers and T7 DNA polymerase (Sequenase).

In situ hybridization

In situ hybridization was performed essentially as previously described (10). Briefly, 7–10 μm ovarian or testis sections were hybridized at room temperature overnight with ^{35}S [α–dATP] tailed gene–specific kallikrein oligonucleotide probe. Sections were then washed at room temperature, dehydrated and air–dried. Following exposure to Kodak XAR film overnight, the slides were processed for liquid emulsion autoradiography. Slides were developed after 3–6 weeks and counterstained with haematoxylin–eosin.

RESULTS AND DISCUSSION

RT PCR Analysis

Southern blot analysis of RT–PCR products, generated with the universal exon 2–4 kallikrein primers, derived from the ovary, testis or heart was first performed with a rKlk1 (kallikrein; rGK1/PS) cRNA probe under non–stringent conditions to determine expression of any member(s) of the rat kallikrein gene family in these tissues. Figure 2A depicts auto-radiograms from a representative Southern blot of such RT–PCR – derived products from the rat salivary gland, prostate, heart and ovary. As shown in this figure, a kallikrein gene family PCR product of the appropiate size (426 bp) was detected with the rKlk1 cRNA probe not only in the salivary gland and prostate, as expected (9), but also in the ovary and heart. The subsequent hybridization of the same blot (left panel) to an oligonucleotide probe derived from the gene–specific region in exons 3/4 of the rKlk3 (S1) gene also demonstrated the presence of a rKlk3 or rKlk3 – like mRNA in the rat ovary as well as the salivary gland control. In this case, the prostate was appropriately negative since rKlk3 gene expression has not been demonstrated in this tissue (9). A rKlk3 gene–derived RT–PCR product was also detected using an exon 2 rKlk3 derived oligonucleotide probe in the rat testis (Fig 2B).

rKlk1 gene expression was also detected on Southern blot analysis of rat heart, ovary and testicular exon 2–4 universal RT–PCR products with the exon 3/4 derived gene–specific rKlk1 oligonucleotide probe (see Table 1). The expression of rKlk1 in the rat heart is not surprising since an enzyme immunochemically and enzymatically identical to true kallikrein (k1) has been identified in this tissue (3). The ovarian and testicular kallikrein–like activities have not been so fully characterized. On further analysis of these Southern blots with other gene – specific oligonucleotide probes derived from the same exon 2 or 3/4 dyshomologous regions,

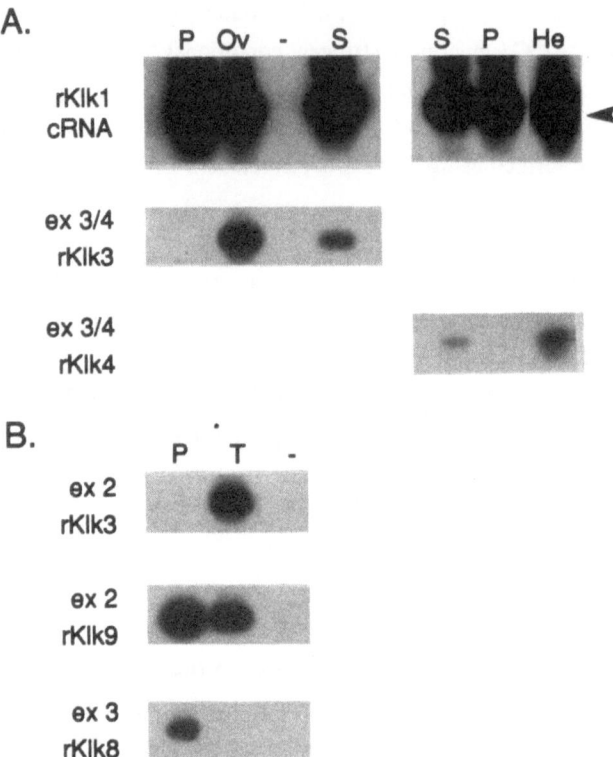

Figure 2. Southern blot analysis of universal exon 2–4 kallikrein RT–PCR products from rat prostate (P), ovary (Ov), salivary gland (S), heart (He) and testis (T). The negative control (–) indicates a RT–PCR reaction with no RNA added. Hybridization was performed successively to the same Southern blot with an rKlk1 cRNA probe (upper panels A) and an exon 3/4 rKlk3 or rKlk4 oligonucleotide probes (lower panels A). Panel B depicts successive hybridizations of the same Southern blot with exon 2 rKlk3/rKlk9 and exon 3 rKlk8 oligonucleotide probes. The arrow indicates a RT–PCR product of the appropiate size (426 bp).

rKlk4 (rGK4) and rKlk9 (S3, SEV) gene expression was detected in the rat heart and testis respectively (Fig 2A/B). The expression of rKlk4 in the rat heart correlates with the immunolocalization to rat atriocytes of arginine esterase A (4), a kallikrein–like enzyme first isolated from the rat kidney.

The above data would suggest that several kallikrein gene family members are expressed in a variety of tissues where their respective mRNAs have not been previously detected. This may simply reflect the increased sensitivity of detection afforded by the RT–PCR method. In order to confirm this expression sequence analysis of the RT–PCR products was performed after molecular cloning. This analysis has demonstrated one or more clones with sequences identical to rKlk1 (ovary, testis, heart), rKlk3 (ovary, testis), rKlk4 (heart) and rKlk9 (testis) over the region sequenced (codons 10–152) thus confirming the expression of these genes in the respective tissues.

Hybridization of the rat testis RT–PCR products with an exon 3 rKlk8 (P1) derived oligonucleotide probe, however, has not detected a similar mRNA species to that observed previously on Northern blots (Fig 2B). In accordance with these results, we have not yet detected any clones bearing any similarity to rKlk8 in the testicular RT–PCR products. It is not clear whether this negative result reflects a low level of expression of an rKlk8–like gene. This would seem unlikely given that expression was previously observed on Northern blot analysis and one would expect the more sensitive RT–PCR method to amplify such a signal accordingly. Alternatively, the previous data may simply reflect the aberrant hybridization of this probe to an unrelated gene product.

Additional confirmation of the expression of a these kallikrein gene family members was obtained from RT–PCR generated from gene–specific primers. We have demonstrated the expression of rKlk3 in the rat ovary and testis using this protocol and confirmed our previous findings from RT–PCR with universal primers. Similarly, we have verified with gene–specific primed RT–PCR that rKlk1 is expressed in the testis and ovary and rKlk9 is expressed in the rat testis.

In situ hybridization

As shown in Figure 3, hybridization of an exon 3/4 derived rKlk12 (RSKG3) probe with rat testis sections has given a cell–specific pattern of expression in the seminiferous tubule. Only those tubules with developing germ cells (round spermatids) at a particular stage of development (see arrowed tubules) have hybridized with the rKlk12 probe. A similar pattern of hybridization, although fainter, was also observed with an exon 2 derived rKlk9 probe. This pattern of hybridization is similar to that observed for nerve growth factor in the rat and mouse testis where a role in the maturation and/or motility of spermatozoa has been suggested (11). Given these similar patterns of hybridization, it is possible that rKlk9 or 12 may encode the rat homologue of the NGF processing enzyme, γ–NGF, previously described in the mouse (12), but this remains to be established.

In the rat ovary, hybridization was observed with an exon 2 rKlk7 probe to the granulosa cells of the ruptured follicles , post ovulation, in the gonadotrophin treated immature female rat (Clements, JA, et al: unpublished observation). Whether this kallikrein gene family member or others detected in this tissue by RT–PCR will be important in the inflammatory response at ovulation as has been previously suggested (5) or another aspect of local ovarian function is yet to be determined.

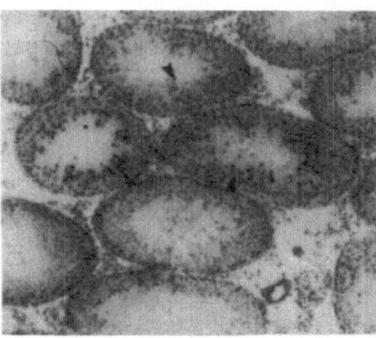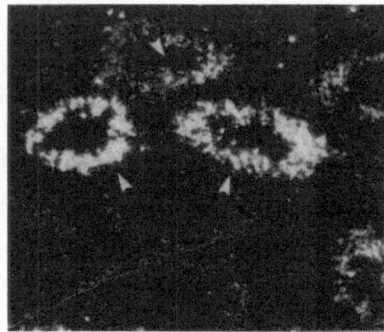

Figure 3. In situ hybridization of rat testis sections with an exon 3/4 rKlk12 oligonucleotide probe. The left and right panels show bright and dark field illumination respectively of the same field of view. Tubules at a similar stage of development and exhibiting kallikrein hybridization are arrowed. (magnification x 20)

CONCLUSION

From the data presented here, we have expanded the known pattern of tissue–specific expression of some members of the rat kallikrein gene family (see Table 1). In light of the possibility of amplification with our universal RT–PCR protocol of potential new family members which may hybridize with what we currently consider to be gene–specific oligonucleotide probes, we have been cautious in assigning expression of a particular gene family member to a new tissue site. Thus, only where we have been able to provide evidence from several sources – Southern blot and sequence analysis data from universal and/or gene–specific RT–PCR – have we been certain of expression of a given gene. The suggested cell specific expression of some family members from insitu–hybridization (rKlk7/ovary; rKlk12/testis) is yet to be verified by all the methods outlined above.

Similarly from the observations made here some caution is needed in using Northern blot analysis as the only index of kallikrein gene family expression. Although mRNA levels which would only be identified by RT–PCR and not Northern blot analysis indicates a relatively low level of expression of a particular gene, and/or high mRNA turnover, this may still be important physiologically, perhaps indicating a local action by a particular sub–population of cells and specific to the microenvironment of that tissue.

The determination of the definitive pattern of tissue and cell–specific expression of all members of the rat kallikrein gene family, using the approach outlined above, will help to elucidate the potential physiological functions of this large and diverse family of enzymes.

ACKNOWLEDGEMENTS

We thank Dr Ray MacDonald, Dept of Biochemistry, University of Texas South Western Medical Center, 5323 Harry Hines Boulevard, Dallas, Texas, USA, for his generous gifts of some of the oligonucleotide probes/primers used in this study. We also thank him for his valued advice and critically reading of this manuscript.

REFERENCES

1. Clements JA. The glandular kallikrein family of enzymes: tissue–specific expression and hormonal regulation.Endocrine Rev 1989; 10:393–419.

2. Macdonald RJ, Margolius HS, Erdos HG. Molecular biology of tissue kallikrein. Biochem J 1988; 253:313–321.

3. Xiong W, Chen L–M, Woodley–Miller C, Simson JAV, Chao J. Identification, purification and localization of tissue kallikrein in rat heart. Biochem J 1990; 267:639–646.

4. Simson JAV, Currie M, Chao L, Chao J. Colocalization of a kallikrein–like serine protease (arginine esterase A) and atrial natriuretic peptide in rat atrium. J Histochem Cytochem 1989; 37:1913–1917.

5. Espey LC, Tanaka N, Winn V, Okamura H. Increase in ovarian kallikrein activity during ovulation in the gonadotrophin–primed immature rat. J Reprod Fert 1989; 87: 503–508.

6. Clements JA, Matheson BA, Funder JW. Tissue–specific developmental expression of the kallikrein gene family in the rat. J Biol Chem 1990; 265:1077–1081.

7. Brady JM, Wines DR, Macdonald RJ. Expression of two kallikrein gene family members in the rat prostate. Biochemistry 1989; 28:5203–5210.

8. Maniatis T, Fritsch EF, Sambrook J. A laboratory manual. Cold Spring Harbor, New York: Cold Spring Harbor Laboratory 1989.

9. Clements JA, Matheson BA, Wines DR, Brady JM, Macdonald RJ, Funder JW. Androgen dependence of specific kallikrein gene family members expressed in rat prostate. J Biol Chem 1988; 263:16132–16137.

10. Fuller PJ, Clements JA, Funder JW. Localization of arginine vasopressin–neurophysin II messenger ribonucleic acid in the hypothalamus of control and Brattleboro rats by hybridization histochemistry with a synthetic pentadecamer oligonucleotide probe. Endocrinology 1985; 116:2366–2368.

11. Ayer–LeLievre C, Olsen L, Ebendad T, Hallbrook F, Persson H. Nerve growth factor mRNA and protein in the testis and epididymis of the mouse and rat. Proc Natl Acad Sci USA 1988; 85:2628–2632.

12. Evans BA, Richards RI. Genes for the α and γ subunits of mouse nerve growth factor are contiguous. EMBO J 1985; 4:133–138.

AAS 38/I
Recent Progress on Kinins
© 1992 Birkhäuser Verlag Basel

FUNCTIONAL DIVERSITY OF PROTEINASES ENCODED BY GENES OF THE RAT TISSUE KALLIKREIN FAMILY

F. GAUTHIER, T. MOREAU, N. GUTMAN, A. EL MOUJAHED, M. BRILLARD-BOURDET

Laboratoire d'Enzymologie et Chimie des Protéines, URA 1334 du Centre National de la Recherche Scientifique, Université François Rabelais, Faculté de Médecine, 2bis Bd Tonnellé F37032 TOURS Cedex (France)

Summary: A group of proteinases closely related to tissue kallikrein was purified from the rat submandibular gland. Physicochemical characterization of these proteinases, including amino terminal sequencing, allowed correlation with the genes of the rat kallikrein family. In spite of their similar structure, these proteinases have different substrate specificities and different susceptibilities to inhibitors which suggest that they do not share the same biological function. Kallikrein-like proteinases also have restricted specificities that are probably related to their extended substrate binding site. This makes them good candidates for processing inactive protein or peptide precursors into biologically active peptides. A general approach to identifying the putative biological substrates of individual proteinases based on analysis of the specific cleavage of synthetic and natural peptide substrates by kallikrein-related proteinases is described.

Introduction

Kallikrein-related proteinases are encoded by the genes of a multigene family which includes at least 15 closely related members in the rat (1). This makes the identification and characterization of the protein products of these genes somewhat difficult since they have up to 89 % primary amino-acid sequence identity (1). Many kallikrein-related proteinases have been described in the rat (Table 1), but their characterization has often been too preliminary to allow clear identification and correlation with other members of the gene family. Until recently, only true tissue kallikrein (kallikrein rK1) and tonin (rK2) were unambiguously correlated with their genes (2, 3). Since then however, sequence data have been obtained for at least 9 kallikrein-related proteinases (4-12), some of which were found to be identical, so that a total of 6 proteinases including rK1 and rK2, have been unambiguously identified in the rat submandibular gland. We have purified and characterized these 6 proteinases (7, 8, 11) and studied their enzymatic properties. The demonstration that these proteinases had different substrate specificities led to the conclusion that they also had different biological substrates, which may be identified by determining the nature of amino acids around the cleavage sites in synthetic and natural peptide substrates.

Protein products of the rat kalikrein gene family

Table 1 lists most of kallikrein-related proteinases so far isolated from the rat. Unless sequence data are available, the physicochemical characterization of these proteinases is often too preliminary to allow clear comparison between all varieties.

Table 1. Tissue kallikrein-related proteins in the rat

Kallikrein	*Ekfors et al.. 1967* (13)	Antigen γ	*Berg et al.. 1987* (22)
Salivain	*Riekkinen et al.. 1966* (14)	T-kininogenase	*Barlas et al. 1987* (23)
Glandulain	"		*Xiong et al. 1990* (5)
Esterase A	*Nustad and Pierce 1974* (15)	Endopeptidase k	*Gutman et al. 1988* (24)
Esterases B1-B4	"	Prostatic protease	*Winderickx et al. 1989* (6
Tonin	*Boucher et al. 1974* (16)	Kallikrein k7	*El Moujahed et al. 1990* (7)
Esterases C1-C4	*Brandtzaeg et al. 1976* (17)	Kallikrein k8	"
Esterase A1, A2	*Mc Partland et al. 1981* (18)	Kallikrein k10	*Gutman et al. 1991* (8)
Esterase B	*Khullar et al. 1986* (19)	SEV	*Yamaguchi et al. 1991* (9)
RSP-V	*Ikeno et al. 1986* (20)	rSMT 3, 4	*Araujo et al. 1991* (25)
Arginyl esteropeptidase	*Catalioto et al. 1987* (21)	· rPT1	"
Proteinase A	*Kato et al. 1987* (4)	KLP-S3	*Berg et al. 1992* (10)
Proteinase B	"	Kallikrein rK2, rK9	*Moreau et al. 1992* (11)

Nevertheless, it remains that the information available on each of them is sufficient to predict or to demonstrate that several of them are identical, and to correlate those of known sequence with the corresponding genes of the multigene kallikrein family. Six different kallikrein-related proteinases may be clearly identified in the rat submandibular gland (Table 2).

Table 2. Rat tissue kallikrein family

Gene	mRNA	Encoded Protein	Homology or identity
rKlk1 (rGK1)	PS	**rK1**	Tissue kallikrein = renal kallikrein
rKlk2 (rGK2)	S2	**rK2**	Tonin
(RSKG5)			
rKlk3 (rGK3)	S1	**?**	
rKlk4 (rGK4)			
rKlk5 (rGK5)			
rKlk6 (rGK6)			
rKlk7 (RSKG7)	K1	**rK7**	Proteinase A = Esterase B
rKlk8 (rGK8)	P1	**rK8**	Esterase A2 ?
rKlk9 (?)	S3	**rK9**	Prostatic protease = SEV
			= KLP-S3 = Esterase A1 = rSMT3 ?
rKlk10 (?)	?	**rK10**	Antigen γ = Endopeptidase k,
			= Proteinase B ? = T-kininogenase ?
rKlk11 (rGK7)	?	?	?
rKlk12 (RSKG3)	?	?	?
rKlk....			

Gene (rKlkx) and protein (rKx) names are according to the rules of nomenclature proposed at this meeting and based on the gene numberings previously defined (26, 27). Previous names of genes are indicated in parentheses; genes reported in italics have not yet been identified.

As indicated in Table 2, kallikrein-like proteinases were correlated with already known genes or mRNA, with the notable exception of rK10 though this proteinases is quantitatively a major kallikrein-like component in the rat submandibular gland (24). rK10 has been also reported as antigen γ (22), which has an identical sequence (12). It may also be identical to Proteinase B (4) and T-kininogenase (5, 23), both have similar properties, but differ by a few residues. The five other kallikreins correspond to a known gene or mRNA of the family, with the amino-acid sequences obtained by peptides sequencing and predicted from nucleotide sequences being identical. In addition to the proteases formerly described as tissue kallikrein and tonin, now called rK1 and rK2 respectively, rK7 and rK8 have been characterized (7); rK7 is identical to Proteinase A (4) or esterase B(19) while rK8 is probably esterase A2 (18). The newly described rK9 (11) is the protein product of the S3 mRNA (28), and partial protein sequence data have recently been reported under different protein names by several laboratories (9, 10).

Purification and characterization of kallikrein-related proteinases from the rat submandibular gland

The electrical properties of individual kallikreins may be exploited to fractionate submandibular gland homogenates by DEAE A50 chromatography to separate individual proteinases. This chromatographic step, which was first used for this purpose by Brandtzaeg et al. (17) has been used in our laboratory and others (6, 12, 25) as the initial step for purifying 6 different kallikrein-related proteinases from a single tissue. Another critical feature used for fractionating and purifying these proteinases is their differing susceptibilities to inhibitors. Some were strongly inhibited by aprotinin (rK1, rK7, rK8, rK10), while others were only slightly (rK2), or not at all (rK9) susceptible to this inhibitor (11). SBTI can be used in a similar fashion, as it does not inhibit rK1 and rK8; this feature was applied to the separation of rK8 from rK7. The complete purification procedure is summarized in Fig.1.

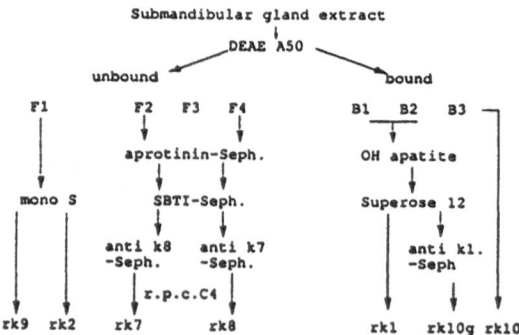

Fig 1. Scheme of purification of 6 proteinase members of the rat tissue kallikrein family from the submandibular gland. Complete information on the specific procedures for individual proteinases are given in (11) for rK2 and rK9, (7) for rK7 and rK8, and (8) for rK1 and rK10.

4 proteinases were purified from the DEAE-unbound material. This material probably contains at least one additional, so far unidentified, proteinase. rK10 was separated from rK1 by chromatography on hydroxyapatite and appears to be heterogeneous (8).

Table 3. Physicochemical properties of kallikrein-like proteinases

	pHi	Mr (kDa)	
		Non reduced	Reduced (heavy chain)
rK1	3.8-4	27	38
rK2	6.2	25	35
rK7	5.2	27	19
rK8	5.1	27	18
rK9	6.85	25	20
rK10	4.3	27.5 +26.5 +26	21

Kallikrein-related proteinases were also identified by their N-terminal sequences. Sequence data for the light and heavy chains of all six proteinases allowed correlation with the corresponding genes when they were known (Table 4). They also demonstrated the microheterogeneity of rK10, which is due to alternative processing of the peptide chain to generate N-terminal and C-terminal light and heavy chains, and to a different glycosylation of the light chain (8).

Table 4 . Amino terminal sequences of kallikrein-like proteinases

```
     Light chains                        Heavy chains
     1        10        20               90        100
rK1:  VVGGYNCEMNSQPWQVAVYYFGEYL...   -LIWNHTRQPGDDYSNDLMLLHLSQPADITD...
rK2:  IVGGYKCEKNSQPWQVAVIN--EYL...   -IVTNDTEQPVHDHSNDLMLLHLSEPADITG...
rK7:  VIGGYKCEKNSQ...                 KPGDDHSNDLMLLHLSQPADITD...
rK8:  IIGGFNCFKNSQPWQVAVYHFNE...      KPGNDYSNDLMLLHLKTPADITD...
rK9:  VVGGYNCETNSQPWQVAVI--GTxF...    AYDHNNDLMLLHLSKPADITG...
rK10: IVGGYKCEKNSQPWQVAIIN--EYL...    GDDYSNDLMLLHLSEPADITD...
                                      QRGDDYSNDLMLLHLSEPADITD...
```

The proteinases of the kallikrein family can also be discriminated by their tissue localization. Studies on the expression of the genes in different tissues have shown significant differences between kallikrein family members in human, mouse and rat tissues (reviewed in 29). Preliminary experiments on proteinase immuno-localization in the kidney and prostate gland using polyclonal antibodies which were made specific by immunoadsorbtion with cross reacting antigens confirmed those previously reported (10, 30, 31) and agreed with the results of gene expression (32-34). Among the 6 purified proteinases, only immunoreactive rK1 and rK7 were found in whole kidney extracts, whereas the prostate contained large amounts of rK9 or rK9-like material (10) as well as trace amounts of rK8. Several other tissues have also been reported to express one or several kallikrein-related genes (33, 35, 36).

Enzymatic properties of kallikrein-related proteinases

Preliminary investigations of the biological function of kallikrein-related proteinases in the rat showed that most of them were not involved in the release of kinin from kininogens. This may be due to the specificity of each kallikrein, but also to the specific control exerted by physiological inhibitors on individual proteinases. Kallikrein-like proteinases however, all seem to have restricted specificities, which makes them good candidates for processing peptide precursors. Identification of the preferential cleavage sites in various peptide chains represents therefore an exciting task which may result in the discovery of new biologically active peptides and of their precursors. Several putative precursor proteins have been shown to be processed *in vitro* at the bond hydrolysed *in vivo* by one or more members of the kallikrein family (reviewed in 29). However the biological relevance of these phenomena often remained questionable due to the experimental conditions used to obtain the response. The approach we have used to identify the biological substrates of individual kallikreins has been to determine substrate specificities using synthetic, fluorogenic and chromogenic peptide substrates in addition to protein substrates. The combined results can be used to define consensus sequences that would fit each enzyme binding pocket, and to look for such sequences in protein data banks. This approach is particularly appropriated for kallikreins which are known to have an extended interacting site; this extended site probably gives rise to their restricted specificity. Commercially available synthetic substrates with fluorescent or chromogenic leaving groups only provide information on the P1 and P2 specificities, and to a lesser extent on P3 and P4 specificities. Intramolecularly quenched fluorescent substrates, which include residues downstream to the scissile bond in positions P1' to P3' in addition to those in P1 to P3, have been recently introduced (37). These substrates are more appropriate for defining kallikrein specificities. For the reasons cited above, denatured proteins are particularly powerful tools for investigating kallikrein specificities, but identification of the cleavage sites in these substrates requires more sophisticated analysis, i.e. peptide fractionation and amino-acid sequencing, than is needed for synthetic chromogenic and fluorogenic peptides.

The specificity of each kallikrein variety may be determined by measuring kcat/Km values for synthetic substrates (7) or by identifying the position of scissile bonds in protein substrates (11). Some representative results obtained with synthetic substrates are shown in Table 5. Most of kallikrein-related proteinases have a strong amidolytic activity and a marked specificity for arginyl residues at position P1. This was not the case however for rK2 and rK9 which have poor amidolytic activity whatever the P1 residue (11).

Unlike the P1 specificity, the P2 specificity clearly differs from one kallikrein to another.

Whereas the restricted specificity of rK1 for releasing a kinin from kininogen is explained by its ability to accomodate only bulky and hydrophobic residues in P2, several other proteinases can hydrolyse substrates with small, uncharged residues at that position (Table 5). For example, rK7 hydrolysed the synthetic substrate Boc-F-R-S-R-NHMec more rapidly than other kallikreins. Interestingly, the prokallikrein sequence in rat and human also has a seryl residue in P2 (2, 38). We demonstrated that human urinary kallikrein was activated from its precursor 30 to 40 times faster by rK7 than by trypsin, which is generally used for in vitro activation of prokallikrein (unpublished data).

Short peptide substrates cannot always be used to discriminate between kallikreins activities. That is the case for rK2 and rK9 for example which hydrolyse synthetic amide substrates poorly, so that denatured proteins were used to identify their preferential cleavage sites (11). These studies on P3 to P3' specificity show that these two proteinases differ only by their P1 specificity and that both prefer a prolyl residue in P2 and an hydrophobic residue in P2'. They also let suppose that other residues far from the scissile bond could be important in determining the substrate specificity, as was previously reported for rK2, thus confirming the presence of an extended interacting site for these proteinases (39).

Table 5. Kinetic properties of kallikrein-like proteinases

	k_{cat} / Km (1/ mM.s)					
	Kallikreins					
	rK1	rK2	rK7	rK8	rK9	rK10
P-F-R-NHMec	171	<5	474	34	<5	64
Z-F-R-NHMec	57	<5	424	56	<5	64
Boc-F-S-R-NHMec	<5	<5	223	<5	<5	48
Z-R-R-NHMec	<5	<5	<5	<5	<5	<5
Boc-V-P-R-NHMec	<5	<5	345	20	<5	36
Boc-L-G-R-NHMec	<5	<5	129	6	<5	<5
Boc-F-V-R-NHMec	17	<5	709	79	<5	79
Boc-L-S-T-R-NHMec	n.d	<5	n.d	n.d	5.5	n.d
Abz-F-R-S-R-EDDnp	n.d	21	90	100	6	179
Abz-F-R-L-V-R-EDDnp	n.d	<5	14	128	<5	1100

Even though the P2-prolyl specificity does not allow discrimination between rK2 and rK9, it may help in identifying the biological target of these two proteinases. It has been reported that a proline-directed arginyl cleavage is important in the processing of peptide precursors (40). rK2 and rK9 may therefore be candidates for this function. Work is now in progress to identify biological substrates that have this structure at their processing site.

Acknowledgements

We are indebted to Dr Eline Prado (University of Sao Paulo, Brazil) for the gift of intramolecularly quenched fluorogenic substrates.

References

1. Wines, D.R., Brady, J.M., Southard, E.M., MacDonald, R.J. Evolution of the rat kallikrein gene family: gene conversion leads to functional diversity. J. Mol. Evol. 1991; 32, 476-492.

2. Swift, G.H., Dagorn, J-C., Ashley, P.L., Cummings, S.W., MacDonald, R.J. Rat pancreatic kallikrein mRNA : nucleotide sequence and amino acid sequence of the encoded preproenzyme. Proc. Natl Acad. Sci. USA 1982; 79, 7263-7267.

3. Lazure, C., Leduc, R., Seidah, N.G., Thibault, G., Genest, J., Chretien, M. The complete amino acid sequence of rat submaxillary gland tonin does contain the aspartic acid at the active site: confirmation by protein sequence analyses. Biochem. Cell Biol 1987; 65, 321-337.

4. Kato, H., Nakanishi, E., Enjyoji, K., Hayashi, I., Oh-Ishi, S., Iwanaga, S. Characterization of serine proteinases isolated from rat submaxillary gland: with special reference to the degradation of rat kininogens by these enzymes. J. Biochem 1987; 102, 1389-1404.

5. Xiong, W., Chen, M.L., Chao, J. Purification and characterization of a kallikrein-like T-kininogenase. J. Biol. Chem 1990; 265, 2822-2827.

6. Windericks, J., Swinnen, K., Van Dijck, P., Verhoeven, G., Heyns, W. Kallikrein-related protease in the rat ventral prostate: cDNA cloning and androgen regulation. Mol. Cell. Endocrinol 1989; 62, 217-226.

7. El Moujahed,A., Gutman,N., Brillard,M.,Gauthier,F. Substrate specificity of two kallikrein family gene products isolated from the rat submaxillary gland. FEBS Lett 1990; 265,137-140.

8. Gutman N., El Moujahed, A., Brillard, M., Monegier du Sorbier, B., Gauthier, F. Microheterogeneity of rat submaxillary gland kallikrein k10, a member of the kallikrein family. Eur. J. Biochem 1991; 197, 425-429

9. Yamaguchi, T., Carretero, O.A., Scicli, G. A novel serine protease with vasoconstrictor activity coded by the kallikrein gene S3. J. Biol. Chem. 1991; 266, 5011-5017.

10. Berg, T., Schoyen, H., Wassdal, I., Hull, R., Gerskowitch, V.P., Toft, K. Characterization of a new kallikrein-like enzyme (KLP-S3) of the rat submandibular gland. Biochem. J. 1992; in press.

11. Moreau, T., Brillard-Bourdet, M., Bouhnik, J., Gauhtier, F. Protein products of the rat kallikrein gene family : substrate specificity of kallikrein rK2 (Tonin) and kallikrein rK9. J. Biol. Chem 1992; in press.

12. Berg, T., Wassdal, I., Mindroiu, T., Sletten, K., Scicli, G., Carretero, O.A., Scicli, A.G. T-kininogenase activity of the rat submandibular gland is predominantly due to the kallikrein-like serine protease antigen γ. Biochem. J. 1991; 280, 1-25.

13. Ekfors, T.O., Riekkinen, P.J., Malmiharju, T. Four isozymic forms of a peptidase ressembling kallikrein purified from the rat submandibular gland. Hoppe Seyler' s Z Physiol Chem 1967; 348, 111-118.

14. Riekkinen, P.J., Ekfors, T.O. Demonstration of a proteolytic enzyme, salivain in rat saliva.   Acta Chem Scand 1966; 20, 2013-2018.

15. Nustad, K., Pierce, J.V. Purification of rat urinary kallikreins and their specific antibody. Biochemistry 1974; 13, 2312-2319.

16. Boucher, R., Asselin, J., Genest, J. A new enzyme leading to the direct formation of angiotensin II. Circ. Res 1974; 35, I-203-I-209

17. Brandtzaeg, P., Gautvik, K.M., Nustad, K., Pierce, J.V. Rat submandibular gland kallikreins: purification and cellular localization. Br. J. Pharmacol 1976; 56, 155-167.

18. Mc Partland, R.P., Sustarsic, D.L., Rapp, J.P. Evidence for an androgen-dependent urinary arginine esterase in the rat : separation from other urinary arginine esterases including kallikreins. Endocrinology 1981; 108, 1634-1638.

19. Khullar, M., Scicli, G., Carretero, O.A. Scicli, A.G. Purification and characterization of a serine protease (Esterase B) from rat submandibular gland. Biochemistry 1986; 25, 1851-1857.

20. Ikeno, K., Ikeno, T., Kuzuya, H., Ishiguro, I. Purification and characterization of a trypsin-like protease in the submandibular gland of rats. J. Biochem 1986; 99, 1219-1226.

21. Catalioto, R.M., Négrel, R., Gaillard, D., Ailhaud, G. Growth promoting activity in serum-free medium of kallikrein like arginylesteropeptidases from rat submaxillary gland. J Cell Physiol 1987; 130, 352-360.

22. Berg, T., Holck, M., Johansen, L. Isolation, characterization and localization of antigenγ, a serine proteinase of the "kallikrein-family " in the rat submandibular gland. Biol. Chem. Hoppe-Seyler 1987; 368, 1455-1467.

23. Barlas, A., Gao, X., Greenbaum, L.M. Isolation of a thiol-activated T-kininogenase from the rat submandibular gland. FEBS Lett 1987; 218, 266-270.

24. Gutman, N., Moreau, T., Alhenc-Gelas, F., Baussant, T., El Moujahed, A., Akpona, S., Gauthier, F. T-kinin release from T-kininogen by rat submaxillary gland endopeptidase k. Eur. J. Biochem 1988; 171, 577-582.

25. Araujo, G.W., Pesquero, J.B., Lindsey, C.J., Paiva, A.C.M., Pesquero, J.L. Identification of serine proteinases with tonin-like activity in the rat submandibular and prostate glands.Biochim. Biophys. Acta, 1991, 1074, 167-171.

26. Wines, D.R., Brady, J.M., Pritchett, D.B., Roberts, J.L., MacDonald, R.J. Organization and expression of the rat kallikrein gene family. J. Biol. Chem 1989; 13, 7653-7662.

27. Chen, Y.P., Chao, J., Chao, L. Molecular cloning and characterization of two renal kallikrein genes. Biochemistry 1988; 27, 7189-7196.

28. Ashley, P.L., MacDonald, R.J. Kallikrein-related mRNAs of the rat submaxillary gland: nucleotide sequences of four distinct types including tonin. Biochemistry 1985; 24, 4512-4520.

29. MacDonald, R.J., Margolius, H.S., Erdös, E.G. Molecular biology of tissue kallikrein. Biochem. J 1988; 253, 313-321.

30. Johansen, L., Berg Orstavik, T., Nustad, K., Holck, M. Excess antibody immunoassays for rat glandular kallikreins. Measurement of kallikrein from different organs in the presence of cross-reacting antigens. Journal of Immunological Methods 1983; 59, 315-326.

31. Chao, J., Chao, L. Identification and expression of kallikrein gene family in rat submandibular and prostate glands using monoclonal antibodies as specific probes. Biochim. Biophys. Acta 1987; 910, 233-239.

32. Clements, J.A., Matheson, B.A., Wines, D.R., Brady, J.M., MacDonald, R.J.,Funder, J.W. Androgen dependence of specific kallikrein gene family members expressed in rat prostate. J. Biol. Chem 1988; 263, 16132-16137.

33. Clements, J.A., Matheson, B.A., Funder, J.W. Tissue specific developmental expression of the kallikrein gene family in the rat. J. Biol. Chem 1990; 265, 1077-1081.

34. Brady, J.M., Wines, D.R., MacDonald, R.J. Expression of two kallikrein gene family members in the rat prostate. Biochemistry 1989; 28, 5203-5210.

35. Chao, J., Woodley, C., Chao, L., Margolius, H.S. Identification of tissue kallikrein in brain and in the cell-free translation product encoded by brain mRNA. J. Biol. Chem 1983; 258, 15173-15178.

36. Xiong, W., Chen, L.M., Woodley-Miller, C., Simson., J.A.V., Chao, L. Identification, purification, and localization of tissue kallikrein in rat heart. Biochem. J 1990; 267, 639-646.

37. Chagas, J.R., Juliano, L., Prado, E.S. Intramolecularly quenched fluorogenic tetrapeptide substrates for tissue and plasma kallikrein. Anal. Biochem 1991; 192, 419-425.

38. Fukushima, D., Kitamura, N., Nakanishi, S. Nucleotide sequence of cloned cDNA for human pancreatic kallikrein. Biochemistry 1985; 8037-8043.

39. Fujinaga, M., James, M.N.G. Rat submaxillary gland serine protease, tonin. Structure solution and refinement at 1.8 A resolution. J. Mol. Biol 1987; 195, 373-396.

40. Schwartz, T.W. The processing of peptide precursors 'Proline-directed arginyl cleavage' and other monobasic processing mechanisms. FEBS Lett 1986; 200, 1-10.

AAS 38/I
Recent Progress on Kinins
© 1992 Birkhäuser Verlag Basel

IDENTIFICATION OF PROTEINS OF THE KALLIKREIN FAMILY BY ISOELECTROFOCUSING AND IMMUNOBLOTTING

T. Berg, H. Schøyen, I. Wassdal, and A. Bjørnstad-Østensen

Institute of Physiology, Medical Faculty, University of Oslo, Box 1103, Blindern, 0317 Oslo, Norway

SUMMARY: We have found that kallikrein-like proteins differ in their isoelectric point but share antigenic determinants. For identification of kallikrein-like proteins an initial separation was carried out in flat-bed isoelectrofocusing gels. The kallikrein-like nature was demonstrated by an immunological similarity to kallikrein-like proteins by immunoblotting using antiserum against a kallikrein family member for staining. We used this system to identify different kallikrein-like proteins during purification of both known as well as new enzymes.

INTRODUCTION

A group of closely related serine proteases has been shown to be encoded by a group of genes showing a high degree of sequence similarity (1). This group of genes is referred to as the kallikrein gene family since one of the genes encodes tissue kallikrein. Although it appears that each enzyme of the kallikrein family has one particular substrate of preference, other enzymes of the kallikrein family often show some activity against the same substrate (2) which may result in a low but false positive reading. Selective enzyme inhibitors for these proteins are not yet available, and little variation is observed in molecular weight. Morover, as expected from their high degree of sequence homology, several of these proteins are immunologically related often showing a high degree of immunological cross-reactivity (2 - 5).

Due to the great similarities between kallikrein-like proteins, a robust method for easy identification was needed. We have observed that proteins of the kallikrein family differ in their isoelectric point. This fact combined with their immunological similarities, allowed us to develop a method to detect and identify kallikrein-like proteins by separation in flat-bed isoelectrofocusing followed by immunoblotting.

MATERIALS AND METHODS

Reagents: Bovine serum albumin was obtained from Sigma Chemical Company, St. Louis, MO. Swine antirabbit immunoglobulin G antiserum and peroxidase-antiperoxidase reagent were from Boehringer, Mannheim, Germany, and 3,3'-diaminobenzidin tetrahydrochloride was obtained from Ega-Chemie, Steinheim am Albuch, Germany. PhastGel[R,] IEF 3-9 and PhastGel[R] Gradient 8-25 were from Pharmacia LKB Biotechnology, Uppsala, Sweden.

Tissue: Male Wistar rats, 3-4 months of age, were anesthetized with pentobarbitone (Nembutal, 60 mg/kg b.w., *i.p.*) and anterior prostate glands and submandibular glands (SMG) were extirpated. Tissue homogenates were made in phosphate buffered saline (PBS; 0.01 M Na-phosphate, pH 7.4, 0.14 M NaCl) in a Potter Elvehjem homogenizer (20 strokes, 4°C) at a ml volume : g gland wet weight of 10 : 1. The homogenate was centrifuged at 13,000 g for 30 min (4°C), and the supernatant was collected. For SMG, the procedure was repeated on the precipitate and the two supernatants combined.

Purified SMG kallikrein, antigen γ, esterase B, tonin, KLP-S3, and polyclonal rabbit antisera against these enzymes were obtained as previously described (2 - 7). Prostate KLP-S3 was purified with the same method as that described for SMG KLP-S3 as indicated in Figure 4 legend (2).

Flat-bed isoelectrofocusing (IEF): Tissue homogenate and enzyme fractions were run in flat-bed isoelectrofocusing gels (PhastGel[R] IEF 3-9) with a pH range from 3 to 9 in the Pharmacia Fast System as described in the manufacturer's manual. Isoelectric point (pI) was determined by the use of the Pharmacia Isoelectric focusing calibration kit (pH 3-10) as standard. The gels were stained with the silver staining technique as described in the manufacturer's manual or blotted on to nitrocellulose membrane (0.2 μm) and immunostained as described below.

SDS-polyacrylamide gelelectroforesis (SDS-PAGE): Proteins were run in PhastGel[R] Gradient 8-25 using the Pharmacia Phast System as described in the manufacturer's manual. Proteins were treated with SDS (25 g/l) without or with beta-mercaptoethanol (5 % final concentration, 2 min, 100°C). Pharmacia electrophoresis calibration kit (low molecular weight proteins) was used as standard for determination of molecular weights. The gels were stained with silver as described in the manufaturer's manual or used for immunoblotting as described below.

Immunostaining: After blotting, the nitrocellulose membrane was moistened with transfer buffer (0.025 M Tris, 0.192 M glycine, 20 % methanol, pH 8.3), placed onto the Fast System gel, wrapped in layers of filter paper stabilized with a perforated polyacrylamide frame, and incubated for 30 min during shaking in a buffer-containing chamber (37°C). The nitrocellulose membrane was subsequently immersed (22°C) in: 1) 6 % bovine serum albumin (BSA) in phosphate-buffered saline (60 min), 2) rabbit primary antiserum (1-2:5000::v:v), 3) swine antirabbit immunoglobulin G antiserum (1:1000::v:v), and 4) peroxidase antiperoxidase reagent (1:1000::v:v). Polyclonal rabbit antisera against rat SMG kallikrein, antigen γ, esterase B, tonin, or KLP-S3 (1-2:5000::v:v) were used in the primary layer. Antisera were diluted in PBS containing 0.1 % BSA, and incubations lasted 45 min with the protein side of the membrane facing downwards. Between each incubation, the membrane was washed in PBS containing 0.1 % Tween 20 for 3 x 15 min. Staining was developed with 3,3'-diaminobenzidin tetrahydrochloride (8).

Amino acid sequence: Purified proteins were run in SDS-PAGE in Excel[TM]Gel (SDS gradient 8-18) (Pharmacia LKB Biotechnology, Uppsala, Sweden) and transferred electrophoretically to Immobilon PVDF transfer membrane (Millipore, Bedford, MA) in a Pharmacia Multiphor II Novablot System as previously described (4). After staining with Coomassie blue, protein bands were cut out and used for N-terminal amino acid analyses, performed in an automatic 477A Protein/Peptide Sequencer with an on-line 120A PTH amino acid analyser from Applied Biosystems (Foster City, CA) (9).

RESULTS

The IEF-migration pattern of purified SMG kallikrein-like proteins, *i.e.*, tissue kallikrein, antigen γ, esterase B, tonin, and KLP-S3, was demonstrated by staining the IEF-gels with silver (Figure 1) or, after blotting the proteins on to a nitrocellulose membrane, with homologous antiserum (not shown). Clear differences were observed in the pI of these proteins (Table 1). Their molecular weights were determined in SDS-PAGE-gels stained with silver or with antiserum after blotting (not shown). Kallikrein and tonin ran as one band after reduction with mercaptoethanol, whereas the others were split into two chains (Table 1). Little variation was found in their molecular weights (Table 1). With the exception of esterase B, all proteins showed microheterogeneities in charge, and for tissue kallikrein heterogeneities were also observed in molecular weight (Table 1).

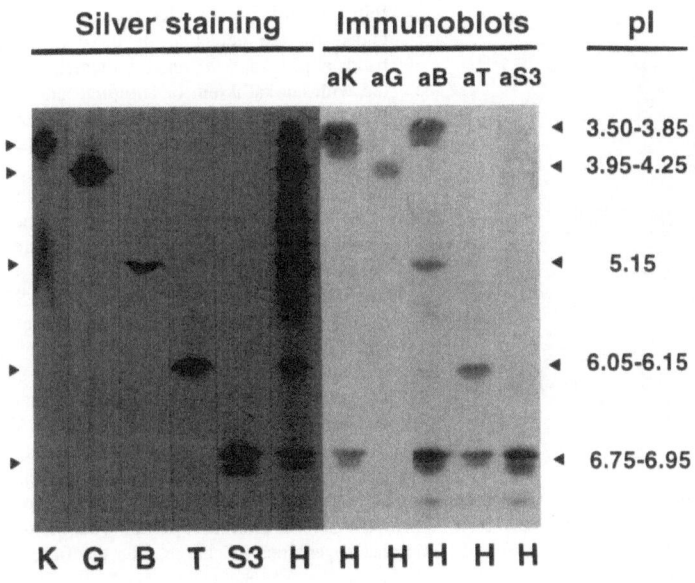

Figure 1. Demonstration of proteins of the kallikrein family by IEF and immunoblotting

Purified SMG proteins of the kallikrein family and SMG homogenate were run in IEF gels and stained with silver. The same antigens were demonstrated in homogenate with homologous antiserum. In addition, cross-reactivity to other family members was demonstrated. Polyclonal antisera with reactivity against common antigenic epitopes were needed to demonstrate such cross-reactivity. The antiserum used for staining of the immunoblots are indicated above the figure; against kallikrein = aK, antigen γ = aG, esterase B = aB, tonin = aT, and against KLP-S3 = aS3. The proteins applied to the wells are indicated below each column (kallikrein = K, antigen γ = G, esterase B = B, tonin = T, kallikrein-like protein S3, KLP-S3 = S3, and SMG homogenate = H). Isoelectric point (pI) is indicated to the right. Microheterogeneities in charge were observed for all except for esterase B.

Table 1. Isoelectric point and molecular weight of submandibular gland proteins of the kallikrein family

	Isoelectric point	Molecular weight		
		Nonreduced	Reduced	
kallikrein	3.50 - 3.85	25,400 - 28,200	31,400	-
antigen γ	3.95 - 4.25	28,400	19,000	10,000
esterase B	5.15	25,100	17,200	13,100
tonin	6.05 & 6.15	25,700	29,200	-
KLP-S3	6.75 - 6.95	24,600	16,200	12,600

Isoelectric point and molecular weight was determined in flat-bed isoelectrofocusing gels and in SDS-PAGE without or with reduction with mercaptoethanol as described in Materials and Methods.

The sensitivity of the IEF-staining techniques was found by dilution of the antigens, and was for the silver- and the immunostaining technique 0.01-0.02 g/l (3-6 ng applied per well) and 0.02-0.04 g/l, respectively. The technique thus also allowed for the detection of contaminating proteins down to this low level of concentration, and, through demonstration of their pI, to some extent also identify such proteins during enzyme purification.

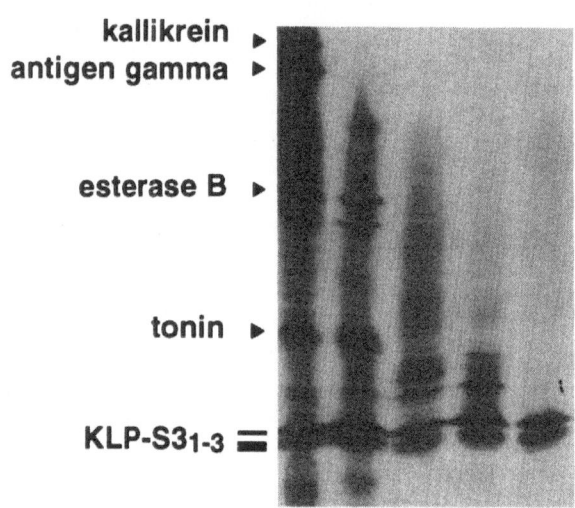

kallikrein ▶
antigen gamma ▶

esterase B ▶

tonin ▶

KLP-S3₁-₃ ▤

Figure 2. Purification of SMG KLP-S3 followed by IEF

Initial identification of KLP-S3$_{1-3}$ was obtained by the detection of three protein bands at pI 6.75, 6.90, and 6.95 which reacted with antikallikrein or antitonin antisera (Figure 1). During purification, the presence of KLP-S3 in column fractions was monitored by flat-bed isoelectrofocusing-gels stained with silver as shown above. Identity of KLP-S3 was also confirmed by immunoblotting with antiKLP-S3 antiserum (not shown). The lanes contained: lane 1 = SMG homogenate; lane 2 = the KLP-S3 fraction from a DEAE-cellulose anionexchange column (equilibrated with 0.05M ammonium-acetate buffer, pH 5.8, and eluted with a 0.05-0.5M ammonium acetate gradient, pH 5.8); lane 3 = the KLP-S3 fraction after cationexchange chromatography (equilibrated with 0.05M sodium-acetate buffer, pH 5.0, and eluted with a 0.05-0.5M sodium acetate gradient, pH 5.0); lane 4 = the KLP-S3 void fraction after chromatofocusing (pH 7.4-4.0); and lane 5 = purified KLP-S3 after a repeated run on the cationexchange column. The purified KLP-S3 fraction showed microheterogeneities in charge. The purification procedure is described in detail elsewhere (2).

By comparison with purified standards, the same proteins were easily detected in a SMG homogenate (Figure 1). The method thus allowed detection of kallikrein-like proteins in tissue homogenates or in impure preparations. The high resolution of protein bands in silver-stained gels made it easy to follow one protein band during the purification procedure (Figure 2). Enzyme identification was always confirmed during the purification procedure by immunoblotting (not shown).

When tissue homogenate was stained by immunoblotting using antiserum against tissue kallikrein, antigen γ, esterase B, tonin, or KLP-S3, cross-reactivity with other members of the kallikrein family was demonstrated (Figure 1). Variation in the cross-reactivity pattern was also observed among antisera raised in different rabbits against the same antigen; the number of protein bands stained in addition to the homologous antigen varied considerably from giving an almost monospecific reaction to multiple band staining (not shown). Thus, the system did not only allow detection and identification of kallikrein-like antigens but was also useful for characterization of an antiserum cross-reactivity pattern. Monospecific antisera were made as previously (10) by absorption with insolubilized cross-reacting antigens (not shown).

When immunostaining was performed with polyclonal antiserum not made monospecific by absorption with cross-reacting antigens, i.e., with antiserum reacting against antigenic epitopes shared by several kallikrein-like proteins, previously unidentified family members were demonstrated. New immunoreactive proteins were more easily detected when enriched fractions were applied to the gels (not shown). We used this procedure to detect (Figure 1) and purify KLP-S3 (Figure 2), a SMG kallikrein-like protein with vasoconstrictory properties (2). Other properties characteristic of proteins of the kallikrein family members, were confirmed after KLP-S3 had been purified such as demonstration of immunological partial identity to SMG kallikrein, and enzymatic classification as a serine protease by being inhibited by phenylmethylsulphonyl fluoride (I_{50} = 0.73 mM, 1 µM KLP-S3) (2). The kallikrein-like nature of KLP-S3 was confirmed by amino acid sequence analysis which also revealed sequence homology with the kallikrein-like mRNA S3 (Figure 3).

Light chain:

```
                 1    5    10   15   20   25   30   35
PS (Kallikrein)  VVGGYNCEMNSQPWQVAVYYFGEYLCGGVLIDPSWVITAA
S2 (Tonin)       IVGGYKCKKNSQPWQVAVIN   EYLCGGVLIDPSWVITAA
Esterase B       VIGGYKEKNSQPWQV
Kallikrein k7    VIGGYKCKKNSQ
RSKG-7           VIGGYKCKKNSQPWQVALYSFTKYLCGGVLIDPSWVITAA
K1                             YSFSKYLCGGVLIDPSWVITAA
S3 (KLP-S3, SEV) VVGGYNCETNSQPWQVAVIGTTF  CGGVLIDPSWVITAA
Ant γ = kallikrein 10  IVGGYKCKKNSQPWQVAIIN  EYLXGGVLIDPSXVITAA
T-kininogenase   IVGGYKCKKNSQPWQVAIIIETEYL
Proteinase A     VIGGYKCKKNDQPWQVALYSFSKYLCGGVLIDPSWVITAA
Proteinase B     IVGGYKCKKNSQPWQVAIIN   EYLCGGVLIDPSWVITAA
S1
P1 (kallikrein k8)  IIGGFNCKKNSQPWQVAVY
RSKG-3           VVGGYKCKKNSQPWQVAVIN   RYLCGGVLIDPSWVITAA
RSKG-50
```

Heavy chain:

```
                   90        100       110       120
PS (Kallikrein)  QPGDDYSNDLMLLHLSQPADITDGVKVIDLPIEEP
S2 (Tonin)       QPVHDHSNDLMLLHLSEPADITDGVKVIDLPTKE
Esterase B       KPGDDXSNDLMLLXL
Kallikrein k7    KPGDDHSNDLMLLHLSQPADITDGVKV
RSKG-7           KPGDDHSNDLMLLHLSQPADITDGVKVIDLPTEEPKVGST
K1               KPGADHSNDLMLLHLSQPADITDGVKVIDLPTEEPKVGST
S3 (KLP-S3, SEV) QRAYDHNNDLMLLHLSKPADITGGVKVIDLPTEEPKVGSI
Ant γ = kallikrein 10  GDDYSNDLMLLHLSEPADITDGVKVIDLPTKE
T-kininogenase       GDDYSNDLMLLHLSEPADITDGVKVIDLPTE
Proteinase A         GDDHSNDLMLLHLSQPADIT
Proteinase B         GDDYSNDLMLLHLSEPADDSD
S1                 G DYSNDLMLLHLSEPADITDGVKVIDLPTKE
P1 (kallikrein k8)  KPGNDYSNDLMLLHLKTPADITDGVKVIDLPTEEPKVGST
RSKG-3           FPGDDHSNDLMLLHLSEPADITDGVKVIDLPTEEPKVGST
RSGK-50            K DYSNDLMLLHLSEPADITDGVKVIDLPTKEPKVGST
```

Figure 3. Partial amino acid sequence of kallikrein, antigen gamma, esterase B, tonin, and KLP-S3 in comparison to that of other kallikrein-like proteins, mRNA's and genes The name of the homologous protein when known is indicated in parenthesis after the name of the gene or the mRNA. Complete homology was found between the sequenced amino acids of KLP-S3 (2) and the mRNA S3 (11) as well as the vasoconstrictory protein SEV (12). The T-kininogenase antigen γ (4) was found to have the same sequence as kallikrein k10 (13) and with the exception of one amino acid also Proteinase B (14) both shown to have T-kininogenase activity, whereas the T-kininogenase isolated by Xiong et al. (15), showed more variation in the first variable region. Complete homology was also detected between esterase B and kallikrein k7 (16) as well as the gene RSKG-7 (17), whereas minor differences were observed between esterase B/RSKG-7 and K1 (18). The figure also shows the sequence of the proteins proteinase A (14) and tonin (19), the mRNAs kallikrein, and S1 (11), and P1 (20) which has the same sequence as kallikrein k8; and the genes: RSKG-3 (17) and RSKG-50 (21).

X - unidentified amino acid. Open space was used to allienate identical sequences.

IEF and immunoblotting was also used for identification of kallikrein-like proteins in other organs without enzyme purification or knowing the specific substrate to demonstrate activity. In the rat prostate gland, several immunoreactive bands were detected when staining with antiserum against SMG kallikrein, tonin, or KLP-S3. Of these, only one, *i.e.*, KLP-S3, was identical to any of the SMG kallikrein-like proteins (Figure 4). The presence of KLP-S3 was not so clearly demonstrated in tissue homogenate as it was in more enriched fractions. Purification of prostate KLP-S3 revealed that this enzyme behaved chromato-graphically the same as the SMG enzyme, and an identical migration pattern was observed in IEF-gels stained with silver (Figure 4).

Silver staining **Immunoblots**

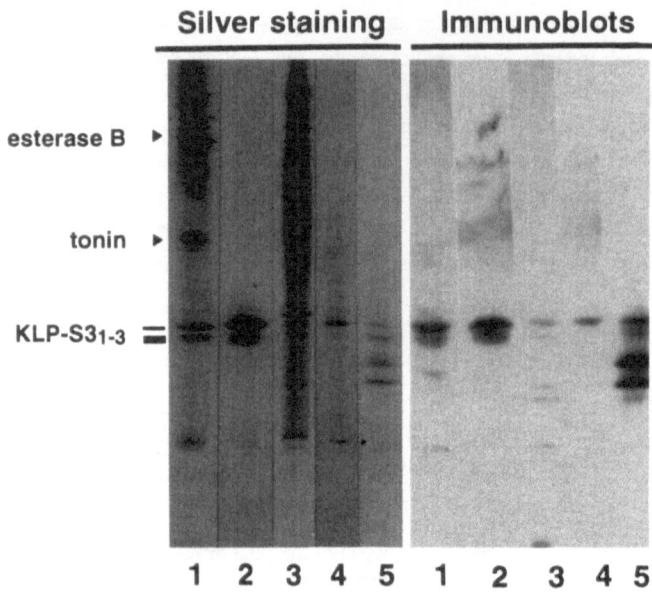

esterase B ▸

tonin ▸

KLP-S3₁-₃ ═

1 2 3 4 5   1 2 3 4 5

Figure 4. Demonstration of KLP-S3 in the rat prostate

KLP-S3 was by IEF and immunoblotting with antiserum against KLP-S3 demonstrated in the rat prostate gland homogenate (lanes marked 3) by comparison with the migration pattern of KLP-S3 in SMG homogenate (lanes marked 1) and purified SMG KLP-S3 (lanes marked 2). KLP-S3 was purified from the prostate gland by DEAE-cellulose anioexchange chromatography (0.05M ammonium-acetate equilibration buffer, pH 5.8, 0.05-0.5M ammonium acetate gradient, pH 5.8) followed by chromatofocusing (pH 7.4 - 4.0) where $KLP-S3_1$ adhered to the column. By this procedure only $KLP-S3_1$ was obtained (lanes marked 4) whereas both $KLP-S3_{1 \text{ and } 2}$ were obtained when the chromatofocusing-(pH 7.4 - 4.0)-void subsequently was run on a chromatofocusing column now using a pH range of 9.3 to 6.0 (lanes marked 5). This fraction also contained other prostate immunoreactive proteins which presently were not further studied. By the identical migration pattern in IEF and the immunoreactivity it was concluded that KLP-S3 was present not only in the SMG but also in the rat prostate.

DISCUSSION

Although kallikrein-like proteins seem to have one preferred natural substrate, overlap in substrate as well as inhibitor specificity has been observed for members of the rat SMG kallikrein family (2). Due to similarities in their amino acid sequence, these enzymes also share antigenic epitopes. Identification of kallikrein-like proteins is therefore hampered by the close relationship between these enzymes, particularly when the natural substrate is not known. During purification of proteins of the rat SMG kallikrein family we observed that kallikrein-like enzymes differed in their pI and thus could easily be separated in flat-bed isoelectrofocusing gels (2, 4, 5). After separation, three-dimensional structures common to kallikrein-like enzymes could be demonstrated by an antiserum with reactivity against common antigenic epitopes. We have previously used a similar principle to identify antigen γ as a kallikrein-like protein (6), where antigen γ was defined as one of the SMG proteins which in immunoelectrophoresis reacted with antikallikrein antiserum in a pattern of partial immunological identity to SMG kallikrein. Similarly, the kallikrein-like nature of tonin was also detected by the demonstration of immunological partial identity between tonin and kallikrein (3). However, flat-bed isoelectrofocusing gives a far better resolution and separation of the different kallikrein-like enzymes than immunoelectrophoresis. Moreover, the technique was sensitive and thus allowed protein identification during the purification procedure without prior concentration, and cross-reacting antigens were easier to detect than with precipitating techniques. Due to the high sensitivity of the technique, contaminating proteins were easily detected during the purification procedure, and based on the determination of their pI, a method for their removal was more adequately determined.

By this method, we were able to detect and purify new SMG kallikrein-like enzymes such as the kallikrein-like protein encoded by the S3 kallikrein family mRNA (2), a protein with vasoconstrictory properties probably identical to SEV isolated by Yamaguchi et al. (12). The method allowed us by identical IEF-migration pattern and immunoreactivity also to demonstrate the presence of this protein in the rat prostate, another organ known to contain members of the kallikrein family. The present results agree with observations at the mRNA level demonstrating the presence of S3 mRNA in the rat prostate (20). Furthermore, by IEF and immunoblotting we were unable to demonstrate the presence of kallikrein, esterase B, tonin, or antigen γ in the prostate. These results are in agreement with studies by Chao & Chao (22) who also did not detect tissue kallikrein and tonin but the presence of esterase A or an esterase A-like protein in the rat prostate.

CONCLUSION

Rat kallikrein-like proteins differ in isoelectric point but share antigenic determinants. Flat-bed isoelectrofocusing combined with immunoblotting thus offered a robust and easy method for identification of kallikrein-like proteins. By immunological cross-reactivity new members of the kallikrein family could be detected. The high resolution and sensitivity of this technique made it useful for protein monitoring during purification of both known and new enzymes. The method was also useful for characterization of antiserum cross-reactivity pattern, and for demonstration of a kallikrein-like protein in other organs without enzyme purification or knowing a specific substrate..

ACKNOWLEDGEMENTS

We are grateful to Ms. Ingunn Brusevold Fjeld for her excellent technical assistance. This study was supported by *The Norwegian Research Council for Science and the Humanities* and The Norwegian Council on Cardiovascular Diseases.

REFERENCES

1. Wines DR, Brady JM, Southard EM, MacDonald RJ. Evolution of the rat kallikrein gene family: Gene conversion leads to functional diversity. J Mol Evol 1991; 32:476-492.

2. Berg T, Schøyen H, Wassdal I, Hull R, Gerskowitch VP, Toft K. Characterization of a new kallikrein-like enzyme (KLP-S3) of the rat submandibular gland. Biochem J 1992; 281:819-828.

3. Ørstavik TB, Carretero OA, Hayashi H, Scicli AG, Johansen L. Immunohistochemical localization of tonin and its relation to kallikrein in rat salivary glands. J Histochem Cytochem 1982; 30:1123-1129.

4. Berg T, Wassdal I, Mindroui T, Sletten K, Scicli G, Carretero OA, Scicli AG. T-kininogenase activity of the rat submandibular gland is predominantly due to the kallikrein-like serine protease antigen gamma. Biochem J 1991; 280:19-25.

5. Berg T, Wassdal I, Sletten K. Immunhistochemical localization of rat submandibular gland esterase B (homologous to the RSKG-7 kallikrein gene) in relation to other serine proteases of the kallikrein family. J Histochem Cytochem 1992; 40:83-92.

6.   Berg T, Holck M, Johansen L. Isolation, characterization, and localization of antigen γ, a serine protease of the "kallikrein-family" in the rat submandibular gland. Hoppe-Seyler's Z Physiol Chem 1987; 368:1455-1467.

7.   Johansen L, Bergundhaugen H, Berg T. Rapid purification of tonin, esterase B, antigen gamma, and kallikrein from rat submandibular gland by fast protein liquid chromatography. J Chromatography 1987; 387: 347-

8.   Taylor CR. The nature of Reed-Sternberg cells and other malignant "reticulum" cells. Lancet 1974; Oct.:802-806.

9.   Cornwell GG, Sletten K, Johansson B, Westermark P. Evidence that the amyloid fibril protein in senile systemic amyloidosis is derived from normal prealbumin. Biochem Biophys Res Comm 1988; 154:648-653.

10. Berg T. Immunohistochemical viewing of kallikrein in tissues. Methods in Enzymol 1988; 163:143-159.

11. Ashley PL, MacDonald RJ. Kallikrein-related mRNAs of the rat submaxillary gland: Nucleotide sequences of four distinct types including tonin. Biochemistry 1985; 24:4512-4520.

12. Yamaguchi T, Carretero OA, Scicli AG. A novel serine protease with vasoconstrictor activity coded by the kallikrein gene S3. J Biol Chem 1991; 266:5011-5017.

13. Gutman N, Elmoujahed A, Brillard M, Monegier Du Sorbier B, Gauthier F. Microheterogeneity of rat submaxillary gland kallikrein k10, a member of the kallikrein family. Eur J Biochem 1991; 197:425-429.

14. Kato H, Nakanishi E, Enjyoji K-i, Hayashi I, Oh-ishi S, Iwanaga S. Characterization of serine proteinases isolated from rat submaxillary gland: With special reference to the degradation of rat kininogens by these enzymes. J Biochem 1987; 102:1389-1404.

15. Xiong W, Chen L-M-, Chao J. Purification and characterization of a kallikrein-like T-kininogenase. J Biol Chem 1990; 265:2822-2827.

16. Elmoujahed A, Gutman N, Brillard M, Gauthier F. Substrate specificity of two kallikrein family gene products isolated from the rat submaxillary. FEBS Lett 1990; 265:137-140.

17. Chen Y-P, Chao J, Chao L. Molecular cloning and characterization of two rat renal kallikrein genes. Biochemistry 1988; 27:189-7196.

18. Brady JM, MacDonald RJ. The expression of two kallikrein gene family members in the rat kidney. Arch Biochem Biophys 1990; 278:342-349.

19. Lazure C, Leduc R, Seidah NG, Thibault G, Genest J, Chretien M. The complete amino acid sequence of rat submaxillary gland tonin does contain the aspartic acid at the active site: confirmation by protein sequence analysis. Biochem Cell Biol 1987; 65:321-337.

20. Brady JM, Wines DR, MacDonald RJ. Expression of two kallikrein gene family members in the rat prostate. Biochemistry 1989; 28:5203-5210.

21. Shai S-Y, Woodley-Miller C, Chao J, Chao L. Characterization of genes encoding rat tonin and a kallikrein-like serine protease. Biochemistry 1989; 28:5334-5343.

22. Chao J and Chao L. Identification and expression of kallikrein gene family in rat submandibular and prostate glands using monoclonal antibodies as specific probes. Biochim. Biophys. Acta 1987; 910:233-239.

AAS 38/I
Recent Progress on Kinins
© 1992 Birkhäuser Verlag Basel

COMPARATIVE STUDIES ON P2 SPECIFICITY OF WILD-TYPE RAT TISSUE KALLIKREIN, Y99H:W215G MUTANT AND TONIN

Jing Wang, Julie Chao, Luiz Juliano[*] and Lee Chao

Department of Biochemistry and Molecular Biology, Medical University of South Carolina, Charleston, SC 29425, USA, and [*]Department of Biophysics, Escola Paulista de Medicina, Caixa Postal 20388, 04034 Sao Paulo, Brazil

SUMMARY

To probe residues responsible for P2 specificity, we have recently created a mutant enzyme from rat tissue kallikrein with Tyr99 to His and Trp215 to Gly exchange (Y99H:W215G) using site-specific mutagenesis. In the present study, additional characterization of substrate specificities of both wild-type tissue kallikrein, Y99H:W215G mutant and native tonin was performed using synthetic Ac-X-Arg-pNA substrates especially designed for testing P2 specificity. Kinetic analyses of K_m and k_{cat} demonstrate a clear correlation between dramatically reduced affinity for hydrophobic P2 side-chain and the loss of the Tyr99-Trp215 hydrophobic pair. Analyses of rat tonin reveal a correlation between increased reaction rate and P2 hydrophilicity although tonin displays similar pattern in P2 affinity as compared with tissue kallikrein, suggesting a less hydrophobic environment in the substrate-binding pocket of rat tonin. The results strongly support the hypothesis that Tyr99-Trp215 interaction is the major determinant for P2 specificity and that the presence of a hydrophobic side-chain in P2 position substantially facilitates substrate hydrolysis of tissue kallikrein-like enzymes.

INTRODUCTION

Kallikreins are a group of highly homologous serine proteinases comprising a multigene family[1]. Different members of the kallikrein family specifically cleave different peptide precursors to release biologically active peptides, and these members are expressed in a tissue-specific fashion[2]. As a result of this diversity, kallikreins have been implicated in a variety of physiological and pathophysiological processes[1,2].

One of the most intriguing features of the kallikrein family is the distinct substrate specificity among individual members despite their high degree of sequence identity (70-90%) at the protein level[3,6] and very similar tertiary structures[4,5]. A famous example is the comparison between rat tissue kallikrein and tonin. With 74% sequence identity at the protein level and highly conserved tertiary structures[4,5], these two enzymes differ significantly in substrate selection. Rat tissue kallikrein selectively cleaves between Arg-Arg and Arg-Ala in both low molecular weight and high molecular weight rat kininogens[7], liberating bradykinin. Tonin, however, also cleaves between Phe-X[9,10]. It convert angiotensinogen to angiotensin II, by cleaving between Phe-His[9]. Their specificity difference is also reflected on their preference for different P2 side-chains[8,11].

When comparisons were made between the key residues of kallikreins in the substrate binding pocket (Table 1), the S1 subsite Asp189 is conserved throughout the family and most of the members have also conserved the Gly216 and Gly226 located at the opening of the binding pocket. This led us to believe that alternative residues must be responsible for the specificity difference. X-ray diffraction study has suggested the role of Tyr99 and Trp215 in P2 specificity toward a bulky hydrophobic side chain[4,12]. When sequences are compared at these two positions, a very interesting difference is observed[1-3,13]. Both tonin and the S3 enzyme have replaced the Tyr99-Trp215 pair with His99 and Gly215, respectively. Whereas the majority of the kallikrein-like members have conserved the hydrophobic pair. Among the remaining members, RSKG7 and RSKG3 have a tonin-like Tyr99 to His substitution but conserved the Trp215. The recently purified protein counterpart of RSKG7 (k7) displays a different specificity from true tissue kallikrein by favoring a Val residue in stead of Phe in the P2 position[13]. Two human members, hGK1 and PSA, have also replaced Tyr99 with a Ser residue while conserving the Trp215. These seem to indicate that the Tyr99-Trp215 pair plays an important role in the function of the enzyme. To probe the function of this hydrophobic pair, we have recently created a Tyr99 to His and Trp215 to Gly mutation on rat tissue kallikrein enzyme to generate the Y99H:W215G mutant[11]. In this study, we have compared wild-type, mutant kallikreins and tonin using a set of Ac-X-Arg-pNA substrates specially designed for testing P2 specificity.

Table 1. Comparison of key amino acids in the substrate-binding pocket of kallikrein-like enzymes

	189	216	226	99	215
PS (rat)	Asp	Gly	Gly	Tyr	Trp
P1 (rat)	Asp	Gly	Ser	Tyr	Trp
PPK (porcine)	Asp	Gly	Ser	Tyr	Trp
kallikrein (human)	Asp	Gly	Ser	Tyr	Trp
kallikrein (monkey)	Asp	Gly	Ala	Tyr	Trp
hGK1 (human)	Asp	Gly	Gly	Ser	Trp
PSA (human)	Asp	Gly	Gly	Ser	Trp
RSKG7 (rat)	Asp	Gly	Ala	His	Trp
RSKG3 (rat)	Asp	Ser	Ala	His	Trp
S3 (rat)	Asp	Gly	Ala	His	Gly
Tonin (rat)	Asp	Gly	Ala	His	Gly

MATERIALS AND METHODS

Materials The following materials were obtained from commercial sources: Affi-Gel 10, low molecular mass protein standards, prestained molecular mass protein standards (Bio-Rad); DEAE-Sepharose CL-6B (Pharmacia); bovine serum albumin, Coomassie Blue, rifampicin (Sigma); DTT (Aldrich). All other reagents used were of analytical grade.

<u>Vectors and Bacterial Strains</u> *E. coli* HB101 [hsdS20, (rB-, mB-) recA13, ara-14, proA2, lacY, galK2, rps (smr), xyl-5, mtl-1, supE44, λ-/F-/-] is from S. Tabor (Harvard Medical School). pGP1-2, provided by S. Tabor, is a derivative of pACYC177 that contains gene 1 of phage T7 under the control of the inducible λ PL promoter, and the gene for the heat-sensitive λ repressor, cI857.

<u>Expression of Kallikrein Mutants in *E. coli* Cells</u> *E. coli* HB101/pGP1-2 carrying recombinant plasmids were grown with aeration at 30°C in 2YT medium containing 50 μg/ml-ampicillin and kanamycin. At A590 of 1.0, the cells were induced at 42°C for 25 min. Rifampicin was then added to a final concentration of 100 μg/ml. The temperature was reduced to 37°C for an additional 2 h, and the cells were harvested.

<u>Purification of Kallikrein Mutant</u> *E. coli* HB101/pGP1-2 harboring the mutant expression plasmid was cultured as described above. The cells were harvested by centrifugation at 4,000 x g for 30 min. The pellets were combined and washed with 10 mM-Tris-HCl (pH 8.0) and resuspended in 1/50 volume of buffer [10 mM-Tris-HCl (pH 8.0), 1mM-EDTA, 1μg/ml DNase I, 1 mM-MgCl$_2$]. The cells were lysed by two passages through a French pressure cell (Amicon) at 110.4 MPa (16,000 lbf/in2). The homogenate was then centrifuged at 27,000 g for 30 min and the supernatant fraction was used as the starting material for mutant purification. The purification procedures were essentially as described[14] except that the activity of chromatographic fractions was monitered by the amidolytic activity using D-Pro-Phe-Arg-AMC (7-amino-4-methyl coumarin) as the substrate as measured by fluorescence spectrophotometry with the excitation wavelength at 380 nm and the emission wavelength at 460 nm. Rat tonin[15] was purified from submandibular gland using the procedure essentially as described. Concentrations of wild-type and mutant kallikreins were determined by a direct radioimmunoassay[16].

<u>Kinetic Analyses</u> Steady state kinetic studies were performed at 25°C in reaction buffer [50 mM-Tris-HCl (pH 9.0), 1 mM EDTA, 100 μg/ml BSA, 0.02% (w/v)NaN$_3$]. Synthetic Ac-X-Arg-pNA substrates were used for each of the three enzymes: wild-type recombinant kallikrein, tonin, and mutant Y99H:W215G. The concentrations of enzymes used ranged from 20 nM to 100 nM depending on the level of activity. The concentrations of substrates ranged from 5 times less than K$_m$ to 5 times greater than K$_m$ when possible (the highest concentration used was 2.0 mM and the lowest concentration was 10 μM). The initial velocity was measured by a Cary 3 Spectrophotometer with the wavelength at 405 nm. Five to eight initial velocities were recorded for each substrate. Values of K$_m$ and k_{cat} were determined by linear regression analysis of the Line Weaver-Burk equation.

RESULTS AND DISCUSSION

<u>Purification of Mutant Enzymes From *E. coli*</u>

The wild-type and mutant kallikreins have been purified from *E. coli* lysate (HB101/pGP1-2 harboring recombinant plasmids) to homogeneity with DEAE-Sepharose CL-6B and aprotinin-affinity column chromatography. The purity of each enzyme was analyzed by reduced SDS-PAGE to contain one single band of approximately 36 kDa and the recombinant proteins were recognized by specific anti-rat tissue kallikrein antibodies[14]. Concentrations of purified enzymes were measured by direct radioimmunoassay for rat tissue kallikrein as we have shown that the mutant displays immunological identities with both the native and the wild-type kallikrein[11].

Kinetic Analyses of Wild-type and Mutant Kallikreins and Native Tonin

The substrate specificity of the wild-type and mutant kallikreins were examined using synthetic Ac-X-Arg-pNA substrates. The substrates used were designed such that the P1 residue, the protecting and the leaving groups are all identical with only the P2 side-chains differing from each other. The purpose of our experiment is to probe residues responsible for P2 specificity. Hydrolysis of peptidyl pNA substrates by these enzymes followed Michaelis-Menten kinetics under a wide range of substrate concentrations. The kinetic parameters, k_{cat}, K_m and k_{cat}/K_m, of these enzymes toward different substrates are presented in Table 2.

Table 2. Steady state kinetics of Ac-X-Arg-pNA substrate hydrolysis by wild-type tissue kallikrein (wt-kallikrein), Y99H:W215G mutant and native tonin

Substrate		Enzyme		
		wt-kallikrein	Y99H:W215G	tonin
	K_m (mM)	0.796	1.39	7.10
Ac-Glu-Arg-pNA	k_{cat} (s⁻¹)	1.30	0.38	21.67
	k_{cat}/K_m (mM⁻¹s⁻¹)	1.63	0.27	3.05
	K_m (mM)	0.738	1.38	7.39
Ac-Ser-Arg-pNA	k_{cat} (s⁻¹)	5.94	0.46	4.59
	k_{cat}/K_m (mM⁻¹s⁻¹)	8.05	0.33	0.62
	K_m (mM)	0.202	2.64	0.382
Ac-Leu-Arg-pNA	k_{cat} (s⁻¹)	54.55	4.88	0.55
	k_{cat}/K_m (mM⁻¹s⁻¹)	270.05	1.85	1.44
	K_m (mM)	0.079	3.52	0.674
Ac-Phe-Arg-pNA	k_{cat} (s⁻¹)	46.56	40.23	0.33
	k_{cat}/K_m (mM⁻¹s⁻¹)	590.11	11.43	0.49

Wild-type tissue kallikrein has the highest affinity toward Ac-Phe-Arg-pNA (K_m=79 μM) which has the highest hydrophobicity score among all the P2 residues tested while its lowest affinity is toward Ac-Glu-Phe-pNA (K_m=796 μM) which has the lowest hydrophobicity score. Its affinity toward P2 Phe is 2.6-fold higher than toward the slightly less hydrophobic P2 Leu and is 9.3- to 10.1-fold higher than with P2 Ser or Glu. There is a perfect correlation between its increased affinity and greater P2 hydrophobicity.

When the P2 affinity is compared with the wild-type tissue kallikrein, the Y99H:W215G mutant has drastically reduced affinity toward hydrophobic side-chain as its K_m value toward the P2 Leu is 13.1-fold higher than that of the wild-type and toward Phe is nearly 44.6-fold higher than that of the wild-type. However, its P2 affinity toward hydrophilic side-chains remains comparable with the wild-type enzyme (Table 2). An amazing fact is that despite the loss of affinity toward Phe, the reaction rate of the mutant toward Ac-Phe-Arg-pNA remains essentially the same as that of the wild-type enzyme. These results clearly indicate that the Tyr99-Trp215 pair is critical to the high-affinity binding of the rat tissue kallikrein toward hydrophobic side-chains at P2 position.

In addition, when the reaction rates (k_{cat} value) are compared between the wild-type and the mutant kallikrein, another relationship can be observed. That is the correlation between the increase of k_{cat} value and the hydrophobicity of the P2 residue. The wild-type enzyme has comparably high reaction rates toward substrates with either Phe and Leu as P2 while it has much lower (1/168 to 1/8) rates toward P2 Ser and Glu. The mutant displays an almost perfect correlation between its k_{cat} value and P2 hydrophobicity. This phenomenon suggests that some other factors in addition to Tyr99 and Trp215 may contribute to efficient catalysis of substrates with hydrophobic P2 residues and that the presence of a hydrophobic side-chain in P2 position substantially facilitates the hydrolysis of substrates. This is not unlikely considering the highly hydrophobic environment in the substrate-binding pocket of kallikrein-like enzymes.

When tonin is analyzed using these substrates, a rather complex picture was revealed (Table 2). As affinity is compared, tonin somewhat resembles the wild-type kallikrein with dramatically elevated K_m value toward both Ser and Glu as P2. On the other hand, its affinity toward hydrophobic Leu and Phe as P2 is significantly lower than that of the wild-type due to the lack of Tyr99-Trp215 sandwich, suggesting that some secondary factors may contribute to the affinity toward hydrophobic P2 residues. When the reaction rate is examined, however, tonin is to the contrary of both the wild-type and the mutant tissue kallikrein. There is a perfect correlation between the increase of k_{cat} value and P2 hydrophilicity in stead of hydrophobicity. The reaction rates of tonin toward hydrophilic P2 Glu is 4.7-fold higher than toward the less hydrophilic P2 Ser and is 39.4- to 65.7-fold higher than toward hydrophobic P2 Leu and Phe, respectively. Since tonin has a considerably different compostion of the binding pocket[5], this is not entirely unexpected. Despite the higher affinity toward a hydrophobic P2, the overall environment of the substrate-binding pocket in tonin is much less hydrophobic than that of tissue kallikrein. A likely possibility is that a hydrophobic P2 may be bound more favorably through alternative residues, it is the substrate with a hydrophilic P2 which is positioned more favorably for hydrolysis. This is not unusual considering that specific peptide inhibitors bind with very high affinity with the enzyme while are left completely uncleaved.

Our studies support the hypothesis by Chen and Bode that Tyr99 and Trp215 dictates a P2 specificity toward hydrophobic side-chain. Based on the X-ray diffraction study of Chen and Bode[12], Tyr99 and Trp215 are located closely to each other (approximately 4 Å apart) in the binding pocket. In the structure of free porcine kallikrein, these two residues are interacting with each other through hydrophobic interaction and they form a 30° angle that opens toward the binding pocket[4]. In the binary complex of PPK-BPTI, this hydrophobic pair is located closely (4.8 to 6 Å) with the P2 side chain of the inhibitor (Cys14) (Figure 1). This has led to the proposal by Chen and Bode[12] that Tyr99 and Trp215 form a hydrophobic sandwich responsible for the P2 specificity toward a bulky hydrophobic side chain. In the mutant kallikrein, the hydrophobic Tyr99-Trp215 pair was replaced with a less hydrophobic His99-Gly215. Our kinetic analyses of the Y99H:W215G strongly support the above hypothesis that Tyr99 and Trp215 are major determinants for the P2 specificity of rat tissue kallikrein.

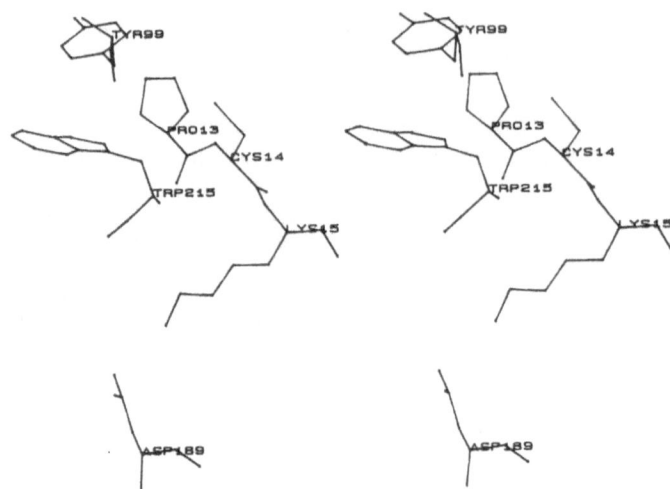

Figure 1. Substrate-binding area of porcine pancreatic kallikrein bound with bovine pancreatic trypsin inhibitor. Residue Asp189 corresponds to the S1 subsite, Tyr99 and Trp215 correspond to the S2 subsite, residues 13 to 15 represent the P3 to P1 positions of the inhibitor with the pseudocleavage site between Lys15 and Ala16 (Chen and Bode, 1983).

ACKNOWLEDGEMENTS

We thank Dr. S. Hazard for excellent technical assistance in computer modelling. This work was supported by NIH grant HL 29397.

REFERENCES

1.   Clements, J. A. (1989) "The glandular kallikrein family of enzymes: Tissue-specific expression and hormonal regulation." Endocrine Reviews 10, 393-418.
2.   Murray, S. R., Chao, J., Lin, F. K., and Chao, L. (1990) "Kallikrein multigene families and the regulation of their expression." J. Cardiovascular Pharmc. 15, S7-S16.
3.   MacDonald, R. J., Margolius, H. S., and Erdos, E. G. (1988) "Molecular biology of tissue kallikrein." Biochem. J. 253, 313-321.
4.   Bode, W., Chen, Z., Bartels, K., Kutzbach, C., Schmidtkastner, G., and Bartunik, H. (1983) "Refined 2 Å X-ray crystal structure of porcine kallikrein A." J. Mol. Biol. 164, 237-282.

5. Fujinaga, M., and James, M. N. G. (1986) "Rat submaxillary gland serine protease, tonin: Structure solution and refinement at 1.8 Å resolution." J. Mol. Biol. 195, 373-396.
6. Ashley, P. L., MacDonald, R. J. (1985) "Kallikrein-related mRNAs of the rat submaxillary gland: Nucleotide sequences of four distinct types including tonin." Biochem. 24, 4512-4520.
7. Kato, H., Enjyoji, K., Miyata, T., Hayashi, I., Oh-ishi, S., and Iwanaga, S, (1985) "Demonstration of arginyl-bradykinin moiety in rat HMW kininogen: direct evidence for liberation of bradykinin by rat glandular kallikreins." Biochem. Biophys. Res. Commun. 127, 228-295.
8. Fiedler, F. (1987) "Effects of secondary interactions on the kinetics of peptide and peptide ester hydrolysis by tissue kallikrein and trypsin." Eur. J. Biochem. 163, 303-312.
9. Schiller, P. W., Demassieux, S., Boucher, R. (1976) "Substrate specificity of tonin from rat submaxillary gland." Circ. Res. 39, 629-632.
10. Chretien, M., Lee, C. M., Sandberg, B. E. B., Iversen, L. L., Boucher, R., Seidah, N. G. and Genest, J. (1980) "Substrate specificity of the enzyme tonin: Cleavage of substance P." FEBS Lett. 113, 173-176.
11. Wang, J., Chao, J., and Chao, L. (1992) "Specificity determinants of rat tissue kallikrein analyzed by site-specific mutagenesis." Biochemistry. submitted.
12. Chen, Z., and Bode, W. (1983) "Refined 2.5 Å X-ray crystal structure of the complex formed by porcine kallikrein A and the bovine pancreatic trypsin inhibitor." J. Mol. Biol. 164, 282-311.
13. Elmoujahed, A., Gutman, N., Brillard, M., and Gauthier, G. (1990) "Substrate specificity of two kallikrein family gene products isolated from the rat submaxillary gland." FEBS Lett. 265, 137-140.
14. Wang, J., Chao, J., and Chao, L. (1991) "Purification and characterization of recombinant rat tissue kallikrein from *Escherichia coli* and yeast." Biochem. J. 276, 63-71.
15. Shih, H. C., Chao, L., and Chao, J. (1986) "Age and hormonal dependence of tonin levels in rat submandibular gland as determined by a new direct radioimmunoassay." Biochem. J. 238, 145-149.
16. Shimamoto, K., Margolius, H. S., Chao, J., and Crosswell, A. R. (1979) "A direct radioimmunoassay of rat urinary kallikrein and comparison with other measures of urinary kallikrein activity." J. Lab. Clin. Med. 94, 172-179.

AAS 38/I
Recent Progress on Kinins
© 1992 Birkhäuser Verlag Basel

EXPRESSION OF HUMAN SALIVARY-GLAND KALLIKREIN IN INSECT CELLS BY A BACULOVIRUS VECTOR

H.-P. Rahn, A. Angermann, T. Hektor, M. Klöppinger and M. Kemme

Institut für Biochemie, Technische Hochschule Darmstadt, Petersenstr. 22,
W-6100 Darmstadt, FRG

SUMMARY: A cDNA fragment encoding human salivary-gland kallikrein, including the kallikrein-owned signal peptide, was inserted into a baculovirus vector adjacent to the polyhedrin promoter and expressed in transfected insect cells. Biologically active kallikrein was isolated to homogeneity from serum-free culture supernatant using a four-step protocol. The N-terminal amino acid sequence of the insect-derived kallikrein was identical to that of the natural proteinase, thus indicating the proper removal of the mammalian signal peptide.

INTRODUCTION

Tissue kallikreins (EC 3.4.21.35) belong to a closely related subfamily of trypsin-like glycoproteins synthesized by exocrine glands which are characterized by their ability to release vasodepressor peptides from kininogens upon cleavage at two selected sites (1). The principal determinants of this kallikrein specificity are explained by unique structural features with protruding surface loops surrounding the active site and an extended hydrophobic substrate binding cavity. The enzyme scaffold is covalently cross-linked by five disulfide bridges (2), suggesting that correct disulfide bond-mediated folding is essential for its biological function.

Heterologous gene expression turned out to be a major prerequisite for a detailed study of kallikrein structure-function relationships. Efforts have been made to overproduce human and rat tissue kallikreins in different *Escherichia coli* (3, 4) and *Saccharomyces cerevisiae* (4) expression systems, which resulted in low yields of active enzymes and considerable amounts of insoluble aggregates and improperly folded recombinant material. Recently, the baculovirus *Autographa californica* nuclear polyhedrosis virus (AcNPV) was shown in our laboratory to be suitable as an efficient expression vector for the production of human tissue prokallikrein in mg-amounts using infected *Spodoptera frugiperda* (Sf9) insect cells (5). Correct processing of the exported proenzyme and post-translational glycosylation was demonstrated and proved the versatility of the baculovirus-based expression system.

In the present study, we describe the expression of biologically active human salivary-gland kallikrein in recombinant AcNPV-infected Sf9 cells cultivated under different medium conditions. The isolated enzyme has been purified to homogeneity and characterized by proteinchemical data.

MATERIALS AND METHODS

The recombinant transfer vector pVLKA30 based upon pVL1392 (generous gift of M. Summers, College Station, Texas) was constructed using fragments of the human salivary-gland preprokallikrein cDNA (3) according to established cloning protocols (6). Co-transfection into Sf9 cells and purification of recombinant virus were performed as described by Summers and Smith (7).

Sf9 cells were plated in 175-cm^2 flasks at a density of 2 - 3 x 10^5 cells/ml in TC100 medium (5) supplemented with 5 % fetal calf serum (FCS) and maintained at 27 °C. After 4 days, infection with recombinant virus occured at a rate of 1 plaque forming unit/cell and 5 days post-infection the cell supernatant was harvested by centrifugation at 2000 g for 20 min. Alternatively, Sf9 cells were rinsed twice with TC100 prior to infection and transfected cells were propagated in the same medium without serum.

Secreted kallikrein was purified by a modification of the procedure described previously (5). Culture supernatant (100 ml) was diluted 10-fold with 20 mM sodium phosphate buffer, pH 6.0 and applied to a DEAE-cellulose DE52 column (12 x 2 cm, Whatman) equilibrated with the same buffer. The column was washed with 1 l of the above buffer und elution was performed by two isocratic steps (1 l each) using the same buffer with 0.1 M NaCl and then with 1.0 M NaCl. Kallikrein containing fractions of the second elution step were pooled, concentrated by ultrafiltration (YM-10 membrane, Amicon) to a volume of 10 ml and further fractionated on a Sephacryl S-200 column (110 x 4 cm, Pharmacia) equilibrated with 50 mM sodium phosphate buffer, pH 7.0, 750 mM NaCl. Enzymatically active fractions were collected, dialysed overnight against 20 mM sodium phosphate buffer, pH 6.0 and applied to a Fractogel EMD-TMAE 650 (S) column (Superformance 150-10, Merck) fitted to FPLC equipment (Pharmacia). Kallikrein was eluted with a 45 ml linear NaCl gradient (0 - 0.5 M) in dialysis buffer and the volume was reduced to 200 µl in a microconcentrator (Centricon-10, Amicon). Final purification was achieved on a Superose 12 HR 10/30 column (Pharmacia) with 10 mM sodium phosphate buffer, pH 7.2, 100 mM NaCl.

All purification steps were performed at 4 °C. Chromatography fractions were monitored at 280 nm and protein concentrations calculated by the standard protocol of the BCA protein assay kit (Pierce) using bovine serum albumin for calibration.

The purity of the kallikrein preparation was controlled by SDS/PAGE according to Laemmli (8) and immunological identification achieved by Western blot analysis (9) using a rabbit antiserum against human urinary kallikrein (kind gift of U. Gröschel-Stewart, Darmstadt).

For detection of kallikrein distribution an indirect enzyme immunosorbent assay (ELISA) was developed on the basis of established procedures (10) with the above mentioned polyclonal antiserum. Specific antibody-binding was quantified by monitoring p-nitrophenol release at 405 nm with goat anti-rabbit IgG, alkaline phosphatase conjugated.

Esterolytic kallikrein activity was measured by a two enzyme coupled assay introduced by Fiedler (11).

The N-terminal amino acid sequence of kallikrein (150 pmol) was determined employing a model 470A gas-phase sequencer with on-line HPLC 120A system (Applied Biosystems).

RESULTS AND DISCUSSION

The construction of the baculovirus transfer vector pVLKA30 (Fig. 1) was based upon a human salivary-gland kallikrein cDNA fragment comprising only the mature enzyme-coding region from the first N-terminal Ile-codon to the opal stop signal (3). A synthetic adaptor encoding the kallikrein-owned signal peptide was ligated to the 5´-end of the cDNA and the hybrid gene was inserted downstream of the strong polyhedrin promoter in the expression plasmid pVL1392 generating an artificial kallikrein precursor.

After co-transfection of Sf9 cells with pVLKA30 and AcNPV DNA, a recombinant virus strain was purified and used to infect Sf9 expression cultures. Parallel approaches in FCS-containing and serum-free medium resulted in constitutive expression and secretion of recombinant kallikrein into the fermentation broth. The cell-free supernatant was subjected to a purification protocol which is based upon the isolation procedure for tissue prokallikrein (5).

The purification scheme involved two alternating anion exchange chromatography and gel filtration steps which allowed the separation of very low kallikrein amounts displaying enzymatic activity in the case of FCS-containing cultures. The ELISA data of the S-200 gel filtration profile (Fig. 2A) exhibited two peaks with major protein content in the high-molecular fraction which indicated a kallikrein complex formation. This speculation was

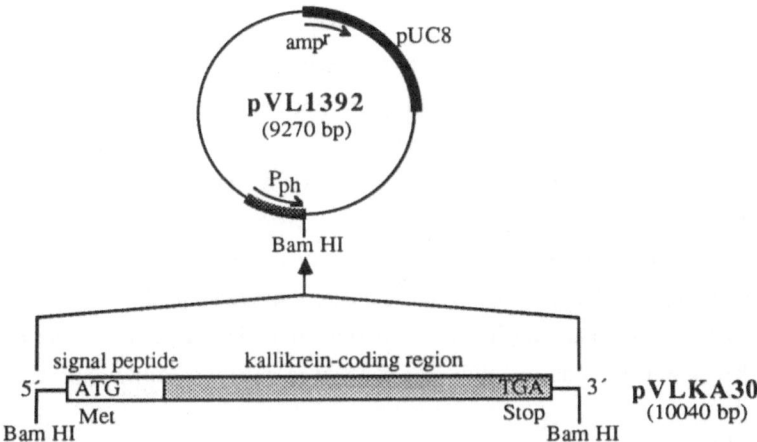

Figure 1. Construction of the transfer vector pVLKA30.
The kallikrein cDNA fragments were inserted into the Bam HI site of pVL1392 downstream the polyhedrin promoter (P_{ph}) which is flanked by wild-type AcNPV DNA sequences. In addition, the vector contains the pUC8 plasmid carrying the ampicillin resistence gene (amp^r).

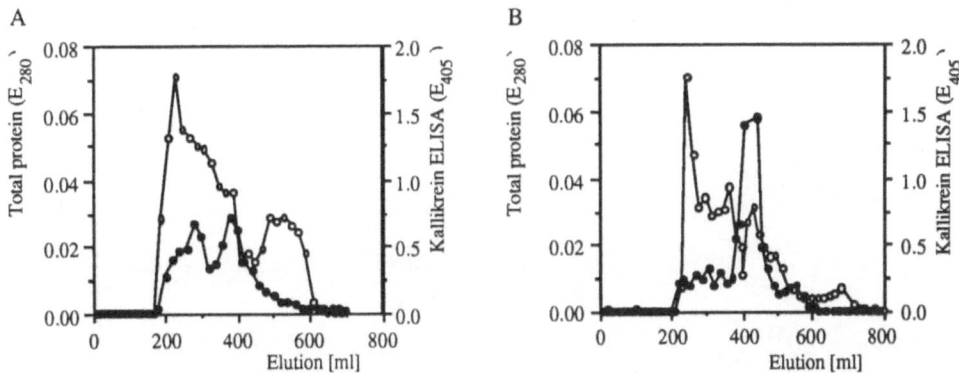

Figure 2. Sephacryl S-200 gel filtration chromatography of (A) FCS-containing and (B) serum-free transfected Sf9 culture medium after DEAE-cellulose preseparation. Total protein content was monitored spectrophotometrically (O) while kallikrein was detected by an indirect ELISA (●).

confirmed by Western blot analysis (Fig. 3A) of both peaks showing a distinct pattern with a 95 kDa kallikrein immuno-reactive protein band and a low-molecular product identical with purified kallikrein from serum-free cultures. Together, these results strongly indicate that the secreted kallikrein forms SDS-stable, high-molecular weight complexes with protein components of the fetal calf serum and was therefore removed during purification. It remains to be elucidated whether α_1-proteinase inhibitor or a hitherto unknown specific kallikrein-binding protein from bovine serum acts as complex partner shown in the case of tissue kallikrein-binding proteins from humans and rats (12).

To increase the level of kallikrein recovery we employed the well introduced purification protocol (5) for fermentation cultures propagating recombinant Sf9 cells in serum-free medium post-infection. Due to the reduction of contaminating protein by-products the chromatography profiles exhibited fewer and better separated peaks as for instance shown in the S-200 gel filtration pattern (Fig. 2). In contrast to the FCS-containing sample, only one prominent kallikrein immuno-reactive maximum was detected in the expected molecular mass-range

Fig. 3B represents the proteins obtained at various stages in the isolation process. The majority of Sf9-derived insect proteins released as a result of cell lysis in the late fermentation phase were effectively separated during S-200 gel filtration and TMAE anion exchange chromatography. The purified recombinant kallikrein (lane 9) migrated as a single, broad band indicating microheterogeneity, possibly due to a variation in carbohydrate content. The same phenomenon has been observed in the corresponding baculovirus expression system of tissue

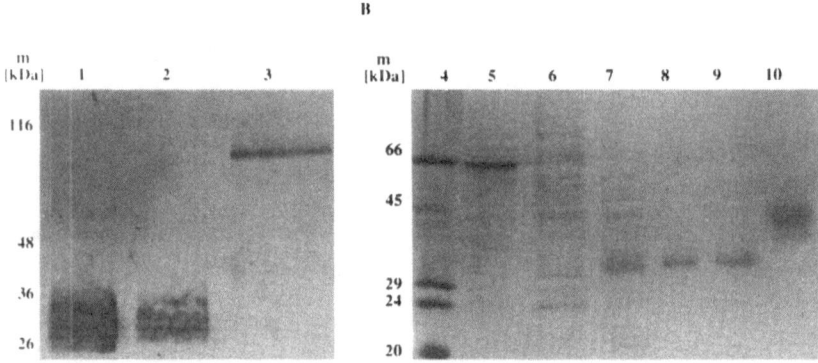

Figure 3. SDS-PAGE and Western blot analysis of recombinant Sf9 supernatant proteins. Electrophoresis was performed on 12.5 % polyacrylamide slab gels. (A) Immunoblotting of kallikrein complex formation; lane 1, purified kallikrein from serum-free culture; lane 2 and 3, low-molecular-mass and high-molecular-mass fractions of S-200-eluate isolated from FCS-containing medium. (B) SDS-PAGE of the isolation products from serum-free culture. Protein was stained with Coomassie Blue; lane 4, low-molecular mass-markers; lane 5, supernatant of pVLKA30/Sf9-culture; lane 6; DEAE-cellulose eluate; lane 7, pooled S-200 column fractions; lane 8, kallikrein from TMAE-separation; lane 9, purified kallikrein eluted from Superose 12; lane 10, human urinary kallikrein.

prokallikrein (5) suggesting the different recognition of all three potential N-glycosylation sites. The apparent molecular mass of the kallikrein band was about 33 kDa which was confirmed by gel filtration on a calibrated Superose 12 column (data not shown).

Table 1 summarizes a representative purification of recombinant kallikrein from serum-free culture supernatants. A 700-fold purification was achieved in four steps, giving a kallikrein yield of 12 % with regard to esterolytic activity and a total amount of 100 μg homogenous protein per litre fermentation broth which corresponds to an initial concentration of 1 mg kallikrein per litre supernatant as calculated from the activity. The kallikrein isolate exhibited a specific esterolytic activity of 280 U/mg, which is comparable to the value of trypsin activated prokallikrein produced in the previously described baculovirus-infected Sf9 cell line (5).

Table 1. Purification of recombinant salivary-gland kallikrein from serum-free Sf9 culture.

Purification step	Volume [ml]	Total protein[a] [mg]	Activity[b] [U]	Specific activity [U/mg]	Yield [%]	Purification [-fold]
supernatant	100	54.5	23.0	0.4	100	1
DEAE-cellulose	218	6.2	8.2	1.3	36	3
Sephacryl S-200	180	1.8	6.8	3.8	30	10
TMAE-Fractogel	6	0.07	3.9	56	17	140
Superose 12	1	0.01	2.8	280	12	700

[a] BCA method. [b] 1 esterolytic unit equals 1 μmol Ac-Phe-Arg-OEt hydrolysed/min at 25 °C.

The enzymatic activity of the secreted material should not obscure the fact that the expression level revealed a dramatic drop compared to the secretion of 10 mg recombinant prokallikrein per litre fermentation broth in the analogous baculovirus system. It seems unlikely that this significant difference is attributable to a low transcription/translation competence of the constructed expression plasmid pVLKA30 since both cDNA fragments encoding the proenzyme and mature kallikrein were inserted in the same cloning site of pVL1392. In either baculovirus transfer vectors the genetic elements driving heterologous protein expression (13) are identical with respect to promoter strength, integrity of the polyhedrin mRNA leader and codon usage.

N-terminal sequencing allowed detection of the first six amino acids Ile-Val-Gly-Gly-Trp-Glu, which match perfectly with the amino acid sequence deduced from the salivary-gland kallikrein cDNA (3). This result supported the purity of the isolated material and proved the accurate cleavage of the original kallikrein signal peptide.

Both findings, kallikrein processing and secretion, demonstrated the ability of the insect cells to recognize a human signal sequence, to separate the prepeptide at the correct position and release the recombinant material along a secretory pathway. However, the reason for the low efficiency of this process remains unclear and the reduced secretion of active kallikrein compared to prokallikrein may be due to an obstruction within the processing mechanism. Further experiments are planned to investigate the prospective accumulation of recombinant kallikrein in the transport pathway of the insect cells after removal of the signal sequence indicating a slow cleavage of the artificial Ala-Ile-link by means of the signal peptidase (14).

Although the level of expression for mature recombinant tissue kallikrein is significantly lower than that for the proenzyme, the reported data demonstrate the utility of recombinant baculovirus-infected insect cells for the *in vitro* production of defined and biologically active members of the kallikrein gene family.

ACKNOWLEDGEMENTS

The authors wish to thank H. G. Gassen for stimulating discussions and his continuous interest in our work and H. G. Miltenburger for his encouragement. We thank M. Requardt for help in kallikrein purification and our appreciation is extended to B. Möckel for critical reading of the manuscript.

REFERENCES

1. MacDonald RJ, Margolius, HS, Erdös, EG. Molecular biology of tissue kallikrein. Biochem J 1988; 253: 313 - 321.

2. Chen Z, Bode W. Refined 2.5 Å X-ray Crystal Structure of the Complex Formed by Porcine Kallikrein A and the Bovine Pancreatic Trypsin Inhibitor. J Mol Biol 1983; 164: 283 - 311.

3. Angermann A, Bergmann C, Appelhans H. Cloning and expression of human salivary-gland kallikrein in *Escherichia coli*. Biochem J 1989; 262: 787 - 793.

4. Wang J, Chao J, Chao L. Purification and characterization of recombinant tissue kallikrein from *Escherichia coli* and yeast. Biochem J 1991; 276: 63 - 71.

5. Angermann A, Rahn HP, Hektor T, Fertig G, Kemme M. Purification and characterization of human salivary-gland prokallikrein from recombinant baculovirus-infected insect cells. Eur J Biochem 1992; in press.

6. Sambrook J, Fritsch, EF, Maniatis T. In: Molecular cloning, a laboratory manual. New York: Cold Spring Harbor Press, 1989.

7. Summers MD, Smith GD. In: Manual of Methods for Baculovirus and Insect Cell Culture Procedures. Texas Agricultural Experiment Station Bull. 1555, 1987.

8. Laemmli U. Cleavage of structural proteins during assembly of the head of bacteriophage T4. Nature 1970; 227: 680 - 685.

9. Matsudeira P. Sequence from Picomole Quantities of Proteins Electroblotted onto Polyvinylidene Difluoride Membranes. J Biol Chem 1987; 262: 10035 - 10038.

10. Harlow E, Lane D. In: Antibodies, a laboratory manual. New York: Cold Spring Harbor Press, 1988.

11. Fiedler F, Geiger R, Hirschauer C, Leysath G. Peptide Esters and Nitroanilides as Substrates for the Assay of Human Urinary Kallikrein. Hoppe-Seyler's Z Physiol Chem 1978; 259: 1667 - 1673.

12. Chao J, Chai KX, Chen LM, Xiong W, Chao S, Woodley-Miller C, Wang L, Lu HS, Chao L. Tissue Kallikrein-binding Protein is a Serpin. J Biol Chem 1990; 265: 16394 - 16401.

13. Krieger J, Raming K, Prestwich GD, Frith D, Stabel S., Breer H. Expression of a pheromone-binding protein in insect cells using a baculovirus vector. Eur J Biochem 1992; 203: 161 - 166.

14. Gunne H, Hellers M, Steiner H. Structure of preproattacin and its processing in insect cells infected with a recombinant baculovirus. Eur J Biochem 1990; 187: 699 - 703.

AAS 38/I
Recent Progress on Kinins
© 1992 Birkhäuser Verlag Basel

DETERMINANTS OF TISSUE KALLIKREIN CLEAVAGE SPECIFICITY IN THE LIMITED PROTEOLYSIS OF KININOGENS

E.S. Prado, J. Chao*, J.R. Chagas, M.A. Juliano and L. Juliano

Department of Biophysics, Escola Paulista de Medicina,
Rua Tres de Maio 100, São Paulo-04044, SP, Brazil, and *Department
of Biochemistry and Molecular Biology, Medical University of South
Carolina, Charleston, SC29425. USA

SUMMARY: Further evidence for interactions at tissue kallikrein
extended binding sites, as determinants of the kininogen cleavage
specificities is presented. Differences in the cleavage sites in
kininogen hydrolysis by rat and other tissue kallikreins is related
to subsite S1' specificity, while the low susceptibility of rat
kininogen to horse tissue kallikrein is explained by the difference
in their subsite S3'.

INTRODUCTION

Rat tissue kallikrein (TKK) presents a different kininogen cleavage
specificity from human, porcine and horse TKK.In the hydrolysis
of bovine kininogen (Kng), rat TKK releases bradykinin (BK) by
cleavage of a Lys-Arg bond (1) while the other TKK split a Met-Lys
bond, releasing Lys-BK (2). The cleavage of the Met-Lys bond by
horse and porcine TKK has also been demonstrated in the hydrolysis
of peptides with partial Kng sequence, Gly-(orSer)-Leu-Met-Lys-BK
(3,4). From studies on the hydrolysis of Arg or Lys bonds in
oligopeptides (5,6) and from the X-ray structure of the complex
porcine pancreatic KK-aprotinin (7), the cleavage specificities of
TKK have been attributed to secondary interactions at their
extended binding sites.
In the present work, we have investigated whether differences in
the subsite specificities of rat and horse TKK could explain their
different Kng cleavage specificities. The kinetic parameters for
the hydrolysis, by rat TKK, of a series of peptidyl p-nitroanilides
(pNA) were determined and compared to those previously reported for
horse TKK (8,9).Differences in the susceptibilities of rat Kng to

rat and other TKK have been reported (1). To find out if this species specificity results from differences in subsite interactions, we synthesized fluorogenic peptides having rat Kng partial sequence at the C-terminal side of the BK moiety, and containing ortho-aminobenzoic acid (Abz) and ethylenodiamino dinitrophenyl (EDDnp) as amino and carboxyl blocking groups.In order to exclude a possible effect of other interactions outside the extended binding site on TKK cleavage specificities, we studied the hydrolysis of Abz-Leu-Met-Lys-Arg-Pro-EDDnp. In this peptide, with partial bovine Kng sequence, the two susceptible bonds, Met-Lys and Lys-Arg are present.

MATERIALS AND METHODS

Enzymes. Homogeneous horse urinary and rat submandibular kallikrein preparations were obtained by the previously described procedures (10,11). The molar concentrations of the enzymes were determined by active site titration with 4-dinitrophenyl-4-guanidinobenzoate (12). Samples of porcine pancreatic kallikrein (1374 KU/mg) were kindly supplied by Dr. Schmidt-Kastner,from Bayer AG. We also thank Dr. W. Xiong, University of South Carolina USA, for samples of rat submandibular and human urinary kallikreins and T-kininogenase, and Dr. C.A.M. Sampaio, Escola Paulista de Medicina, Brazil, for human plasma kallikrein.

Synthetic substrates. D-Val-Leu-Arg-pNA and D-Val-Leu-Lys-pNA were purchased from Kabi Peptide Research, Sweden. Previously described procedures were used for synthesis, purification and analyses of other peptidyl-pNA (13) and of intramolecularly quenched fluorogenic substrates (9).

HPLC analysis of the synthetic substrates and their enzymatic hydrolysis products. The peptide solutions (80 to 150 uM) in 20 mM Tris-HCl, pH 8.0 or 9.0 were incubated with the different proteinases at 30°C. Samples (20 ul) of the substrate and enzyme controls, and of the enzymic digests, were removed for analysis until 100% of the substrate hydrolysis was reached. The HPLC conditions were: 0.1 M NaH_2PO_4 (pH 4.2) as solvent A; acetonitrile-H_2O (9:1) as solvent B; gradient 10-80% of B in 15 min; flow rate, 1 ml/min; Novopack C-18 column 3.2 x 150 mm; detection by ultraviolet at 214 nm and by fluorescence with λ em = 420 nm and λ ex = 320 nm.The hydrolysis products were identified from their elution times and/or from amino acid analysis of the HPLC fractions.

Enzyme assays. Hydrolysis of peptidyl-pNA and of fluorogenic peptide substrates were measured and the kinetic parameters calculated as previously described (9,8).

RESULTS AND DISCUSSION

<u>Hydrolysis of peptidyl-pNA by rat and horse TKK : Interactions at subsites S1, S2 S3</u>

The preference of rat and horse TKK for Arg over Lys in position P1 was demonstrated by the k_{cat}/K_m values for D-Val-Leu-X-pNA (X= Arg or Lys) hydrolysis (Table 1).

TABLE 1. Specific constant (k_{cat}/K_m) for the hydrolysis of peptidyl-pNA by rat and horse TKK

Substrates	k_{cat}/K_m $(mM^{-1}s^{-1})$	
	TKK	
	Rat	Horse
P1		
D-Val-Leu-<u>Arg</u>-pNA	1323	31.0
D-Val-Leu-<u>Lys</u>-pNA	156	0.6
P2		
Ac-<u>Gly</u>-Arg-pNA	10	0.2
Ac-<u>Pro</u>-Arg-pNA	241	2.8
Ac-<u>Leu</u>-Arg-pNA	1925	6.0
Ac-<u>Phe</u>-Arg-pNA	2485	37.0

Hydrolysis conditions : 30°, 50 mM Tris/HCl,1 mM EDTA, 10% MeSO$_4$v/v pH 9.0

Data for the hydrolysis of dipeptidyl-pNA (Ac-X-Arg-pNA) demonstrate a strong preference of both TKK for hydrophobic residues at P2 (Table 1). This specificity for TKK subsite S2, first described for porcine TKK (14), has been considered as a determinant for kinin release in the limited proteolysis of Kng (5). In favor of this proposal, is the presence of hydrophobic residues at the P2 position of the two bonds split for BK or Lys-BK release from different Kng. As this specificity was shown to be a common feature for rat and other TKK, it cannot explain the differences in their Kng cleavage specificities.

Regarding subsite S3, it is interesting to remark that for kinin release from Kng the P3 residue at the C-terminal cleavage site is Pro; at the N-terminal site it is Leu and Ser, respectively, for BK and Lys-BK release from bovine Kng. At the present time, we only have data showing that Ac-Pro-Phe-Arg-pNA is a slightly better substrate than Ac-Phe-Arg-pNA for both rat and horse TKK.

Hydrolysis of fluorogenic peptide substrates by TKK : Interactions at subsites S1',S2' and S3'

As observed previously with horse and porcine TKK (9) and in accordance with the demonstrated specificity of rat TKK subsite S2, only the Arg-X bond, in the peptides listed in Table 2, were cleaved. The k_{cat}/K_m values show that peptides I and II, having Pro at P2' and Ala and Ser at P1', were the poorest substrates for both TKK. Substitution of Pro in peptide II by Val (peptide III) and by Arg (peptide IV) increased the k_{cat}/K_m values for both TKK. The k_{cat}/K_m values for the hydrolysis of peptide Abz-Phe-Arg-Ser-Arg-EDDnp by rat, pig and horse TKK (9) are very similar and show that the strong specificity of subsite S2' for Arg is a common feature for TKK. On the other hand, the marked differences in k_{cat}/K_m for rat and horse TKK in the hydrolysis of peptides having Arg-Val and Arg-Pro as leaving groups (P1'-P2') indicate a difference in the interactions S1'-Arg for these enzymes. In a previous paper (3), we have also demonstrated that the peptide Ac-Phe-Lys-Arg-Pro-NH$_2$ was a good substrate for rat TKK and resistant to horse TKK. These data on subsite specificities of rat TKK are consistent with the conclusion that cleavage of the Lys-Arg and Arg-Arg bonds in bovine and in rat Kng, respectively, results from the favourable overall interactions at subsites S2 to S2'. Therefore, the resistance to other TKK may be explained by the unfavourable interactions S1-Arg and S2'-Pro, as has been demonstrated in our studies.

TABLE 2. Specific constants (k_{cat}/K_m) for the hydrolysis of fluorogenic peptide substrates, Abz-Phe-Arg-X-Y-Z-EDDnp, by rat and horse TKK[a]

Substrates Abz-Phe-Arg - X - Y - Z- EDDnp	k_{cat}/K_m (mM^{-1}s^{-1}) TKK	
P1' P2' P3'	Rat	Horse[b]
I Ala-Pro	26	nd[c]
II Ser-Pro	116	91
III Ser-Val	3930	1000
IV Ser-Arg	40833	38000
V Arg-Pro	4630	170
VI Arg-Val	20960	4630
VII Ala-Pro-Arg	506	nd[c]

[a]Hydrolysis conditions: 30°C, 50 mM Tris-HCl, 1 mM EDTA pH 9.0
[b]Data from reference (8)
[c]nd = not determined since for peptide VII the specific activity for horse TKK was 2 orders of magnitude lower than for rat TKK

Regarding the Met-Lys bond cleavage, favourable interactions for Leu at P2 and Arg at P2', and unfavourable for Met at P1' are known, while no information regarding Lys at P1' has been reported. Release of kinin from bovine and rat Kng implies the cleavage of Arg-Ser and Arg-Ala bonds in the sequences Phe-Arg-Ser-Val and Phe-Arg-Ala-Pro in bovine and rat Kng, respectively. Data in Table 2 show that the Arg-Ser bond in peptide III, having Val as P2' residue, is susceptible to both kallikreins, while Arg-Ala is resistant. However, peptide VII having, like rat Kng, an Arg residue at P3', was susceptible to rat but not to horse TKK. These results explain the species specificity of horse TKK, demonstrated in the hydrolysis of rat Kng.

Hydrolysis of Abz-Leu-Met-Lys-Arg-Pro-EDDnp

The cleavage sites in the hydrolysis of this peptide by different proteinases was determined by HPLC analysis of the hydrolysis products. As shown below, Met-Lys cleavage was a unique feature of the horse, human and porcine TKK, but not of the rat TKK.

Abz-Leu-Met-Lys-Arg-Pro-EDDnp

Tissue Kallikreins	Rat Tissue Kallikrein
(Human, Porcine, Horse)	Trypsin, Plasma Kallikrein
	T-kininogenase

These results indicate that interactions at TKK subsites S2-S2' are sufficient for determining the cleavage specificities of TKK. In our previous work on Met-Lys cleavage by horse TKK (3), the k_{cat}/K_m for hydrolysis of the peptide Gly-Leu-Met-Lys-BK was three orders of magnitude lower than for Lys-BK release from horse Kng (10). A similar ratio was found for Met-Lys bond cleavage in Ser-Met-Lys-BK and in HMW-des-Arg-Kng by porcine TKK (15). These data indicate that further interactions outside the extended binding site are essential for the efficiency of TKK in the cleavage of the Met-Lys bond in Kng. In preliminary kinetic studies on Abz-Leu-Met-Lys-Arg-Pro-EDDnp hydrolysis by horse and human TKK, the k_{cat}/K_m values were two orders of magnitude higher than for Gly-Leu-Met-Lys-BK. Thus apparently, blocking the N-terminal amino group or the C-terminal carboxyl group by Abz and EDDnp, respectively, and/or shortening of the BK chain led to a favourable effect on the susceptibility to TKK. Studies with peptides, having at the N-terminal side an extended peptide chain with partial Kng sequence, are in progress for further understanding of the high susceptibility of the Met-Lys bond in Kng to the kallidin liberating TKK.

ACKNOWLEDGMENTS

This research was supported by the following Brazilian research agencies: FINEP, CNPq and FAPESP.

REFERENCES

1. Kato H, Nakanishi E, Enjyoji K, Hayashi I, Ohishi S., Iwanaga S. Characterization of serino proteinases isolated from rat submaxillary gland:With special reference to the degradation of rat kininogens by these enzymes. J Biochem 1987; 102:1389-1404.

2. Fiedler, F. In: Handbook of Experimental Pharmacology. Erdos, E.G. editor. Berlin: Springer-Verlag, 1979; 25:103-161.

3. Araujo-Viel MS, Juliano L, Prado ES. The cleavage of the Met-Lys bond in a bradykinin derivative by glandular kallikreins. Hoppe-Seyler's Z Phys Chem 1981; 362:337-345.

4. Fiedler F. Enzymology of porcine tissue kallikrein. Adv Exp Med Biol 1983; 156A:263-274.

5. Fiedler F. Effects of secondary interactions on the kinetics of peptide and ester hydrolysis by tissue kallikrein and trypsin. Eur J Biochem 1987; 163:303-312.

6. Prado ES, Araujo-Viel MS, Juliano MA, Juliano L, Stella RCR, Sampaio CAM. Tetrapeptide substrates for the discrimination among kallikreins and other trypsin-like serine proteinases. Biol Chem Hoppe-Seyler 1986; 367:199-205.

7. Chen Z , Bode W. Refined 2.5 A X-ray crystal structure of the complex formed by porcine kallikrein A and the bovine pancreatic trypsin inhibitor. J Mol Biol 1983; 164:283-311.

8. Araujo-Viel SM, Juliano MA, Oliveira L, Prado ES. Horse urinary kallikrein,II. Biol Chem Hoppe-Seyler 1988; 369:397-401.

9. Chagas JR, Juliano L, Prado ES. Intramolecularly quenched fluorogenic tetrapeptide substrates for tissue and plasma kallikreins. Anal Biochem 1991; 192:419-425.

10. Giusti EP, Sampaio CAM, Michelacci YM, Stella RCR, Prado ES. Horse urinary kallikrein,I. Biol Chem Hoppe-Seyler 1988; 369:387-396.

11. Chao J, Margolius HS. Isozymes of rat urinary kallikrein. Biochem Pharmacology 1979; 28:2071-2079.

12. Sampaio CAM, Sampaio MU,   Prado ES. Active-site titration of horse urinary kallikrein. Biol Chem   Hoppe-Seyler's   1984; 365:297-302.

13. Juliano MA,   Juliano L. Synthesis and kinetic parameters of hydrolysis by trypsin of some acyl-arginyl-p-nitroanilides and peptides containing arginyl-p-nitroanilide. Braz J Med Biol Res 1985; 18:435-445.

14. Fiedler F, Leysath. In: Kinins-II: biochemistry, patholology, and   clinical   aspects.   Setsuro   F,   Moriya   H,   Suzuki   T, editors.Plenum Pbl Corp, 1979: 261-271.

15. Fiedler F, Hinz H, Lottspeich F. Individual reaction steps in release of kallidin from kininogen by tissue kallikrein. Adv Exp Biol 1986; 198 A: 283-289.

AAS 38/I
Recent Progress on Kinins
© 1992 Birkhäuser Verlag Basel

KINETICS OF BOND CLEAVAGES AT KALLIDIN RELEASE BY TISSUE KALLIKREIN: CLEAVAGE OF TWO PEPTIDE BONDS IN A SINGLE ENZYME-SUBSTRATE COMPLEX ?

F. Fiedler and H. Hinz

Abtg. Klin. Chem. Klin. Biochem., Chirurg. Klinik Innenstadt d. Universität,
Nussbaumstr. 20, D-8000 München 2, Germany

SUMMARY: The kinetics of the release of kallidin, L- and KL-chains from bovine L-kininogen by porcine tissue kallikrein were followed and individual kinetic constants for cleavage of the Met-360 and the Arg-370 bond determined. The results suggest that both these bonds in L-kininogen r are hydrolyzed "simultaneously" without appearance of a free singly-nicked intermediate. Kallidin release in the human analogous system is also compatible with such a mechanism.

INTRODUCTION

The characteristic property of a typical tissue kallikrein is the release of kallidin from kininogens. This requires the cleavage of two peptide bonds, one Arg- and one Met-bond in bovine and human kininogens.

Efficient cleavage at the neutral amino acid Met by Arg-specific tissue kallikrein is a most puzzling reaction. Model peptides with partial sequences as occurring around the Arg cleavage site of bovine kininogen were easily hydrolyzed by tissue kallikrein from porcine pancreas (1). In contrast, a model peptide of the Met cleavage site was a poor substrate (2) with a specificity constant k_{cat}/K_m 3500 times lower than that for kallidin release from kininogen (3). How does the enzyme then achieve efficient cleavage at Met in kininogen?

Attempts to determine in a first approach the sequence of the two cleavage steps in kallidin release had been made using bovine high molecular weight kininogen (H-kininogen) and tissue kallikrein from porcine pancreas (3). Surprisingly, that work provided evidence that both the Met-360 and the Arg-370 bonds might be hydrolyzed in a single enzyme-substrate complex, without involvement of a singly-nicked free intermediate. (The numbering scheme used is that of mature bovine H-kininogen I (4)).

To obtain more evidence for such a unique reaction course, bovine low molecular weight kininogen (L-kininogen) has now been used as substrate. Primary attack at Met-360 will produce a fragment composed of kallidin linked to the L-chain, called here KL-chain. Primary attack at Arg-370 will produce L-chains. These fragments, in addition to kallidin, could be quantitated by HPLC. Formation of singly-nicked intermediates should reveal itself by transient appearance of either KL-chains or an excess of L-chains over kallidin.

Furthermore, kinetic constants for the release of kallidin from native single-chain L-kininogen and for the hydrolysis of the Met-360 and the Arg-370 bonds in nicked L-kininogens have been determined. First experiments on the autologous system human tissue kallikrein/human L-kininogen are also reported.

MATERIALS AND METHODS

Bovine L-kininogen was isolated as described (5) with several modifications. Arg-370-cleaved L-kininogen was prepared by the action of endoproteinase Arg-C from mouse submaxillary glands (Boehringer), and Lys-361-cleaved L-kininogen by means of endoproteinase Lys-C from Lysobacter enzymogenes (Boehringer). To obtain des-Lys-361-L-kininogen, this material was treated with carboxypeptidase B. Neuraminidase-treated porcine pancreatic ß-kallikrein B obtained as generous gift from Bayer AG, Wuppertal, was rechromatographed (6).

For determination of kinetic constants, kallidin and other kinins released by tissue kallikrein were quantitated by RP-HPLC in the pH3 system (7). Kinins, L-, KL- and BL-chains (the latter consisting of bradykinin linked to the L-chains and derived from Lys-361-cleaved kininogen) were separated and quantitated at 200 nm with a linear or stepwise gradient of acetonitrile in the pH3 buffer after reduction with DTT in 6N guanidinium chloride.

RESULTS AND DISCUSSION

Composition of the preparations of bovine L-kininogen and multiplicity of L-chains.
The preparations of bovine L-kininogen obtained contained several nicked molecular species. 10-20% of the L-chains were already preformed (mainly as kinin-free or des-Arg-370-kininogen), but at least 94% of the kallidin was anchored at both ends

(single-chain kininogen). L-chains preexisting or released by porcine tissue kallikrein occur in multiple forms. L_1 probably carries C-terminal Ala, L_2 Leu. Two further kininogen preparations contained in addition an L_2'-chain, presumably an L_2-variant. The contents of KL-chains, mainly KL_2 (authentic material obtained by partial BrCN cleavage), and BL-chains were maximally 1% of each.

Determination of kinetic constants of kinin release from native and nicked bovine L-kininogens. Initial rates of kinin release from L-kininogens (0.5 to 4 μM) by porcine tissue kallikrein were determined and were evaluated for the present on the basis of simple Michaelis-Menten kinetics. Complications as the presence of multiple molecular species in the kininogen preparations may require a more sophisticated final analysis.

Table 1. Preliminary kinetic constants for kinin release by porcine pancreatic ß-kallikrein B from various molecular species of bovine L-kininogen (0.1 M Tris/HCl, 0.4 M NaCl, 0.04 M NaAc, 0.1 mM EDTA, pH 9.0, 25°C).

L-kininogen species	k_{cat} (s^{-1})	K_m (μM)	k_{cat}/K_m (μM^{-1}s^{-1})
single-chain	0.96	0.71	1.36
Lys-361-cleaved	1.96	0.80	2.11
des-Lys-361	1.75	0.84	2.08
Arg-370-cleaved	0.99	1.2	0.83

The kinetic constants obtained (Table 1) are remarkably similar for the hydrolysis of such dissimilar bonds as those at Arg-370 (in Lys-361-cleaved and des-Lys-361 kininogens) and at Met-360 (in Arg-370-cleaved kininogen). They are also similar for native single-chain L-kininogen where both the bonds have to be cleaved. The inhibition constant for kallidin-free L-kininogen seems to be of a magnitude comparable to the K_m values. The kinetic constants resemble those previously determined for bovine H-kininogen (3).

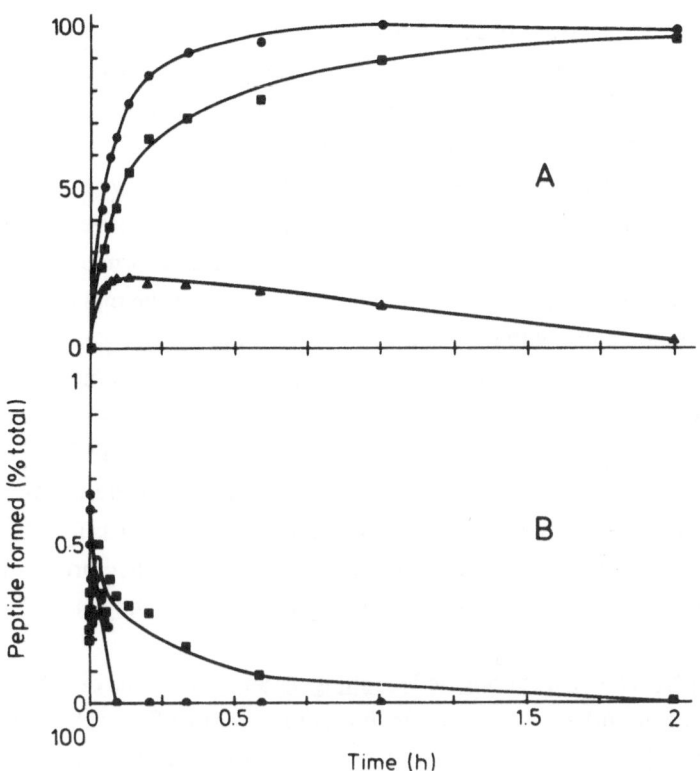

Figure 1. Kinetics of the release of kallidin, L-chains and KL-chains from bovine L-kininogen (10 μM) by porcine pancreatic ß-kallikrein B (0.1 M Tris/HCl, 0.4 M NaCl, 0.04 M NaAc, 0.1 mM EDTA, pH 9.0, 25°C).
A) Formation of L-chains (●) and kallidin (■) and their difference (▲) representing Arg-370-cleaved kininogen.
B) Behaviour of BL (●)- and Kl (■)-chains.

<u>Kinetics of the release of kallidin and L-chains from bovine L-kininogen</u>. When the release of L-chains from bovine L-kininogen by porcine tissue kallikrein is followed simultaneously with that of kallidin, the chains are found to be formed more rapidly than is the kinin (Fig. 1A). Arg-370-cleaved kininogen accumulates and is slowly further attacked to release more kallidin. However, this Arg-370-cleaved kininogen cannot repesent the intermediate of the initial rapid main phase of kallidin release: Its disappearance is much too slow to account for the fast formation of kallidin in the earlier phases. (Control experiments showed that the low rate is due neither to

enzyme inactivation nor to massive product inhibition). Kallidin formation does not exhibit the initial lag period to be expected if such large amounts of an obligatory intermediate should accumulate. Different kininogen preparations furnish different maximum amounts (15-26%) of Arg-370-cleaved kininogen.

Arg-370-cleaved kininogen prepared by complete conversion of native bovine L-kininogen is rapidly cleaved by tissue kallikrein (Table 1). So the Arg-cleaved kininogen only slowly attacked must have been derived from a minor form of bovine L-kininogen, called here L-kininogen s. One possibility is identity of the main form, L-kininogen r, and L-kininogen s with bovine L-kininogens I and II (8), respectively.

From the values of the kinetic constants (Table 1) follows that large amounts of Arg-370-cleaved kininogen r would have to be formed transiently if this nicked species should be a free intermediate in the process of kallidin release. This is contrary to observations. Addition of Arg-370-cleaved kininogen r to single-chain kininogen did only marginally increase the rate of kallidin formation by tissue kallikrein. Consequently, Arg-370-cleaved kininogen r (of the kind as obtained preparatively) is not an intermediate in kallidin release from single-chain L-kininogen r.

Kinetics of release of KL-chains from bovine L-kininogen. Small amounts of KL-chains (0.5% at the maximum) are formed in the initial phases of kallidin release by tissue kallikrein (Fig. 1B). This indicates formation of Met-360-cleaved kininogen as an intermediate. According to a relationship derived for the moment of maximum accumulation of an intermediate (3), k_{cat}/K_m would have to be 140fold higher for Met-360-cleaved than for single-chain kininogen, if this nicked species should be an intermediate in the main pathway of kallidin release. However, k_{cat}/K_m for L-kininogen nicked at Lys-361 juxtaposed to Met-360, as well as for des-Lys-361-kininogen, is similar to that for single-chain kininogen (Table 1). It appears most improbable that the similar Met-360-cleaved kininogen should have a 100fold higher specificity constant. Met-360-cleaved kininogen seems consequently to be located only on a minor side pathway.

Conclusions from the experiments with bovine L-kininogens. Neither Met-360-cleaved nor Arg-370-cleaved kininogens r (of the kind as can be isolated) are free intermediates in the main pathway of the release of kallidin by porcine ß-tissue kallikrein from bovine L-kininogen.

Either, kininogen with a single cleavage site at Met-360 or Arg-370 is formed transitorily in a highly reactive conformation (leading to only very low concentrations of the intermediate) which rearranges to a more tissue kallikrein-resistant conformer on isolation.

Alternatively, both peptide bonds of kininogen are cleaved in one enzyme-substrate complex which does not dissociate between the two events - a most unusual reaction. This second interpretation is supported by two further observations: k_{cat}/K_m for L-chain release from kininogen s is 3fold higher than for kininogen r. In addition, the rate of L-chain (but not kallidin) formation is higher at pH 6.5 than at pH 9, contrary to other tissue kallikrein-catalyzed reactions. These might be related phenomena: when cleavage at Met is prevented - either by the structure of kininogen s or by low pH - the rate of formation of the Arg cleavage product is increased.

An analogous reaction mechanism has only been reported for bradykinin release from human H-kininogen by human plasma kallikrein (9), though other authors described cleavage of the kininogen molecule prior to kinin release (10, 11).

Experiments with human tissue kallikrein and human L-kininogen. In cooperation with W. Müller-Esterl and R. Geiger, kinetic experiments on this autologous system were begun. The preparation of human L-kininogen used released on exhaustive treatment with human urinary kallikrein mainly kallidin besides hydroxyprolyl-4-kallidin (12,13) (22% of the kinins) and des-Arg-10-kallidin (9%).It furnished essentially one L-chain (27% existing already in the kininogen preparation), besides a minor (<5%) component, possibly an L-chain derivative.

Human L-kininogen (3.2 μM) was treated with human urinary kallikrein and the reaction followed by HPLC until termination of kinin liberation. Hyp-4-kallidin was released strictly in parallel with kallidin, implying similarity of kinetic constants. The transient maximum of KL-chains formed amounted to less than 1% of the kininogen. Kinins and L-chains were released in parallel. In further contrast to the results with bovine L-kininogen, their release followed an integrated Michaelis-Menten rate equation.

No evidence for the existence of kinetically different forms of human L-kininogens was obtained, possibly because only one gene for human kininogen exists (14). Species of L-kininogen singly-nicked at Met or Arg are formed during the reaction at most in low concentrations. The situation resembles that on kallidin release from bovine L-kininogen r.

REFERENCES

1.   Fiedler F. Effects of secondary interactions on the kinetics of peptide and
      peptide ester hydrolysis by tissue kallikrein and trypsin. Eur J Biochem 1987;
      163:303-312

2.   Fiedler F. Enzymology of porcine tissue kallikrein. Adv Exp Med Biol 1983;
      156A:263-274

3.   Fiedler F, Hinz H, Lottspeich F. Individual reaction steps in the release of
      kallidin from kininogen by tissue kallikrein. Adv Exp Med Biol 1986;
      198A:283-289

4.   Sueyoshi T, Miyata T, Hashimoto N, Kato H, Hayashida H, Miyata T,
      Iwanaga S. Bovine high molecular weight kininogen. J Biol Chem 1987;
      262:2768-2779

5.   Kato H, Nagasawa S, Iwanaga S. HMW and LMW kininogens. Methods
      Enzymol 1981; 80:172-198

6.   Fiedler F, Fink E, Tschesche H, Fritz H. Porcine glandular kallikreins.
      Methods Enzymol 1981; 80:493-532

7.   Fiedler F, Geiger R. Separation of kinins by high-performance liquid chro-
      matography. Methods Enzymol 1988; 163:257-262

8.   Nawa H, Kitamura N, Hirose T, Asai M, Inayama S, Nakanishi S. Primary
      structures of bovine liver low molecular weight kininogen precursors and
      their two mRNAs. Proc Natl Acad Sci USA 1983; 80:90-94

9.   Wiedler J, Dutler H. Hydrolysis of human high-molecular-mass kininogen by
      human plasma kallikrein. Biol Chem Hoppe-Seyler 1987; 368:1203-1213

10.   Mori K, Nagasawa S. Studies on human high molecular weight (HMW) kini-
      nogen. II. J Biochem 1981; 89:1465-1473

11.   Scott CF, Silver LD, Purdon AD, Colman RW. Cleavage of human high
      molecular weight kininogen by factor XIa in vitro. J Biol Chem 1985;
      260:10856-10863

12.   Maier M, Reissert G, Jerabek I, Lottspeich F, Binder BR. Identification of
      (hydroxyproline-3)-lysylbradykinin released from human kininogens by
      human urinary kallikrein. FEBS Lett 1988; 232:395-398

13.   Mindroiu T, Carretero OA, Proud D, Walz D, Scicli AG. A new kinin moiety
      in human plasma kininogens. Biochem Biophys Res Commun 1988; 152:519-
      526

14.   Kitamura N, Kitagawa H, Fukushima D, Takagaki Y, Miyata T, Nakanishi S.
      Structural organization of the human kininogen gene and a model for its
      evolution. J Biol Chem 1985; 260:8610-8617

AAS 38/I
Recent Progress on Kinins
© 1992 Birkhäuser Verlag Basel

KINETICS OF LYS-BRADYKININ RELEASE BY PORCINE PANCREATIC KALLIKREIN FROM RABBIT LOW MOLECULAR WEIGHT KININOGEN

L.G. Makevnina, G.O. Levina and A.K. Yatzimirsky*

Institute of Biological and Medical Chemistry, Moscow 119832,
Pogodinskaya str. 10, and *Moscow State Lomonosow University, Chemical
Department, Moscow 119899, G.U.S.

SUMMARY: The initial rates of Lys-bradykinin release by porcine pancreatic kallikrein from rabbit low molecular weight kininogen are found to follow the Michaelis-Menten kinetics with k_c=0.62 sec^{-1} and K_m=1.93 μM at substrate concentrations 0.3-1.3 μM, but at higher ones the Michaelis dependence is broken. Inhibition of the reaction by its product(s) with $K_p < K_m$ is revealed with integral analysis methods in a range of 4.5-270 μM kininogen.

INTRODUCTION

The enzymic hydrolysis of low molecular weight kininogen by tissue kallikreins resulting in Lys-bradykinin (kallidin) release is a highly specific reaction of limited proteolysis. Only two peptide bonds, which bind kinin within the polypeptide chain, are hydrolyzed in the course of this reaction [1,2,3]:

$$\text{LMW KININOGEN} \xrightarrow{\text{Tissue kallikrein}} \text{KININ-free LMW KININOGEN + Lys-BRADYKININ}$$

Kinetics of the kinin releasing reaction monitored by the bioactive product has been studied with high and low molecular weight kininogens as substrates [4,5]. In all cases, however, only initial rates of the reaction in a limited range of substrate concentrations have been analyzed. Furthermore, kinetic characteristics found by the different authors differ within an order of magnitude. In the present study the kinetic investigation

of the kinin release from rabbit plasma low molecular weight
kininogen catalyzed by porcine pancreatic kallikrein has been
carried out both by the initial rates and the integral analysis
methods in a wide range of enzyme and substrate concentrations.

MATERIALS AND METHODS

The preparation of two-chain porcine β-kallikrein B of 1480 Frey
U/mg (a gift from Dr.F.Fiedler, Munich University) was found to
contain 100% of active enzyme according to its titration with
aprotinin [6]. The M_r value 28000 was used for calculations of
kallikrein molar concentrations in solutions.

Low molecular weight kininogen was purified from rabbit
plasminogen-free blood plasma [2] as a single-chain protein with
an apparent M_r 69000. Kinin released from kininogen by pancreatic
kallikrein was identified with kallidin by means of SP-Sephadex
C-25 gradient chromatography [7]. Its amount measured in rat
uterus test [8] was 8.5±0.9 μg bradykinin equivalents per 1 mg of
kininogen preparation corresponding to 82±9% content of native
kininogen. In this biotest kallidin has 67% of activity of
equimolar concentrations of bradykinin.

Initial rates of kallidin release by kallikrein from
0.27-1.30 μM kininogen were determined as follows: stock solution
of 1.3 μM kininogen in 0.05 M Tris-HCl, pH 8.0, 6 mM EDTA, 0.1 mM
dithioerithritol was diluted by the same buffer to the final
concentrations 0.27, 0.33, 0.50, 0.70, 0.90, 1.1 and 1.3 μM in 1.0
ml volume;each sample was incubated with 25 ng (1 μl) of
kallikrein at 37°. Aliquots (0.40 ml) were removed at 5 and 7 min
and mixed with 20% trichloroacetic acid (0.08 ml),then heated
(98°,10 min), neutralized and bioassayed.

In the range 4.4-270 μM kininogen the initial rates were
determined from a linear parts of complete kinetic curves,
obtained as described in the legend to Fig.3.

The examination of kallikrein activity in initial solutions
and in incubation mixtures with kininogen was carried out with
D-Val-Leu-Arg-pNA (Serva) as a substrate according to [9].

RESULTS

ANALYSIS OF THE INITIAL REACTION RATES. The dependence of the initial rates v_o of kinin release on the initial kininogen concentrations $[S]_o$, presented in Fig.1 in semi logarithmic coordinates, allows to reveal two distinctly different regions. In the region of low substrate concentrations (0.27-1.3 μM) the dependence fits the Michaelis-Menten equation (2) for the stationary phase of the reaction (1):

$$E + S \xrightleftharpoons{K_m} ES \xrightarrow{k_c} E + P \qquad (1)$$

$$v_o = \frac{k_c[E]_o[S]_o}{K_{m(app)} + [S]_o} \qquad (2)$$

Using the graphic Lineweaver-Burk method [10], the kinetic constants of the reaction have been calculated: $k_c = 0.62$ sec^{-1}, $K_m = 1.93$ μM, $k_c/K_m = 320$ μM^{-1}sec^{-1} (Fig.2). These data compare well with those of F.Fiedler [5] for the reaction of kallidin release by the same enzyme from 0.5-5.0 μM bovine high molecular weight kininogen.

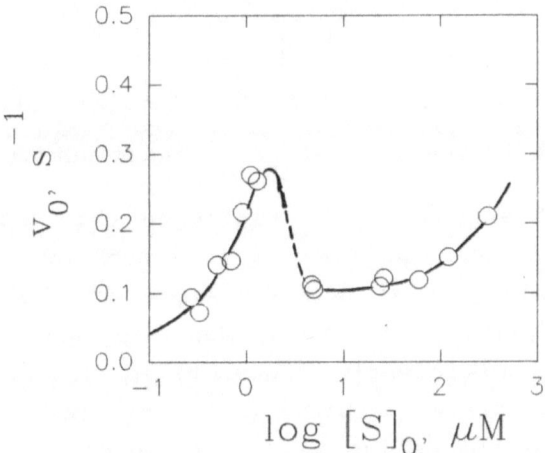

Figure 1. The semi logarithmic dependence of the initial reaction rates on initial concentrations of kininogen (0.27-307 μM).

As seen from Fig.1, with the increase of kininogen concentration up to 4.4 μM and higher, the constant rate V_m, corresponding to the saturation of enzyme with substrate, is not achieved, because the initial reaction rates markedly decrease in this concentration region. However, as substrate concentration becomes higher up to 270 μM v_o again gradually increases. The dependence of v_o on $[S]_o$ in this latter region has the appearance typical for an initial part of the Michaelis-Menten curve.

Based on kinetic data, such an unusual dependence may be accounted for by certain changes in substrate affinity for

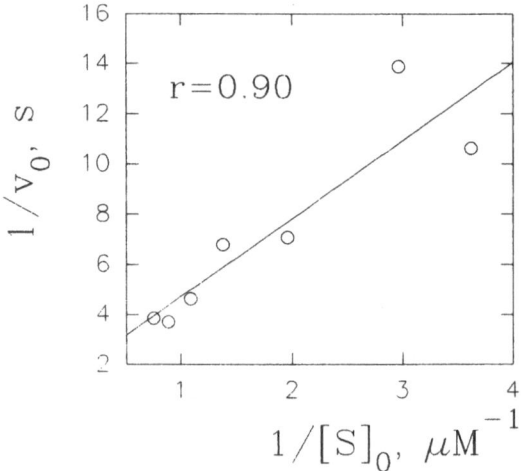

Figure 2. Lineweaver-Burk analysis of the initial rates of kinin release by pancreatic kallikrein from low molecular weight kininogen. Each point is the mean of two determinations.

the active center of enzyme. As to kininogen this dependence is explainable in view of the ability of both the low and the high molecular weight kininogens to autoaggregate in the absence of dissociating agents [11,12]. It seems that di- and oligomers of kininogen formed in sufficiently concentrated solutions act as major kallikrein substrates exhibiting lower (as compared to monomers) affinity for the active center of the enzyme.

INTEGRAL ANALYSIS OF KINETIC DATA. To determine kinetic parameters characterizing time course of the kinin releasing reaction under the action of tissue kallikrein, we have obtained complete kinetic curves in the substrate concentration range 4.4-270 μM and have analyzed them with integral analysis methods.

The typical curve for $[S]_o = 109$ μM is shown in Fig.3. The analysis using the Michaelis-Menten equation in the integral form (3) shows

$$[P] = V_m t - K_{m(app)} \ln \frac{[S]_o}{[S]_o - [P]} \qquad (3)$$

that the reaction rate, determined as a slope of the curve at every given moment, is lowered much faster than it would have to be expected according to Michaelis-Menten kinetics. Formally, these data comply with the assumption of the enzyme inactivation in the the reaction: the concentration of the unreacted substrate under the maximal retardation of the reaction $([S]_o - [P]_{max})/[S]_o$ is exponentially connected with the initial concentration of the enzyme $[E]_o$ according to equation (5) describing the inactivation scheme (4).

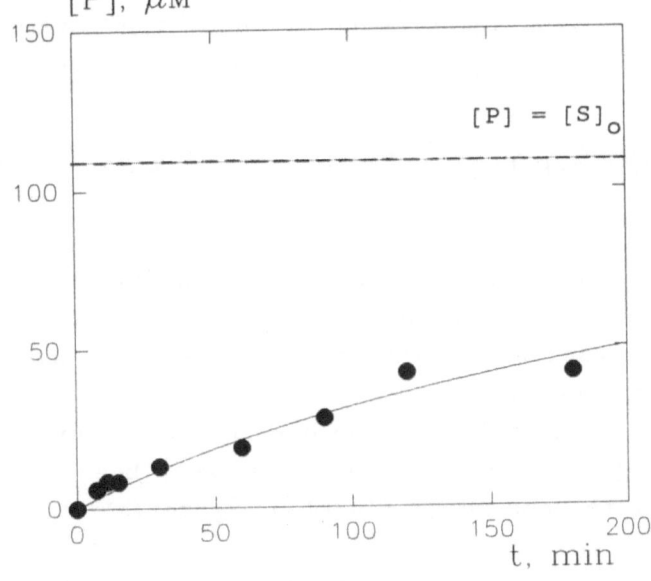

Figure 3. Time course of kallidin release by porcine pancreatic β-kallikrein B (64.9 nM) from rabbit low molecular weight kininogen (109 μM) at pH 8.0, 37° (●).

12.0 nmol of kininogen were incubated with 0.2 μg of kallikrein in 0.11 ml of 0.05 M Tris-HCl, pH 8.0, 6 mM EDTA, 0.1 mM dithioerythritol at 37°. Samples of 0.02 to 0.005 ml were removed at the times indicated, then added to 0.50 ml 3% trichloroacetic acid and immediately heated at 95° for 10 min. Kinins were quantified by bioassay.

Theoretical curve (——) is drawn according to eq. (7) with $V_m = 0.47$ $\mu M/min$ and $K_m/K_p = 2.9$.

$$E + S \xrightleftharpoons{K_m} ES \xrightarrow{k_c} E + P \tag{4}$$

$$k_{in} \downarrow$$

inactive enzyme

$$([S]_o - [P]_{max})/[S]_o = \exp(-k_c[E]_o/k_{in}K_m) \tag{5}$$

In coordinates $\ln\{([S]_o-[P]_{max})/[S]_o\}$ and $[E]_o$ it is a straight line with the negative slope. However, the control experiments have shown that kallikrein activity determined with the synthetic substrate D-Val-Leu-Arg-pNA does not change either in the course or upon termination of the kinin release from kininogen.

If the inhibition of the enzyme is connected with some admixture in the substrate preparation the concentration of which is equal to $\alpha[S]_o$, the concentration of the unreacted substrate must depend on the $[E]_o/[S]_o$ ratio according to equation (6):

$$\frac{[S]_o - [P]_{max}}{[S]_o} = \exp\left\{-\frac{k_c}{K_m k_{in}^* \alpha [S]}[E]_o\right\} = \text{const.} \times \exp\left(-\frac{[E]_o}{[S]_o}\right) \tag{6}$$

It has been shown that the experimental data do not fit the dependence (6) and, consequently, the assumption concerning the presence of kallikrein inhibitor in the substrate preparation cannot be substantiated.

We have studied the complete kinetic curves data using the equation (7) which quantitatively describes a scheme of the inhibition of the enzyme by reaction product(s) [13]:

$$\frac{[P]}{t} = \frac{V_m}{1 - K_{m(app)}/K_p} - \frac{K_{m(app)}(1+[S]_o/K_p)}{1 - K_{m(app)}/K_p} \ln\frac{[S]_o}{[S]_o-[P]} \times \frac{1}{t} \tag{7}$$

Linearization of the kinetic curves in coordinates of equation (7) according to Walker & Schmidt [14] (Fig.4) confirms our suggestion that the enzyme is inhibited by the reaction product(s). As seen from Fig.4, the straight line has a positive slope. According to equation (7) this is possible when $K_p < K_m$, i.e. if the enzyme forms a tighter complex with the product than with the substrate. As equation (7) contains 3 independent magnitudes V_m, K_m and K_p in different combinations, we succeeded in finding only the K_m/K_p ratio assuming that $[S]_o/K_m \gg 1$ and, consequently, $[S]_o/K_p \gg 1$ for the considered region of substrate concentrations. The results of application of equation (7) to all kinetic data are summarized in Table 1, which demonstrates a good coincidence of the K_m/K_p values obtained from different curves with each other in a wide range of enzyme and substrate concentrations.

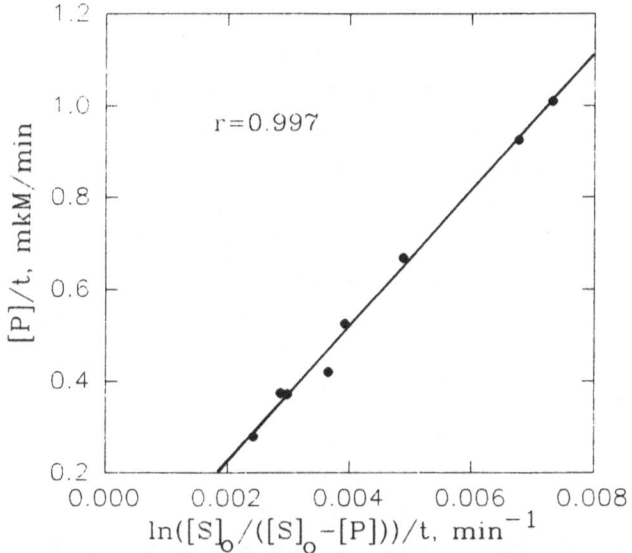

Figure 4. Analysis of the kinetic curve presented in Fig.3 by means of eq.(7) in Walker-Schmidt coordinates.

Table 1. Calculation of K_m/K_p values from complete kinetic curves data by the Walker-Schmidt integral method

$[S]_o$ µM	$[E]_o$ nM	K_m/K_p
4.4	2.6	6.50
21.8	65.0	6.70
23.5	14.0	6.30
54.4	32.5	6.30
108.8	64.9	5.36

Mean±SD=6.21±0.5

Kinetic curves were also analyzed by the non-linear regression method using the standard Sigma Plot program. Based on this method, we have obtained $K_m/K_p > 1$ for all cases but an average K_m/K_p value of 2.8±1.2 was found to be lower than that obtained by the Walker-Schmidt method.

CONCLUSIONS

The kinetic study of kinin release by porcine pancreatic kallikrein from rabbit low molecular weight kininogen has revealed two novel features of this enzyme-substrate system.

Firstly, the continuous Michaelis dependence v_o on $[S]_o$ is interrupted upon transition from the low substrate (kininogen) concentration (0.3-1.3 μM) to the higher ones. There is every reason to suggest that this effect is caused by changes in the affinity of kininogen for the enzyme due to di- and oligomerization of kininogen molecules in sufficiently concentrated solutions. For the region of $[S]_o$ 0.3-1.3 μM the kinetic constants of the reaction are close enough to those obtained for the same enzyme with 0.5-5.0 μM bovine high molecular weight kininogen [5].

Secondly, kallikrein is inhibited by the product(s) of the reaction in a wide range of kininogen concentrations, but this effect is observed only in the kallikrein-kininogen system. There is no inhibition of kallikrein by the products of kinin releasing reaction when a low molecular weight tripeptide p-nitroanilide is used as a substrate.

Both effects are observed at kininogen concentration equal to and higher (by an order of magnitude) than its concentration in plasma, but the latter does not make them out of physiological sense. It cannot be excluded that local concentrations of kininogen in certain tissues (interstice) may substantially exceed its plasma concentration. These new observations point to the existence of yet unknown mechanisms of regulation (or auto regulation) of tissue kallikreins in the systems with their natural protein substrates.

ACKNOWLEDGEMENT

We would like to thank Dr. F.Fiedler for the fruitful discussion
at the KININ Conference (Munich, 1991).

REFERENCES

1.Makevnina   LG,   Levina   GO,   Sherstjuk   SF,   Paskhina   TS.
   Fragmentation of rabbit low molecular weight kininogen by pig
   pancreatic kallikrein. Adv Biosci 1979; 17:151-159.
2.Levina   GO,   Makevnina   LG,   Sherstjuk   SF,   Paskhina   TS.
   Single-stranded low molecular weight kininogen of rabbit blood
   plasma: purification and nature of fragmentation by porcine
   pancreatic   kallikrein.   Biokhimiya   (Engl.transl.)   1985;
   50:277-287.
3.Müller-Esterl W,Rauth G, Lottspeich F,Kellermann J,Henschen A.
   Purification   and   properties   of   human   low   molecular   weight
   kininogen. Eur J Biochem 1985; 149:15-22.
4.Maier M, Austen KF, Spragg J. Kinetic analysis of the
   interaction of human tissue kallikrein with single-chain human
   high and low molecular weight kininogens. Proc Natl Acad Sci
   USA 1983; 80:3928-3932.
5.Fiedler F, Hinz H, Lottspeich F. Individual reaction steps in
   the release of kallidin from kininogen by tissue kallikrein.
   Adv Exp Med Biol 1986; 198A:283-289.
6.Larionova   NI,   Makevnina   LG,   Nartikova   VF,   Paskhina   TS.
   Influence of covalent binding of aprotinin to a polysaccharide
   carrier on its inhibition of human blood plasma kallikrein,
   porcine pancreatic kallikrein and trypsin. Biokhimiya (Engl.
   transl.) 1987; 52:709-715.
7.Makevnina LG, Levina GO, Filatova MP, Utkina EA, Paskhina TS.
   A method for purification, separation and quantification of
   kinins in multi component mixtures. Bioorg Chem (Russ) 1982;
   8:1607-1614.
8.Wilkens HJ, Steger R. In: Screening methods in pharmacology.
   Turner RA, Hebborn P, editors. New York, London: Acad Press,
   1971; 11:61-73.
9.Dietl T, Huber C, Geiger R, Iwanaga S, Fritz H. Inhibition
   of porcine glandular kallikreins by structurally homologous
   proteinase inhibitors of the Kunitz (trasylol) type. Biol Chem
   Hoppe-Seyler 1979; 360:67-71.
10.Lineweaver H, Burk D. The determination of enzyme dissociation
   constants. J Amer Chem Soc 1934; 56:658-666.
11.Müller-Esterl W, Vohle-Timmermann M, Boos B, Dittman B. Purification and properties of human low molecular weight kininogen.
   Biochim Biophys Acta 1982; 706:145-152.
12.Dittman   B,   Steger   A,   Wimmer   R,   Fritz   H.   A   convenient
   large-scale preparation of high molecular weight kininogen from
   human plasma. Biol Chem Hoppe-Seyler 1981; 362:919-927.
13.Fersht A. Enzyme structure and mechanism.San Francisco:Freeman,
   1977.
14.Walker AC,Schmidt CLA. Studies on histidase. Arch Biochem 1945;
   5:445-467.

98

AAS 38/I
Recent Progress on Kinins
© 1992 Birkhäuser Verlag Basel

CHARACTERIZATION OF KALLIKREIN ISOLATED FROM RAT SUBMANDIBULAR GLANDS BY A SIMPLE AND RAPID PURIFICATION PROCEDURE

T.S.H. El-Thaher, G.M. Saed†, A.A.A. Al-Hamidi* and G.S. Bailey

Department of Chemistry and Biological Chemistry,
University of Essex, Colchester, Essex CO4 3SQ, UK

SUMMARY: Numerous biochemical properties (e.g. Mr, carbohydrate content, pI) were determined for kallikrein isolated from rat subsmandibular glands by a simple, rapid purification procedure. The kinetic behaviour of the enzyme towards various inhibitors and synthetic substrates was investigated. The effects of different salts and detergents on the esterolytic activity of the rat tissue kallikrein were recorded.

INTRODUCTION

The richest source of tissue kallikrein yet discovered is the submandibular gland of the male rat (1). Although various multiple-step purifications of kallikrein from rat submandibular gland have been published (2-7) relatively few biochemical properties of the enzyme have been reported. This paper provides a description of some of the biochemical data of the tissue kallikrein isolated by a simple purification procedure (8).

---

†Present address: Hypertension Research Division, Henry Ford Hospital, Detroit, Michigan 48202, USA

*Present address: King Khalid Military Academy, Department of Science, P.O. Box 22140, Riyadh 11495, Saudi Arabia

MATERIALS AND METHODS

The purification procedure for tissue kallikrein consisted of sequential anion-exchange and hydrophobic interaction chromatographies of an initial crude homogenate of rat submandibular glands (8). The catalytic activity of the enzyme towards a number of arginine esters was measured at pH 8.0 and 25°C by a titrimetric assay (9). Initial rates were determined in triplicate for each substrate concentration (range 0.03 to 0.23 mM). Activity towards D-Val-Leu-Arg-p-nitroanilide (range 0.025 to 0.070 mM) was measured at pH 8.2 and 25°C (10). Estimates of Km and V_{max} were made from Hanes-Wolf plots (11) and an Mr of 38000 was assumed (8) in the calculations of kcat. In evaluation of inhibitors of tissue kallikrein, the type of inhibition and value of Ki were determined using Dixon plots (12) with Bz-Arg-OEt as substrate. Carbohydrate analysis was carried out using chemical methods. Neutral hexoses were measured by the method of Roe (13) using glucose as standard, sialic acids by the method of Jourdian and co-workers (14) and hexosamines by the method of Blix with glucosamine as standard as described by Gardell (15).

RESULTS AND DISCUSSION

As can be seen from Table 1 kallikrein was purified in a very high recovery by the simple, three-stage procedure.

TABLE 1. Purification of tissue kallikrein from rat submandibular glands[a]

Purification Step	Protein (mg)	Kallikrein[b] (mg)	Purification[b] (fold)	Recovery[b] (%)
1) Homogenate	851	187.3	(1)	(100)
2) Anion-exchange	222	184.7	3.7	98.6
3) Hydrophobic	158	158.0	4.6	84.4

[a] 13 g tissue was processed
[b] measured by radioimmunoassay (9)

The purification scheme was simpler and faster than other published procedures (2-7). The final preparation was shown to be pure by various types of analytical gel electrophoresis (8). It was seen on gel isoelectric focusing to consist of six isoenzymes of isoelectric points in the range pH 3.4 to 4.2. It eluted as a single symmetrical peak of constant specific esterolytic activity from a column of Sephadex G100 resin. The Mr was estimated to be 30000. Earlier Orstavik and co-workers (4) reported a value of Mr of 34000 for gel filtration on a Biogel 150 column whilst Matsuda *et al.*(6) recorded a value of 38000. However, as rat submandibular kallikrein is a glycoprotein (8) those estimates of Mr are likely to be less reliable than for a non-conjugated protein. Carbohydrate analyses by chemical means gave a 6% (w/w) content of neutral hexoses, a 3.3% (w/w) content of sialic acids and a 4.3% (w/w) content of hexosamines. We are not aware of any other reports of the carbohydrate content of rat submandibular kallikrein.

The kinetic behaviour of the rat tissue kallikrein towards a number of synthetic substrates is summarized in Table 2.

TABLE 2. Kinetic constants for kallikrein-catalysed hydrolysis

Substrate	V_{max} (μ mole/min per mg)	Km (mM)	kcat (s^{-1})	kcat/Km (s^{-1} mM^{-1})
Cbz-Arg-O-Me	173.0	0.26	109.6	421.5
Bz-Arg-OEt	156.3	0.23	99.0	430.4
Tos-Arg-OMe	15.2	0.14	9.6	68.6
S2266	15.6	0.031	9.9	320.0

Similar values of Km for the hydrolysis of Tos-Arg-OMe and S2266 have been reported earlier (16).

It used to be thought that soyabean trypsin inhibitor (SBTI) does not inhibit tissue kallikreins (17). However, in the present study SBTI was found to act as a non-competitive inhibitor of rat submandibular kallikrein with a Ki of 2.3×10^{-5}M. Indeed positive, neutral and negative effects have been noted for SBTI on rat tissue kallikreins (6,16,18,19).

As expected aprotinin was seen to be a competitive inhibitor of rat submandibular kallikrein (17). The Ki of 4.8 x 10⁻⁷M found in this work is higher than the corresponding values recorded for several other tissue kallikreins (20). In contrast, no inhibition of the esterolytic activity of the rat enzyme towards Bz-Arg-OEt was seen for amiloride, tosyl lysyl chloromethyl ketone (TLCK), lima bean trypsin inhibitor (LBTI) or benzamidine (all at 5 mM). Previously amiloride has been reported to have no effect (21) or to inhibit (6) rat urinary kallikrein. In general, it is believed that TLCK is inactive towards tissue kallikreins (17) but Chao has reported (22) inhibitory activity towards rat urinary kallikrein.

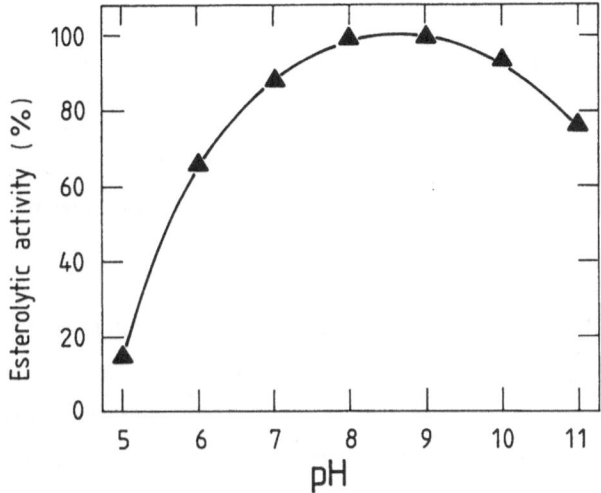

Figure 1. Influence of pH on the esterolytic activity of rat submandibular kallikrein

As can be seen in Figure 1 rat submandibular kallikrein showed maximum activity towards Bz-Arg-OEt in the pH range 8-9. A relatively wide pH optimum may be characteristic of tissue kallikreins (6,23).

The thermal stability of rat submandibular kallikrein was examined by incubating aliquots for one hour at various temperatures before assessing activity towards Bz-Arg-OEt. From the results presented in Figure 2 it can be seen that the enzyme is very stable. The stability of the enzyme was also checked by measuring activity after storage at various temperatures. Aliquots stored at -70°C and -20°C showed no loss of esterolytic activity after two months. There was a 20% loss of activity for aliquots stored at 4°C for two months.

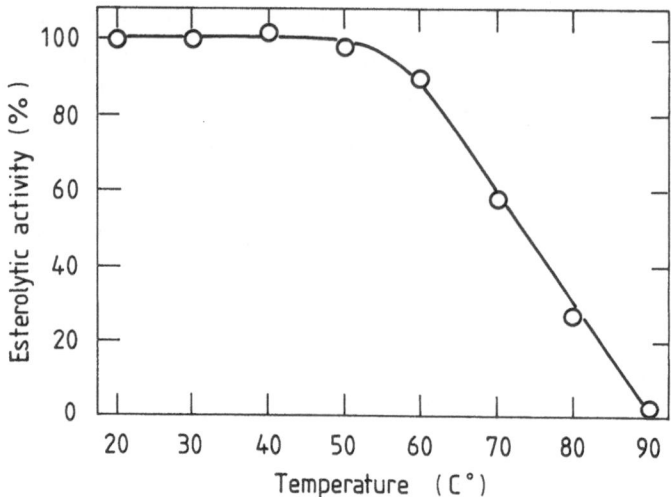

Figure 2. Influence of temperature on the esterolytic activity of rat submandibular kallikrein

A similar level of stability has been reported for rat urinary kallikrein (24).

To check for the effects of salts on catalytic activity, rat submandibular kallikrein was thoroughly dialyzed against de-ionized water and aliquots were incubated with various concentrations of salts for 20 minutes at 25°C. The esterolytic activity of the incubated samples was measured by the normal titrimetric assay using Bz-Arg-OEt as substrate in the presence of the appropriate concentration of salt. From the results presented in Figure 3 it can be seen that NaCl, KCl, CaCl$_2$ and MgCl$_2$ all greatly increased the activity of the enzyme. It could be argued that the observed effects are due to the increase in ionic strength of the medium (25). However, no effects were seen for NH$_4$Cl or (NH$_4$)$_2$SO$_4$ over the same range of concentration.

Other workers have noted various effects of cations on the activity of tissue kallikreins but the literature is rather contradictory. The magnitude and type of effect appear to depend on the nature of the substrate and type of assay employed (26,27,28).

The effects of detergents on the catalytic activity of rat submandibular kallikrein were investigated in an analogous way to the effects of salts. As can be seen from the results given in Figure 4A one anionic detergent, sodium deoxycholate, and two non-ionic detergents, Triton

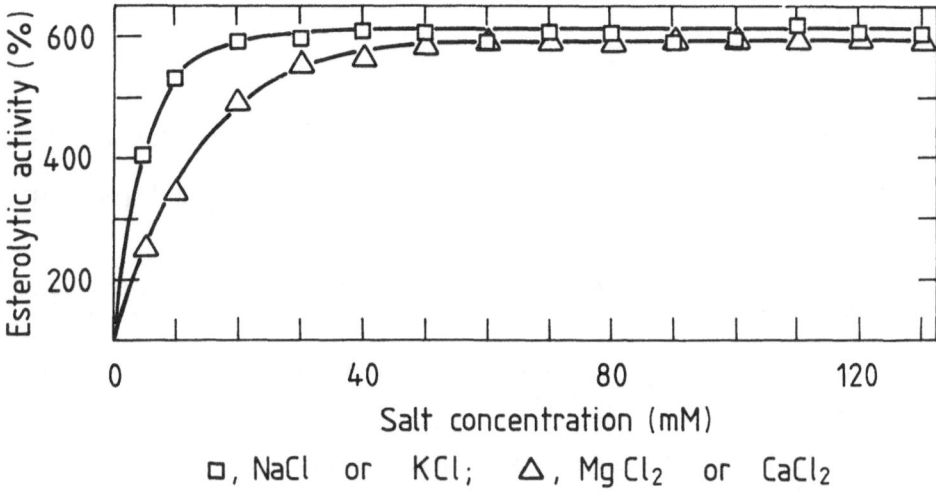

Figure 3. Influence of salts on the esterolytic activity of rat submandibular kallikrein

X-100 and Tween 20, greatly increased the esterolytic activity of the enzyme. In contrast, a cationic detergent, hexadecyltrimethylammonium bromide, significantly decreased the esterolytic activity of the enzyme as shown in Figure 4B. Similar results have been reported for rat urinary kallikrein (29). The mechanisms by which detergents influence the catalytic activity of rat tissue kallikreins are unknown and warrant further study but almost certainly they involve the relatively high hydrophobicity of the enzymes.

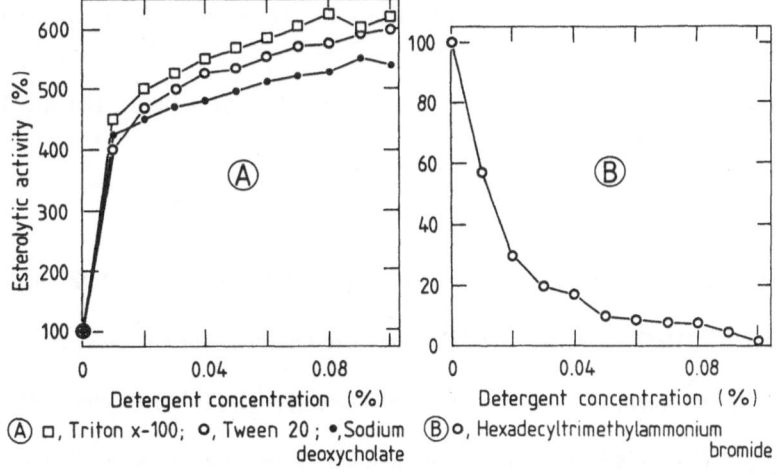

Figure 4. Influence of detergents on the esterolytic activity of rat submandibular kallikrein

REFERENCES

1. Werle, E., Vogel, R. and Lentrodt, J. (1960) Arch. Int. Pharm. Ther. 126, 187-193.

2. Ekfors, T.O., Riekkinen, P.J., Malmiharju, T. and Hopsu-Havu, V.K. (1967) Hoppe-Seyler's Z. Physiol. Chem., 348, 111-118.

3. Brandtzaeg, P., Gautvik, K.M., Nustad, K. and Pierce, J.V. (1976) Br. J. Pharmacol. 56, 155-167.

4. Orstavik, T.B., Carretero, O.A., Hayashi, H., Scicli, A.G. and Johansen, L. (1982) J. Histochem. Cytochem. 30, 1123-1129.

5. Gutkowska, J., Thibault, G., Cantin, M., Garcia, R. and Genest, J. (1983) Can. J. Physiol. Pharmacol. 61, 449-456.

6. Matsuda, Y., Akihama, S. and Fujimoto, Y. (1986) Jap. J. Clin. Chem. 15, 131-139.

7. Kato, H., Nakanishi, E., Enjyoji, K., Hayashi, I., Oh-Ishi, S. and Iwanaga, S. (1987) J. Biochem. 102, 1389-1404.

8. El-Thaher, T.S., Saed, G.M. and Bailey, G.S. (1990) Biochim. Biophys. Acta 1034, 157-161.

9. Bailey, G.S. (1988) in Methods in Enzymology (Di Sabata, G. ed.) Vol. 163, pp115-128, Academic Press, San Diego.

10. Amundsen, E., Putter, J. Friberger, P., Knos, M., Larsbraten, M. and Glaeson, G. (1979) Adv. Exp. Med. Biol. 120A 83-95.

11. Wharton, C.W. and Giesenthal, R. (1981) Molecular Enzymology, Blackie, London.

12. Dixon, M. (1953) Biochem. J. 55, 170-171.

13. Roe, J.H. (1955) J. Biol. Chem. 212, 335-343.

14. Jourdian, G.W., Dean, L. and Roseman, S. (1971) J. Biol. Chem. 246, 430-435.

15. Gardell, S. (1957) in Methods of Biochemical Analysis Vol.VI pp289-317.

16. Khullar, M., Scicli, G., Carretero, O.A. and Scicli, A.G. (1986) Biochem. 25, 1851-1857.

17. Vogel, R. (1979) in Handbook of Experimental Pharmacology (Erdős, E.G. ed.) Vol.XXV Supplement, pp163-225, Springer-Verlag, Berlin.

18.   Hojima, Y., Yamashita, M., Ochi, N., Moriwaki, C. and Moriya, J. (1977) J. Biochem. 82, 599-610.

19.   Chao, J., Woodley, C., Chao, L. and Margolius, H.S. (1983) J. Biol. Chem. 258, 15173-15178.

20.   Fritz, H. and Wunderer, G. (1983) Drug. Res. 33, 479-494.

21.   Scicli, A.G., Diaz, M.A. and Carretero, O.A. (1983) Am. J. Physiol. 245, F198-F203.

22.   Chao, J. (1981) Hoppe-Seyler's Z. Physiol. Chem. 362, 1113-1118.

23.   Geiger, R. and Fritz, H. (1981) in Methods in Enzymology (Lorand, L., ed.) Vol.80, pp466-492, Academic Press, San Diego.

24.   Chao, J. and Chao, L. (1988) in Methods in Enzymology (Di Sabato, G. ed.) Vol. 163, pp128-143, Academic Press, San Diego.

25.   Dixon, M. and Webb, E.C. (1979), Enzymes, 3rd Edition, Academic Press, New York.

26.   Wieberthal, W., Oza, N.B., Bernard, D.B. and Levinsky, N.G. (1982) J. Biol. Chem. 257, 10827-10830.

27.   Worthington, K.J. and Cushieri, A. (1974) Clin. Chim. Acta 52, 129-136.

28.   Friedler, F. and Werle, E. (1968) Eur. J. Biochem. 7, 27-33.

29.   Chao, J. (1978) Arch. Biochem. Biophys. 85, 549-556.

Author for correspondence: Dr. G.S. Bailey, Department of Chemistry and Biological Chemistry, University of Essex, Wivenhoe Park, Colchester CO4 3SQ, UK.

AAS 38/I
Recent Progress on Kinins
© 1992 Birkhäuser Verlag Basel

KALLIKREIN-LIKE ACTIVITY IN NONPREGNANT AND PREGNANT RAT UTERUS,
FETAL MEMBRANES, PLACENTA AND AMNIOTIC FLUID

R. M. Miatello, M. C. Lama, E. S. González and H. L. Nolly

Laboratory of Experimental Hypertension and Vasoactive Peptides.
Argentine Council of Research (CONICET). Mendoza. Rep. Argentina

SUMMARY: SBTI-resistant kininogenase activity was found in nonpregnant and
pregnant rat uterus, placenta, amniotic fluid and fetal membranes. After
trypsin treatment the kininogenase activity increased 2-3 fold. Total kininogenase (active plus inactive) was completely blocked by kallikrein antibodies. The physiological role of these kallikrein-like enzymes is unknown.
It is speculated that these enzymes play a local role, perhaps in the
processing of polypeptide hormones of through the release of kinins in the
regulation of uterine blood flow.

INTRODUCTION

Uteroplacental ischemia has been postulated as the cause of toxemia in

pregnancy (1). Some investigators have suggested that the ischemic utero-

placental-fetal complex releases a humoral factor in the maternal circulation

that produces an increase of the blood pressure, proteinuria, and edema (2).

It has also been postulated that increased local production of vasodepressor

hormones like kinins, EDRF(s) and prostaglandins (PGs) are needed to counter-

act the vasopasm that characterize the discase. Kinins are potent vasodilator

peptides released from kininogen by kininogenases. There is now clear evidence

that part of the hemodynamic effect of kinins is mediated by PGs and EDRF.

The best known and most potent kininogenases, the glandular or tissue kallikrein has been implicated in the regulation of uteroplacental blood flow. However, whether or not kallikrein can be found within the uteroplacental complex is not known. Study of this system during pregnancy have received little attention. Although kinin forming activity has been reported in human myometrial, placental tissues and amniotic fluid(3 , 4)further characterization is needed because proteases other than glandular kallikrein can also release kinins.

To study the characteristics of kininogenases of the uteroplacental complex, we examine: a) the relative concentration of kininogenase activity in these tissues and b) the sensitivity of these kininogenases to kallikrein-antibodies and to protease inhibitors. The present data demonstrates that kininogenase enzymes with the characteristics of glandular kallikrein are present in nonpregnant and pregnant rat uterus, amniotic fluid, placenta and fetal membranes.

MATERIAL AND METHODS

Young adult female Wistar rats between 14 and 15 days gestation (term rat pregnancy, 22 days) weighing 200-250 g were anesthetized with sodium pento-barbital (50 mg/kg i.p). A catheter was introduced into the aorta and the uteri were perfused by hydrostatic pressure with saline until the fluid flowing out of the inferior vena cava appeared free of blood (usually 5 min). Uteri from pregnant and nonpregnant rats were dissected free of placenta, fetal material or extraneous tissue and washed thoroughly to remove all blood. Amniotic fluids were obtained without blood contamination by amniocentesis. Placentas and fetal membranes were also removed, and placed in a Petri dish containing saline, washed by renewing the buffer several times and then minced, rinsed further and frozen at -20°C until used.

Preparation of rat tissue extracts: The homogenate (200 mg wet tissue/ ml) was centrifuged at 1,000 G for 10 min to eliminate debris and the super-natant dialyzed overnight at 4°C against 0.01M Tris-HCl buffer (pH 7.4).

Incubation procedure: The homogenate supernatant (400 μl) from different tissue extract (80 mg wet tissue weight) was incubated for 5 hr at 37°C with 200 μl partially purified dog kininogen (2,000 ng kinin-releasing capability) in the presence of 1,000 μl fresh 0.1M Tris-HCl buffer (pH 8.5) containing

EDTA (15 mg/ml), 1-10 phenanthroline (1mg/ml), 8-OH-quinoline (1 mg/ml) and
soybean trypsin inhibitor (SBTI) (100 μg/ml). SBTI was used to inhibit plasma
kallikrein or trypsin-like enzymes that might contaminate the preparations.
The kinins generated during the 5-hour incubation period were measured by
radioimmunoassay (RIA) (5). Bradykinin recovery was 80 ± 5% (n = 6).
Results are expressed as pg bradykinin per mg protein per min incubation. To
determine the optimum pH, aliquots of the homogenates were incubated with
kininogen and peptidase inhibitors at pH levels ranging from 5 to 9 using
different buffers (0.1 M acetate, 0.1 M phosphate and 0.1 M Tris-HCl).

Trypsin activation: To determine whether inactive kallikrein was present,
the homogenates were trypsinized. To establish the best radio between trypsin
and tissue homogenate for activation of inactive kininogenase, a fixed amount of
tissue was preincubated for 30 min at 37°C with varying concentrations of trypsin
ranging from 0.05 to 1.0 μg/mg tissue in 500 μl 0.1M Tris-HCl buffer (pH 8.5).
A ratio equal to 0.2 μg trypsin per mg tissue was found to be optimal for our
use. In short, the equivalent of 100 mg tissue homogenate in 500 μl Tris was
incubated with trypsin (20 μg) in 0.5 ml 0.1M Tris-HCl buffer (pH 8.5) for 30
min at 37°C, after which the reaction was stopped by adding SBTI (100 μg).

Immunological characterization: Inhibition of kininogenase activity was
assessed by incubating the tissue homogenates with globulin purified from rabbit
antiserum against rat urinary kallikrein or from non-immunized rabbits (5).
Prior to incubation with kininogen, 400 μl of the homogenate supernatant from the
tissues (equivalent to 80 mg tissue) was incubated with 200 μg of either
globulin, after which kininogenase activity was measured.

Gel filtration on Ultrogel AcA$_{54}$: 2 ml of the supernatant homogenate (35
mg protein) was applied to an Ultrogel AcA$_{54}$ column (100 x 1 cm) equilibrated and
eluted with 0.1M phosphate buffer (pH 7.4). The column was eluted at a rate of
18 ml/hr; 3-ml fractions were collected and kininogenase activity monitored. To
determine molecular weight, the elution volume of the present enzyme was compared
with standards of known molecular weight, namely gamma globulin (MW 158,000),
ovalbumin (MW 43,000), chymotrypsinogen (MW 25,000) and myoglobin (MW 17,000).
Rat submandibular gland kallikrein, used as a control, was purified using a
modification of a previous method (5). Purified rat kallikrein was homogeneous
on 12% alkaline polyacrylamide gel electrophoresis and released 1.2 μg of kinin
per 1 μg protein per min when incubated with 2,000 ng semipurified dog kininogen.

Inhibition studies: Homogenates (equivalent to 80 mg wet tissue in
400 μl Tris) were preincubated at 37°C for 30 min together with SBTI   (100 μg/
ml final concentration), phenylmethylsulfonyl fluoride (PMSF, 2mM), aprotinin
(1000 KIU), and D-Phe-Phe-Arg-chloromethyl ketone (D-PPACK, 10^{-6} M).   The
inhibitors were dissolved in 0.1M Tris-HCl (pH 7.4), except for PMSF which was
dissolved in methanol. After the preincubation period, samples were incubated
with kininogen for 5 hr at 37°C to assay kininogenase activity. As a control,
we used a dilution of purified rat submandibular kallikrein which gave kinin-

ogenase activity similar to that observed with the kininogenase under study. Proteins were determined by Bradford's method (5).

Reagents: Molecular weight markers (BioRad, NY) Ultrogel (LKB, NJ), Trypsin and SBTI (Worthington Biochemical Corp., NJ), captopril (Squibb), aprotinin (Bayer), and polyacrylamide (Eastman Kodak, NY) were all analytical grade.

Statistics: Two-sided, two sample t tests were used to assay kininogenase activity. Bonferroni's adjustment for multiple comparisons was employed. Unless otherwise noted, all results are expressed as mean ± SEM.

RESULTS AND DISCUSSION

The rat uterus contained kininogenase activity. Most of the enzyme was present in an inactive form. Only 5% was already active; the rest required activation by trypsin. After trypsin activation the enzyme was completely inhibited by kallikrein antibodies, whereas it was resistant to soybean trypsin inhibitor (SBTI) (Table 1).

Table 2 compares sensitivity of kininogenases from maternal tissues and fetal membranes to several proteinase inhibitors.

Figure 1 shows that the kininogenase activity present in amnions was blocked by kallikrein antibodies and almost unaffected by incubation with SBTI.

Figure 2 shows that the kininogenase activity in placenta was partially blocked by incubation with SBTI. The kininogenase activiy increased 2-3 fold by incubation with trypsin. Kallikrein antibodies completely inhibited the kininogenase activity of trypsin-treated placenta.

Figure 3 shows low but detectable amounts of kininogenase activity in amniotic fluid. The kininogenase activity increased 3 fold by incubation with trypsin. Total kininogenase (active plus inactive) was resistant to SBTI. In contrast, it was completely inhibited by incubation with kallikrein antibodies.

TABLE 1. Kininogenase activity in rat uterus

	Total Kininogenase pg Bk / mg wt / hr	n	% Inhibition KK-Ab	SBTI
. nonpregnant	240 ± 15	(6)	86	4
. pregnant (14th day)	182 ± 22	(5)	88	5

n = number of experiments; KK-Ab = glandular kallikrein antibodies; SBTI = soybean trypsin inhibitor (100 μg/ml); mean ± S.E.; total kininogenase (active plus trypsin-activatable) is expressed per mg wet tissue per hour of incubation.

TABLE 2. Effects of proteinase inhibitors on the kininogenase activity of fetal membranes and maternal tissues.

Inhibitor	Percent inhibition			
	Uterus	Placenta	Amnion	Amniotic Fluid
Phenylmethylsulfonyl Fluoride (3) (2 mM)	94 ± 3	88 ± 5	96 ± 3	92 ± 2
D-Phe-Phe-Arg-Chloromethyl ketone (3) (10^{-6} M)	89 ± 4	90 ± 4	92 ± 2	90 ± 4
Soybean Trypsin Inhibitor (100 μg/ml) (6)	5 ± 3	18 ± 5	4 ± 2	6 ± 2
Aprotinin (100 KIU) (3)	91 ± 2	93 ± 5	94 ± 3	96 ± 2

Values between parenthesis indicate number of experiments.

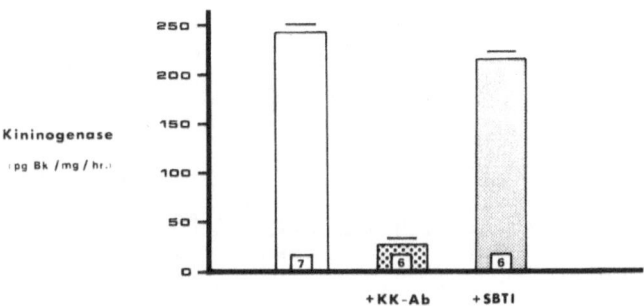

FIGURE 1. Kininogenase activity in rat fetal membranes

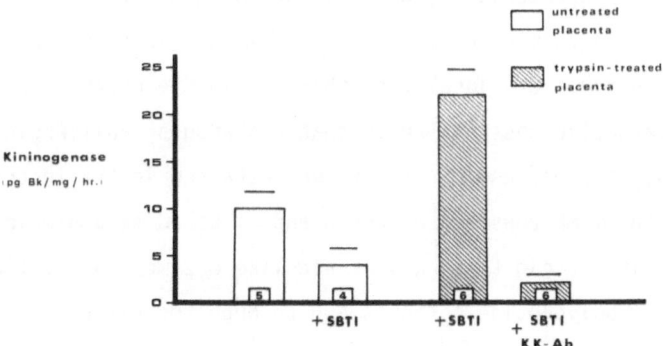

FIGURE 2. Kininogenase activity in rat placenta

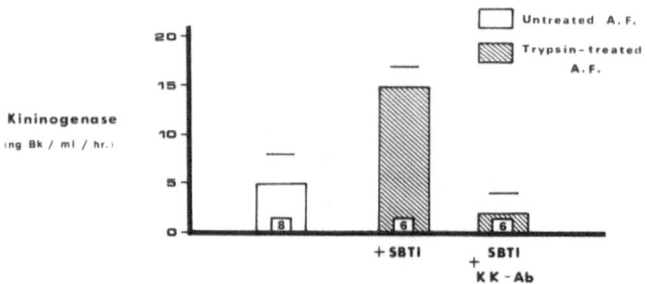

FIGURE 3.   Kininogenase activity in rat amniotic fluid

The present study demonstrates the presence of a kinin-forming enzyme in rat maternal tissues and fetal membranes. The insensitivity of this kininogenase to SBTI readily distinguishes it from trypsin and plasma kallikrein. This enzyme is present in both active and inactive form and its isoelectric point, molecular weight between 32,000 and 34,000 daltons (data not shown), and immunological characteristics are similar to those of glandular kallikrein. The finding of kinin forming enzyme in these tissues suggest, but does not prove, that the enzymes are locally synthesized in the uterus-placental complex. An alternative possibility is that a glandular kallikrein from salivary glands, pancreas and/or kidney were retained in the intersticial space of the fetal membranes and placenta and filtered to amniotic fluid. Irrespective of its origin these kallikrein-like enzymes may participate in the processing of polypeptide hormones and through the release of kinins may contribute to the regulation of utero placental blood flow during pregnancy and labor. Kinin is a powerful systemic vasodilator but has been shown to cause vasoconstriction in isolated blood vessels preparations (6). Kinins released in the proximity of the uterine smooth muscle would be oxytocic and stimulate prostaglandin production. Placenta is known to produce large amounts of prostaglandins that may have local actions on the feto placental circulation which is the only route for providing needs of the growing fetus. Fetoplacental blood flow is predominantly controlled by circulating or locally produced hormones since the placental vasculature lacks innervation.

In summary, a protease(s) which resembles glandular kallikrein is present in rat maternal tissues and fetal membranes.

REFERENCES

1. Abitol M M, Gallo G R, Pirani C L and Ober W B. Production of experimental toxemia in the pregnant rabbit. American Journal of Obstetrics
   and Ginecology 1976a; 124: 460.

2. Cavanagh D, Rao PS, Tsai CC and O'Connor TC. Experimental toxemia in
   the pregnant primate. American Journal of Obstetrics and Gynecology
   1977 ; 128 : 75 .

3. Malofiejew M. Kallikrein-like activity in human myometrium, placenta
   and amniotic fluid. Biochem. Pharmacol. 1973 ; 22: 123-127.

4. McCormick JT and Senior J. Plasma kinin and kininogen levels in the
   female rat during the oestrous cycle, pregnancy, parturition and the
   puerperium. Br. J.Pharmacol. 1974 ; 50 : 237-241 .

5. Nolly HL, Scicli AG, Scicli G, Carretero OA. Characterization of a
   kininogenase from rat vascular tissue resembling tissue kallikrein.
   Circ. Res. 1985 ; 56: 816-821.

6. Fasciolo JC, Vargas L, Lama MC, Nolly HL. Bradykinin induced vasoconstriction of the rat mesenteric arteries precontracted with
   noradrenalina. Br. J. Pharmacol. 1990 ; 101: 344-348.

AAS 38/I
Recent Progress on Kinins
© 1992 Birkhäuser Verlag Basel

DYNAMICS OF KALLIKREIN ACTIVITY IN DIFFERENT BIOLOGICAL FLUIDS OF PREGNANT ANIMALS

K.Helili, B.Somlev, V.Karcheva*

Institute of Biology and Immunology of Reproduction, Sofia 1113, *Institute of Animal Breeding, Kostinbrod, Bulgaria

SUMMARY: Kallikrein activity was measured in urine, saliva and blood plasma samples from pregnant cows by using the chromogenic substrates S-2266 and S-2302 (Kabi, Sweden). It was found that the kallikrein activity in these biological fluids showed a trend to an increase with a peak prior to parturition. At the same time the plasma prekallikrein levels decreased during pregnancy reaching the lowest values at the end of the gestation period.

INTRODUCTION

It has been already found that the components of the kallikrein-kinin system are actively involved in the reproductive processes occurring in the female organism. In the last years reports were published that these components undergo considerable changes during the pregnancy of women and some female laboratory mammals(1, 2, 3). By using RIA it has been revealed that there are also changes in the amount of ewe's blood plasma kallikrein at different stages of reproduction (4).Most of these studies demonstrated that the kallikrein activity manifested a trend to an increase with the advance of pregnancy. It has been suggested that these changes in the levels of kallikrein-kinin system components are mainly related to the participation of kinins in uterine contractions and dilation of the cervix from the onset of labor to delivery, as well as to other physiological processes occurring at the final stages of pregnancy. These investigations are of considerable interest either from theoretical point of

view to elucidate the role of kallikrein-kinin system in reproduction and of clinical point of view. In contrast to the numerous papers treating this problem in women, the data on domestic
animals are rather scanty. Taking into consideration these cir-
cumstances, the aim of this study was to follow up the dynamics of kallikrein activity in urine, saliva and blood plasma
samples, as well as prekallikrein level in blood plasma samples
from pregnant cows.

MATERIALS AND METHODS

A total of 200 clinically healthy multiparous cows at ages from 3
to 5 years were used as donors of urine, saliva and blood
samples. The animals were divided into six groups according to
their reproductive state: (1) non-pregnant, (2) up to 20 days
after insemination, (3) pregnant in the first trimester, (4)
pregnant in the second trimester, (5) pregnant in the third trimester, (6) up to 20 days after parturition.

All biological fluids tested in this study were
analysed with the aid of the spectrophotometric methods developed
by the firm "KabiVitrum", Sweden (5) for measurement of glandular
and blood plasma kallikreins and prekallikrein. Urine and saliva
samples were assayed for glandular kalikrein activity by using
the specific chromogenic substrate S-2266, and the blood plasma
samples were analysed by the application of the substrate S-2302.
The blood plasma prekallikrein was converted into the active
enzyme form by adding prekallikrein activator. All these products
were obtained from "KabiVitrum", Sweden. The urine and saliva
blanks were prepared by using Trasylol (Bayer, Germany), while
the blood plasma blanks were performed by adding the reagents in
reverse order without incubation. The absorbances of the samples
against their blanks were read in a spectrophotometer at 405 nm.

The enzyme activity was calculated in kat/l. For the
purpose of comparison the prekallikrein and kallikrein activities
in blood plasma samples were also recalculated in mU/ml protein
(1 mU was the amount of enzyme which changed the absorbance by

0.001 at 405 nm). The total protein content was measured by the
method of Lowry et al. (6). All data were statistically analysed
by the Student's t-test.

RESULTS

Pooled urine samples from 25 cows analysed for glandular kallikrein activity showed 9.387 ± 1.314 nkat/l (1.91 ÷ 28.62 nkat/l),
on an average. The results from measurements made during the
different reproductive stages are given in Fig.1.

        Pooled cow's saliva samples manifested an activity of
4.09 µkat/l, on an average. Data on the glandular kallikrein
activity in saliva samples from pregnant cows are presented in
Fig.2.

        The analysis of blood plasma prekallikrein and
kallikrein activity in pregnant animals expressed in kat/l and in
mU per 1 mg total protein, are given in Fig. 3 and 4, resp.

        As seen from the graphs, there were similar trends in
the dynamics both of the glandular and of plasma kallikrein activity in the pregnant cows. In all fluids this activity gradually
increased with the advance of pregnancy reaching its maximum just
prior to parturition. Afterwards the activity dropped to attain
the levels before conception within a period of about 20 days.
Similar tendency was also recorded when the data on blood plasma
kallikrein activity were recalculated per mg total protein regardless of the fact that the total protein level varied during the
different periods of pregnancy.

        At the same time the prekallikrein level in cow's blood
plasma samples showed an opposite tendency. It gradually
decreased with the advance of pregnancy, and the lowest values
were found in the period near the delivery.

        All differences recorded both in the prekallikrein and
in the glandular and blood plasma kallikrein activity between the
various periods, as well as between the pregnant and non-pregnant
animals were statistically significant.

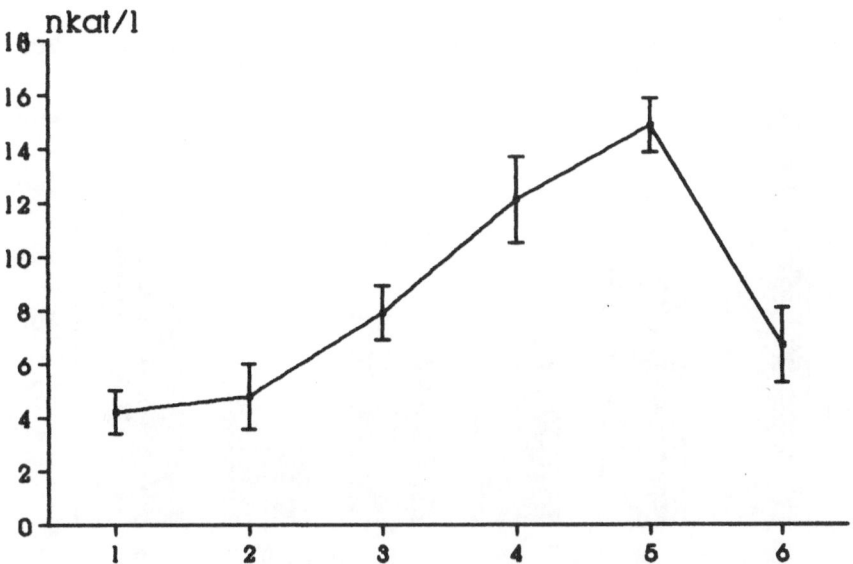

Fig.1. Kallikrein activity in cow's urine samples:
1 - non-pregnant; 2 - after insemination;
3 - 1st trimester; 4 - 2nd trimester; 5 -
3rd trimester; 6 - after parturition

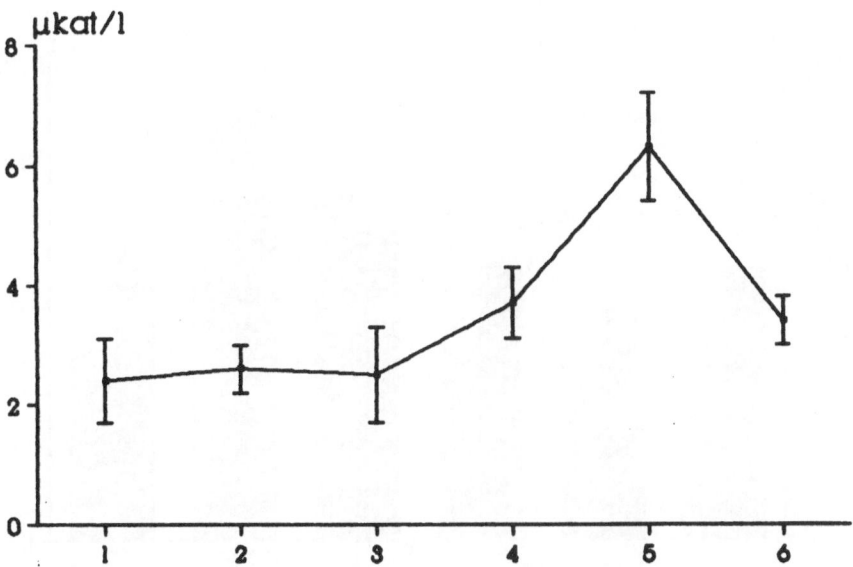

Fig.2. Kallikrein activity in cow's saliva samples:
1 - non-pregnant; 2 - after insemination;
3 - 1st trimester; 4 - 2nd trimester; 5 -
3rd trimester; 6 - after parturition

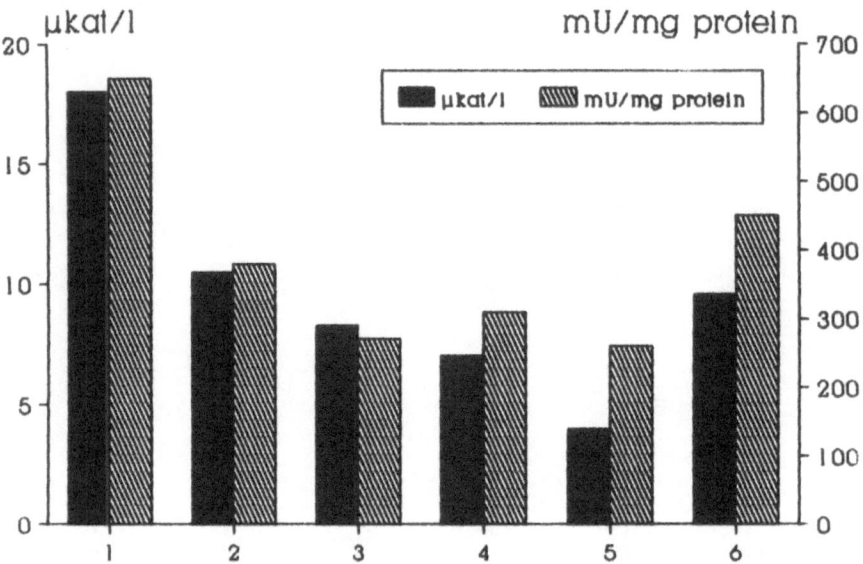

Fig.3. Prekallikrein level in cow's blood plasma:
1 - non-pregnant; 2 - after insemination;
3 - 1st trimester; 4 - 2nd trimester; 5 -
3rd trimester; 6 - after parturition

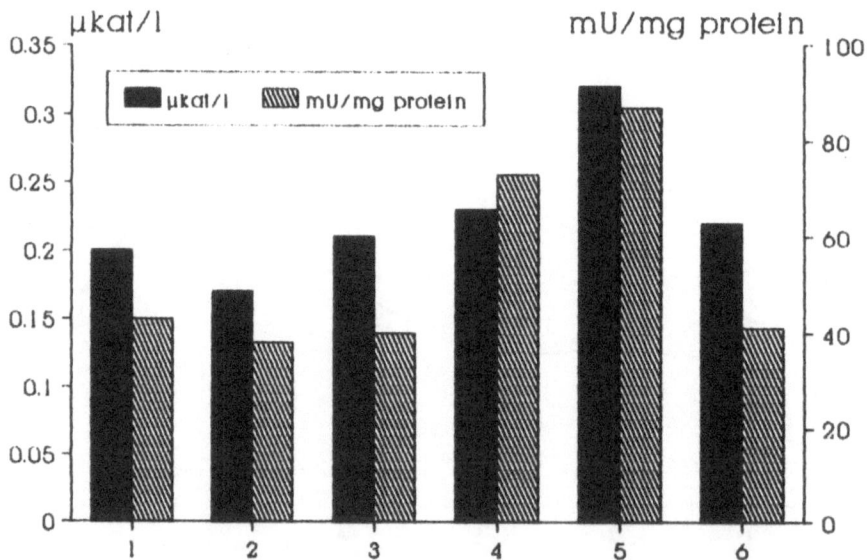

Fig.4. Kallikrein activity in cow's blood plasma:
1 - non-pregnant; 2 - after insemination;
3 - 1st trimester; 4 - 2nd trimester; 5 -
3rd trimester; 6 - after parturition

DISCUSSION

The results obtained from the present study carried out to determine the glandular and blood plasma kallikrein activity both in non-pregnant and pregnant cows revealed a clearly expressed curve. The highest values of glandular and blood plasma kallikrein activity in the pregnant animals were recorded near the period of parturition. These trends were similar to those demonstrated in amniotic fluid (7) and urine samples (8) from pregnant women. At the same time the trends in the prekallikrein levels observed in this investigation resembled those in women published by other authors (1, 2), revealing a marked decrease in the period of delivery. It was demonstrated that there was also a drop of the kininogen levels during parturition (7). This indicates that at this final stage of the pregnancy it is likely that the female organism requires greater amounts of kinins needed, as it has been suggested by a number of investigators (1, 7), for the direct participation of the kallikrein-kinin system in the processes of delivery such as contractions of the uterus and dilation of the cervix. It was also assumed that the components of this system might be involved in other vitally important physiological processes occurring during the delivery. Miatello et al. (9) assaying the kallikrein activity in uterine tissue and placenta suggested that the role of the kallikrein-kinin system is probably to generate kinins locally and to take part in the circulatory homeostasis during pregnancy. Salas et al. (3) assumed that the physiological reduction of blood pressure at the end of the pregnancy in rats is probably due to the enhanced vasodilation activity of the renal kallikrein-kinin system. In additon to the concept of the direct effect of the kinins on the uterine activity during delivery, it is possible that there is also an indirect involvement of the kallikrein-kinin system through an interaction with the prostaglandin metabolism (2).

ACKNOWLEDGEMENTS

The authors are grateful to Mr.Leif Aurell (KabiVitrum, Sweden)
for the generous supply of plasma prekallikrein activator and the
substrates S-2266 and S-2302.

REFERENCES

1. Suzuki S, Murakoshi T, Sakamoto W. Studies on the various
   causal factors related to hypercoagulability in the field of
   obstetrics - with special reference to the onset of DIC as
   viewed from the changing of kinin-kallikrein system and fibri-
   nopeptide A. In: KININ-III, part B. Fritz H, Back N, Dietze G,
   Haberland GL, editors. New York - London: Plenum Press, 1983:
   1055-1065.

2. Ito R, Statland BE, Sher G, Knutzen V. Assaying plasma prekallikrein (PPK) by a chromogenic based method: analytical consi-
   derations and reference values in healthy adults, the pregnant
   and the neonate. In: KININ-III, part A. Fritz H, Back N, Dietze G, Haberland GL, editors. New York - London: Plenum Press,
   1983: 205-223.

3. Salas SP, Roblero JS, Godoy JE. Urinary kallikrein activity in
   pregnant hypertensive rats. In: KININ-IV. Greenbaum LM, Margolius HS, editors. New York - London: Plenum Press, 1986: 297-
   303.

4. Somlev B, Stankov B. RIA of kallikrein in blood plasma of ewes
   at different reproductive stages. C R Acad bulg Sci 1985; 38:
   1219-1221.

5. KabiVitrum AB (Sweden). Determination of prekallikrein in
   plasma, kallikrein activity in blood plasma, urine and saliva.
   Laboratory instructions 1985.

6. Lowry DH, Rosenbrough NJ, Farr AL, Randall RJ. Protein measurement with the folin phenol reagent. J Biol Chem 1951; 193:
   265-275.

7. Mutoh S, Yaoi Y, Saitoh M, Aoki N, Abe T, Ohno Y, Itoh N. Studies of coagulation-fibrinolytic and kallikrein-kinin system
   in amniotic fluid. In: Abstract Volume. Int Congress Kinin'87.
   Tokyo: 1987: p.149.

8. Kovatz S, Arber I, Korzet G, Rathaus M, Aderet NB, Bernheim J.
   Urinary kallikrein in normal pregnancy, pregnancy with hypertension and toxemia. Nephron 1985; 40: 48-51.

9. Miatello R, Cristina Lama M, Nolly H. Kallikrein-like enzymes
   in rat amniotic fluid, fetal membranes and maternal tissues.
   In: Abstract Volume. Int Conf Kinin'91, Munich: 1991: p.249.

AAS 38/I
Recent Progress on Kinins
© 1992 Birkhäuser Verlag Basel

BOVINE PANCREATIC KALLIKREIN: PURIFICATION AND RADIOIMMUNOASSAY

A.A.A. Al-Hamidi[*], M.A.S. Al-Tufail[+] and G.S. Bailey

Department of Chemistry and Biological Chemistry,
University of Essex, Colchester, Essex CO4 3SQ, UK

SUMMARY: Kallikrein was isolated from bovine pancreatic tissue by a sequential procedure of anion-exchange, hydrophobic interaction and gel filtration chromatographies. A monospecific polyclonal antiserum to the pure enzyme was raised in rabbits and was used to set up a specific radioimmunoassay for bovine tissue kallikrein.

INTRODUCTION

During the last 50 years or so tissue kallikreins have been studied following their isolation from numerous organs and fluids of a variety of species (1). As kallikreins are often described as trypsin-like proteases and bovine trypsin is a well characterised enzyme (2) it is rather surprizing that there have been no reports of the complete purification of a tissue kallikrein from any bovine tissue or fluid. This paper gives an account of the isolation of kallikrein from bovine pancreas and describes the establishment of a specific radioimmunoassay for the enzyme.

---

[*]Present address: King Khalid Military Academy, Department of Science, P.O. Box 22140, Riyadh 11495, Saudi Arabia

[+]Present address: King Faisal Specialist Hospital and Research Centre, Toxicology Laboratory, P.O. Box 3354, Riyadh 11211, Saudi Arabia

MATERIALS AND METHODS

Kallikrein was isolated from fresh bovine pancreatic tissue by a sequential procedure consisting of batch and column anion-exchange, hydrophobic interaction and gel filtration chromatographies. Samples were concentrated by ultrafiltration using membranes of Mr cut-off of 10,000. The purification was monitored by means of a kininogenase assay in which the kinin released from bovine kininogen was measured by a specific radioimmunoassay (3). The assay was carried out in the presence of sufficient soyabean trypsin inhibitor (SBTI) to inhibit endogenous trypsin. Slab gel electrophoresis was performed under non-denaturing conditions at pH 8.9 on 10% and 16% acrylamide gels (4). SDS-polyacrylamide gel electrophoresis was carried out using a discontinuous Tris-glycine buffer system (4). A monospecific, polyclonal antiserum to bovine pancreatic kallikrein was produced in rabbits using a conventional procedure (5). The specificity of the antiserum was tested by double immunodiffusion. Protein concentrations were measured by the method of Bradford with bovine serum albumin as standard (6). Radioactive labelling of an aliquot of pure bovine pancreatic kallikrein with ^{125}I was carried out using the protocol previously described for rat pancreatic kallikrein (7).

RESULTS

Purification of kallikrein from bovine pancreas

All steps were carried out at 4°C.

Step 1: A crude homogenate (10% w/v) was produced in a Waring blender using washed, chopped pancreatic tissue (40 g) in 0.05 M Tris-HCl/0.1 M NaCl pH 7.4 (buffer A). The initial homogenate was clarified by filtration through muslin, centrifugations at 300 g for 7 minutes followed by 18000 g for 30 minutes and a second filtration.

Step 2: The clarified homogenate (250 ml) was subjected to batch adsorption on to DEAE-Sephadex A-50 anion-exchange resin (250 ml) equilibrated with buffer A. After washing the resin with buffer A (about 2000 ml) the adsorbed material was removed by application of 0.05 M Tris-HCl/1.0 M NaCl pH 7.4 (buffer B, 200 ml). The salt concentration of the eluted samples was reduced to 0.1 M NaCl by ultrafiltration.

Step 3: The sample from batch adsorption (150 ml) was applied to a column (5 x 11 cm) of DEAE-Sephadex A-50 resin equilibrated with buffer A. After washing with buffer A (100 ml) the bound material was removed by application of a linear salt gradient (600 ml buffer A to 600 ml 0.05 M Tris-HCl/0.7 M NaCl pH 7.4) at a flow rate of 45 ml/hour with fractions collected every 10 minutes. The elution profile is shown in Figure 1.

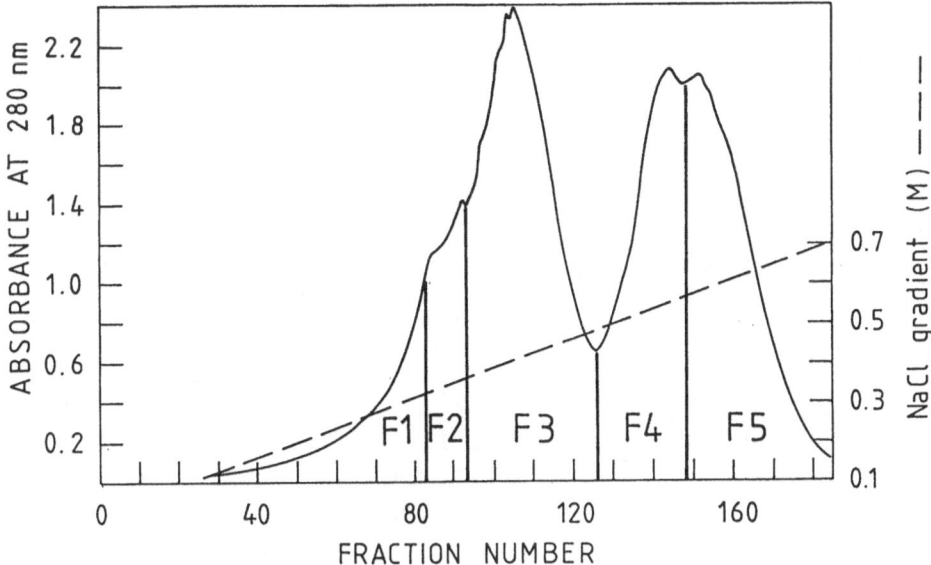

Figure 1. Step 3 Anion-exchange Chromatography

Step 4: The major kallikrein-containing fraction (F$_3$) from step 3 was made into aliquots and each aliquot in turn was subject to hydrophobic interaction chromatography. Typically an aliquot of F$_3$ (46.8 mg/6 ml) was brought to 1 M (NH$_4$)$_2$SO$_4$ and was applied to a column (1.3 x 8 cm) of Phenyl-Sepharose CL-4B resin equilibrated in 0.05 M Tris-HCl/1 M (NH$_4$)$_2$SO$_4$ pH 7.0 (starting buffer). The column was washed with starting buffer (30 ml) at a flow rate of 6.8 ml/hour and collecting fractions every 15 minutes. Bound material was eluted by application of a linear negative gradient consisting of starting buffer (100 ml) and 0.05 M Tris-HCl pH 7.0 (finishing buffer, 100 ml). Strongly bound material was removed from the resin by washing with 50% (v/v) ethylene glycol in finishing buffer (25 ml). A representative elution profile is shown in Figure 2. The major kallikrein-containing fraction (AF$_2$) from each run was combined, concentrated and made into aliquots.

Step 5: An aliquot of AF$_2$ (1.8 mg/2 ml) was applied to a column (1.6 x 87 cm) of Sephadex-G150 resin and was eluted with 0.05 M Tris-HCl/0.15 M NaCl pH 7.4 at a flow rate of 7.6 ml/hour and collecting fractions over 15 minute periods. A representative elution profile is shown in Figure 3.

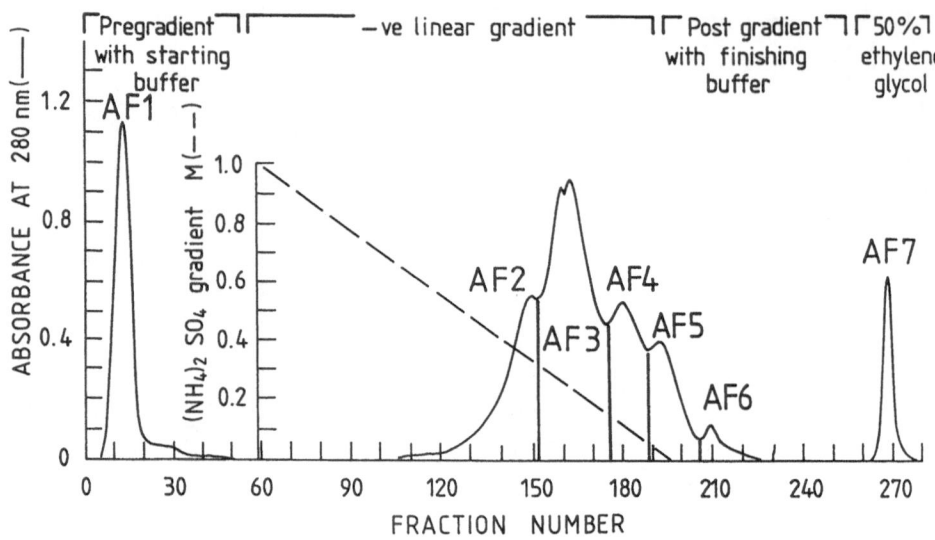

Figure 2. Step 4 Hydrophobic Interaction Chromatography

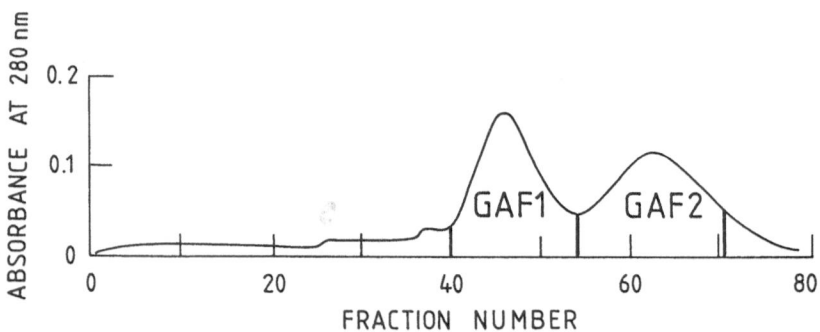

Figure 3. Step 5 Gel Filtration

The major kallikrein-containing fraction (GAF$_2$) from gel filtration eluted at a position corresponding to Mr 25000 and was seen to consist of a single component on gel electrophoresis under native conditions. The single component on SDS gel electrophoresis corresponded to Mr 27000. A summary of the purification procedure is shown in Table 1.

TABLE 1. Purification of kallikrein from bovine pancreas

Fraction	Protein (mg)	Specific Activity (units/mg)[a]	Purification (n-fold)	Recovery (%)
Homogenate	2325.0	38.0	(1)	(100)
Batch adsorption	640.0	93.0	2.4	67.3
Ion-exchange F$_3$	218.0	200.0	5.3	49.3
Hydrophobic AF$_2$	26.6	1127.5	29.7	33.9
Gel filtration GAF$_2$	6.5	3565.0	93.8	26.2

[a] units/mg = ng kinin per minute per mg protein

Radioimmunoassay for bovine pancreatic kallikrein

Antiserum to bovine pancreatic kallikrein was raised in rabbits by initially injecting each rabbit with the pure kallikrein (100 µg) followed by a first booster injection (50 µg kallikrein) after 2 weeks and a second booster injection (30 µg kallikrein) after 12 weeks. The specificity of the antiserum for kallikrein was confirmed by double immunodiffusion.

The procedure for radioimmunoassay consisted of setting up incubation tubes as outlined in Table 2.

TABLE 2. Radioimmunoassay for bovine pancreatic kallikrein

Tube	RIA buffer[a] (μl)	Standard[b] or Sample (μl)	^{125}I-labelled[c] kallikrein (μl)	Antiserum[d] (μl)
Total Count (Tc)	-	-	100	-
Non-specific binding (NSB)	300	-	100	-
Maximum binding (MB)	200	-	100	100
Standard or unknown	-	200	100	100

[a]   RIA buffer is 0.1 M sodium phosphate buffer pH 7.4 containing 0.15 M NaCl, 0.01% NaN3 and 0.1% bovine serum albumin.

[b]   standard kallikrein ranged from 76 ng/200 μl to 1.2 ng/200 μl.

[c]   labelled kallikrein was used at 10000 counts/min.

[d]   antiserum was used at 1/5000 dilution (i.e. final dilution was 1/20000).

The tubes were incubated at 25°C for 18 hours. Bound and free radioactivities were separated at 4°C by the addition to each tube except Tc of 30% polyethylene glycol 6000/1% KI in RIA buffer lacking BSA (1 ml) and 1% bovine γ globulin in forementioned buffer (0.2 ml). The tubes were vortexed and left to stand at 4°C for 15 minutes before centrifugation at 5000 g for 30 minutes. The supernatants were aspirated at a water pump and the radioactive sediments were counted. A standard curve was constructed using the logit-log transformation (8) and a typical curve is shown in Figure 4 with the limits of linearity being 1.2 ng kallikrein and 76 ng kallikrein. A value of 7.7% was found for the inter-assay coefficient of variation determined by measuring the same sample in a number of separate assays. A value of 4.5% was found for the intra-assay coefficient of variation determined by measuring identical aliquots of the same sample in a single assay. Under the described conditions the minimal detection limit was 0.6 ng kallikrein.

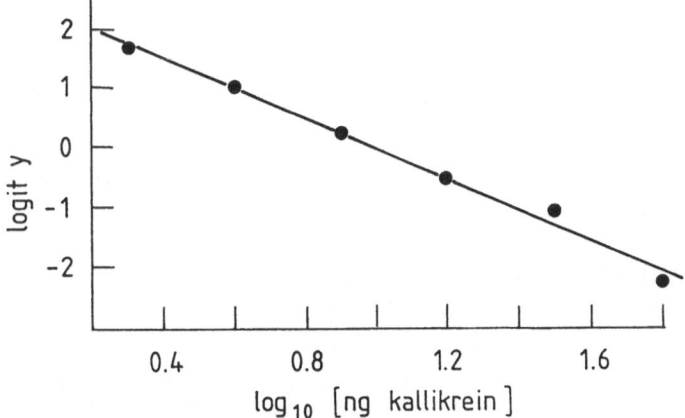

Figure 4. Standard curve of radioimmunoassay of bovine pancreatic kallikrein

DISCUSSION

This paper describes the first ever purification of a bovine tissue kallikrein. The overall degree of purification, based on the release of kinin from kininogen, has been calculated to be 94-fold (Table 1). However, that is almost certainly an underestimate since the assay used to monitor the purification is not specific for kallikrein; the kininogen substrate will be cleaved by any kinin-releasing enzyme that is not inhibited by SBTI. The final sample (GAF₂) was shown to be pure by analytical gel electrophoresis.

A monospecific, polyclonal antiserum to bovine pancreatic kallikrein was raised in rabbits. That antiserum was used to set up a radioimmunoassay for bovine pancreatic kallikrein. Bearing in mind that tissue kallikreins within a given species are immunologically very similar (9) the radioimmunoassay should prove to be very useful for the measurement of any bovine tissue kallikrein.

REFERENCES

1.   Fiedler, F. (1979) Enzymology of glandular kallikreins in Handbook of
     Experimental Pharmacology (Erdos, E.G., ed.), vol. XXV Supplement, pp103-
     161, Springer-Verlag, Berlin.

2.   Walsh, K.A. (1970) Trypsinogens and trypsins of various species in Methods in
     Enzymology (Perlman, G.E. and Lorand, L., eds) vol. XIX, 41-63, Academic
     Press, San Diego.

3.   Bailey, G.S., Al-Joufi, A., Rawat, S. and Smith, D.C. (1991) Neutralization of
     kinin-releasing enzymes of crotalid venoms by monospecific and polyspecific
     antivenoms.Toxicon 29, 777-781.

4.   Blackshear, P.J. (1984) Systems for polyacrylamide gel electrophoresis in Methods
     in Enzymology (Jakoby, W.B., ed.), vol. 104, 237-255, Academic Press, San
     Diego.

5.   Bailey, G.S. (1984) The production of antisera in Methods in Molecular Biology
     (Walker, J.M., ed.), vol. 1, 295-300, Humana Press, Clifton, New Jersey.

6.   Bradford, M.M. (1976) A rapid and sensitive method for the quatitation of
     microgram quantities of protein utilizing the principle of protein-dye binding. Anal.
     Biochem. 72, 248-254.

7.   Bailey, G.S. (1988) Rat pancreas kallikrein in Methods in Enzymology (Di Sabata,
     G., ed.), vol. 163, 115-128, Academic Press, San Diego.

8.   Bailey, G.S. (1984) Radioimmunoassay in Methods in Molecular Biology (Walker,
     J.M., ed), vol. 1, 335-347.

9.   Proud, D., Bailey, G.S., Nustad, K. and Gautvik, K.M. (1979) The
     immunological similarity of rat glandular kallikrein. Biochem. J. 167, 835-838.

AAS 38/I
Recent Progress on Kinins
© 1992 Birkhäuser Verlag Basel

PURIFICATION AND CHARACTERIZATION OF NEW ARGININE ESTEROPEPTIDASE FROM THE SOLUBLE FRACTION OF HUMAN SUBMAXILLARY GLANDS*

Y. Fujimoto, M. Suzuki and Y. Watanabe

Hokkaido Institute of Pharmaceutical Sciences, Katsuraoka-cho, Otaru-shi, Hokkaido, 047-02, Japan

SUMMARY: An arginine esteropeptidase was completely purified from the soluble fraction of human submaxillary glands. The molecular weight was calculated to be 12,000, having 2 species of subunits. The study of the effect of inhibitors confirmed the enzyme's serine protease-like characteristics. The best ester and amide substrates were Tos-Arg-OMe and D-Ile-Pro-Arg-pNA, respectively.

INTRODUCTION

The concept of kallikrein multigene family has been widely accepted recently (1). Tissue kallikrein and the related proteases, equally liable to cleavage of synthetic peptide substrate after arginine residue, designated here as arginine esteropeptidase, are members of a family of very similar genes. As in the mouse, it is reported the gene family consists of 24 genes of which at least 10 are expressed (2). In the rat, the gene family consists of 17 genes (2). In view of the fact that the human kallikrein gene family consists of at least 4 distinct genes, the encoded proteins are less than murine ones.

Recently, we reported that a major arginine esteropeptidase present in soluble fraction of human submaxillary glands was identical to tissue kallikrein (3). Moreover, we found a new latent arginine esteropeptidase in the microsomal membrane of the gland tissues (4).

---

*We dedicate this paper to the late Professor Dr. Hiroshi Moriya.

On the other hand, detecting another arginine esteropeptidase in the soluble fraction, we then proceeded to focus
our attention on this new enzyme. In this report, we deal with
the purification and characterization of new arginine esteropeptidase from the soluble fraction of human submaxillary glands.

MATERIALS AND METHODS

Human submaxillary glands tissues were kindly provided by the
Department of Pathology, Sapporo Medical College, as described
(3-5). Nα-p-Tosyl-L-arginine methyl ester (Tos-Arg-OMe) was
purchased from the Protein Research Foundation (Osaka). D-Iso-
leucyl-prolyl-arginine-p-nitroanilide (D-Ile-Pro-Arg-pNA: S-2288)
and D-Val-Leu-Lys-pNA (S-2251) were obtained from Daiichi Pure
Chemical Co., Ltd. (Tokyo). Other synthetic substrates were
obtained as described previously (4). Sources of the chromatographic resins and inhibitors were as illustrated (4). All other
unspecified chemicals were of the best quality available
commercially.

      General enzyme assay, Kininogenase activity and Plasminogen
activator activity   Tos-Arg-OMe was used as the substrate to
monitor the activity during the purification procedures, and
the esterolytic activity was measured by colorimetry as described
(5). Amidolytic activity was assayed as illustrated (5). These
activities were expressed in terms of micromoles of substrate
hydrolyzed per minute. Kinin liberation by the purified enzyme
was assayed with purified kininogen, the generated kinins being
assayed with the Markit-A bradykinin (3). Plasminogen activator
activity was determined by a photometric assay using S-2251 as
a substrate (6).

      Electrophoresis   Unless otherwise stated, sodium dodecyl
sulfate (SDS)-polyacrylamide gel electrophoresis was performed
as described (3).

      Protein assay   Effluent from chromatographic column were
monitored at 280 nm. The protein concentration was determined,
by use of BCA protein assay reagents (3).

RESULTS

All operations for the purification were performed at 0-4 °C.
Step 1: Extraction   Human submaxillary glands tissues (100 g)
were chopped into small pierces, after being washed in cold
saline of the frozen-stored (-80 °C) raw-materials, and then
homogeneized with an Ultra-Turrax homogeneizer in 400 ml-10 mM
phosphate buffer, pH 8.0.   The post microsomal supernatant was
used for the enzyme purification.
Step 2: Chromatography on Benzamidine-Sepharose 6B   The soluble
fraction was loaded to a Benzamidine-Sepharose column (2.5 x
8 cm) preequilibrated with the above buffer.   The column was
washed with the buffer and then eluted with a 180 ml of 0.2 M
guanidine-HCl in the buffer.   And then, the column was further
eluted with a 120 ml of the buffer containing 1.0 M guanidine-
HCl (Fig. 1).   The eluted active preparations were separately
pooled, and tentatively named them as pool A (0.2 M guanidine-
HCl effluent) and as pool B (1.0 M of elution), and then the
A and B were dialyzed against 10 mM phosphate buffer, pH 8.0.
The pool A was identified as kallikrein fraction.

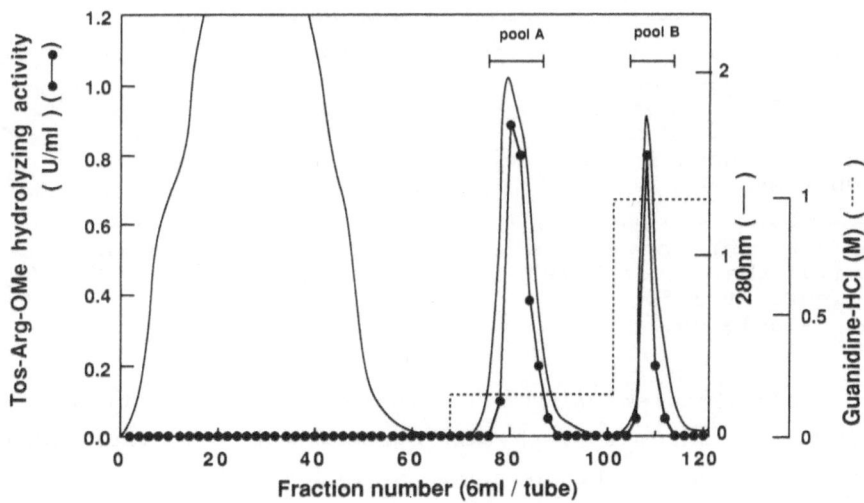

Figure 1.   Separation on benzamidine-sepharose 6B of
enzyme active on Tos-Arg-OMe.

Step 3: Chromatography on butyl-Toyopearl 650S   The solution
of pool B was adjusted to 40% saturation with ammonium sulfate
and then applied to a column of butyl-Toyopearl (1 x 5 cm) being
equilibrated with 40% ammonium sulfate-saturated 10 mM phosphate
buffer, pH 8.0.   After washing with the buffer, the proteins
were eluted with a 200 ml linear gradient of ammonium sulfate
from 40% - 0%.

Step 4: Chromatography on Sepharose 6   The pooled active fraction
was concentrated to 200 µl by means of a Centricut (Kurabo KK.,
Mr. 20,000).   The resulted solution was applied to a column of
Sepharose 6 (1 x 30 cm), which has been equilibrated by 10 mM
phosphate buffer, pH 8.0, containing 1 M NaCl.

The results of a typical purification of the enzyme from
soluble fraction of human submaxillary glands tissues are
summarized in Table 1.

Table 1. Summary of purification of the enzyme

Step	Protein (mg)	Tos-Arg-OMe		
		Total act. (U)	Spec. act. (mU/mg)	Yield (%)
1. Soluble fraction	2676	137	51.2	100
2. Benzamidine-Sepharose				
Pool A	218	39.9	183	29.1
Pool B	6.60	14.9	226	10.9
3. Butyl-Toyopearl	0.27	8.50	31500	6.20
4. Superose	<0.05	2.30	-*	1.67

Note: One unit of enzyme activity is defined as the amount of
activity that hydrolyzed 1 micromole substrate, Tos-Arg-OMe,
per minute at 37°C.
* Not calculated.

The molecular weight of the enzyme was estimated to be
120,000 from chromatography on Sepharose 6.   Polyacrylamide gel
electrophoresis in the presence of SDS was employed for further
estimate of the molecular weight of the enzyme.   The experiment
revealed the presence of two species with apparent molecular
weight of 30,000 and 32,000.

The relative activities of the enzyme obtained in this study, and of the purified kallikrein (3) are shown in Table 2. The enzyme readily hydrolyzes Tos-Arg-OMe, Ac-Lys-OMe and Tos-Lys-OMe. As the amidolytic substrate, D-Ile-Pro-Arg-pNA (S-2288) was hydrolyzed well, but the other substrates tested were very poorly degraded. The hydrolysis of S-2288 by the enzyme showed a sigmoid pH-velocity profile over the pH range 7.2 - 8.8, with maximum activity at pH 8.4. The purified enzyme had negligible activity of kinin-generation and that of plasminogen activator.

Among the microbial inhibitors examined (10 μg of each), antipain and leupeptin were found effective, while bestatin, chymostatin and elastatinal were no effect. Naturally occuring trypsin inhibitors such as aprotinin, soybean trypsin inhibitor and α_1-antitrypsin were found no inhibitory. The enzyme activity was depressed strongly by DFP (100 μM) and effectively by TLCK (100 μM), but not by EDTA (10 mM) and by PCMS (100 μM).

Table 2. Substrate specificity of the enzyme

Substrate	Relative Activity (%)	
	This enzyme	Kallikrein*
Esterolytic activity		
Tos-Arg-OMe	100	100
Bz-Arg-OMe	34.1	70.7
Ac-Arg-OMe	43.2	N.D.**
Tos-Lys-OMe	82.8	51.7
Ac-Lys-OMe	43.3	Nil
Ac-Phe-Arg-OMe	90.0	324
Amidolytic activity		
D-Ile-Pro-Arg-pNA	100	100
D-Val-Leu-Arg-pNA	15.9	505
D-Val-Leu-Lys-pNA	15.8	387
D-Pro-Phe-Arg-pNA	3.7	42.1

Note:The substrate concentrations of reaction mixtures were 25 mM for esterolytic activities and 1 mM for amidolytic activities.
* From reference 3.
** Not determined.

DISCUSSION

Our recent study has revealed that through the purification and characterization of an enzyme a major arginine esteropeptidase present in the soluble fraction of human submaxillary glands is kallikrein (3). However, as the result obtained in preliminary study suggested the presence of unknown arginine esteropeptidase(s) other than kallikrein, we focused our attention on this enzyme. The attempts to purify the unknown enzyme were difficult task, because this activity varies from batch to batch of stocked raw-materials. Table 1 is a record of the preparation made with a batch stocked weighing 100 g of glands tissues.

The best ester and amido substrates for the purified enzyme were Tos-Arg-OMe and D-Ile-Pro-Phe-Arg-pNA, respectively (Tab. 2). This enzyme had the substrate specificities similar to the latent arginine esteropeptidase newly purified from microsomal membranse of human submaxillary glands (4). However, the study of the effect of synthetic and natural inhibitors on the enzyme disclosed those properties different from that of membrane enzyme. The most effective inhibitor for the purified enzyme was DFP. Although the enzyme exhibited the serine protease-like characteristics, aprotinine and soybean trypsin inhibitor are incapable of diminishing the activity of enzyme. Furthermore, the molecular nature of the enzyme is quite different from that of the latent enzyme (4).

The submaxillary glands of murines are known to be the most abundant sources of arginine esteropeptidases. In the mouse at least seven different trypsin-like arginylesteropeptidase activities have been identified in its glands (2,7). Among them, γ-subunit of nerve growth factor (γ-NGF), β-NGF-endopeptidase (identical to submaxillary tissue kallikrein) and epidermal growth factor binding protein (EGF-BP) are members of the tissue kallikrein family (8). Meanwhile, it has been reported that the glands contain at least four enzyme proteins capable of hydrolyzing Tos-Arg-OMe (9). Later, Boesman et al. has illustrated that the alleged enzyme-D is identical to EGF-BP (10).

Furthermore, Schenkein et al. explained that enzyme-A became enzyme-D as a result of sponteneous cleavage (11). A number of proteases with remarkably high esterolytic activity have been recognized in the rat salivary gland, and Riekkinen et al. partially purified and characterized two of these enzymes, namely salivain and glandualin (12). Salivain was found to be a mixture of kallikrein and unidentified protease (13). Khuller et al. purified a new protease from the submaxillary glands of rat, which has been named esterase-B (not rat urinary B), and characterized as its plasminogen activator. Although it has a weak kininogenase activity, it is not to be identified as tissue kallikrein, glandualin, salivain nor tonin (14).

In this study, as the purified enzyme had neglible activity as far as kinin-generation and plasminogen activator are concerned, its function seemed to be different from that of kallikrein and/or plasminogen activator. It is possible that the new enzyme has a unique function of processing precursors as yet unknown. The kallikrein subfamily of serine proteases is implicated in the generation of a number of biologically active peptides while their precursors are being processed. Precise physiological role of the purified enzyme is now under study.

REFERENCES

1. MacDonald RJ, Margolius HS, Erdös EG. Molecular biology of tissue kallikrein. Biochem J 1988; 253:313-321.

2. Angermann A, Bergmann C, Appelhans H. Cloning and expression of human salivary-gland kallikrein in Escheria coli. Biochem J 1989; 262:787-793.

3. Fujimoto Y, Suzuki C, Watanabe Y, Matsuda Y, Akihama S. Purification and characterization of kallikrein from human submaxillary gland. Biochem Med Metab Biol 1990; 44:218-227.

4. Watanabe Y, Suzuki C, Fujimoto Y. A new latent arginine esteropeptidase from human submaxillary gland. Biochem Intl 1991; 23:669-677.

5. Matsuda Y, Fujimoto Y, Watanabe Y, Obara T, Akihama S. Human salivary kallikrein and submaxillary glands kallikrein. In: KININ V Part B. Abe K, Moriya H, Fujii S, editors. New York: Plenum Press, 1989: 169-175.

6. Overwien B, Neumann C, Sorg C. Detection of plasminogen activator in macrophage culture supernatants by a photometric assay. Hoppe-Seyler's Z Physiol Chem 1980; 361:1251-1255.

7. Schachter M. Kallikrein (Kininogenases)-A group of serine proteases with bioregulatory actions. Pharmacol Rev 1980; 31:1-17.

8. Bothwell MA, Wilson WH, Schooter M. The relationship between glandular kallikrein and growth factor processing proteases of mouse submaxillary gland. J Biol Chem 1979; 254:7287-7294.

9. Levy M, Fishmann L, Schenkein I. Mouse submaxillary gland proteases. In: Methods Enzymol. Perlmann GE, Lorand L. editors. New York: Academic Press, 1970: 672-681.

10. Boesman M, Levy H, Schenkein I. Esteroproteolytic enzymes from the submaxillary gland. Arch Biochem Biophys 1981; 175:463-476.

11. Schenkein I, Franklin EC, Fragione B. Proteolytic enzymes from the mouse submaxillary gland: A partial sequence and demonstration of sponteneous cleavages. Arch Biochem Biophys 1981; 209:57-62.

12. Riekkinen PJ, Ekfors TO, Hopsu VK. Purification and characteristics of an alkaline protease from rat-submandibular gland. Biochem Biophys Acta 1976; 118:604-620.

13. Brandtzaeg P, Gautvik KM, Nustad K, Pierce JV. Rat submandibular gland kallikreins: Purification and cellular localization. Br J Pharmacol 1976; 56:155-167.

14. Khullar M, Scicli, Carretero OA, Scicli AG. Purification and characterization of a serine protease (Esterase B) from rat submandibular glands. Biochemistry 1986; 25:1851-1857.

15. Mason AJ, Evans BA, Cox DR, Shine J, Richards I. Structure of mouse kallikrein gene family suggests a role in specific processing of biologically active peptides. Nature 1983; 303:300-307.

AAS 38/I
Recent Progress on Kinins
© 1992 Birkhäuser Verlag Basel

MOLECULAR DIVERSITY OF TISSUE KALLIKREIN IN HUMAN SALIVA

Joyce W. Jenzano, Hsieh-wing Su, Gerald L. Featherstone and Roger L. Lundblad[1]

Dental Research Center and the Departments of Dental Ecology and Periodontics, School of Dentistry and the Departments of Pathology and Biochemistry, School of Medicine, University of North Carolina at Chapel Hill, Chapel Hill, NC 27599-7455

SUMMARY: The present study was conducted to explore the extent of heterogeneity of tissue kallikrein in saliva using immunological analysis and to demonstrate that such heterogeneity resulted from secretory phenomena and not degradation secondary to secretion. Human mixed saliva was collected by paraffin-stimulation and centrifuged at 10,000 rpm for 10 minutes. Special collectors were used to obtain parotid and submandibular/sublingual saliva using citric acid stimulation. Western blot analysis of human mixed saliva demonstrated major immunoreactive species with molecular masses of <20 KD, 45 KD, 60 KD, 90 KD and >200 KD. The polyclonal antibody used for these blotting studies was monofunctional with respect to reaction with purified salivary tissue kallikrein. Only the <29 KD and 45 KD species were active using an enzyme overlay technique. While a similar distribution of molecular weight material was observed in both parotid and submandibular saliva, the amount of immunoreactive material was markedly less in parotid secretion. In addition, the <20 KD material was essentially absent in parotid saliva. Treatment of the saliva with thermolysin eliminated the immunoreactive band at 60 KD while treatment with various glycosidases also eliminated some heterogeneity. These results demonstrate considerable variation in tissue kallikrein expression in salivary gland secretions.

INTRODUCTION

Tissue kallikrein(TK) is a well-recognized component of human saliva(1-3). Most work suggests that the salivary protein is either identical or closely related to the tissue kallikrein found in urine and other biological fluids(4,5). As with most regulatory tryptic-like proteases, tissue kallikrein is synthesized as a preprotein which is processed to the proprotein which in turn is activated

---

[1] Present Address: Baxter Healthcare-Hyland Division, 1710 Flower Avenue, Duarte, CA 91010

to active enzyme by limited proteolysis. Our laboratory has demonstrated the
presence of a tissue prokallikrein in human mixed saliva(6) indicating the
possibility of at least two immunoreactive forms of TK in saliva, mature TK and
tissue prokallikrein. Our demonstration of the presence of tissue prokallikrein
in human saliva is contrary to general opinion(c.f. reference 7) which states
that prokallikrein is not found in either saliva or salivary glands.

The present study was initiated to obtain more information regarding the
various molecular forms of tissue kallikrein found in human saliva. The results
clearly demonstrate the presence of at least two prokallikrein fractions and a
number of other immunologically reactive forms of tissue kallikrein.

METHODS AND MATERIALS

The peptide nitroanilide substrate, H-$\underline{D}$-Val-Leu-Arg-$\underline{p}$-nitroanilide(S-2266)
was a product of Kabi Laboratories obtained from Helena Laboratories, Beaumont,
Texas. A 1 mM stock solution in deionized water was prepared from a 25 mg bottle
and stored in 1 mL portions at -20°C. The assay for tissue kallikrein was
performed essentially as previously described(6,8) in the presence of soybean
trypsin inhibitor. Enzyme overlay membranes for TK were obtained from Enzyme
System Products, Dublin, CA, and used in accordance with the manufacturer's
instructions and published reports in the literature(9,10). The substrate in the
enzyme overlay membranes is $\underline{D}$-Val-Leu-Arg-4-trifluoromethyl-coumarin-7-amide.
Hydrolysis of substrate was determined by the appearance of a fluorescent band.
Specificity of reaction was obtained by comparing the hydrolysis in the presence
and absence of soybean trypsin inhibitor(inhibits non-TK proteases in saliva) and
aprotinin(a relatively specific inhibitor of TK under our reaction conditions.
Human mixed saliva, parotid saliva and submandibular saliva was collected as
previously described(6,8,11).

Tissue kallikrein was purified from human mixed saliva by chromatography
on DEAE-Cellulose(DE-52, Whatman) as described by Ole-Moiyoi et al(12) for the
urinary enzyme followed by affinity chromatography on aprotinin-agarose(Sigma
Chemical Company, St. Louis, MO)(13). The resulting protein was homogeneous on
polyacrylamide gel electrophoresis in the presence of sodium dodecyl sulfate(14).
This protein was used to immunize four rabbits for the preparation of polyclonal

antibodies.   Antibodies were purified by chromatography on protein G columns(Genex) prior to use. Western blot analysis was performed essentially as described by Towbin et al(15) using equipment and reagents obtained from BioRad Laboratories, Richmond, CA. The reaction product between rabbit anti-human TK and salivary proteins was detected by the use of goat anti-rabbit IgG labeled with alkaline phosphatase. Detection was accomplished by the use of 5-bromo-4-chloro-3-indoyl phosphate coupled with nitro blue tetrazolium.

RESULTS AND DISCUSSION

Our first experiments were designed to explore the possible existence of multiple forms of TK in human saliva using Western Blot analysis(15). This is a powerful technique which allows for the identification of immunological identical materials(16). Figure 1 shows the Western Blot analysis of parotid saliva, submandibular saliva and mixed saliva. It is observed that there is a distribution of immunoreactive material ranging from greater than 200 KD to less than 20 KD. Control experiments(data not shown) with normal rabbit IgG showed the absence of reactivity in this system. Evaluation with enzyme overlay analysis(data not shown) demonstrated two major areas of activity. There was substantial activity (inhibited by aprotinin but not by soybean trypsin inhibitor) at approximately 20 KD and 40 KD but not at the higher molecular weight regions. The diffusion of fluorescent product prevents a more exact assignment of mass. The pattern of inhibition with aprotinin and soybean trypsin inhibitor is consistent with that expected for human TK(7). The molecular mass characteristics observed are consistent with those observed by other investigators for human TK(7).

In an attempt to identify one of the immunoreactive fractions as prokallikrein, human mixed saliva was treated with a variety of proteolytic enzymes. As shown in Figure 2, the disappearance of both the 60 KD, the 80-90 KD, and the approximate 150 KD materials was observed upon treatment with thermolysin. Thermolysin has been shown to be an effective activator of human prokallikrein(17). Neither trypsin nor chymotrypsin had an effect on the distribution of the immunoreactive materials. The disappearance of these bands was not associated with the appearance of immunoreactive material in the 40-45

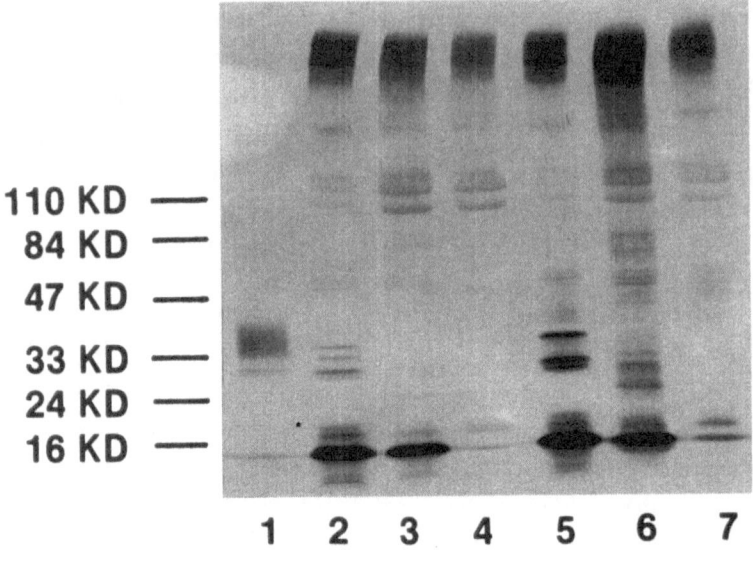

Figure 1. Western Blot Analysis of Human Mixed and Glandular Saliva for Tissue Kallikrein. Lane 1 contains purified salivary tissue kallikrein. Lanes 2, 3 and 4 and 5, 6 and 7 contain submandibular, mixed and parotid saliva, respectively, from two different individuals.

KD region but there was an increase in immunoreactive material migrating in the 16 KD region. In data not shown, treatment of any of the saliva samples with thermolysin was associated with an increase in catalytic activity toward the peptide nitroanilide substrate. These observations confirm our earlier demonstration of the presence of prokallikrein in human saliva(6) which is contrary to previous studies(7).

The above experiments allow the identification of two of the immunoreactive components as active tissue kallikreins and two as prokallikreins. There are, however, a number of other immunoreactive species detected by Western blot analysis as shown in Figures 1 and 2. Various possibilities for these forms include a complex with alpha-1-antiprotease inhibitor(18), a complex with a recently described serpin interacting with tissue kallikrein(19,20) or complexes with immunoglobulin(s)(21), In order to further characterize these species, the stability of the immunoreactive bands to reduction in sodium dodecyl sulfate(with

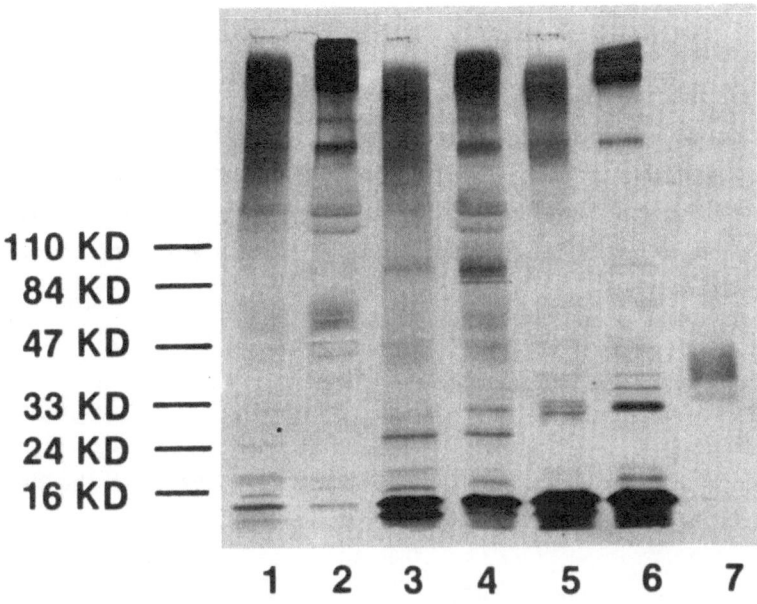

Figure 2.   Effect of Thermolysin Treatment on the Distribution of Tissue Kallikrein Antigen in Human Saliva. Lanes 1, 3 and 5 contain submandibular, mixed and parotid saliva, respectively, all treated with thermolysin(10 ug/mL., 30 min, 37° C). Lanes 2, 4 and 6 are untreated matching control samples. Lane 7 is purified salivary kallikrein. Tissue kallikrein was detected by Western Blot analysis as described under Figure 1.

boiling) prior to electrophoresis was investigated. Only bands at approximately 60 KD, 35 KD and 16 KD materials were completely stable. A portion of the high molecular weight material remained possibly reflecting the presence of a membrane-bound precursor. This data does not support the presence of tissue-serpin complexes but rather suggests the presence of noncovalent complexes

While tissue sources are likely the major source of tissue kallikrein in saliva(7), there is evidence that tissue kallikrein can be in a membrane-bound form on epithelial cells(22) and epithelial cells are found in saliva(23). While there is no data directly comparing the structure of membrane-bound TK to solution TK, data has been presented which suggest that there may be functional differences between the membrane bound-TK and solution TK(24,25). Thus, membrane-bound forms of TK can possibly contribute to the heterogeneity of immunologically reactive TK in saliva.

CONCLUSION

The present data demonstrates significant protein heterogeneity of tissue kallikreins in human saliva. This heterogeneity appears to relate more to protein secretion patterns rather than degradation occurring after secretion. More information regarding the molecular heterogeneity of this protein is required before changes in salivary levels can be used as a satisfactory index of systemic or oral disease.

ACKNOWLEDGEMENTS

This research was supported in part by grant DE-06997 from the National Institutes of Health.

REFERENCES

1. Werle, E., and P. von Roden. Uber das Vorkommen von Kallikrein in den Speicheldrusen und im Mundspeichel und uber eine bludrucksteigernde Substanz in der Submaxillarisdruse des Hundes. Biochem Zeitschrift 1939; 301:328.

2. Sakmoto, W., and O. Nishikaze. Alpha-1-antitrypsin and alpha-2-macroglobulin do not inhibit the kinin-releasing activity of kallikreins from human urine and saliva. Biochim Biophys Acta 1980; 633:305.

3. Sakamoto, W., K. Yoshikawa, S. Uehara, and O. Nishizaze. 1983. Characterization of human salivary kallikrein: Reactivities to human plasma kininogens and proteinase inhibitors. J Biochem 1983;93:833.

4. Geiger, R., W. Hofmann, M. Franke, and X. Baur. Biochemistry of Human tissue kallikrein. Adv Exptl Med Biol 1983; 156A:275.

5. Kellermann, J., F. Lottspeich, R. Geiger, and R. Deutzmann. Human urinary kallikrein: Amino acid sequence and carbohydrate attachment sites. Adv Exptl Med Biol 1990; 247A:519.

6. Jenzano, J.W., Coffey, J.C., Heizer, W.D., Lundblad, R.L., and Scicli, A.G. The Assay of tissue kallikrein and prekallikrein in human mixed saliva. Archs Oral Biol 1988: 33:641.

7. Geiger, R. and Fritz, H. Human urinary kallikrein. Methods in Enzymology 1981; 80:466-492.

8. Jenzano, J.W., Daniel, P.W., Kent, R.T., Leal, J.L., and Koth, D.L. Evaluation of kallikrein in human parotid and submandibular saliva. Archs Oral Biol 1986;31:627.

9. Garret,J.R., Smith, R.E., Kidd,A., Kyriacou, K. and Grabske, R.J. Kallikrein-like activity in salivary glands using a new tripeptide substrate, including preliminary secretory studies and observations on mast cells. Histochem J 1982; 14:967.

10. Garrett,J.R., Kidd,A., Kyriacou,K., and Smith,R.E., 1985. Use of different derivatives of D-Val-Leu-Arg for studying kallikrein activities in cat submandibular glands and saliva. Histochem J 1985; 17:805.

11. Jenzano, J.W., N.F. Courts, D.A. Timko, and R.L. Lundblad. 1986. Levels of tissue kallikrein in whole saliva obtained from patients with solid tumors remote from the oral cavity. J Dent Res 1986; 65:67.

12. Ole-MoiYoi, O., Austen, K.F., and Spragg, J. Kinin-generating and esterolytic activity of human urinary kallikrein (urokallikrein). Biochem Pharmacol 1977; 26:1893.

13. Ole-Moiyoi, O., Spragg, J., and Austen, K.F. Inhibition of human urinary kallikrein(urokallikrein) by anti-enzyme FAB. J Immunol 1978; 121:66-71.

14. Laemmli, U.K. Cleavage of structural proteins during the assembly of the head of bacteriophage T4. Nature 1970; 227:680.

15. Towbin, H., Staehelin, T., and Gordon, J. Electrophoretic transfer of protein from polyacrylamide gels to nitrocellulose. Procedure and some applications. Proc Nat Acad Sci USA 1979; 76:4350.

16. Wakefield, L.M., Smith, D.M., Flanders, K.C. and Sporn, M.B. Latent transforming growth factor-beta from human platelets. A high molecular weight complex containing precursor sequences. J Biol Chem 1988; 263:7646.

17. Takada, Y., Skidgel, R.A. and Erdos, E.G. Purification of human urinary prokallikrein. Identification of the site of activation by the metalloproteinase thermolysin. Biochem J 1985; 232:851.

18. Geiger, R., Stuckstedle, U., Clausnitzer, B., and Fritz, H. Progressive inhibition of human tissue(urinary) kallikrein by human serum and identification of the progressive antikallikrein as alpha-1-antitrypsin(alpha-1-antiprotease inhibitor). H -S Z Physiol Chem B 1981; 362:5317.

19. Chao,J., Tillman,D.M., Wang, M., Margolius, H.S., and Chao, L. Identification of a new tissue kallikrein-binding protein. Biochem J 1986; 239:325.

20. Chao,J., Chai,K.X., Chen,L.-M., Xiong, W., Chao, S., Woodley-Miller, C., Wang, L., Lu, H.S. and Chao, L. Tissue kallikrein-binding protein is a serpin. I. Purification, characterization, and distribution in normotensive and spontaneously hypertensive rats. J Biol Chem 1990; 265:16394.

21.Chao, L., Mayfield, R.K. and Chao, J., 1988. Circulating
   autoantibodies to mammalian tissue kallikrein. Proc Soc Exptl Biol Med 1988;
   187:320.

22.Baird, A., Miller, D.H., Schwartz, D.A. and Margolius, H.
   Enhancement of kallikrein production and kinin sensitivity in T84 cells by
   growth in the nude mouse. Amer J. Physiol 1991; 261:C822.

23.Sindt-Pedersen, Gram, J., and Jespersen, J., The possible role
   or oral epithelial cells in tissue-type plasminogen activator-related
   fibrinolysis in human saliva. J Dent Res 1980; 69:1283.

24.Chao, J., Tanaka, S. and Margolius, H.S. Inhibitory Effects of
   Sodium and Other Monovalent Cations on Purified versus Membrane-bound
   Kallikrein. J Biol Chem 1983; 258:6461.

25.Lieberthal, W., Oza, N.B., Bernard, D.B., and Levinsky, N.G.,
   1982, The Effects of Cations on the Activity of Human Urinary Kallikrein. J
   Biol Chem 1982; 257:10827.

AAS 38/I
Recent Progress on Kinins
© 1992 Birkhäuser Verlag Basel

DETECTION AND SEPARATION OF SOME ARGININE AMIDASES INCLUDING TISSUE KALLIKREIN FROM HUMAN SEMINAL PLASMA

Y. Matsuda[a], S. Kaneko[b], K. Miyazaki[c], T. Kobayashi[b],
Y. Fujimoto[d] and S. Akihama[a]

Department of Biochemistry, Meiji College of Pharmacy (a), Nozawa, Setagaya-ku, Tokyo. Department of Obstetrics and Gynecology, School of Medicine, Keio University (b), Shinanomachi, Shinjuku-ku, Tokyo. Department of Biochemical Sciences, Tokyo Institute of Seikagaku Kogyo Co. (c), Higashiyamato-shi, Tokyo and Department of Clinical Biochemistry, Hokkaido Institute of pharmaceutical Sciences (d), Otaru-shi, Hokkaido, Japan.

Summary: A plasminogen/plasmin like substance (AHSAA-1), with affinity to lysine column was separated from DEAE-cellulose adsorbed human seminal plasma. Two forms of acidic arginine amidase with different affinities to LBTI (AHSAA-2) and aprotinin columns (AHSAA-3) were separated from the DEAE-cellulose adsorbed preparation and AHSAA-3 was identified as tissue kallikrein. Two basic arginine amidase preparations having affinity to LBTI (BHSAA-1) and aprotinin column were also separated from the CM-cellulose adsorbed human seminal plasma. Three basic arginine amidases with different molecular mass (BHSAA-2 to 4) were separated by Cellulofine GCL-2000 gel filtration from aprotinin adsorbed material and some of their properties were examined.

INTRODUCTION

Tissue kallikrein (E.C. 3.4.21.35) is a serine proteinase which releases kinin through the cleaving of kininogen as substrate. It in seminal plasma was first purified by Geiger et al. (1) using immunoaffinity chromatography in human and other esterases (amidases) in seminal plasma, such as seminin (2) and arginine amidase in dog (3) have also been detected. Recently, we identified and separated three arginine amidases with different molecular mass from human seminal plasma using Cellulofine GCL-2000 gel filtration (4). We purified and characterized a basic arginine amidase from human seminal plasma (5) and the properties of this enzyme differed from those of tissue kallikrein and human acrosin (E.C. 3.4.21.10).

In this paper we report the separation of some acidic and basic arginine amidases including tissue kallikrein, from human seminal plasma.

MATERIALS AND METHODS

Human Seminal Plasma.   Human semen was collected by masturbation after four days of sexual abstinence.   A seminal plasma preparation was separated from mixed human semen by the percoll density gradient method (6).   This preparation was removed to the centrifugation to eliminate cell debris, bacterias and other insoluble materials and the supernatant was stored at -40°C until use.

Materials.   All chemicals, proteins and chromatographic materials used were of analytical grade.

Enzyme Assay and Protein Determination.   Amidolytic activity was measured by the method of Amundsen et al. (7) with a slight modification at pH 8.5 for 37°C with substrate concentration of 0.5 mM and the amidolytic activity was expressed as n mol of substrate hydrolyzed per min (n mol/min) under the above conditions.   Enzyme activity was monitored by amidolysis of Val-Leu-Arg-pNA during the separation of arginine amidases from human seminal plasma.   Human kallikrein was determined by the enzymeimmunoassay of Moriya's group (8) using anti-human urinary kallikrein (HUK).

The protein concentration was estimated spectrophotometrically assuming that the absorbance of 1 mg per ml of protein in a1 cm width cuvette at 280 nm was 1.0.

RESULTS

Enzyme Separation.   The separation procedure of acidic and basic arginine amidases from human seminal plasma was summarized in Fig. 1, and the detailed procedures for separating acidic (A) and basic (B) enzymes from human seminal plasma are shown below.

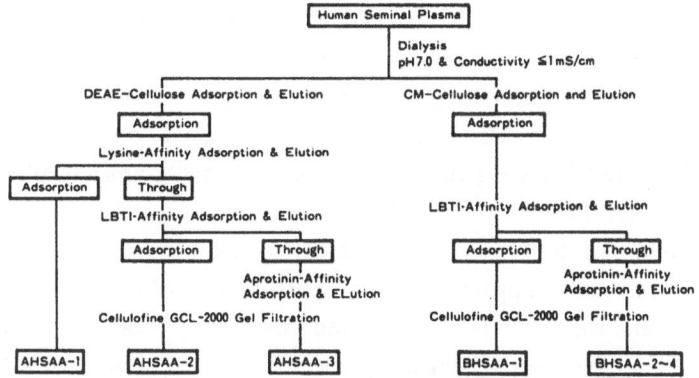

Fig. 1. Scheme of separation procedure for acidic and basic arginine amidases from human seminal plasma

A) Separation of Acidic Arginine Amidases. Human seminal plasma was dialyzed against deionized water and 0.02 M Tris-HCl buffer at pH 7.5, then diluted by deionized water with a conductivity of 2.0 mS/cm or less. The dialyzed solution was adjusted to pH 7.5, DEAE-cellulose was added then the mixture was stirred for 2 hr. DEAE-cellulose was then parked in a column and washed with the above mentioned buffer. Acidic arginine amidases were eluted with same buffer containing 0.6 M NaCl and the eluates were adjusted to pH 8.5. This preparation was applied to a lysine Cellulofine column which was then washed with 0.05 M Tris-HCl buffer at pH 8.5 (Buffer A). A small amount of protein with affinity to a lysine column (Plasminogen/plasmin (EC 3.4.21.7) -like enzyme, tentatively called acidic human seminal plasma arginine amidase-1 : AHSAA-1) was detected in this eluates.

The through and wash solutions from the above were applied to a lima bean trypsin inhibitor (LBTI) column and weak arginine amidase activity with affinity to a LBTI column was detected. An arginine amidase activity having affinity to an aprotinin column was also found in the wash and through solutions from the LBTI affinity column.

These two enzymes were separately applied to a Cellulofine GCL-2000 gel filtration column and the enzyme activities detected were tentatively called AHSAA-2 (from LBTI column) and AHSAA-3 (from aprotinin column).

Fig. 2 shows the elution profiles of the acidic arginine amidases as described above.

B) Separation of Basic Arginine Amidases.   CM-cellulose adsorbed human seminal plasma at pH 8.5 was applied to a LBTI column and the column was washed with buffer A.   The fractions eluted with 0.01 N HCl which contained arginine amidase activity were applied to gel filtration on Cellulofine GCL-2000.   An arginine amidase activity with an approximate molecular mass of 3.8 x 10⁴ daltons was detected and this enzyme was homogeneous on SDS-PAGE (5)(called basic human seminal plasma arginine amidase-1 : BHSAA-1).

The wash and through solution containing arginine amidase activity from the LBTI column was applied to an aprotinin column and an adsorbed enzyme was detected.   The adsorbed enzyme was also applied to a Cellulofine GCL-2000 gel filtration column as described above, and three arginine amidase activities with different molecular masses were separated.   They were tentatively called BHSAA-2 to BHSAA-4 from high to low molecular masses.

The elution profiles of basic arginine amidases from human seminal plasma by LBTI and aprotinin affinity adsorption and gel filtrations are shown in Fig. 3.

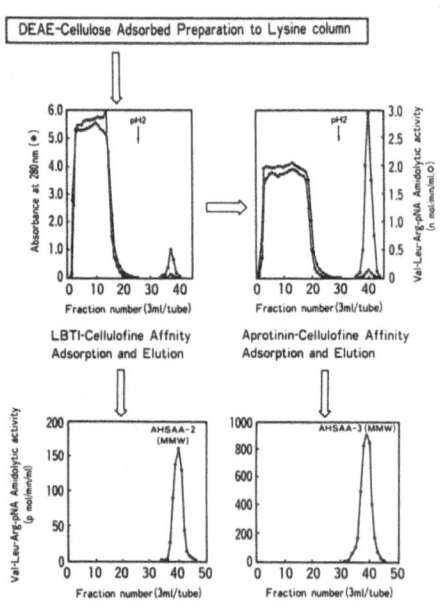

Fig. 2.   Cellulofine GCL-2000 Gel Filtration of LBTI- and Aprotinin-Affinity Adsorbed Acidic Arginine Amidases in Human Seminal Plasma

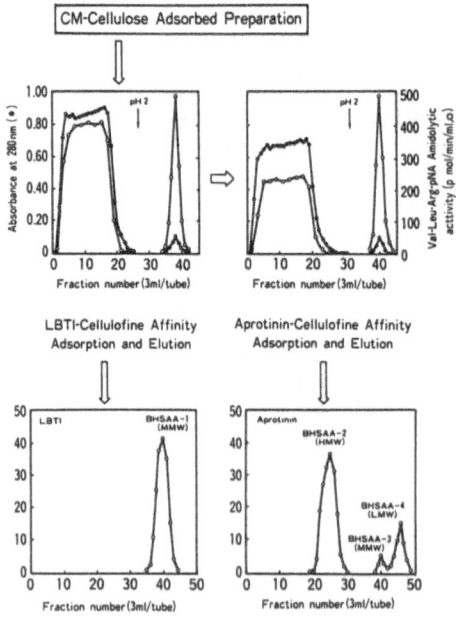

Fig. 3.   Cellulofine GCL-2000 Gel Filtration of LBTI-and Aprotinin-Affinity Absorbed Basic Arginine Amidases in Human Seminal Plasma

Specific Activity. The acidic enzymes, AHSAA-2 and -3 had 2.7 and 38.4 n mol/min/A_{280} of Val-Leu-Arg-pNA amidolytic activity, respectively. Kinin-releasing activity was found qualitatively in AHSAA-3, but the other two acidic enzymes had no activity. AHSAA-3 contained 45 ng kallikrein protein/ml as determined by enzymeimmunoassay using anti-HUK. The others showed no response to anti-HUK. As for the basic arginine amidases, the specific Val-Leu-Arg-pNA amidolytic activity of BHSAA-1, -2, -3 and -4 were 5.2, 9.2, 1.9 and 11.4 n mol/min/A_{280}, respectively, and they had no affinity for human kallikrein as determined by the enzyme-immunoassay.

Substrate Specificity. The amidolytic substrate specificity of the main arginine amidases in human seminal plasma; AHSAA-3, BHSAA-1, -2 and -4 were summarized in Table I, and the activity is shown as the ratio of activity relative to that against standard Val-CHA-Arg-pNA as the substrate for tissue kallikrein. The best substrate for AHSAA-3 (tissue kallikrein) was Val-CHA-Arg-pNA in the tested, whereas Tos-Gly-Pro-Arg-pNA and Bz-Leu-Pro-Arg-pNA were the best substrate for BHSAA-1, -2 and -4, respectively. The Val-CHA-Arg-pNA were further good substrate for basic arginine amidases from human seminal plasma. The profiles of substrate specificity differed among the four arginine amidases of human seminal plasma.

Table I. Substrate Specificity of Acidic and Basic Arginine Amidases in Human Seminal Plasma

Substrate	Enzyme			
	Acidic	Basic		
	AHSAA-3	BHSAA-1	BHSAA-2	BHSAA-4
Val-CHA-Arg-pNA	1	1	1	1
Val-Leu-Lys-pNA	0.03	0.40	0.02	0.12
Tos-Gly-Pro-Arg-pNA	0.22	3.8	1.5	0.79
Bz-Phe-Val-Arg-pNA	0.08	1.4	0.36	0.08
Boc-Leu-Pro-Arg-pNA	0.16	3.2	2.0	0.74
Suc-(Ala)$_2$-Pro-Leu-pNA	—	0.61	1.3	0.49

Retio of activity was given relative to standard Val-CHA-Arg-pNA

Inhibitor Action .   The effects of some proteinase inhibitors towards Val-Leu-Arg-pNa amidolytic activity of AHSAA-3, BHSAA-1 and -2 were tested and the results are summarized in Table II.   All basic arginine amidases were strongly inhibited by Leupeptin and Antipain, but AHSAA-2 was not affected.   BHSAA-1 was inhibited by LBTI and α_1-antitrypsin and weakly effects were observed by EGTA and t-ACA.   The effect of calcium chloride on the enzyme activity of AHSAA-2, AHSAA-3, BHSAA-1 and -2 are shown in Fig. 4.   The activity of all enzymes were not increased by addition of calcium chloride.

Table II.

Effect of Some Inhibitors on Val-Leu-Arg-pNA Amidolytic Activity of Human Seminal Plasma Arginine Amidases

Inhibitor		Acidic enzyme	Basic enzymes	
		AHSAA-3	BHSAA-1	BHSAA-2
			(% of Inhibition)	
Leupeptin	30μM	30	96	100
Antipain	30μM	28	92	100
EGTA	30μM	15	20	60
t-ACA	30μM	16	—	28
LBTI	15μg	10	92	30
α_1-AT	15μg	—	76	26

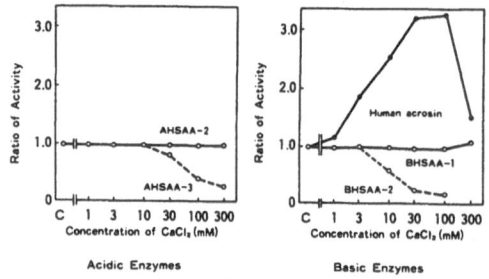

Fig. 4. Effect of Calcium Chloride on Val-Leu-Arg-pNA Amidolytic Activity of Human Seminal Plasma Arginine Amidases

DISCUSSION

Three acidic arginine amidases, including plasminogen (or plasmin) like substance (AHSAA-1) and tissue kallikrein (AHSAA-3), with different affinities to Lysine, LBTI and aprotinin affinity columns, were detected in DEAE-cellulose adsorbed human seminal plasma (Fig. 1,2), as well as four basic arginine amidases with different affinities to LBTI and aprotinin columns from basic arginine amidase preparation were also detected in this investigation (Fig. 3).

Our recent report (4) has shown that three arginine amidases preparations with different molecular masses, which were tentatively named high, middle and low molecular weight (HMW-, MMW- and LMW-) types were separated from human seminal plasma.   All those of them contained trypsin-like basic arginine amidase with affinity to LBTI column.

Furthermore, we have purified and characterized a basic arginine amidase which was classified as MMW-type (5). We consider that the BHSAA-1 in this report is the same enzyme as that report to above (5) because the properties of substrate specificity, behavior in the presence of inhibitors including calcium chloride and the molecular mass are in good agreement. This enzyme seemed to be the origin of basic arginine esterases (amidases) in human male urine, similar to Esterase A-1 in rat male urine (9,10). Some properties, including behavior in respense to calcium chloride (Fig. 5), of all the basic arginine amidases separated in this study, are clearly different from human acrosin (11) which is trypsin-like basic arginine amidase from sperm with affinity to LBTI column.

In this investigation we also detected the three acidic arginine amidases, only one of which had affinity to aprotinin column, AHSAA-3 therefore, is tissue kallikrein. The enzyme having affinity to lysine column was thought to be plasminogen and/or plasmin in seminal plasma (Fig. 2). Tissue plasminogen activator has also been detected from seminal plasma (12,13). These results suggest that the blood coagulation and thrombosis systems exist in the seminal plasma. Two acidic arginine amidase with affinity to LBTI or aprotinin column have also been detected in boar sperm (14) and the substrate specificity as well as behavior in the presence of calcium chloride of those enzymes seemed to be of a different quality from the two acidic enzymes having affinity to LBTI or aprotinin column described here. This result indicates that the arginine amidase in sperm with affinity to aprotinin column is not tissue kallikren.

The functional role of these acidic and basic arginine amidases including tissue kallikrein and plasminogen remain unknown. The enzymatic properties and functions of these acidic and basic enzymes in human seminal plasma are well make further study, which we plan to undertake when sufficient amount of human seminal plasma is available.

We dedicated this paper to the late Professor Dr. Hiroshi Moriya.

REFERENCES

1.   Geiger R. Clausnitzer B.   Isolation an enzumatically active tissue kallikrein from human seminal plasma by immunoaffinity chromatography.   Hoppe Seyler's Z Physiol Chem 1981; 362: 1279.

2.   Syner FN.   Moghissi K.   Purification and properties of a human seminal proteinase. Biochem J 1972; 126:1135.

3.   Frenette G.   Dube JY.   Tremblay RR.   Enzymatic characterization of arginine esterase from dog seminal plasma.   Biochim Biophys Acta 1985; 838: 270.

4.   Kobayashi T. Matsuda Y. Park J-Y. Kaneko S. Oshio S. Nozawa S. Fujimoto Y. Akihama S.   Amidase activity : Arginine amidase in human seminal plasma.   Mol Androl 1991; 3:307.

5.   Kobayashi T. Park J-Y. Matsuda Y. Hara I. Kaneko S. Oshio S. Akihama S. Fujimoto Y.   Basic arginine amidase from human seminal plasma : Purification and some properties.   Arch Androl 1991; 27: 196.

6.   Kaneko S. Oshio S. Kobanawa K. Kobayashi T. Mohri H. Iizuka R.   Purification of human sperm by a discontinuous Percoll density gradient with an inner column.   Biol Reprod 1986; 35: 1059.

7.   Amundsen E. Putter J. Firberger P. Knos M. Larsbraten M. Claseson G.   In : Method for the determination of glandular kallikrein by means of chromogenic substrate. Fujii S. Moriya H. Suzuki T. editors.   New York: Plenum Press, 1979: 83-90.

8.   Suzuki S. Inaba T. Ikekita M. Kizuki K. Moriya H.   Tissue kallikrein in human plasma. Jpn. J. Clin. Chem. 1987; 16: 194.

9.   McPartland RP. Sustarsic DL. Rapp JP.   Evidence for an androgen dependent urinary arginine esterase in the rat : Separation from other urinary arginine esterases including kallikrein.   Endocrinol. 1981 ; 108: 1634.

10.   Nakamura M. Takaoka M. Nishii N. Morimoto S.   Purification and characterization of rat urinary esterase A-1.   Biochim. Biophys. Acta 1986; 884: 311.

11.   Kobayashi T. Matsuda Y. Oshio S. Kaneko S. Mohri S. Akihama S. Fujimoto Y. Human acrosin : Purification and some properties.   Arch Androl. 1991; 27: 9.

12.   Van Dreden P. Gonzales J. Richard P.   Determination of tissue plasminogen activator antigen in seminal plasma by modified enzyme-linked immunosorbant assay. Andrologia 1988; 20: 48.

13.   Maier U. Kirchheimer JC. Hienert G. Christ G. Binder BR.   Fibrinolytic parameters in spermatozoas and seminal plasma.   J. Urol. 1991; 146: 906.

14.   Kobayashi T. Hara I. Matsuda Y. Park J-Y. Oshio S. Kaneko S. Umeda T. Akihama S. Detection and separation of two kinds of acidic arginine amidases from boar sperm using lima bean trypsin inhibitor and aprotinin affinity adsorptions.   Arch Androl. 1992; in press.

AAS 38/I
Recent Progress on Kinins
© 1992 Birkhäuser Verlag Basel

IMMUNOASSAYS FOR THE DETERMINATION OF HUMAN TISSUE KALLIKREIN (TK) IN DIFFERENT BODY FLUIDS BASED ON MONOCLONAL ANTIBODIES

K. Witzgall, G. Godec, K. Shimamoto* and E. Fink

Department of Clinical Chemistry and Clinical Biochemistry,
University of Munich, Nussbaumstr. 20, D-8000 Munich 2, Germany
and *2nd Department of Internal Medicine, Sapporo Medical
College S-1 W-16 Chuo-ku, Sapporo 060, Japan

SUMMARY: A monoclonal antibody produced against human tissue kallikrein was used to develop solid phase immunoassays for the determination of total immunoreactive tissue kallikrein, of the complex of tissue kallikrein with α_1-proteinase inhibitor, and of enzymatically active tissue kallikrein. The assays permit the specific determination of various forms of tissue kallikrein in body fluids and should be very useful in studies on the biological function of tissue kallikrein-kinin systems.

INTRODUCTION

The determination of tissue kallikrein (TK) in body fluids and tissues can be achieved by a number of methods, e. g. radioimmunoassays, enzyme immunoassays, determination of kinin-releasing activity, or hydrolysis of synthetic substrates. Due to the fact that TK is present in the organism in different forms, such as enzymatically inactive proenzyme, active TK or complexes with inhibitors, no single assay technique alone can accomplish the specific quantification of each of the TK species.

Here we present assays which are based on a monoclonal antibody for capturing the TK antigen and various detection systems permitting the specific determination of different forms of TK.

MATERIALS AND METHODS

Materials

Human urinary kallikrein (HUK) isolated according to (1) and rabbit polyclonal antibodies to HUK were gifts of Dr. R. Geiger (Me-

dor, Herrsching, Germany). Polyclonal antibodies to human α_1-pro-
teinase inhibitor (α_1PI): Calbiochem, Frankfurt, Germany; alkaline phosphatase labeled anti-rabbit IgG: BioRad, Munich, Germany; substrate for kallikrein: H-D-ValLeuArg-p-nitroanilide (S-
2266): KABI, Freiburg, Germany. Microplate reader MR 700: Dynatech, Denkendorf, Germany.

Buffers. A: 0.015 M sodium carbonate, 0.035 M sodium bicar-
bonate, pH 9.6;
B: 0.01 M monosodium phosphate, 0.15 M sodium chloride, pH 7.4;
C: 25 g/l casein in buffer B;
D: 20 g/l bovine serum albumin, 0.5 ml/l Tween 20 in buffer A;
E: 0.01 M monosodium phosphate, 0.14 M sodium chloride, 0.03 M
EDTA, 3 mM o-phenanthroline, pH 7.4;
F: 0.01 M monosodium phosphate, 0.14 sodium chloride, 0.03 M
EDTA, 3 mM o-phenanthroline, 0.5 g sodium azide/l, 0.2 g thimero-
sal/l, 0.4 ml Tween 20/l, pH 7.4;
G: 1.0 M diethanolamine/HCl, 100 mg/l $MgCl_2*6$ H_2O, pH 9.6.

Standards. The protein concentration of a stock solution of
highly purified human urinary kallikrein was determined by amino
acid analysis. Standard solutions of TK were prepared by diluting
the stock solution appropriately. A stock solution of TK-α_1PI was
prepared by incubating an aliquot of the TK stock solution with
an excess of α_1PI for 24 h at room temperature.

Murine monoclonal antibodies against human tissue kallikrein
were developed using human urinary kallikrein (1) as antigen by
employing conventional hybridoma techniques. Antibodies of six
different clones were produced, isolated and characterized, one
of them was used for the immunoassays.

Coating of solid phase with monoclonal antibody. The wells
of microtiter plates (Immunolon F, Dynatech, Denkendorf, Germany)
were coated with monoclonal antibody by incubation (16 h, 4 °C)
with 0.2 ml of a solution containing 3 μg/ml monoclonal antibody
in buffer A. After washing the plate six times with 30 ml buffer
B the remaining protein-binding sites in each well were blocked
by incubation with buffer C for 1 h. After removing the buffer
the plate was ready for use.

Capturing of immunoreactive TK. 0.2 ml of TK standard solutions or unknown samples containing TK and/or TK-α_1PI, diluted in

buffer D, were pipetted into the wells, then the microtiter plate was incubated for 2 h at 37 °C and washed.

Determination of captured antigen by second antibody. For the determination of total immunoreactive TK 0.2 ml of a solution of a rabbit anti-TK antibody, 1 μg/ml in buffer D, was added, the plate was incubated for 2 h at 37 °C and washed. Then 0.2 ml of alkaline phosphatase labeled anti-rabbit IgG (diluted 1:3000 in buffer D) was pipetted into each well. After washing 0.2 ml 4-nitrophenylphosphate, 1-2 g/l in buffer G was added and after 10-30 min incubation at 37 °C the absorbance at 405 nm was read. The complex of TK with α_1-proteinase inhibitor (TK-α_1PI) captured by the monoclonal antibody was determined by the same technique but using as second antibody a rabbit antiserum to α_1PI diluted 1:3000 with buffer D.

Determination of captured enzymatically active tissue kallikrein with a synthetic substrate. After the capturing step 0.2 ml of freshly prepared substrate solution, 0.4 mM H-D-Val-Leu-Arg-p-nitroanilide in 0.01 M Tris, pH 8.2 were pipetted into each well. After 24 h incubation at 37 °C absorbance at 405 nm was read using the microplate reader.

Determination of captured enzymatically active tissue kallikrein with kininogen as substrate. Into each well with TK bound to the coating monoclonal antibody 0.2 ml of a solution of dog kininogen (Marin-Grez and Carretero, 1972), 2 mg/ml in buffer E, was pipetted. After 4 h at 37 °C 0.1 ml of the solution was removed and mixed with 1.0 ml ethanol, the mixture was centrifuged for 10 min at 10,000 x g and 1.0 ml of the supernatant was dried in a SpeedVac concentrator. The dry residue was dissolved in buffer F and the kinin was determined by radioimmunoassay (2).

RESULTS AND DISCUSSION

A system of assays based on one monoclonal antibody was developed by which various forms of tissue kallikrein present in body fluids can be determined.

The antibody is bound to a solid phase and captures the TK present in the sample. By using different detection systems different species of TK, i. e. total (= free + complexed) tissue kallikrein, the complex of the enzyme with α_1-proteinase inhibitor and enzymatically active TK can be determined. Total TK and

the TK-α_1PI complex captured by the monoclonal antibody are detected using polyclonal antibodies to TK and α_1PI, respectively
as second antibody in a sandwich ELISA.

    Enzymatically active TK captured by the monoclonal antibody
was determined either by using the synthetic substrate H-D-Val-
Leu-Arg-p-nitroanilide or by incubation with kininogen and subsequent measuring of released kinin by a radioimmunoassay.

    The lower levels of detection and the inter- and intraassay
coefficients of variation are given in Table 1 for all assay systems. The activity determination with S-2266 as substrate is by a
factor of 25-50 less sensitive then the other assays. However,
speed and/or sensitivity of this assay can be improved by employing fluorimetric substrates.

	Total TK	TK-α_1PI	Active TK Kininogen	S-2266
Lower limit of detection	0.2 ng/ml	0.2 ng/ml	0.1 ng/ml	5.0 ng/ml
Intraassay variation	3.3 %	4.8 %	13.1 %	4.4 %
Interassay variation	5.2 %	11.6 %	16.4 %	6.7 %

Table 1.   Lower levels of detection and intra- and interassay
           coefficients of variation. Values for TK-α_1PI con-
           centrations represent concentrations of the TK bound to
           α_1PI.

The recovery of tissue kallikrein added to samples of biological
fluids (final concentrations: 2 ng/ml; for the assay with S-2266:
10 ng/ml) was between 92 and 99 % for urine, seminal plasma and
saliva. The recovery in serum of total TK and of the complex of
TK with α_1PI was 79-81 %. Recovery of active TK in serum was in
the range of only 40 % reflecting the inactivation of the added
tissue kallikrein by complex formation with α_1PI and possibly
other plasmatic inhibitors.

The assays were successfully employed to determine the concentrations of the various tissue kallikrein species in human serum,
urine, seminal plasma and saliva (Table 2). In all the fluids the
concentrations of all TK species varied over a wide range. The

lowest concentrations of total TK were found in serum and virtually all of the TK was complexed with α_1PI, enzymatically active
kallikrein could not be detected. In the individual urine samples
the concentrations of total and enzymatically active TK differed
by up to 75 %. This difference could not be explained by the presence of TK-α_1PI since this was found at low concentrations only.
The difference was obviously due to the presence of high portions
of tissue prokallikrein in urine as it disappeared when the urine
samples were treated with trypsin prior to the activity assay
(data not shown).

	Total TK [ng/ml]	TK-α_1PI [ng/ml]	Active TK Kininogen [ng/ml]	S-2266 [ng/ml]
Serum (n = 10)	0.2 - 2.2	0.2 - 2.0	n.d.	n.d.
Urine (n = 5)	195 - 558	4 - 32	56 - 212	71 - 210
Seminal plasma (n = 20)	13 - 201	1 - 32	3 - 204	n.d. - 188
Saliva (n = 5)	1141 - 6116	44 - 1043	798 - 5183	1129 - 5351

Table 2. Contents of total TK, TK-α_1PI and active TK in human
          serum, urine, seminal plasma and saliva.
          Values for TK-α_1PI concentrations represent concentra-
          tions of the TK bound to α_1PI; n.d. = not detectable.

CONCLUSION

The assay system described here is highly suitable for the specific determination of different forms of human tissue kallikrein
in body fluids. In addition, it can be easily adapted to the determination of complexes of TK with proteins other than α_1PI,
such as kallikrein binding protein (3) or protein C inhibitor
(4), by employing as second antibody a specific antibody directed
towards the respective complex-forming protein.

ACKNOWLEDGEMENTS
This work was supported by the Sonderforschungsbereich 207 of the
University of Munich.

REFERENCES

(1) Geiger, R., Stuckstedte, U., Fritz, H. Isolation and characterization of human urinary kallikrein. Hoppe-Seyler's Z. Physiol.
Chem. 1980, 361:1003-1016.

(2) E. Fink, W.-B. Schill, F. Fiedler, F. Krassnigg, R. Geiger and
K. Shimamoto (1985) Tissue kallikrein of human seminal plasma is
secreted by the prostate gland. Biol. Chem. Hoppe-Seyler 366:917-
924

(3) L.-M. Chen, L. Chao, R.K. Mayfield and J. Chao (1990) Differential interactions of human kallikrein-binding protein and α_1-
antitrypsin with human tissue kallikrein. Biochem. J. 267:79-84.

(4) S. Ecke, M. Geiger, I. Resch, I. Jerabek, M. Maier, B. R.
Binder (1991) Possible identity of kallikrein binding protein
with protein C inhibitor. Presented at KININ '91, September 8-14,
1991.

AAS 38/I
Recent Progress on Kinins
© 1992 Birkhäuser Verlag Basel

BIOLOGICAL ASSAY FOR TISSUE KALLIKREIN: COMPARISON WITH THE SYNTHETIC SUBSTRATE S2266

S.K. Campbell, K.G. Marshall, J.G.B. Millar, G. Venkat Raman and J.D.M. Albano

Department of Renal and Endocrine Medicine, University of Southampton, St. Mary's Hospital, Portsmouth PO3 6AD, UK

SUMMARY: A highly sensitive biological assay for tissue kallikrein is described, using human kininogen as substrate; and quantitation, by radioimmunoassay, of generated kinins. Using purified human urinary kallikrein as a reference standard we have correlated the kininogenase activity of kallikrein with amidase activity as measured by cleavage of the synthetic substrate S2266.

INTRODUCTION

The activity of tissue kallikrein is commonly measured using the synthetic tri-peptide substrate S2266 (1). Although this assay is simple to perform, and is readily automated so that large numbers of samples can be processed, it may, in certain biological fluids, lack specificity. In addition, the levels of kallikrein found in some disease states fall at the lower end of detection by this method, making such measurements subject to error. Furthermore, preliminary studies undertaken in our department have shown that using S2266 we are unable to detect basal kallikrein release from superfused renal cortical cells. Hence the need for the development of an assay with increased sensitivity and specificity.

MATERIAL AND METHODS

Synthetic substrate S2266 (Kabi Diagnostica) was obtained from
Quadratech, Epsom, Surrey, and purified human urinary kallikrein
from Channel Diagnostics, Walmer, Kent, UK. The monoclonal
antibody (SKB1) for bradykinin (BK) was a gift from Dr. M. Webb
of the Sandoz Institute, London, UK , and ^{125}I Tyr^8 bradykinin
tracer was obtained from NEN Du Pont Limited, Stevenage, Herts,
UK. All other chemicals were obtained from Sigma Chemicals,
Poole, Dorset, UK and BDH Ltd, Poole, Dorset, UK.

For the assay of BK standard curves (range 0.25 - 128
ng/ml), were constructed in 0.05 M phosphosaline buffer pH 7.5,
containing 6mM captopril (assay buffer). Standards were run in
triplicate and samples assayed in duplicate. Antibody (initial
binding 40%) and tracer solution were prepared in assay buffer.
After overnight incubation at 4°C, separation of free from bound
tracer moieties was effected by addition of 500µl of 30% (w/v)
polyethylene glycol (PEG) containing 0.1% (v/v) bovine gamma
globulin. After mixing, tubes were left at room temperature for
15 min. and then centrifuged at 2000 RPM for 30min. at 4°C. The
supernatents were aspirated and the radioactivity in the
precipitates measured in a gamma counter. Calibration curves
were plotted as the percentage of total radioactivity bound and
results were calculated by spline analysis using a dedicated
computer program. Cross-reactivity studies showed that at 0.5nM
and 16 nM BK, the antibody SKB1 showed a cross reaction of 72%
and 98% respectively with Lysyl bradykinin (LBK) and 58% and
90% respectively with Met-lysyl bradykinin (MLBK). Des arginine^9
bradykinin and 1-7 bradykinin showed no significant cross
reaction. This suggests that SKB1 does not recognise BK from
which the C-terminal arginine has been removed, indicating that
this residue at the carboxyl terminal region of the BK sequence
is the antigenic determinant required for antibody binding.

Kininogen was prepared from human plasma (single source)
from a patient undergoing routine plasmapheresis, using a
modification of a previously described method (2). Freshly

harvested plasma (500ml) was immediately mixed with 50ml of 5mM
Tris-HCl buffer (pH 7.3) containing 60mM EDTA, 10mM benzamidine
HCl, 3mg/ml polybrene, 0.75mg/ml soybean trypsin inhibitor,
280mM glucose and 150 mM NaCl. The plasma was then heated to
60°C for 2h with intermittent gentle mixing. After cooling, the
heat- inactivated plasma was centrifuged at 2,000 RPM for 30 min
and the supernatent subjected to ammonium sulphate fractionation
(30%). The precipitate obtained was resuspended in distilled
water and dialysed for 18h first against distilled water and
then against three changes of 0.05 M Tris-HCl buffer pH 8.5.
Aliquots of this semi-purified substrate were stored at -20°C.

Kininogenase activity was determined by incubation of
either 200µl kallikrein standard or sample with 200µl of
substrate, with the final volume adjusted to 500µl with assay
buffer. All dilutions of samples and standards were made in
assay buffer. After mixing tubes were incubated in a water bath
at 37°C for two hours. The reaction was stopped by the addition
of 25µl Trasylol (1000U/ml). Released kinins were measured by
assay of 50µl of this reaction mixture for BK. In order to
minimise any reagent effects, standard curves were supplemented
with reagent blank mixture (3). Results were expressed as
ng/ml/min BK generated.

The colorimetric assay using S2266 was carried out as
described (1) but with the addition of 0.5mg/ml of soya bean
trypsin inhibitor to the assay buffer. Urine samples (200µl)
were assayed for amidase activity using S2266 and after dilution
(1:50-1:1000) in assay buffer for kininogenase activity.
Superfusates obtained from isolated renal cortical cell
preparations were assayed, without prior dilution, by the
kininogenase assay only.

RESULTS

Using kallikrein standard concentrations over the range 0.0001-
0.01 U/ml, the prepared kininogen was titrated so that kinin

generation was linear with time (0-4hr) as well as substrate
concentration. Measurement of kinins generated from a set
kallikrein standard concentration gave an intra-assay variation
of 5.2% (24.6±2ng/ml, n=10) and an inter-assay variation of 6.6%
(27.1±8ng/ml, n=14). Compared to the amidase assay the
biological assay was approximately 400 times more sensitive,
0.01U/ml being equivalent to 3ng/ml/min of generated kinin.
Fig.1 shows a comparison of urinary kallikrein (UK)
measurements, using S2266 and the biological assay, in control
subjects and patient groups. When compared to control subjects,
reduced UK excretion was seen in the renal transplant recipients
and in psoriatics; both of these patient groups were receiving
the immunosuppressive drug cyclosporin A (CYA). Although
numbers in each group were small, correlation between the two
methods by linear regression analysis was r= 0.91, n=25.

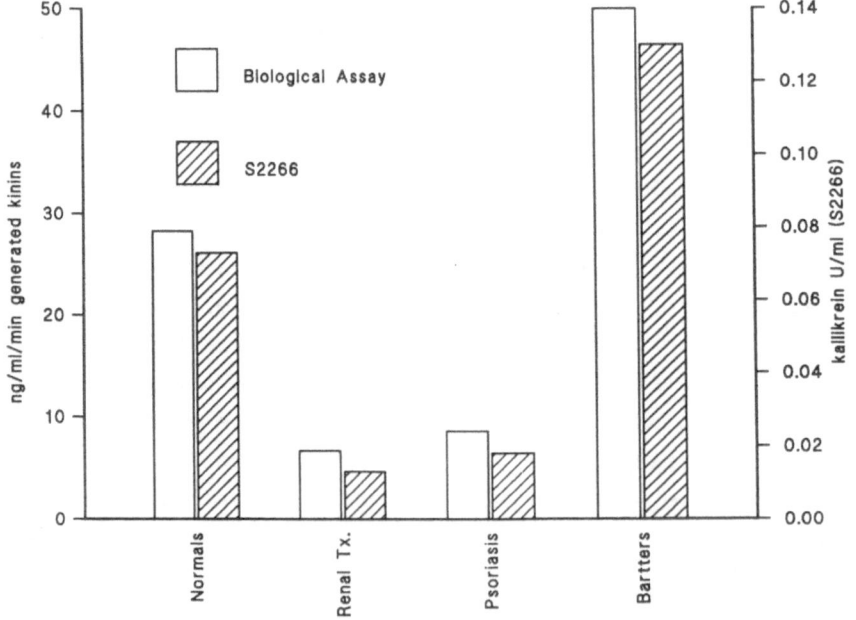

Figure 1. Comparison of urinary kallikrein activity measured by
S2266 and the biological assay. Normal n=8, renal transplant
recipients n=9, psoriatics n=7, Bartter's n=1.

Basal release of kallikrein from superfused isolated renal cortical cell preparations, and the responses to increasing doses of arginine vasopressin (AVP) are shown in Fig.2. Kallikrein concentrations in superfusates from such cell preparations were undetectable using S2266.

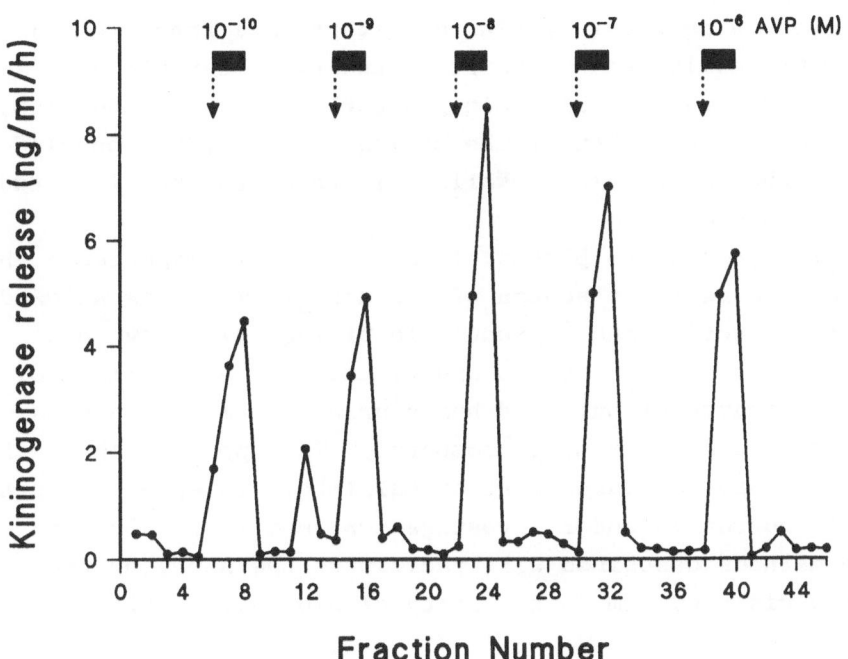

Figure 2. The effect of AVP on kininogenase release from superfused isolated rat renal cortical cells. Dashed arrows represent the beginning of agonist superfusion; solid bars represent the period of agonist superfusion.

DISCUSSION

In this preliminary study with small numbers of patients we have shown that both assays can be applied to the assay of UK in various disease states. However, the biological assay was of particular value in urine samples from renal transplant recipients where kallikrein concentrations were close to the detection limit of the colorimetric assay. The reduced UK excretion seen in the renal transplant group, is in accord with previous reports (4,5). Furthermore, the reduced excretion of UK also seen in psoriasis patients, with normal renal function, receiving CYA would lend support to the view that CYA may directly affect renal kallikrein production (6). In addition, the increased sensitivity of the biological assay has enabled us to measure the low levels of kallikrein released from isolated renal cortical cells.

Single donor human plasma, from routine plasmapheresis, has proved to be a reliable source of kininogen. This has allowed us to run a specific and reproducible biological assay in parallel with the colorimetric assay, and the availability of a commericial source of purified human urinary kallikrein has allowed the two methods to be compared. The application of the biological assay to measurement of kallikrein release from other tissues is currently under investigation, and it is anticipated that the methods described will facilitate the study of the kallikrein-kinin system in a variety of biological milieux.

ACKNOWLEDGEMENTS

We are grateful to Dr. M. Webb for the gift of the monoclonal antibody, and to Mr. J Derrick, our "single source human donor". The National Kidney Research Fund and the Foundation for Nephrology are acknowledged for financial support (KGM).

REFERENCES

1. Amundsen E, Putter J, Friberger P, Knos M, Claeson G. Methods for the determination of glandular kallikrein by means of a chromogenic tripeptide substrate. Adv Exp Biol 1979;120A:83-95.

2. Müller-Esterl W, Johnson DA, Salveson G, Barrett, AJ. Human kininogens. In: Methods in Enzymology 163: Immunochemical techniques: Part M: Chemotaxis and inflammation. Di Sabato GV, London, Academic Press, 1988: 240-256.

3. Albano JDM, Barnes GD, Maudsley DV, Brown BL, Ekins RP. Factors affecting the saturation assay of cyclic AMP in biological systems. Anal Biochem 1974;60:130-141.

4. Martinez L, Vio CP, Valdes G, Kychenthal W , Mendosa S. Decreased kallikrein in renal tranplants treated with cyclosporine. Transplant Proc 1990;22:294-296.

5. Spragg J, Denney DL, Tilney NL, Austen KF. Kallikrein excretion in transplant recipients and uninephrectomised donors. Kidney Int 1985;28:75-81.

6. Vio CP, Martinez L, Gandolfi I, Lenz P. Effect of Cyclosporin A on the distal nephron; the use of kallikrein as a specific morphological marker. Transplant Proc 1990;1730-1732.

AAS 38/I
Recent Progress on Kinins
© 1992 Birkhäuser Verlag Basel

COMPUTERIZED IMMUNOBLOT ANALYSES (CIBA) OF THE DISTRIBUTION OF PREKALLIKREIN AND ITS ACTIVATION PRODUCTS IN VIVO AND IN VITRO

Dulce Veloso and Graham Campbell

Division of Medicine, USAMRIID, Frederick, MD 21702-5011, U.S.A. and The Graduate Hospital, Philadelphia, PA 19146, U.S.A.

SUMMARY: The distribution of prekallikrein and the complexes of kallikrein with C1 inhibitor (C1INH), α_2-macroglobulin and ~58-kDa protein(s) (e.g. antithrombin III), differs in normal and C1INH-deficient human plasma, activated *in vitro*, due to different C1INH levels. Different distribution in the deficient plasma activated *in vivo* or *in vitro*, suggests different rates of complex clearance.

INTRODUCTION

Normal human plasma (NHP) activated *in vitro* shows that kallikrein (KAL) binds mainly to C1 inhibitor (C1INH), followed by α_2-macro-globulin (α_2M) (1-3) and a ~58-kDa protein(s) [antithrombin III (ATIII) (1) or other protein(s) such as protein C inhibitor (PCI) (4,5)]. We developed and characterized five anti-human plasma pre-kallikrein (PK) antibodies, and found that three of them recognize an epitope(s) in PK, KAL and KAL heavy-chains, which overlaps or is placed near the site recognized by factor XIIa (6). One of them (MAb 13G11), selected for further studies, also specifically recognizes complexes of KAL with C1INH, α_2M, α_1-antitrypsin (α_1AT), recombinant α_1AT Pittsburgh, and ATIII in systems of purified proteins and plasma (7,8). It is conceivable, that MAb 13G11 also recognizes complexes of KAL with other proteins. We also showed that MAb 13G11 detects ~45-kDa fragment(s) on immunoblots of all activated plasma samples (7,8).

Using immunoblotting with ^{125}I-MAb 13G11 (7), we confirmed previous reports, which indicated that binding of KAL to α_2M or C1INH depends on inhibitor levels (1,3). In agreement with this fact, KAL binds mainly α_2M and a ~58-kDa protein(s) in kaolin-activated plasma of patients deficient in C1INH (levels about 1/3 of those in NHP) (7,8). Taking advantage of the unique characteristics of MAb 13G11, we were able to develop specific immunoblot and "sandwich" assays to quantify prekallikrein and its activation products in plasma (7,8).

With this information, we quantified relative levels of PK, and its activation products in NHP and C1INH-deficient plasma *in vivo* and *in vitro*, based on the fact that KAL-inhibitor complex levels *in vivo* (and not *in vitro*) depend on their clearance. Thus, complex levels in plasma activated with kaolin were assumed to reflect KAL-inhibitor complexes formation *in vivo* without any clearance.

For quantification, we developed a method, which we have named CIBA. We quantified the intensities of spots on autoradiographs of immunoblots of NHP and C1INH-deficient plasma, before and after their activation with kaolin, with and without $\alpha_2 M$ inactivation. Comparison of the data obtained before and after kaolin-activaton indicates that KAL complexes present in C1INH-deficient plasma, before kaolin-activation, were not formed by surface-activation *in vitro*. An increase in KAL-C1INH complex levels in plasma activated after $\alpha_2 M$-inactivation, indicates that the low binding of KAL to C1INH, in the presence of functional $\alpha_2 M$, was caused by relatively low levels of C1INH, rather than by C1INH inactivation. The results also indicate that, although KAL can bind to other inhibitors such as PCI and ATIII when C1INH and $\alpha_2 M$ are depleted, their low levels, or low affinities for KAL, may cause an increase in the levels and half-life of KAL *in vivo*.

MATERIALS METHODS

Reagents, plasma and MAb 13G11 were obtained as reported (6,8). We stored plasma and MAb 13G11 in aliquots (<-70°C) and kept them on ice during assays. We labeled purified MAb 13G11 with iodine-125 as described (8) and stored it at 4°C. Control and kaolin-activated plasma were prepared for SDS-PAGE as described previously (8). In some experiments, plasma samples were treated with CH_3NH_2 for $\alpha_2 M$-depletion as we have reported (6), except that reagents were

incubated at 24°C. Denatured proteins were resolved in a 3–12%
polyacrylamide gradient using the methods as previously outlined
(8). We used the methods of Towbin et al. (9) for immunoblotting,
as previously outlined (8), with the following exceptions: the
incubation time for blocking non-specific sites was 2 hr;
nitrocellulose (NC) membrane incubation (2 hr, 37°C) with ^{125}I-MAb
13G11 (4 to 7 x 10^5 c.p.m./ml) replaced incubations with unlabeled
MAb 13G11 and secondary antibody; washing of the NC membrane was
followed by rinsing with water, drying with filter paper, and
exposure to CRONEX films (E.I. DuPont Neimours, Wilmington, DE,
U.S.A.) at -70°C. The positions of the autoradiographed antigen-^{125}I-
MAb 13G11 complexes were compared with those of protein standards
immunoblotted similarly, but stained with Amido Black (6).

We determined quantitative distribution of PK and its
activation products by CIBA, which measure the intensity of each
autoradiographed antigen-^{125}I-MAb 13G11 complex. For these analyses,
we used a video chip camera (NEC-180), an IBM PC-AT, an image
grabber (TARGA-M8, ATT) and software developed by Jandel Scientific
(JAVA). The chip camera illuminated and monitored the image. The
software program collected and analyzed the data. We analyzed the
total field of each autoradiograph, first by generating a frequency
histogram of relative intensity. This histogram comprised a multi-
modal distribution, including a distinctive distribution at the
lowest intensity values. The peak of this distribution approximated
one-half the average background intensity. Elimination of pixels
lower than this average value provided an objective perimeter of
the image to be analyzed. We further dissected manually the image
to determine average intensity and area. Antigen intensity was
generated by subtracting the average background intensity values
from the average intensity value of the image and multiplying it by
the area. Quantitative distribution was calculated from the ratios
of the intensity of each antigen-^{125}I-MAb 13G11 complex [PK (or PK
+ KAL) or PK activation products], over the sum of PK plus its
activation products. Intensity of KAL-α_2M complexes was the sum of
the intensities of the three top bands plus that of the lowest
band. For simplification, we grouped the ~140-kDa KAL complexes
together and termed them KAL-ATIII complexes.

RESULTS AND DISCUSSION

PK is the main antigen detectable with ^{125}I-MAb 13G11 on immunoblots of nonactivated NHP (Fig. 1, lane 1). Kaolin-activation of NHP for 3 and 10 min (Fig. 1, lanes 3 and 4) and 20 min (Fig. 2A, lanes 4 and 5), caused a gradual decrease of PK levels (defined 1.0 before activation), and an increase of the levels of KAL-C1INH, KAL-α_2M and KAL-ATIII complexes (values shown in Fig. 3). The relative

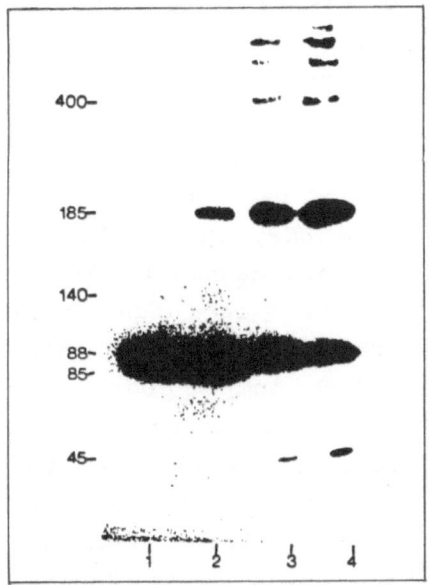

levels of KAL-inhibitor complexes in NHP activated for 20 min (maximum activation), agreed with those determined by other authors using different methods (1-3). Immunoblot patterns were similar to those observed after addition of KAL to NHP (Fig. 1, lane 2). When α_2M was inactivated before NHP activation (20 min), relative levels of PK and of KAL-ATIII and KAL-C1INH complexes were 0.21, 0.13 and 0.66, showing increased KAL binding mainly to C1INH (Fig. 2B, lanes 4 and 5). We show only the values in lane 4 because those in lane 5 are almost identical. CIBA of C1INH-deficient plasma from three patients (P1, P2 and P3) (Fig. 4), containing C1INH levels ~1/3 of those in NHP (8), showed: non-activated PK in P1; activated PK in P2 and P3 with relative levels of PK and complexes of KAL with ATIII, C1INH and α_2M,

Figure 1. Immunoblots of NHP (lane 1), NHP + KAL (lane 2) and NHP activated for 3 or 10 min (lanes 3 and 4). Mr of PK and/or KAL (85-88), of complexes of KAL with ATIII (140), C1INH (185) and α_2M (>400 kDa) and of a ~45-kDa fragment(s) are indicated on left.

0.38, 0.10, 0.002 and 0.50 (P2), and 0.49, 0.15, 0.002 and 0.34 (P3), respectively. KAL-α_2M complexes appeared as four bands

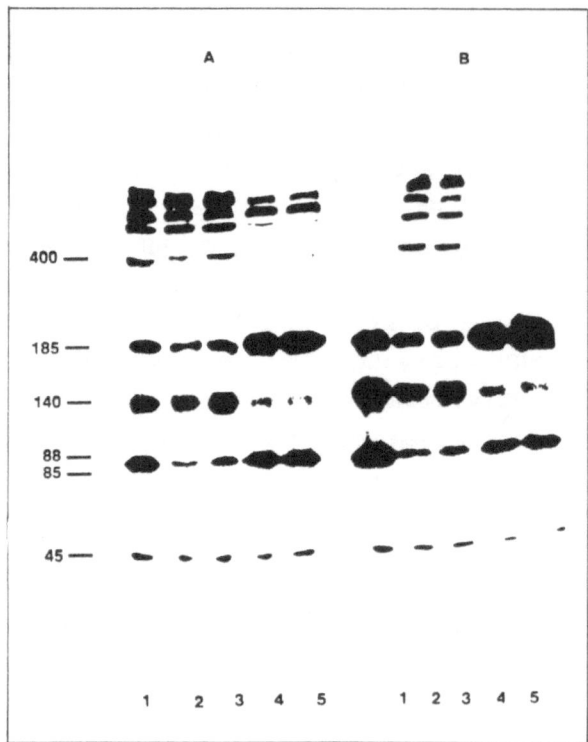

Figure 2. Immunoblots of P1, P2 and P3, lanes 1, 2 and 3, and of two NHP, lanes 4 and 5, kaolin-activated without (A) or with α_2M inactivation (B). (See legend to Fig. 1 and Fig. 4).

(Fig.4), similar to those in activated NHP (Fig. 2A, lanes 4 and 5), in a mixture of purified KAL and α_2M (8), and in a mixture of ^{125}I-KAL and NHP (1). Therefore, the structure of these complexes appear to be similar in NHP and the deficient plasma. To determine whether the differences in the immunoblot patterns of activated NHP, and of P2 and P3 were caused by differences in functional inhibitor levels, KAL-inhibitor complexes clearance, or other reasons, we analyzed the immunoblots of the deficient plasma after its activation with kaolin, as described for NHP. The distribution of KAL among its inhibitors, after deducting the levels of KAL complexes in the plasma before kaolin-activation, was the following: ~0.20 bound to each C1INH and ATIII, and 0.59 to α_2M (P1); 0.33 bound to ATIII, 0.41 to C1INH, and 0.26 to α_2M (P2); and 0.17 bound to ATIII, 0.36 to C1INH and 0.47 to α_2M (P3). PK intensities were similar in kaolin-activated P1, P2 and P3, although the samples had different PK levels before kaolin-activation. This fact indicates the presence of enough levels of inhibitors in P1, P2 and P3 to bind the KAL formed. The absence of KAL-C1INH complexes in P2 and P3 (Fig. 4), and their presence after plasma activation with kaolin (Fig. 2), appears to be caused by

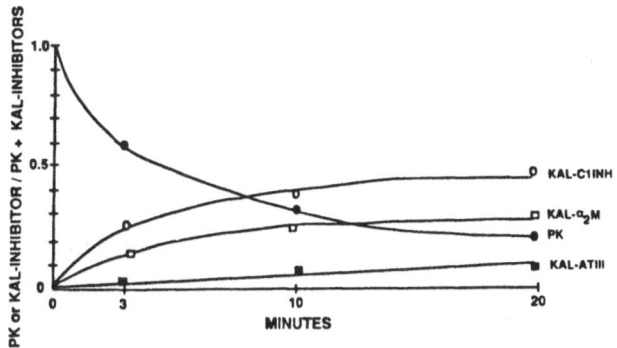

Figure 3. Relative levels of PK and complexes of KAL with its inhibitors in NHP activated for 3, 10 and 20 min.

their faster clearance rather than by inactivation of functional C1INH or formation of SDS-labile complexes (10). Previous reports by other authors (11) also indicate an increased clearance of these complexes in hereditary angio-neurotic patients. It is therefore concluded that the KAL complexes shown in Fig. 4 represent those in plasma *in vivo*. CIBA of the deficient plasma, activated after α_2M inactivation, also showed a value of 0.19 for PK (or PK + KAL) in P2 and P3, but 1.6-fold that of P1. The levels of KAL-α_2M complexes in P2 and P3 - undetectable in P1 - were almost identical to those before kaolin-activation, indicating complete inactivation of the functional α_2M by CH_3NH_2. Distribution of KAL between ATIII and C1INH was 0.57 and 0.43 (P1), 0.40 and 0.60 (P2) and 0.36 and 0.64 (P3). A combination of great PK levels in P1 before kaolin-activation (Fig. 4), reduced C1INH levels and α_2M-depletion, appears to be the cause of the greater levels of the complexes at the position of KAL-ATIII. Under these conditions, the affinity of KAL for these inhibitors or the inhibitor levels were too low to bind all KAL formed. Similar situations *in vivo* will cause prolonged, greater levels of KAL, which may explain the association of the contact system activation with the severity of several diseases. Further research to identify and characterize these inhibitors is necessary, using, for example, "sandwich" assays with MAb 13G11, similar to those previously reported (7).

The presence of 45-kDa fragments in activated plasma (7, 8, and Fig. 2), and in mixtures of purified KAL and inhibitors, and not in purified KAL (8), suggests that their release is facilitated

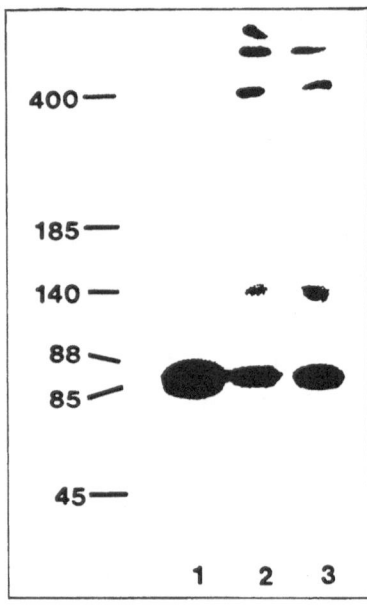

400 —

185 —

140 —

88 —
85 —

45 —

1   2   3

Figure 4. Immunoblots of C1INH-deficient plasma from three patients - P1, P2 and P3, lanes 1, 2 and 3, respectively. (See legend to Fig. 1).

by KAL-inhibitor complexes formation. Whether this release takes place *in vivo* or is an artifact of analysis manipulation deserves further research. Because of their size and recognition by MAb 13G11, the 45-kDa fragments must contain part of or even be the intact KAL heavy-chain. Since 45-kDa fragments appear as faint bands in both NHP activated for 3 min and P2 and P3 *in vivo* (Fig. 4), they do not seem to be useful indicators of plasma activation. Therefore, CIBA of these fragments were not included in our studies. The total intensities [PK (or PK + KAL) + KAL-inhibitor complexes] of the kaolin-activated deficient plasma and NHP shown in Fig. 2A, lanes 1, 2, 3, 4 and 5 were 194, 113, 127, 133 and 154, respectively. These values correlated well (r = 0.95) with those measured in the same plasma samples activated after α_2M inactivation (222, 123, 132, 120 and 183; Fig. 2B, lanes 1, 2, 3, 4 and 5), in spite of different distribution of PK and its activation products in the plasma with and without α_2M inactivation.

These results confirm the validity of our quantitative analyses and also show their usefulness to analyze events *in vivo* associated with activation of the contact system.

ACKNOWLEDGEMENTS

We are grateful to Dr. George Weinbaum (The Graduate Hospital, Philadelphia, PA), for his support. Part of this research was done while D.V. held a National Research Council-USAMRIID Research Associateship.

REFERENCES

1. van der Graaf F, Koedam JA and Bouma BN. Inactivation of kallikrein in human plasma. J Clin Invest 1983; 71:149-58.

2. Schapira M, Scott CF, Colman RW. Contribution of plasma protease inhibitors to the inactivation of kallikrein in plasma. J Clin Invest 1982; 69:462-8.

3. Harpel PC, Lewin MF, Kaplan AP. Distribution of plasma prekallikrein between C1 inactivator and α_2-macroglobulin utilizing a new assay for α_2-macroglobulin complexes. J Biol Chem 1985; 260:4257-63.

4. Meijers JCM, Kanters DHAJ, Vlooswijk RAA, van Herp HE, Hessing M, Bouma BN. Inactivation of human plasma kallikrein and factor XIa by protein C inhibitor. Biochemistry 1988; 27:4231-7.

5. Espana F, Estelles A, Griffin JH, Aznar J. Interaction of plasma kallikrein with protein C inhibitor in purified mixtures and in plasma. Thromb Haemostas 1991; 65:46-51.

6. Veloso D, Silver LD, Hahn S, Colman RW. A monoclonal anti-human plasma prekallikrein antibody that inhibits activation of prekallikrein on a surface. Blood 1987; 70:1053-62.

7. Veloso D, Tseng SY, Craig AR, Colman RW. Binding of a monoclonal anti-human plasma prekallikrein antibody to the complexes of kallikrein with C1 inhibitor and α_2-macroglobulin analyzed by immunoblot and "sandwich' assays. Adv Exp Med Biol 1989; 247 Pt A:499-505.

8. Veloso D, Colman RW. Western blot analyses of prekallikrein and its activation products in human plasma. Thromb Haemostas 1991; 65:382-388.

9. Towbin H, Staehelin T, Gordon J. Electrophoretic transfer of proteins from polyacrylamide gels to nitrocellulose sheets: Procedure and some applications. Proc Natl Acad Sci USA 1979; 76: 4350-4.

10. Donaldson VH, Rosen FS. Action of complement in hereditary angioneurotic edema: The role of C'1 esterase. J Clin Invest 1964; 43:2204-13

11. Nuijens JH, Huijbregts CM, Eerenberg-Belmer AJM, Abbink JJ, van Schijndel RJMS, Felt-Bersma RJF, Thijs LG, Hack CE. Quantification of plasma factor XIIa-C1 inhibitor and kallikrein-C1 inhibitor complexes in sepsis. Blood 1988; 72:1841-48.

AAS 38/I
Recent Progress on Kinins
© 1992 Birkhäuser Verlag Basel

EXPRESSION OF KALLIKREIN-BINDING PROTEIN AND α1-ANTITRYPSIN GENES IN RESPONSE TO SEX HORMONES, GROWTH, INFLAMMATION AND HYPERTENSION

J. Chao, L.M. Chen, K.X. Chai, and L. Chao

Department of Biochemistry and Molecular Biology
Medical University of South Carolina, Charleston, South Carolina 29425, U. S. A.

SUMMARY: We have recently purified rat kallikrein-binding protein (RKBP) and α1-antitrypsin (α1-AT) to homogeneity and isolated, sequenced cDNAs encoding these potential regulators of tissue kallikreins. Characterization of the cDNA and the gene has established the identity of the kallikrein-binding protein as a new member of the serpin (serine proteinase inhibitor) superfamily. Using the cDNA probes in Northern blot hybridization, we found a differential regulation of RKBP and α1-AT gene expression in the liver. Ovariectomy results in a 67% reduction of RKBP mRNA levels but a 30% increase of α1-AT mRNA levels. Estradiol or progesterone treatment of the ovariectomized rats increases RKBP transcripts by 2.5- and 6.5-fold, respectively, but reduces α1-AT mRNA level by 30% and 45%, respectively. In contrast to kininogen expression, both RKBP and α1-AT mRNA levels in the liver are at the lowest at birth and rapidly increase during growth and development. Rats injected with endotoxin from 4 to 24 h show a time-dependent decrease of RKBP mRNA levels while the same treatment induces α1-AT gene expression. RKBP mRNA levels in the normotensive Wistar Kyoto (WKY) rats are higher than those in the spontaneously hypertensive rats (SHR) while there are no differences of α1-AT mRNA levels between SHR and WKY. These studies show that: 1). There is a differential regulation of RKBP vs. α1-AT gene expression by estrogen and progesterone; 2). Both RKBP and α1-AT gene expression are developmentally regulated; 3). RKBP is a negative acute phase reactant while α1-AT is an acute phase protein; 4). RKBP is deficient while α1-AT is normal in the genetically hypertensive rats.

INTRODUCTION

Tissue kallikreins (E.C. 3. 4. 21. 35) are a group of homologous serine proteinases with limited proteolysis. They are encoded by multi-member gene families in mammals including humans, rats and mice. Tissue kallikreins are able to specifically cleave low molecular weight kininogen substrate to release kinin peptides, which mediate a broad spectrum of biological actions including vasodilation, inflammation, pain, and smooth muscle contraction and relaxation. The kallikrein gene family members are known to be regulated at both the transcriptional and the post-translational levels (for reviews, see 1-3).

Geiger *et al.* (4) first reported that human α1-antitrypsin is a progressive tissue kallikrein inhibitor and that α1-antitrypsin forms complex with human urinary kallikrein. We have later shown a novel tissue kallikrein-binding protein distinct from α1-antitrypsin in rat and human plasma (5-7). The tissue kallikrein-binding protein only binds with active kallikrein but does not form complex with inactive (latent) kallikrein or active-site blocked kallikrein (5,6). The identification of endogenously complexed entity of tissue kallikrein and binding proteins (5,7) and *in vivo* clearance studies (8) indicate that kallikrein-binding protein may play a role in regulating the activity and the bioavailability of tissue kallikreins. In order to understand the structure and function of the tissue kallikrein-binding proteins, we have purified and characterized rat kallikrein-binding proteins (RKBP) and α1-antitrypsin and isolated cDNAs encoding these proteins from an expression rat liver cDNA library (9,10). Sequence analysis of the cDNA and the gene encoding RKBP reveals that RKBP is a member of the serpin superfamily and is most homologous to human α1-antichymotrypsin (11). A potential hormone responsive element has also been identified in the promoter region of the RKBP gene. The expression of RKBP gene is regulated by various hormones including growth hormone (12), thyroid hormone (13), and the sex hormones (11). We found a major difference of kallikrein-binding protein levels in the spontaneously hypertensive rats (SHR) vs. the normotensive Wistar Kyoto rats (WKY), and multiple restriction fragment length polymorphisms (RFLP's) associated with the RKBP gene locus in SHR (6,9).

In this study, we showed a differential regulation of RKBP and α1-antitrypsin by the sex hormones and inflammatory agents; and the effect of growth and development on their expression, using Northern blot analysis. We also demonstrated reduced RKBP but not α1-antitrypsin mRNA levels in SHR.

MATERIALS AND METHODS

Animal Treatment

Sprague-Dawley (200-250 g) female rats (Charles River) were either ovariectomized or sham-operated. Three weeks after the surgery, rats began to receive subcutaneous injections of estradiol benzoate (50 μg/kg body weight) or progesterone (5 mg/kg body weight) suspended in sesame oil every 48 hours for 2 weeks. The control group rats were injected with the vehicle (sesame oil).

Sprague-Dawley (250-300 g) male rats (Charles River) received subcutaneous injections of lipopolysaccharide B. (endotoxin) (10 mg/kg body weight, dissolved in 0.9% sodium choloride) and sacrificed 4 h, 8 h, 12 h, 18 h, and 24 h after the injection. The rats of control group were injected with 0.9% sodium choloride.

RNA extractions and Northern Blot Analysis

Livers of treated rats or untreated SHR or WKY male rats (200-250 g, Charles River) were removed, minced and homogenized in GIT buffer (4 M Guanidine thiocyanate, 3 M sodium acetate, pH 6.0, 0.1 M 2-mercaptoethanol). The homogenate was ultracentrifuged (174,000 g at 20°C for 21 h) through a cesium chloride gradient (5.7 M CsCl, 3 M sodium acetate, pH 6.0). Northern blot analyses were performed using cDNA probes of RKBP , rat α1-antitrypsin and kininogen (9,10,14). The blots were quantitated by densitometric scanning of the autoradiograms.

RESULTS

Regulation of Gene Expression by Estrogen and Progesterone

Rat kallikrein-binding protein (RKBP) and α1-antitrypsin gene expression in the liver were analyzed by Northern blot using cDNA probes (9,10). Figure 1 shows that the levels of RKBP mRNA and α1-antitrypsin mRNA in female rats are differentially regulated by estradiol and progesterone. Ovariectomy of female rats resulted in a 67% decrease of RKBP mRMA level (Fig. 1, left panel, lane 2). Progesterone (lane 3) or estradiol (lane 4) replacement in ovariectomized females increased RKBP mRNA levels by 2.5- and 6.5-fold, respectively,

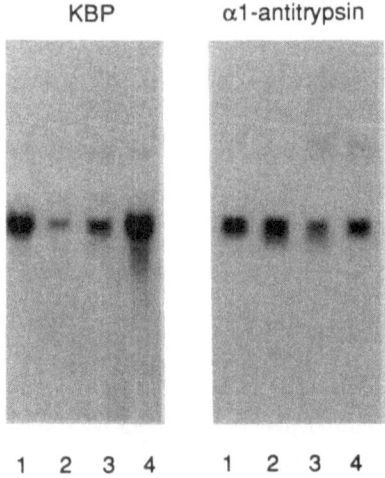

Figure 1. Northern blot analysis of RKBP and α1-antitrypsin mRNA in the female Sprague-Dawley rats. Left panel, liver RNAs (10 μg) probed with a RKBP cDNA. Right panel, liver RNAs (10 μg) probed with an α1-antitrypsin cDNA. Lane 1, sham-operated rat; lane 2, ovariectomized rat; lane 3, progesterone-treated ovariectomized rat; lane 4, estradiol-treated ovariectomized rat.

as compared to ovariectomized rats (Fig. 1, left panel). However, ovariectomy of female rats resulted in a 1.3-fold increase of α1-antitrypsin mRNA level in the liver and either progesterone or estradiol treatment of the ovariectomized rats resulted in 30 and 40% decrease of α1-antitrypsin mRNA level, respectively (Fig. 1, right panel). These results show that estrogen and progesterone up-regulate RKBP expression, but α1-antitrypsin expression is not significantly affected by these sex hormones.

Age-Dependence of Gene Expression

Figure 2 shows the differences in the expression pattern of three rat hepatic genes at different ages analyzed by Northern blot. RKBP and α1-antitrypsin mRNA levels are at their lowest levels at birth and rapidly increase during growth and development (Fig. 2, left and middle panels). In contrast, the expression of the kininogen gene is at its highest level at birth and rapidly decreases during growth to the adult age (Fig. 2, right panel). This result is also consistent with the published results showing that kininogen gene expression is high in new born rats and decreases during growth and development (15).

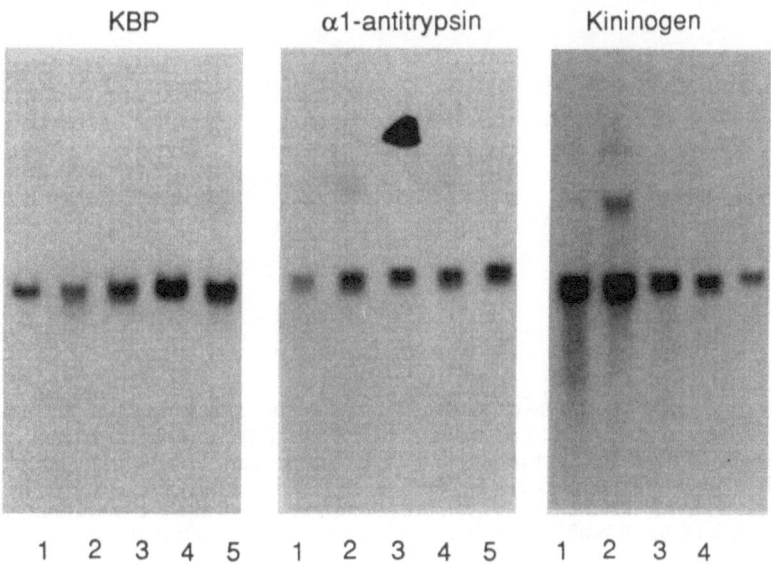

Figure 2. Northern blot analysis of RKBP, α1-antitrypsin, and kininogen mRNA in different ages of male Sprague-Dawley rats. Left panel, liver RNAs (10 µg) probed with a RKBP cDNA. Middle panel, liver RNAs (10 µg) probed with an α1-antitrypsin cDNA. Right panel, liver RNAs (10 µg) probed with a kininogen cDNA. Lane 1, day 1 rat liver; lane 2, days 5 rat liver; lane 3, days 10 rat liver; lane 4, days 20 rat liver; lane 5, adult rat liver.

Differential Regulation During Acute Phase Inflammation

        In order to compare the regulation of RKBP, rat α1-antitrypsin and rat kininogen gene expression following actue phase inflammation, rats were injected with endotoxin for different time periods and the changes of mRNA levels of each gene were analyzed by Northern blots. Figure 3 shows a differential regulation of RKBP vs. α1-antitrypsin gene expression during acute phase inflammation. RKBP mRNA levels (1,8 kb, lower band) showed a time-dependent decrease after endotoxin treatment (Fig. 3, left panel) while α1-antitrypsin mRNA levels increased after the treatment in a time-dependent manner (Fig. 3, middle panel). In consistance to the previous studies (16), rat T-kininogen gene expression was induced by endotoxin treatment (Fig 3, right panel). The results indicate that RKBP is a negative acute phase reactant while rat α1-antitrypsin and T-kininogen are positive acute phase reactants.

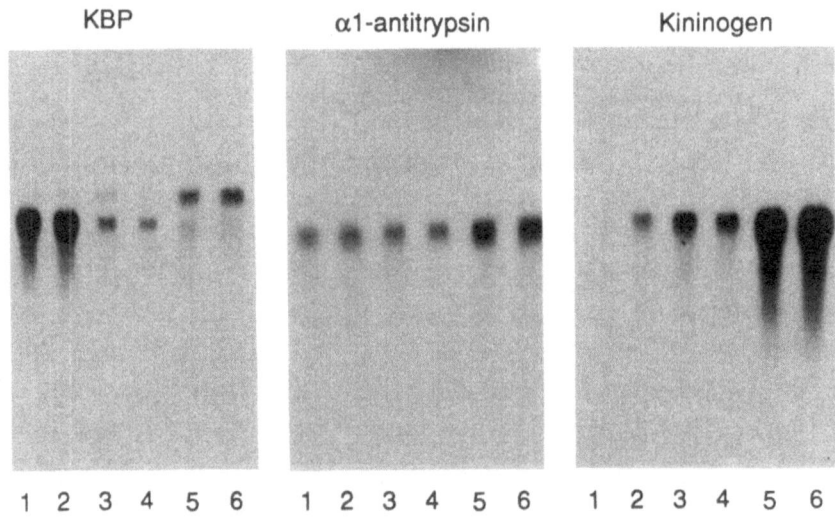

Figure 3. Northern blot analysis of RKBP, α1-antitrypsin, and kininogen mRNAs in the rat liver after endotoxin treatment. Left panel, liver RNAs (10 μg) probed with a RKBP cDNA. Middle panel, liver RNAs (10 μg) probed with an α1-antitrypsin cDNA. Right panel, liver RNAs (10 μg) probed with a kininogen cDNA. Rats were treated with endotoxin for different time intervals. Lane 1, control; lane 2, 4 h after treatment; lane 3, 8 h after treatment; lane 4, 12 h after treatment; lane 5, 18 h after treatment; lane 6, 24 h after treatment.

Expression in the Normotensive vs. Hypertensive Rats

        Figure 4 shows RKBP and α1-antitrypsin mRNA levels in SHR and WKY rats by Northern blots. The result shows that RKBP mRNA level in SHR is lower than that in WKY rats (Fig. 4, left panel), while α1-antitrypsin mRNA level is the same in SHR and WKY rats (Fig. 4, right panel). The results are consistent with our previous studies showing a reduction of immunoreactive RKBP but not α1-antitrypsin levels in SHR (6,9). The difference of the RKBP quantities in SHR vs. WKY rats is reflected at the mRNA level. Therefore, the quantitative difference of RKBP protein in SHR and WKY rats is a result of regulation at the transcriptional rather than the translational level.

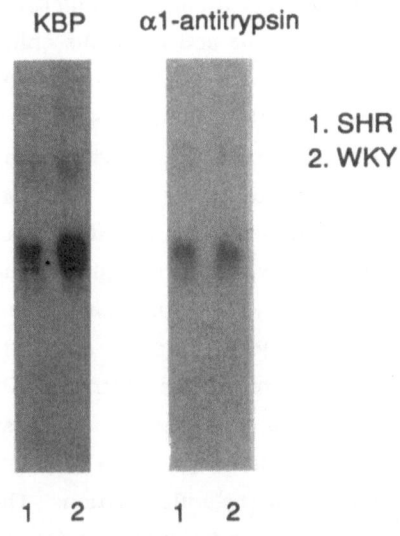

Figure 4. Northern blot analysis of RKBP and α1-antitrypsin mRNA in the male SHR and WKY rats. Left panel, liver RNAs (10 μg) probed with a RKBP cDNA. Right panel, liver RNAs (10 μg) probed with an α1-antitrypsin cDNA. Lane 1, SHR; lane 2, WKY.

DISCUSSION

In this study, we analyzed the regulation of the gene expression of two rat plasma proteinase inhibitors, kallikrein-binding protein and α1-antitrypsin in Sprague-Dawley rats and compared their mRNA levels in SHR and WKY rats. The hepatic expression of a third rat gene, kininogen gene, was also analyzed for comparison. The expression of rat α1-antitrypsin gene and that of the RKBP gene respond differently to the sex hormones. The expression level of both inhibitor proteins increases while that of kininogen decreases with aging from new born to adult. RKBP appears to be a negative acute phase reactant with its expression level being the highest under normal conditions. The expression level of RKBP decreases markedly upon treatment by inflammatory agents. In contrast, the expression of both rat α1-antitrypsin and T-kininogen is inducible by the same inflammatory agents. The expression level of RKBP is lower in SHR than in WKY while the expression level of rat α1-antitrypsin is the same in both strains.

We have previously shown that male rats have higher levels of α1-antitrypsin and kallikrein-binding protein than those of female rats (9,10). Analysis of the RKBP gene has revealed the existence of a potential steroid hormone responsive element in the upstream promoter region of the gene (11). But no such enhancer elements are present in the promoter regions of human α1-antitrypsin gene and human α1-antichymotrypsin gene. In order to carry out *in vitro* analysis to determine the activity of the enhancer element found in the promoter region of the RKBP gene, we tested the response of RKBP gene expression to the treatment of the sex hormones. As a control, the expression of rat α1-antitrypsin was also analyzed, even though the gene encoding rat α1-antitrypsin has not been cloned. The results indicate that estrogen and progesterone up-regulate RKBP gene expression while α1-antitrypsin expression is not significantly affected by estrogen and progesterone. Although both RKBP and rat α1-antitrypsin are expressed at higher levels in male than female rats (9,10), the regulation of their expression by the sex hormones is different.

The different reactions of RKBP and rat α1-antitrypsin expression to the treatment of inflammatory agents may reflect the difference of the functions of these two inhibitor proteins. During inflammation, α1-antitrypsin expression is mobilized so that an increased amount of α1-antitrypsin could be produced to counterbalance the proteinases released by neutrophils in response to the inflammation. The results from the *in vivo* catabolism studies of purified human kallikrein-binding protein and its complex with human tissue kallikrein in rats support the notion that kallikrein-binding protein plays a role in modulating kallikrein's bioavailability (8). The exact physiological function of RKBP in acute-phase inflammation has yet to be established.

In conclusion, although α1-antitrypsin and RKBP are both members of the serpin superfamily and they belong to the same subgroup as evidenced by the homologies in their primary structure and the gene organization (11), the mechanisms governing their expression in rat liver are different. The differential regulation of their expression pattern is very likely a result of the interactions by multiple factors such as enhancer or repressor elements present in the promoter regions of the genes. Furthermore, the differential regulation of their expression may reflect the differences of their physiological functions.

ACKNOWLEDGEMENT

This work was supported by the United States Public Health Service Grant HL 44083.

REFERENCES

1   MacDonald, RJ, Margolius, HS, Erdos, EG. 1988. Molecular biology of tissue kallikrein. Biochem J 253:313-321.

2.   Clements, JA. 1989. The glandular kallikrein family of enzymes: tissue-specific expression and hormonal regulation. Endocrine Reviews 10:393-419.

3.   Murray, SR, Chao, J, Lin, F-K, Chao, L. 1990. Kallikrein multigene families and the regulation of their expression. J Cardiovascular Pharm 15:S7-S16.

4.   Geiger, R, Stuckstedle, U, Clausnitzer, B, Fritz, H. 1981. Progressive inhibition of human glandular (urinary) kallikrein by human serum and identification of the progressive antikallikrein as α1-antitrypsin (α1-protease inhibitor). Hoppe-Seylers Z Physiol Chem B 362:5317-5325.

5.   Chao, J, Tillman, DM, Wang, M, Margolius, HS, Chao, L. 1986. Identification of a new tissue-kallikrein-binding protein. Biochem J 239:325-331.

6.   Chao, J, Chao, L. 1988. A major difference of kallikrein-binding-protein in spontaneously hypertensive versus normotensive rats. J Hypertension 6:551-557.

7.   Chen, L-M, Chao, L, Mayfield, RK, Chao, J. 1990. Differential interactions of human kallikrein-binding protein and α1-antitrypsin with human tissue kallikrein. Biochem J 267:79-84.

8.   Xiong, W, Tang, C, Zhou, XG, Chao, L, Chao,J. 1992. In vivo catabolism of human kallikrein-binding protein and its complex with tissue kallikrein. J Lab Clin Med 94:172-179, in press.

9.   Chao, J, Chai, KX, Chen, LM, Xiong, W, Chao, S, Woodley-Miller, C, Wang, L, Lu, HS, Chao,L. 1990. Tissue kallikrein-binding protein is a serpin: I. Purification, characterization and distribution in normotensive and spontaneously hypertensive rats. J Biol Chem 265:16394-16401.

10. Chao, S, Chai, KX, Chao, J, Chao,L. 1990. Molecular cloning and primary structure of rat α1–antitrypsin. Biochemistry 29:323–329.

11. Chai, KX, Ma, J-X, Murray, SR, Chao, J, Chao, L. 1991 Molecular cloning and analysis of the rat kallikrein-binding protein gene. J Biol Chem 266:16029-16036.

12. LeCam, A, Pages, G, Auberger, P, LeCam, G, Leopold, P, Benarous, R, Glaichenhaus, N. 1987. Study of a growth hormone-regulated protein secreted by rat hepatocytes: cDNA cloning, anti-protease activity and regulation of its synthesis by various hormones. EMBO J 6:1225-1232.

13. Tecce, MF, Dozin, B, Magnuson, MA, Nikodem, VM. 1986. Transcriptional regulation by thyroid hormone of an mRNA homologous to a protease inhibitor. Biochemistry 25:5831-5834.

14. Chao, S, Chao, J, Chao, L. 1990. Immunoscreening of cDNA expression libraries. Methods in Nucleic Acids Research, CRC Press, Chapter 15: 307-320.

15. Sierra, F, Fey, GH, Guigoz, Y 1989. T-Kininogen gene expression is induced during aging. Mol Cell Biol. 9 (12): 5610-5616.

16. Kageyama, R, Kitamura, N, Ohkubo, H, and Nakanishi, S. 1985. Differential expression of the multiple forms of rat prekininogen mRNAs after acute inflammation. J Biol Chem 260(22): 12060-12064.

AAS 38/I
Recent Progress on Kinins
© 1992 Birkhäuser Verlag Basel

POSSIBLE IDENTITY OF KALLIKREIN BINDING PROTEIN WITH PROTEIN C INHIBITOR

S. Ecke, M. Geiger, I. Resch, I. Jerabek, M. Maier and B.R. Binder

Laboratory for Clinical Experimental Physiology, University of Vienna, Schwarzspanierstraße 17, A-1090 Vienna, Austria

SUMMARY: Protein C inhibitor (PCI) inhibits tissue kallikrein by forming stable 1:1 complexes (k_1 = $2.3 \times 10^4 M^{-1}s^{-1}$). Heparin inhibits the tissue kallikrein/PCI-interaction and complex formation of ^{125}I-tissue kallikrein in serum. ^{125}I-tissue kallikrein complexes formed in plasma can be immunoprecipitated with monoclonal anti-PCI IgG suggesting that PCI might be identical to the kallikrein binding protein described previously (J. Chao et al. 1986, Biochem. J. 239, 325-331).

INTRODUCTION

So far no efficient serpin-type inhibitor of tissue kallikrein (TK) has been described. However, a binding protein for TK is present in several biological systems (1, 2). This binding protein interacts with enzymatically active TK by forming SDS-stable complexes with a M_r of 92,000, a process which is abolished in the presence of heparin (2). These data suggest a M_r for the binding protein of ≈50,000 and it should also have affinity for heparin. Kallikrein binding protein might furthermore be a serine protease inhibitor. So far, however, the identity of this protein which might regulate functional activity of tissue kallikrein, has not been defined.

Protein C inhibitor, on the other hand, is a heparin-binding, rather non-specific serine protease inhibitor (M_r = 57,000) (reviews in 3 and 4) the physiological role of which is still unknown. Since urine is not only a major source of TK but also of PCI (5) we analyzed in this study a possible inhibition of urinary TK by PCI.

MATERIALS AND METHODS

Materials: PCI was purified from native human urine by affinity chromatography on a monoclonal anti PCI-IgG(4PCI)-Sepharose 4B followed by affinity chromatography on heparin-Sepharose CL-6B as described in detail elsewhere (6). Urinary TK was obtained from Protogen AG, Switzerland. Radiolabeling of TK and urokinase (uPA; Serono, Germany) was performed using IODO-BEADS iodination reagent (Pierce, USA) and following the manufacturer's instructions. Enzymatically active ^{125}I-labelled TK was further purified by affinity chromatography on aprotinin-Sepharose (7). The purified labeled proteins exhibited a specific activity of 6μCi/nmol (^{125}I-TK) and 4μCi/nmol (^{125}I-uPA), respectively.

Analytical Methods: The concentration of purified urinary PCI was determined from its absorbance at 280nm using an $A_{280,1\%}^{1cm}$ of 14.1 (4). A M_r of 57,000 was used to calculate molar concentrations. The concentration of TK was evaluated from the cleavage of H-D-Val-Leu-Arg-pNA (S-2266, Kabi, Sweden) using a $\triangle A_{405}$/min/cm of 2.75/μM enzyme as given by the manufacturer. Sodium dodecyl sulfate polyacrylamide gel electrophoresis (SDS-PAGE) was performed according to Laemmli (8) using 1.5mm thick slab gels (10% acrylamide). Thereafter gels were fixed with acetic acid/methanol/water (10:50:40), dried, and exposed to X-ray films (Kodak X-Omat AR).

Inhibition of TK by PCI: Inhibition of TK amidolytic activity by PCI was studied by incubating TK (3nM final concentration) without or with PCI (7.5-30nM final concentration) in the absence and presence of heparin at 37°C in wells of a microtiter plate in 50μl 0.01M Tris-HCl, 0.1M NaCl, 0.01% Tween 80, pH 7.4. After 30 min preincubation 50μl S-2266 (0.4mM final concentration) dissolved in 0.05M Tris-HCl, pH 8.3, were added to each well and substrate hydrolysis was determined at 405nm in an ELISA-reader. In order to study the time course of TK inhibition by PCI, PCI and TK were preincubated as above and the reactions were stopped after defined intervals (0-80 min) by adding 10μl heparin (300μg/ml final concentration) since high concentrations of heparin completely abolished the TK/PCI-interactions (Fig. 2, panel A). Data obtained in these experiments were plotted as $\ln[E_t]/[E_0]$ versus incubation time and pseudo first order rate constants were calculated from the slopes of the initial linear parts of these plots. The second order rate constant was calculated by dividing these second order rate constants through the inhibitor concentrations used.

In separate experiments the effect of PCI on kinin generation by TK was also tested using the rat uterus bioassay (9). TK (2.3nM) was preincubated without or with PCI (230nM) in the absence and presence of heparin (5µg/ml final concentration) for 2 hours at 37°C in 0.01M Tris-HCl, 0.1M NaCl, 0.01% Tween 80, pH 7.4. After 2 hours, 5µl of this preincubation mixture were transfered to 100µl heat-inactivated human plasma as a source of kininogens and incubated for 5 min at 37°C. Thereafter, this mixture was applied to the rat uterus bioassay system and kinin generated was quantified using known bradykinin standards (9).

Complex formation of ^{125}I-TK and ^{125}I-uPA with purified PCI: ^{125}I-TK (4.7 nM final concentration) and/or ^{125}I-uPA (3nM final concentration) was incubated without or with PCI (280nM final concentration) in the absence and presence of heparin (30µg/ml final concentration) for one hour at 37°C in 0.01M Tris-HCl, 0.1M NaCl, 0.01% Tween 80, pH 7.4. Reactions were stopped by addition of 35µl 0.26M Tris-HCl buffer containing 2.5% SDS and 25% glycerol and heating the samples in a boiling water bath. Thereafter samples were analyzed by SDS-PAGE and autoradiography as described above.

Complex formation of ^{125}I-TK in plasma: ^{125}I-TK (1.2nM final concentration) was incubated in duplicate tubes for 30min at 37°C either with 1.8ml plasma each or with PCI (400µl, 200nM each). Thereafter either monoclonal anti PCI-IgG (4PCI)-Sepharose 4B (6) or control mouse IgG-Sepharose 4B (500µl settled volume each) were added to each of the four tubes. After 60 min at 22°C supernatants were removed and the Sepharose beads were washed three times with 0.01M Tris-HCl, 1M NaCl, 0.01M benzamidine, 0.01% Tween 80, pH 9.0, and once with 0.01M Tris-HCl, 0.14M NaCl, 0.01% Tween 80, pH 7.4. Thereafter 400µl 10% SDS and 25% glycerol were added to each tube containing the Sepharose beads and the supernatants were removed and analyzed by SDS-PAGE.

RESULTS

Fig. 1 shows the elution profiles of urinary PCI from monoclonal anti PCI-IgG-Sepharose (left panel) and heparin-Sepharose CL-6B (right panel) columns, respectively. By this two step procedure PCI was purified to apparent homogeneity (Inset Fig. 1, right panel). It migrated on SDS-PAGE as a tightly spaced doublet with a major band corresponding to a M_r of 57,000 and a minor band corresponding to a M_r of 54,000 representing cleaved PCI (6).

When TK was incubated with purified urinary PCI the amidolytic activity was inhibited (Fig. 2). This inhibition was PCI-dose dependent (Fig. 2, panel B) and decreased with increasing heparin-concentrations, while heparin had no effect on the amidolytic activity of TK (Fig. 2, panel A). Fig. 2B shows the

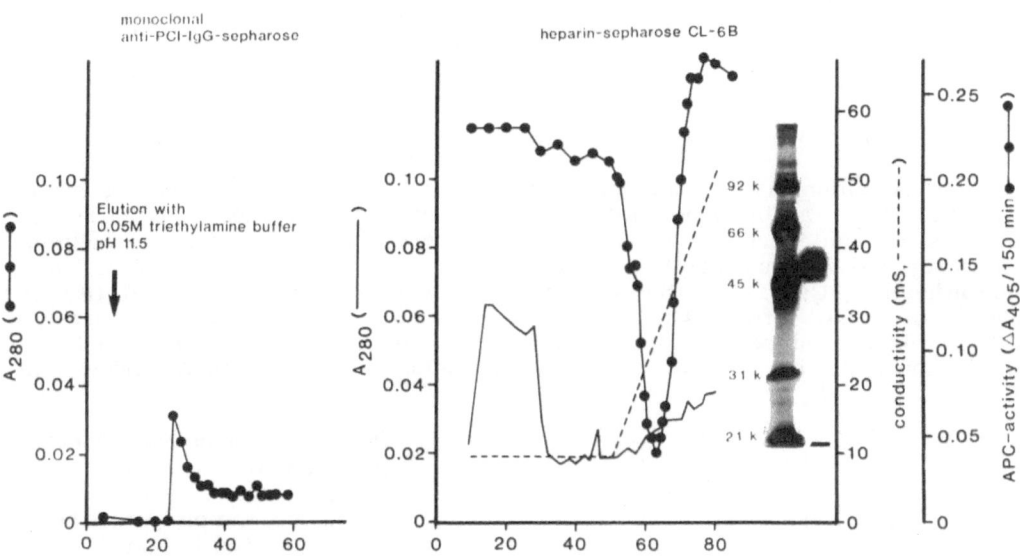

Fig. 1: Elution profiles of urinary PCI from monoclonal anti-PCI-IgG-Sepharose (left panel) and Heparin-Sepharose CL-6B (right panel). The inset in the right panel shows an SDS-PAGE-gel of purified urinary PCI and M_r-markers. Experimental procedures are described in detail elsewhere (6).

time course of TK inhibition by different concentrations of PCI. Heparin (300µg/ml final concentration) was used to stop the reactions after defined intervals, since high heparin concentrations completely abolished TK-inhibition by PCI (Fig. 2, panel A). Data shown in Fig. 2, panel B were used to calculate kinetic constants and revealed an apparent second order rate constant (k_1) of 2.3x10^{4}M^{-1}s^{-1}. Inhibition of TK-activity by PCI was also seen studying kinin formation in the rat uterus bioassay-system (Fig. 3). Also in this assay system heparin abolished TK-inhibition by PCI.

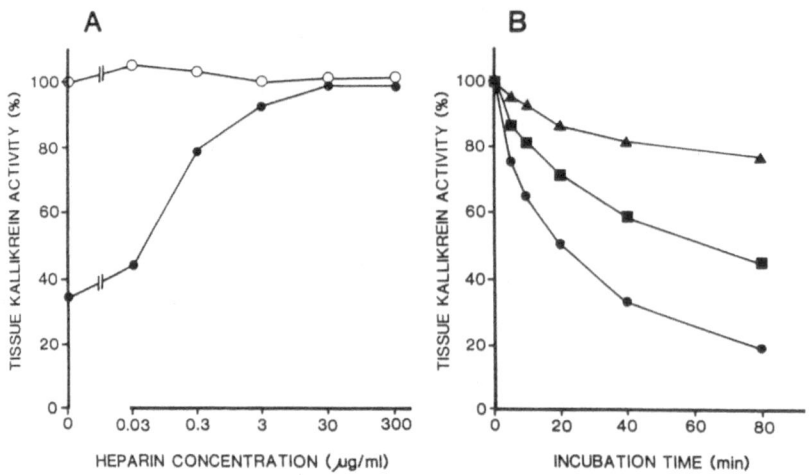

Fig. 2: Inhibition of TK amidolytic activity by PCI. Panel A: Effect of heparin. TK (3nM) was incubated without (o) or with PCI (●, 30nM) for 30 min in the absence and presence of different concentrations of heparin. Remaining enzymatic activity was quantified using S-2266. Panel B: Time course of TK - inhibition by PCI. TK (3nM) was incubated with 7.5nM (▲), 15 nM (■) or 30nM (●) PCI. After the intervals indicated on the abscissa   heparin (300µg/ml) was added to stop the reactions, and remaining enzymatic activity was quantified with S-2266. Experimental details are given in Materials and Methods.

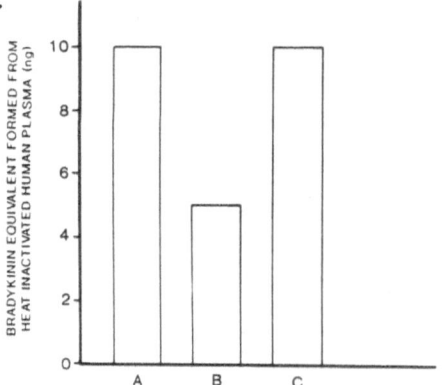

Fig. 3: Effect of PCI on kinin-generation by TK. TK was preincubated without or with PCI in the absence and presence of heparin as described in Materials and Methods. Kinin-formation was analyzed in the rat uterus bioassay-system using heat-indicated human plasma as a source of kininogens.
A: 0.11nM TK; B: 0.11nM TK + 11nM PCI; C: 0.11nM TK + 11nM PCI + 5 µg/ml.

Complex formation of TK was studied using ^{125}I-labeled enzyme (Figs. 4 and 5). As can be seen from these figures ^{125}I-TK formed a complex (M_r = 85,000) with purified PCI. The intensity of this complex was lower in the presence of heparin, while heparin stimulated complex formation of ^{125}I-uPA with PCI (Fig. 4). When both enzymes, ^{125}I-TK and ^{125}I-uPA, were coincubated with PCI, mainly TK/PCI-complexes were formed in the absence of heparin, whereas in the presence of heparin mainly uPA/TK-complexes were observed (Fig. 4).

^{125}I-TK also formed a complex upon incubation in plasma. This complex migrated on SDS-PAGE with the same mobility as TK/PCI-complex (Fig. 5). ^{125}I-TK complex formed in plasma could be immunoprecipitated with monoclonal anti PCI-IgG-(4PCI)-Sepharose but not with control mouse IgG-Sepharose, indicating that this complex consists of ^{125}I-TK and plasma PCI.

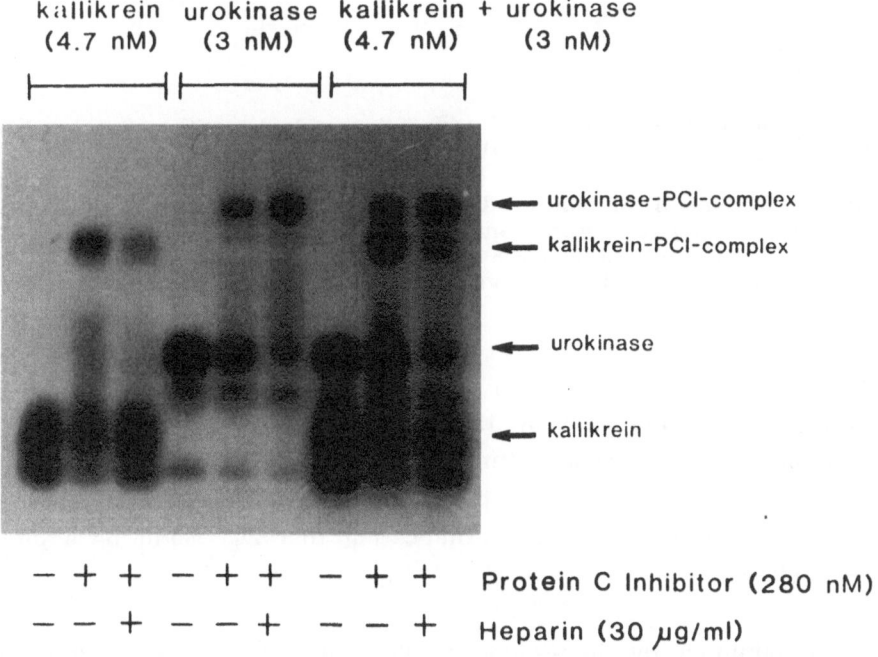

Fig. 4: Complex formation of ^{125}I-TK and/or ^{125}I-uPA with purified PCI, effect of heparin. ^{125}I-TK (4.7nM) and/or ^{125}I-uPA (3nM) were incubated without (-) or with (+) PCI (280nM) in the absence (-) and presence (+) of heparin (30µg/ml) for one hour at 37°C. Thereafter the incubation mixtures were analyzed by SDS-PAGE and autoradiography as described in detail in Materials and Methods.

PURIFIED SYSTEM   PLASMA

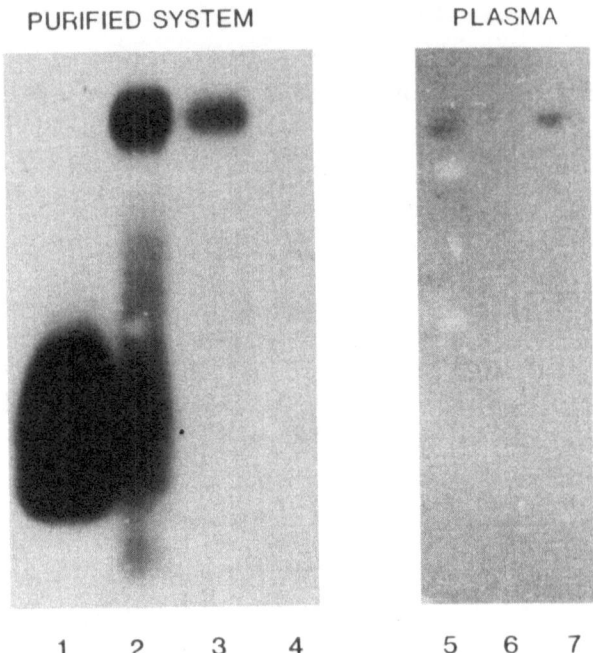

    1   2   3   4   5   6   7

Fig. 5: Immunoprecipitation of ^{125}I-TK complexes with monoclonal anti-PCI-
IgG. ^{125}I-TK was incubated without (lane 1) or with PCI (lanes2-4) or with
plasma (lanes 5-7). Thereafter incubation mixtures were either directly subjected to SDS-PAGE and autoradiography (Lanes 1,2,and 5) or to immunoprecipitation   with either monoclonal anti-PCI-IgG-Sepharose 4B (lanes 3 and 7)
or control mouse IgG-Sepharose 4B (lanes 4 and 6) prior to SDS-PAGE analysis. Experimental details are given in Materials and Methods.

DISCUSSION

In the present study we show that PCI inactivates TK by forming SDS-stable
1:1 complexes. The second order rate constant ($2.3 \times 10^4 M^{-1} s^{-1}$) is in the same
order of magnitude or higher than that observed for the inhibition of other
target proteases by PCI (3, 4), indicating that PCI might be a physiological
TK-inhibitor.

Heparin inhibited the interaction of TK with PCI in a dose dependent way.
This reaction pattern was unexpected since heparin stimulates the interaction
of PCI with most of its target proteases and an inhibiting effect of heparin on
PCI-activity has not been described so far. However, an inhibitory effect of
heparin has been described for the interaction of TK with the so called kallikrein binding protein, a protein which in the meantime has been shown to

be a serine protease inhibitor highly homologous to α_1-antichymotrypsin and α_1-antitrypsin, at least in the rat system (10). These results therefore prompted us to study a possible relationship between PCI and the kallikrein binding protein. We show here that ^{125}I-TK complexes formed in plasma can be immunoprecipitated by monoclonal anti-PCI-IgG. Furthermore, serum immunodepleted of PCI no longer formed complexes with ^{125}I-TK (6). Our data therefore not only suggest that PCI might be the first efficient serpin-type inhibitor of TK but also that PCI and the kallikrein binding protein are very similar, if not identical.

REFERENCES

1. Chao J, Tillman DM, Wang M, Mangolius HS, Chao L. Identification of a new
tissue-kallikrein-binding protein. Biochem J. 1986, 239: 325-331.

2. Chen L-M, Chao L, Mayfield RK, Chao J. Differential interactions of human kallikrein-binding protein and α_1-antitrypsin with human tissue kallikrein. Biochem J 1990; 267:79-84.

3. Geiger M. Protein C inhibitor / plasminogen activator inhibitor 3. Fibrinolysis 1988; 2:183-188.

4. Suzuki, K, Deyashiki, Y, Nishioka, J, Toma K. Protein C inhibitor: structure and function. Thromb Haemostas 1989; 61:337-342.

5. Geiger M, Priglinger U, Griffin JH, Binder BR. Urinary protein C inhibitor. Glycosaminogylcans synthesized by the epithelial kidney cell line TCL-598 enhance its interaction with urokinase. J Biol Chem 1991; 266:11851-11857.

6. Ecke S, Geiger M, Resch I, Jerabek I, Stingl L, Maier M, Binder BR. Inhibition of tissue kallikrein by protein C inhibitor. Evidence for identity of protein C inhibitor with the kallikrein binding protein. J Biol Chem 1992; 267: in press

7. Ole-Moi-Yoi O, Spragg J, Austen KF. Structural studies of human urinary kallikrein (urokallikrein). Proc Natl Acad Sci USA 1979; 76:3121-3125.

8. Laemmli UK. Cleavage of structural proteins during the assembly of the head of bacteriophage T_4. Nature (London) 1970; 227: 680-682

9. Maier M, Jerabek I, Reissert G, Höltzl E, Binder BR. Correlation of two different assays for urinary kallikrein in normotensive and hypertensive subjects. Clin. Chim. Acta 1988;178: 127-140

10. Chai KX, Ma JX, Murray SR, Chao J, Chao L. Molecular cloning and analysis of the rat kallikrein-binding protein gene. J Biol Chem 1991; 266: 16029-16036

AAS 38/I
Recent Progress on Kinins
© 1992 Birkhäuser Verlag Basel

INHIBITION OF GLANDULAR AND PLASMA KALLIKREIN BY BENZAMIDINE DERIVATIVES

Jörg Stürzebecher, Helmut Vieweg[*] and Dagmar Prasa

Institute of Pharmacology & Toxicology, Medical Academy Erfurt
D(O)-5010 Erfurt, FRG
[*]Pentapharm Ltd., CH-4002 Basel, Switzerland

SUMMARY: Besides guanidino compounds and amines structurally related to arginine and lysine, compounds with other cationic groups are inhibitors of trypsin-like serine proteinases. Particularly aromatic ring structures with an amidino moiety have high affinity for these enzymes. In most cases ordinary benzamidine derivatives are no selective inhibitors, however, among derivatives of Nα-arylsulfonyl- ω-amidinophenyl-α-amino-alkylcarboxylic acids selective competitive inhibitors of several enzymes were found. Amides of phenyl-α-aminobutyric acid containing an amidino moiety are inhibitors of plasma kalli-krein. The p-amidinoanilide of 2-tosylamino-4-phenylbutyric acid inhibits selectively plasma kallikrein with a K_i of 0.70 μmol/l. In contrast, potent and selective inhibitors of glandular kalli-krein were hardly found among benzamidines.

INTRODUCTION

Trypsin-like serine proteinases are proteolytic enzymes charac-terized by a reactive serine residue in the catalytic mechanism. They attack at peptide bonds following an arginine or lysine residue. Of special physiological importance are enzymes of this family that are involved in several blood effector systems such as coagulation, fibrinolysis, complement activation and kinin formation.

Kinin is released from kininogen by kallikreins via limited proteolysis. Unfortunately, the kallikreins are assigned to two totally different groups of proteinases: the glandular kallikreins on the one hand, and the plasma kallikrein on the other. The two types differ in molecular and immunological properties, in the type of kinin released, and in susceptibility to inhibition by natural and synthetic inhibitors. Furthermore, plasma kallikrein plays an important role in coagulation and fibrinolysis. This results from the kallikrein-catalysed activation of factor XII.

Selective inhibitors of both types of kallikrein are of great interest to further clarify their physiological function. Moreover, inhibitors of plasma kallikrein are potential anticoagulants. The new conception of anticoagulation is based on the increase in inhibitory potential of plasma by application of inhibitors of enzymes involved in coagulation. In this context, inhibitors of the fibrinogen-converting enzyme thrombin are in the focus of interest (1). However, also other clotting factors are considered points of attack of a protease inhibitor besides thrombin. Two clotting factors are of special interest: factor Xa, where the extrinsic and intrinsic pathways of the coagulation cascade converge, and factor XIIa, which initiates the early phase of clotting together with plasma kallikrein. Several synthetic inhibitors of factor Xa were reported and tested for their anticoagulant efficiency (2). However, there is only little information about inhibitors of plasma kallikrein and factor XIIa. As yet only peptide chloromethyl ketones have been tested systematically for anti-kallikrein activity (3). Among arginine amides derivatives containing N-terminal trans-4-aminomethyl-cyclohexanecarboxylic acid were found which inhibit selectively plasma kallikrein (4). Benzamidine derivatives are reversible inhibitors of these enzymes, however they have not yet been extensively studied (5).

MATERIALS AND METHODS

For inhibitor studies human plasma kallikrein and human coagulation factor XIIa were purchased from Protogen AG (Läufelingen, Switzerland). The glandular kallikrein isolated

from porcine pancreas was a gift of Prof. H. Fritz (München). The
inhibitory activity was determined from the influence of the
inhibitors on the hydrolysis of chromogenic peptide substrates
(Bz-Pro-Phe-Arg-pNA for plasma kallikrein, D-HHT-Gly-Arg-pNA
factor XIIa, D-Val-CHA-Arg-pNA for glandular kallikrein;
Pentapharm AG, Basel, Switzerland) at pH 8 and 25 °C. The
inhibitors were synthesized by the coworkers of Prof. G. Wagner
(Leipzig). They have been described and tested previously for
their inhibitory activity on thrombin, factor Xa, trypsin and
plasmin (2, 6, 7, 8). The K_i values were calculated graphically
according to DIXON (9).

Prothrombin activation was studied in hirudin-stabilized
human plasma. Platelet-rich plasma was prepared from hirudinized
blood (approx. 100 AT-U/ml) and stored in plastic tubes at 37 °C.
Using chromogenic substrate methods the concentrations of hirudin
and the clotting factors VIII, X, XII, prekallikrein and protein
C were determined at different times.

RESULTS AND DISCUSSION

Benzamidine (compound I, Fig. 1) is a weak inhibitor of both
kallikreins. Substitution of benzamidine with hydrophobic
residues and introduction of a carbonyl function caused an
increase in the inhibitory effect. The affinity of the compounds
was generally higher for plasma than for glandular kallikrein.
In most cases, the K_i values differed by about factor ten. Among
the simple compounds 4-amidinophenylpyruvic acid (compound II,
Fig. 1) is of special interest. Some years ago , the compound was
described to discriminate well between plasma and glandular
kallikrein (5). Furthermore, 4-amidinophenylpyruvic acid inhibits
trypsin and thrombin with comparable affinity (Table 1).

Among compounds with two and more benzamidine moieties
potent inhibitors of kallikreins were found (10). We have studied
bis-benzamidines like compound III (Fig. 1). The compounds containing a cycloalkanone linking bridge inhibit plasma kallikrein
with K_i values in the micromolar range as is the case with the

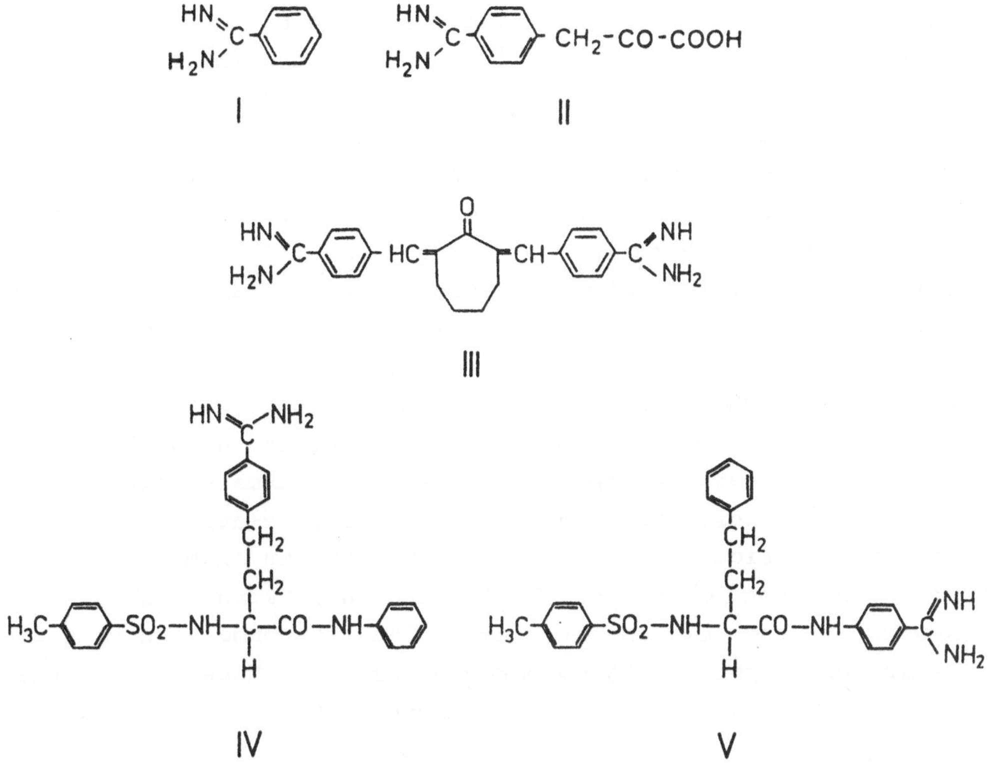

Figure 1. Structures of inhibitors derived from benzamidine (Inhibitor I)

Table 1. Inhibition of Trypsin-like Enzymes by Selected Benzamidine Derivatives

Enzyme	Inhibition constant K_i [μmol/l] for inhibition of several enzymes by compound				
	I	II	III	IV	V
Plasma kallikrein	200	1.4	0.72	0.25	0.70
Gland. kallikrein	2560	610	18	39	101
Factor XIIa	810	86	0.36	1.0	103
Factor Xa	410	9.4	0.022	12	31
Thrombin	220	6.5	0.32	40	170
Trypsin	35	1.6	0.09	0.34	1.3
Plasmin	350	60	6.4	2.3	10

cycloheptanone derivative III (Table 1). The number of C-atoms at
the cycloalkanone ring has no influence on the inhibitory activity. Compound III is a poor inhibitor of glandular kallikrein.
It does not inhibit plasma kallikrein selectively, it inhibits
trypsin and the clotting factors XIIa, Xa and thrombin.

     For designing of selective inhibitors of trypsin-like
enzymes amidinophenylglycine,   amidinophenylalanine,   amidino-
phenyl-α-aminobutyric acid and   amidinophenyl-α-aminovaleric acid
proved to be key building blocks. These amidinophenyl-
α-aminoalkylcarboxylic acids   are   isosteric   derivatives of
arginine in which the basic guanidinoalkyl side chain of arginine
is replaced by a benzamidine moiety. Among the Nα-arylsulfonyl-
ated primary amides potent inhibitors of plasma kallikrein were
found. The Nα-tosylated anilide of phenyl-α-aminobutyric acid
(compound IV, Fig. 1, Table 1), serves as an example. It is a
potent inhibitor of plasma kallikrein and factor XIIa with a
K_i-value in the micromolar range. The compound inhibits also
plasmin and trypsin with comparable potency, however, it has a
relatively weak effect on other clotting factors and glandular
kallikrein.

     To enhance the potency and selectivity, we carried out
several structural variations starting from compound IV. The
transfer of the amidino moiety from the amino acid side chain to
the amide part led to a drastic increase in selectivity. The
compound obtained - the amidinoanilide of phenyl-α-aminobutyric
acid (compound V, Fig. 1) - is a selective inhibitor of plasma
kallikrein (Table 1). It does not influence factor XIIa and other
clotting factors, the fibrinolytic enzymes and glandular
kallikrein.

     Inhibitors of plasma kallikrein are useful tools for
eliminating the undesired enzymatic activity of plasma kallikrein. For example, inhibitor V was used in a chromogenic assay
system for factor XIIa (11). Furthermore, inhibitors of plasma
kallikrein and/or factor XIIa may become important in the
prevention of surface-induced activation of blood coagulation.
This could be demonstrated in blood or plasma anticoagulated with
the thrombin inhibitor hirudin. Hirudin is able to block comple-

tely thrombin-induced fibrin formation. However, the hirudin
concentration in plasma decreased, that means, prothrombin activation occurs. (Fig. 2). In contrast, no significant activation
of clotting factors other than prothrombin was observed (not
shown here).

Obviously, minute amounts of activated clotting factors
provoked prothrombin activation. In this process, the enzymes of
the early phase of clotting, plasma kallikrein and factor XIIa,
play a decisive role. Their influence could be diminished by the
use of selective inhibitors. Thus, consumption of prothrombin in
hirudinized plasma was markedly reduced by the addition of a
synthetic inhibitor of plasma kallikrein like compound V besides

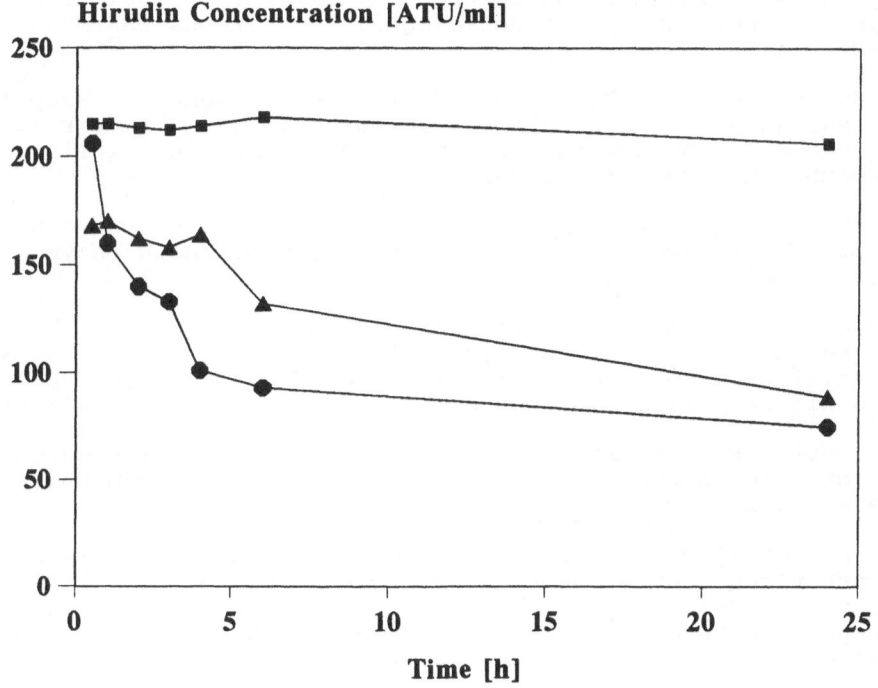

Figure 2. Hirudin concentration in hirudinized plasma of 5
        healthy subjects (100 ATU/ml blood).
        (●) - without inhibitor
        (■) - with an inhibitor of plasma kallikrein
        (▲) - with an inhibitor of factor Xa

hirudin (Fig. 2). However, a factor Xa inhibitor of the 3-amidinophenylalanine type (2) was less effective.

In summary, we have designed potent and selective inhibitor of plasma kallikrein and those that inhibit additionally factor XIIa. Inhibitors V and IV are examples of such types of inhibitors. However, potent and selective inhibitors of glandular kallikrein with benzamidine as key building block have not yet been found.

REFERENCES

1. Markwardt F. Pharmacological control of blood coagulation by synthetic, low-molecular-weight inhibitors of clotting enzymes. A new concept of anticoagulation. Trends Pharmacol Sci 1980; 1:153-157.

2. Stürzebecher J, Stürzebecher U, Vieweg H, Wagner G, Hauptmann J, Markwardt F. Synthetic inhibitors of bovine factor Xa and thrombin. Comparison of their anticoagulant efficiency. Thromb Res 1989; 54:245-252.

3. Kettner C, Shaw E. Inactivation of trypsin-like enzymes with peptides of arginine chloromethyl ketone. Meth Enzym 1981; 80:826-842.

4. Okamoto S, Okamoto U, Hijikata-Okunomiya A, Wanaka K, Okada Y. Recent studies of the synthetic selective inhibitors; with special reference to non-plasmin fibrinolytic enzyme, plasmin and plasma-kallikrein. Thromb Res 1988; Suppl. VIII:131-141.

5. Markwardt F, Drawert J, Walsmann P. Synthetic low molecular weight inhibitors of serum kallikrein. Biochem Pharmacol 1974; 23:2247-2256.

6. Markwardt F, Richter P, Stürzebecher J, Wagner G, Walsmann P. Synthetische Inhibitoren der Serinproteinasen. 6. Mitteilung: Über die Hemmung von Trypsin, Plasmin und Thrombin durch Phenylbrenztraubensäuren mit verschiedenen basischen Substituenten. Acta biol med germ 1974; 33:K1-K7.

7. Walsmann P, Horn H, Markwardt F, Richter P, Stürzebecher J, Vieweg H, Wagner G. Synthetische Inhibitoren der Serinproteinasen. 11. Mitteilung: Über die Hemmung von Trypsin, Plasmin und Thrombin durch neue Bisamidinoverbindungen. Acta biol med germ 1976; 35:K1-K8.

8. Stürzebecher J, Markwardt F, Vieweg H, Wagner G, Walsmann P.
    Synthetische Inhibitoren der Serinproteinasen. 31.Mitteilung:
    Über die Hemmwirkung isomerer Verbindungen von Nα-arylsulfo-
    nylierten ω-Amidinophenyl-α-aminoalkylcarbonsäureamiden ge-
    genüber Trypsin, Plasmin und Thrombin.   Pharmazie 1984;
    39:411-413.

9. Dixon M. The determination of enzyme inhibitor constants.
    Biochem J 1953; 55:170-171.

10. Tidwell RR, Fox LL, Geratz JD. Aromatic tris-amidines. A new
    class of highly active inhibitors of trypsin-like proteases.
    Biochim Biophys Acta 1976; 445:729-738.

11. Stürzebecher J, Svendsen L, Eichenberger R, Markwardt F. A
    new assay for the determination of factor XII in plasma using
    a chromogenic substrate and a selective inhibitor of plasma
    kallikrein. Thromb Res 1989; 55:709-715.

AAS 38/I
Recent Progress on Kinins
© 1992 Birkhäuser Verlag Basel

A FINDING OF HIGHLY SELECTIVE SYNTHETIC INHIBITOR OF PLASMA KALLIKREIN; ITS ACTION TO BRADYKININ GENERATION, INTRINSIC COAGULATION AND EXPERIMENTAL DIC

S. Okamoto, K. Wanaka, A. Hijikata-Okunomiya*, Y. Okada** and Y. Katsuura***

Kobe Research Projects on Thrombosis and Haemostasis, Asahigaoka 3-15-18, Tarumi-ku, Kobe 655, *School of Allied Medical Sciences, Kobe Univ., Kobe 654-01, **Faculty of Pharmaceutical Sciences, Kobe-Gakuin Univ., Kobe 651-21, ***Life Science Research Lab. Showa Denko & Co. Ltd., Tokyo 146, Japan

SUMMARY: We found a novel and highly selective synthetic inhibitor of plasma kallikrein (PK), called PKSI-527; the Ki value was 0.81 µM. PKSI-527 inhibited the bradykinin (BK) generation induced by kaolin and prolonged partial thromboplastin time (PTT). PKSI-527 prevented the decrease of fibrinogen (Fg) levels due to i.v. injection of ellagic acid in mice and ameliorated the endotoxin (ET)-induced DIC in rats.

INTRODUCTION

For the last fifty years, Dr. Shosuke Okamoto has been searching for the highly selective synthetic inhibitors of some target proteinases, and providing some powerful tools to explore the biological significance of the respective proteinases (1). Early in his career, he discovered epsilon-aminocaproic acid (EACA) and tranexamic acid (t-AMCHA), anti-fibrinolysis agents and remedies (2).

Twenty years ago, his goal changed to finding some selective synthetic thrombin inhibitors. Dr. Okamoto and his colleagues identified "arginine derivatives", based on the evidence that thrombin cleaves the C-terminal of arginine of the fibrinogen peptides. Since then, beginning with tosyl arginine methyl ester (TAMe), the Ki of which is approximately 1mM to thrombin, step-by-step chemical modifications of TAMe were made hundreds of times, to reach MD-805, the Ki of which was 1.9×10^{-8}M. They also confirmed MD-805's very high selectivity toward thrombin and satisfactorily low toxicity (3-5). After a number of preclinical and clinical trials (6-8), MD-805 (named argatroban) was officially sanctioned as clinical remedy by the government of Japan, where it was first available for use in 1990.

Very recently, we began a series of studies to design some highly selective synthetic PK inhibitors (9, 10), encouraged by the accumulated evidence concerning the selective synthetic inhibitors of plasmin and thrombin. To determine their inhibitory actions on PK, some representative kinds of arginine derivatives, hundreds of lysine derivatives and also a number of phenylalanine derivatives were checked. Results obtained indicated that a selective synthetic inhibitor of PK assumes a characteristic structure with (i) phenylalanine as a skeleton, (ii) a N-terminal of phenylalanine which is covered with CO of t-AMCHA and (iii) a C-terminal which is covered with 4-carboxymethylaniline NH. Aprotinin, which is an inhibitor to glandular kallikrein and plasmin as well, is not a selective inhibitor to PK (11).

MATERIALS AND METHODS

Inhibitor: PKSI-527 was synthesized in our laboratory. Inhibition constant: Ki values were determined by measuring the effect of the inhibition on the hydrolytic activities of enzymes on synthetic peptide substrates (9). BK generation in plasma: This was reported previously (9). BK generation in synovial fluid: Synovial fluids were obtained from patients with osteoarthritis. Nine parts of the fluid were mixed to one part 3.8 % sodium citrate, and centrifuged 10 minutes at 1,500 g. 0.5 ml of kaolin suspension (0.4 mg/ml) was added to a mixture of 0.40 ml of synovial fluid, 0.05 ml of o-phenanthroline (60 mM) and 0.05 ml of PKSI-527 or borate saline buffer (pH 7.4), and incubated at 37°C. After incubation, reaction of 0.2 ml of the mixture was stopped by adding 0.08 ml of trichloroacetic acid (20 %). The reaction mixture was centrifuged for 10 minutes (1,500 g) at 4°C, and the amount of BK in the supernate was measured using the enzyme immuno assay method (MARKIT-A-Bradykinin kit, Dainippon Pharmaceutical Co., Osaka). Fibrinogen (Fg) decrease induced by ellagic acid (in vivo): 0.15 ml/10g body weight of Actin® (0.028 mg/ml ellagic acid, Kokusai Reagent Co., Kobe) was injected intravenously in ICR-mice, then after 10 minutes, blood was drawn from the posterior vena cava with sodium citrate. Fg levels of the blood were determined according to Ratnoff-Manzie method (12). DIC induced by ET and TP: DIC was induced in male SD-rats by intravenous (i.v.) injection of endotoxin (ET, lipopolysaccharide, E.coli, 0127:B8, Difco, Detroit) at a dose of 10 mg/kg, or i.v. infusion of thromboplastin (TP, Simplastin®, Organon Teknika Co., Turnhout) at a dose of 20 mg/kg/4hr. The inhibitor, PKSI-527, was infused intravenously for 250 minutes, starting 10 minutes prior to DIC induction. After 4 hours, blood was withdrawn and the platelet count, fibrinogen level, GPT and GOT were measured.

RESULTS

Selectivity: PKSI-527 consists of three components, trans-4-aminomethyl-cyclo-hexanecarbonyl (t-AMCHA), phenylalanine residue and carboxymethylanilide (p-APAA), with a rather simple structure (Fig. 1). PKSI-527 inhibited PK with a Ki value of 0.81 μM. By contrast, the Ki values of glandular kallikrein (GK), plasmin (PL), thrombin (TH), urokinase (UK) and factor Xa were >500 μM, 390 μM, >500 μM, 200 μM and >500 μM, respectively, indicating extremely high selectivity of PKSI-527 for PK.

BK generation: The effect of PKSI-527 on BK generation by kaolin was examined using human plasma and synovial fluid. BK generation was induced by the addition of kaolin to human plasma. PKSI-527 clearly suppressed BK generation; about 3 μM of PKSI-527 produced a 50 % inhibition (Fig. 2). As shown in Fig. 3, BK generation was also induced by kaolin in synovial fluid, and PKSI-527 apparently suppressed the BK generation in the fluid.

Coagulation: The effect of PKSI-527 on intrinsic coagulation was examined in vitro and in vivo. PKSI-527 prolonged PTT; the concentration of PKSI-527 which doubles the PTT without inhibitor was about 20 μM, which indicates the inhibition of PKSI-527 for an intrinsic coagulation pathway (Fig. 2). Furthermore, ellagic acid, intravenously injected at a dose of 0.48 mg/kg in a mouse, significantly decreased the plasma Fg levels (Fig. 4). PKSI-527 (3 mg/kg, i.v.) prevented a remarkable decrease in Fg levels. These results suggest that PK is one of the major factors in intrinsic normal coagulation.

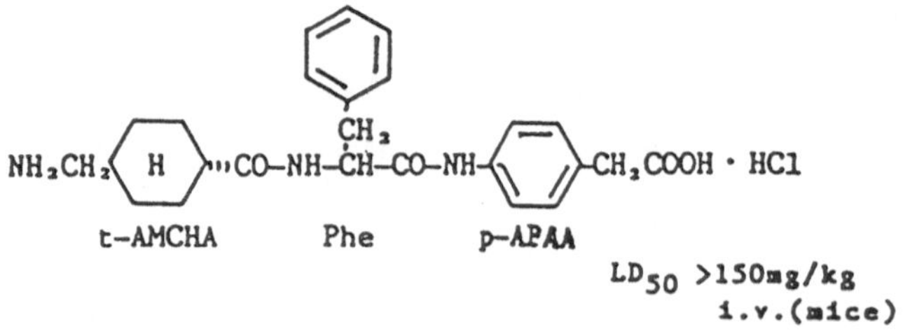

Figure 1. Chemical structure of PKSI-527

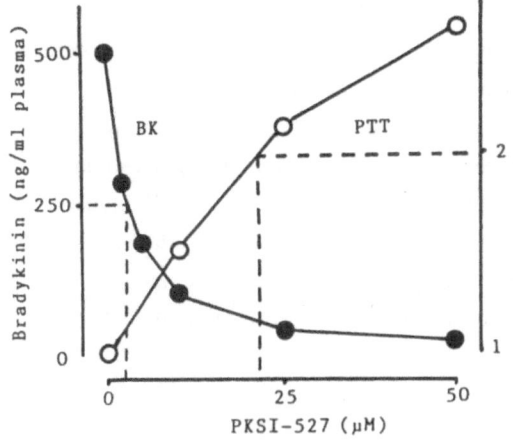

Figure 2. Inhibitory effect of PKSI-527 on BK generation by kaolin and PTT in human plasma. The left ordinate indicates the BK generated, and the right ordinate, the ratio of the clotting time (CT) with PKSI-527 to the CT without PKSI-527. The abscissa indicates the final concentration of PKSI-527.
●: BK generation, ○: PTT

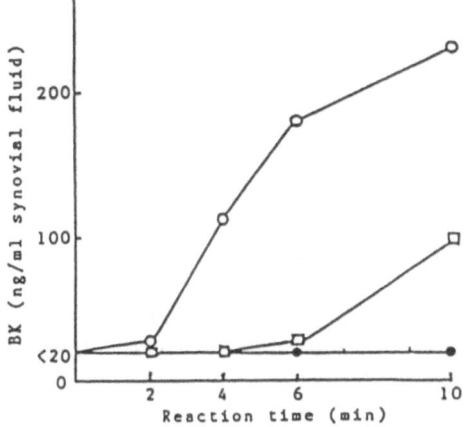

Figure 3. Inhibitory effect of PKSI-527 on BK generation by kaolin in human synovial fluid.
○: control,
□: 20 μM PKSI-527,
●: 100 μM PKSI-527.

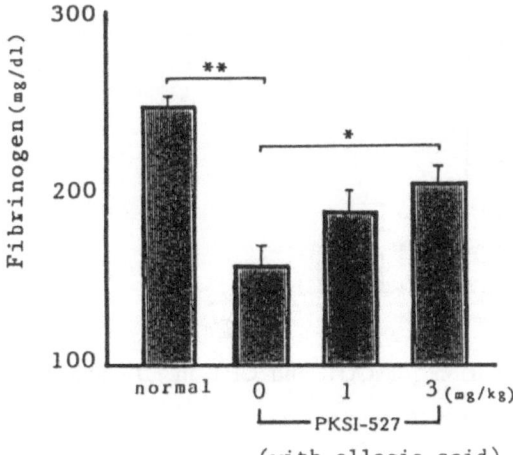

Figure 4. Effect of PKSI-527 on Fg decrease induced by ellagic acid in mice. Ellagic acid (0.42 mg/kg) was intravenously injected into mice. The ordinate indicates the plasma Fg levels after 10 minutes of the ellagic acid injection.
*: $p < 0.05$,
**: $p < 0.01$
vs. control group.

Endotoxin DIC: The effect of PKSI-527 on DIC was examined using the two DIC models, ET- and TP-induced DIC. The respective doses of ET and TP were adjusted to produce nearly the same relative changes in decreasing platelet counts and Fg levels in mice. PKSI-527, intravenously injected at a dose of 0.1 mg/kg/min, clearly prevented the decrease in platelet counts and Fg levels in the ET-induced DIC in rats; while this inhibitory activity was hardly observed in the TP-induced DIC in rats (Fig. 5). Furthermore, GOT and GPT were significantly elevated in the ET-induced DIC in rats, while no elevation was observed in the TP-induced DIC in rats. However, PKSI-527 remarkably prevented the elevation of GOT and GPT levels even in the ET-induced DIC (Fig. 6).

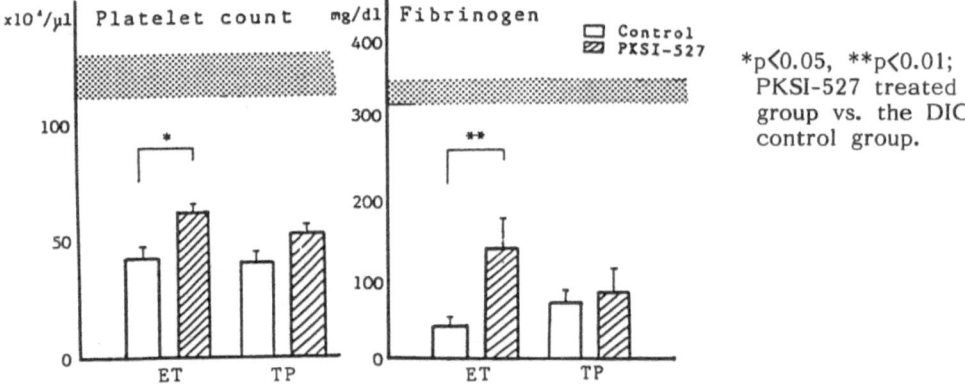

Figure 5. Effect of PKSI-527 on the decreases of platelet counts and Fg levels in ET- and TP-induced DIC. PKSI-527 was intravenously infused at a dose of 0.1 mg/kg/min for 250 minutes.

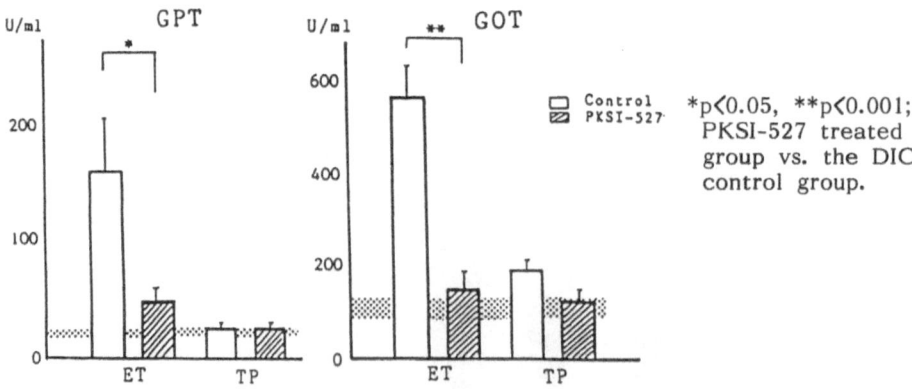

Figure 6. Effect of PKSI-527 on the elevations of GOT and GPT in ET- and TP-induced DIC.

DISCUSSION

During the past 10 years, more than 1,000 kinds of new compounds have been systematically synthesized and examined, with the aim to find highly selective inhibitors of plasmin, PK and serum cholinesterase (13, 10, 14). One of these new compounds, which we have succeeded in designing and synthesizing is PKSI-527, a selective and potent inhibitor for PK (9).

One direct action of PK is the liberation of BK from high molecular weight kininogen (15). We found that PKSI-527 showed the typical inhibitory effect for BK generation by contact activation in both human plasma and synovial fluid. A study of the pathogenesis of joint trouble may be interesting, when PKSI-527 is used to ameliorate the reaction due to BK generation. The effects of PKSI-527 on arthritis are now being investigated.

PKSI-527 prolonged PTT, but not prothrombin time (9). These results indicate that PKSI-527 suppresses the intrinsic coagulation pathway, but not the extrinsic one. Furthermore, PKSI-527 prevented the decrease of Fg, induced ellagic acid in mice. This result indicates that PKSI-527 suppresses the intrinsic coagulation, which implies that PKSI-527 might be a new type of remedy for anticoagulation.

It has been reported that ET stimulates endothelial cells and contact factors (16, 17). Our results showed a qualitative difference between the ET- and TP-induced DIC in rats. Even with nearly the same relative changes in platelet counts and Fg levels found in both kinds of DIC, remarkable elevations of GOT and GPT were observed in the ET-induced DIC, while the elevations were hardly observed in the TP-induced DIC in rats. The elevations of GOT and GPT in the ET-induced DIC are generally understood to be due to multiple organ failure (MOF), in which the effect of PK-kinin system should be considered (18-20). Results obtained indicate that PKSI-527 inhibited the appearance of pathological signs of MOF, which undoubtedly merits our further study regarding preclinical problems, using PKSI-527 as a promising tool.

CONCLUSION

We have identified a highly selective synthetic PK inhibitor, called PKSI-527, with a phenylalanine derivative chemical structure. PKSI-527 inhibited PK with a Ki value of 0.81 μM; PKSI-527 inhibited BK generation by kaolin in both human plasma and synovial fluids, prolonged PTT, and prevented Fg decrease due to ellagic acid in mice. PKSI-527 ameliorated the ET-induced DIC having the involvement of MOF, as GPT and GOT were improved in rats.

ACKNOWLEDGMENTS: The authors express their cordial thanks to Prof. Utako Okamoto for her comments and to Ms. Y. Nakaya for preparing the text.

REFERENCES

1. Okamoto S. Protease inhibitors. In: Proteinase-inhibitors and my life. Takada et al., editors. Amsterdam: Elsevier Science Publishers B.V., 1990; 207-218

2. Okamoto S, Hijikata A. Drug design VI. In: Rational approach to proteinase inhibitors. Ariëns EJ, editor. New York: Academic press, 1975: 143-169

3. Okamoto S, Hijikata A, Kikumoto R, Tonomura S, Hara H, Ninomiya K, Maruyama A, Sugano M, Tamao Y. Potent inhibition of thrombin by the newly synthesized arginine derivative No.805. The importance of stereostructure of its hydrophobic carboxamide portion. Biochem Biophys Res Commun 1981; 101:440-446

4. Kikumoto R, Tamao Y, Tezuka T, Tonomura S, Hara H, Ninomiya K, Hijikata A, Okamoto S. Selective inhibition of thrombin by (2R,4R)-4-methyl-1-[N^2-[(3-methyl-1,2,3,4-tetrahydro-8-quinolinyl)sulfonyl]-L-arginyl)]-2-piperidinecarboxylic acid. Biochem 1984; 23:85-90

5. Hijikata-Okunomiya A, Okamoto S. A strategy for rational approach to design synthetic selective-inhibitors. Seminars Thrombos Hemostas. in press.

6. Tanabe T, Mishima Y, Furukawa K, Sakaguchi S, Kamiya K, Shionoya S, Katsumura T, Kusaba A. Clinical results of MD-805, antithrombin agent, on chronic arterial occulusion. ---Multi-center cooperative study--- J Clin Thr Med 1986; 2:1645-1655

7. Matsuo T, Kario K, Kodama K, Okamoto S. Clinical application of the synthetic thrombin inhibitor, argatroban (MD-805). Seminars Thrombos Hemostas. in press.

8. Fitzgerald DJ, Fitzgerald GA. Role of thrombin and thromboxane A$_2$ in reocclusion following coronary thrombolysis with tissue-type plasminogen activator. Proc Natl Acad Sci USA 1989; 86:7585-7589

9. Wanaka K, Okamoto S, Bohgaki M, Hijikata-Okunomiya A, Naito T, Okada Y. Effect of a highly selective plasma-kallikrein synthetic inhibitor on contact activation relating to kinin generation, coagulation and fibrinolysis. Thrombos Res 1990; 57:889-895

10. Teno N, Wanaka K, Okada Y, Tsuda Y, Okamoto U, Hijikata-Okunomiya A, Naito T, Okamoto S. Development of selective inhibitors against plasma kallikrein. Chem Pharm Bull 1991; 39:2930-2936

11. Fritz H, Wunderer G. Biochemistry and applications of aprotinin, the kallikrein inhibitor from bovine organs. Drug Res 1983; 33:479-494

12. Ratnoff OD, Menzie C. New method for determination of fibrinogen in small samples of plasma. J Lab Clin Med 1951; 37:316-320

13. Teno N, Wanaka K, Okada Y, Tsuda Y, Okamoto U, Hijikata-Okunomiya A, Naito T, Okamoto S. Development of active center-directed inhibitors against plasmin. Chem Pharm Bull 1991; 39:2340-2346

14. Hijikata-Okunomiya A, Okamoto S, Okada Y, Teno N. Structure-activity relationship between arginine derivatives and inhibitory activity of horse serum cholinesterase. Bulletin of Allied Medical Sciences Kobe 1988; 4:39-46

15. Yano M, Nagasawa S, Suzuki T. Partial purification and some properties of high molecular weight kininogen, bovine kininogen-I. J Biochem 1971; 69:471-481

16. Whisler RL, Cornwell DG, Proctor KVW, Downs E. Bacterial lipopolysaccharide acts on human endothelial cells to enhance the adherence of peripheral blood monocytes. J Lab Clin Med 1989; 114:708-716

17. Roeise O, Bouma BN, Stadaas JO, Aasen AO. Dose dependence of endotoxin-induced activation of the plasma contact system: an in vitro study. Circulatory Shock 1988; 26:419-430

18. Katori M, Majima M, Odoi-Adome R, Sunahara N, Uchida Y. Evidence for the involvement of a plasma kallikrein-kinin system in the immediate hypotension produced by endotoxin in anaesthetized rats. Br J Pharmacol 1989; 98:1383-1391

19. Mason JW, Kleeberg U, Dolan P, Colman RW. Plasma kallikrein and hageman factor in gram-negative bacteremia. Ann Inter Med 1970; 73:545-551

20. Gallimore MJ, Aasen AO, Lyngaas KHN, Larsbraaten M, Amundsen E. Falls in plasma levels of prekallikrein, high molecular weight kininogen, and kallikrein inhibitors during lethal endotoxin shock in dogs. Thrombos Res 1978; 12:307-318

AAS 38/I
Recent Progress on Kinins
© 1992 Birkhäuser Verlag Basel

STUDIES ON THE DESIGN OF ORALLY ACTIVE PEPTIDE ANALOGUES

Timothy B. Frigo and James Burton

Unit for Rational Drug Design, Evans Department of Clinical Research, Boston University Medical Center, Boston, MA 02118, U.S.A.

SUMMARY:
Converting peptide inhibitors of tissue kallikrein into drugs requires, among other things, that the compounds be made orally active. Measurement of the rate at which peptides diffuse across model epithelial membranes that mimic the human gut has allowed a quantitative relationship relating lipophilicity and % absorption to be developed. The absorption of simple peptides from the human gut may be predicted with this equation.

INTRODUCTION

Most peptides cannot be used as pharmaceutical agents because of limited bioavailability.[1] Many solutions this problem have been proposed,[2] but none, to date, have found general application.

Poor bioavailability is partly due to lack of understanding of how peptides are absorbed from the gut. Until the rate limiting step which controls absorption is defined,

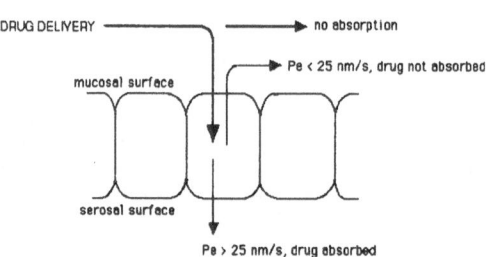

Figure 1. *How P_e is related to absorption of peptides across mucosal surfaces.*

methods of increasing bioavailability will be serendipitous. Amino acids, di- and tripeptides are actively transported from the gut.[3] Larger peptides also cross the gut, but may follow several pathways, the most usual being passive diffusion.[4] By examining a series of model peptides whose properties change in a controlled fashion, the general nature of peptide diffusion across epithelial cells may be established.

RESULTS AND DISCUSSION

The recent development of model epithelial cell lines which mimic the gut allow well controlled studies to be performed. From these studies permeability coefficients (P_e) may be obtained. P_e is the velocity with which a particular drug diffuses into a membrane. In vivo it is a measure of how deep into the epithelial barrier a peptide penetrates before it is swept away by peristalsis (Fig. 1).

Artursson and Karlsson have recently demonstrated that absorption of drugs is related to the transport of drugs across a Caco-2 cell monolayer.[5] When P_e values for various drugs are plotted against % absorption a good relationship is obtained. This data has now been fitted to an equation which relates absorption in humans and P_e (Eq. 1). This equation permits the absorption of drugs in humans to be predicted from the values of P_e observed for a monolayer of human gut cells.

$$\% \, Absorption \; = \; \frac{100}{1 \; + \; 10^{(4.9 \; - \; 3.5 \log P_e)}} \tag{1}$$

A series of six labeled cyclic dipeptides (10 Ci/mol) were synthesized.[6] These have the general form cyclo-[Gly–D–Aaa] where the Gly residue is radiolabelled (10 Ci/mol ^{3}H) and Aaa is glycine, valine, isoleucine, t–butylglycine, 4–methylisoleucine, and cyclohexylglycine. Transport studies of these compounds across T_{84} cell membranes were carried out as previously described.[7]

$K_{o/w}$ values plotted in Figure 2 are the partition coefficients for the peptide between octanol and aqueous buffer (pH 7.4). Including the volumes of the molecules obtained from CHARMm molecular mechanics calculations does not improve the fit between the highly correlated data.

In our experiments, the concentration of peptide for the experiment was varied over a range of 0.05 to 5 mM, and the change in flux of the peptide was shown to be linearly related to the concentration of the peptide. This indicates that the peptide is passed through the membrane by a diffusion controlled mechanism. In another experiment, when the flux of peptide is monitored from the serosal to mucosal sides of the membrane, no significant difference is seen between serosal to mucosal and mucosal to serosal transport rates. These results indicate that the peptide is following a diffusion controlled mechanism for transport across the membrane.

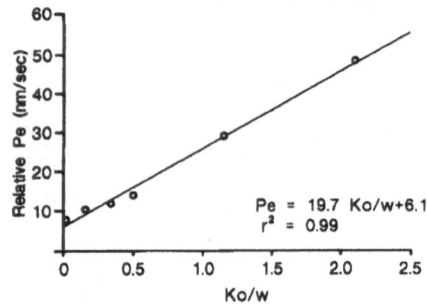

Figure 2.   *Relationship between P_e and lipophilicity for a series of peptides.*

When the permeability for each compound is plotted against the partition coefficient, the resulting graph may be fitted by linear function between lipophilicity and the permeability coefficient shown (Fig. 2). This is consistent with a model of absorption in which a rate limiting equilibrium occurs between peptide in the mucosal chamber and the outer layer of the epithelial followed by unhindered diffusion into the serosal chamber.[8]

When Equation 1 is combined with the equation shown in Figure 2 a relationship between lipophilicity and permeability is obtained (Eq. 2). This relates the measured lipophilicity of a small peptide to the % absorption expected in humans.

$$\%Absorption = \frac{100}{1 + 10^{\,4.3\ +\ 3.5\log(0.051\,K_{o/w}\ -\ 0.32)}} \qquad (2)$$

The relationship shown in Equation 2 predicts that a $K_{o/w}$ value of ~330 will be required for 50% absorption of a small peptide–based tissue kallikrein inhibitor.

REFERENCES

1.   Jackson MJ. Drug transport across gastrointestinal epithelia. In: Physiology of the Gastrointestinal Tract, 2nd Ed. Johnson LR editor. New York: Rava Press, 1987: 1597–1621.

2.   Plattner JJ, Norbeck DW. Obstacles to drug development from peptide leads. In Drug Discovery Technologies. Clark CR, Moos WH, editors. West Sussex, England: Ellis Horwood Ltd., 1991: 92–119.

3.   Matthews DM. Intestinal absorption of peptides. Physiol Rev 1975; 55:537–608.

4.   Burton PS, Conradi RA, Hilgers AR. Transcellular mechanism of peptide and protein absorption: Passive aspects. Advanced Drug Delivery Rev 1991; 7:365–386.

5.   Artursson P, Karlsson J. Correlation between oral drug absorption in humans and apparent drug permeability coefficients in human intestinal epithelial (CACO–2) cells. Biochem Biophys Res Commun 1991; 175:880–885.

6.   Greenstein JP, Winitz M. Chemistry of the Amino Acids. Vol. 2. New York: John Wiley & Sons, 1961: 797.

7.   Madara JL, Dharmsataphorn K. Occluding junctional structure–function relationships in a cultured epithelial monolayer. J Cell Biol 1985; 101:2124–2133.

8.   Frigo TB, Madara JL, Delp C, Burton J. Structure–activity relationships for peptide diffusion across model human intestinal epithelium. J Med Chem 1992; In press.

AAS 38/I
Recent Progress on Kinins
© 1992 Birkhäuser Verlag Basel

A SYSTEMATIC APPROACH FOR DETERMINING MINIMUM INHIBITORY SEQUENCE AND CONTRIBUTION OF INDIVIDUAL RESIDUES IN BINDING OF KININOGEN FRAGMENTS TO TISSUE KALLIKREIN

Milind S. Deshpande[1] and James Burton

Rational Drug Design, E-301, Boston University Medical Center, 88 East Newton Street, Boston, MA 02118, USA

Summary: A systematic approach to evaluate the contribution of individual residues occurring within the sequence Ser[386]-Pro-Phe-Arg-Ser-Val-Gln[392] from bovine kininogen towards binding to tissue kallikrein is developed. Of the 21 sequences which can be formed, no dipeptide and only one tripeptide measurably inhibits the enzyme. Almost 80% of the binding energy of the substrate analogue inhibitors comes from the core sequence Phe-Arg-Ser which occurs between P_2 and P_1'. Molecular models developed from the Chen-Bode coordinates of the aprotinin — β-PPK complex have been used to interpret the results of these studies.

Introduction

Understanding the importance of tissue kallikrein in various biologic processes may depend on development of *specific* tissue kallikrein inhibitors which can be used in vivo. The kinin receptor blockers, protease inhibitors such as aprotinin and its fragments and chloromethyl ketones have been extremely valuable for the study of the biological effects of kinins. The receptor blockers, however, do not identify the source of kinins, and the protease inhibitors do not appear to be specific for tissue kallikrein. Tissue kallikrein is inhibited by peptides which are homologous with the amino acid sequence of the substrate around the cleavage site. Importantly, the substrate analogue inhibitors appear to be reasonably specific for tissue kallikrein. Development of these compounds may lead to specific inhibitors necessary for study of the in vivo function of the enzyme.

In an effort to understand how the various amino acid residues in the substrate analogues interact with tissue kallikrein, all possible peptides which can be formed from residues comprising the $P_4 - P_3'$ sequence were synthesized and tested as inhibitors. Results from these studies were used to quantitate the contributions of the individual amino acid residues of the inhibitor in the enzyme/inhibitor complex.

Materials and Methods

Enzyme Inhibition: Porcine pancreatic kallikrein (β-kallikrein, lot 26F-0197, 50 units/mg protein; 1 unit hydrolyses 1.0 μM BAEE to N-α-benzoyl-L-arginine/min at pH 8.7 at 25°) was purchased from

---

[1]*Current address: Bristol Myers Squibb Pharmaceutical Research Institute, Dept. 203, 5 Research Parkway, Wallingford, CT 06492, USA.*

Sigma (St. Louis, MO). The rate of hydrolysis of BAEE was unaffected in the presence of lima bean trypsin inhibitor indicating that the enzyme preparation contained little, if any, active trypsin. The capacity of the substrate analogues to inhibit β-PPK was examined in an automated assay performed on a Biomek 1000 laboratory workstation (Beckman Instruments) using S-2266 as the substrate. Stability of the inhibitors was evaluated by taking samples of the reaction mixture after 5 min. These were subjected to reversed phase HPLC under conditions used for purification of the peptide. None of the inhibitors were significantly hydrolyzed under the conditions used to determine K_i.

Model Building: Molecular modeling was done on a Silicon Graphics IRIS 4D-70 work station using Quanta 3.0 (Polygen, Waltham, MA) software for creation, manipulation and visualization of molecular structures as previously reported. The coordinates for β-PPK/aprotinin complex were obtained from Brookhaven Protein Data Bank (Brookhaven, NY) and read into Quanta. Residues 12-18 of aprotinin were cut from the rest of the aprotinin molecule by deleting the bonds between Thr[11]-Gly[12], Ile[18]-Ile[19], and the disulfide bond between Cys[14]-Cys[38]. The aprotinin segment devoid of residues 12-18 was deleted to yield the new structure which displayed β-PPK in contact with aprotinin residues 12-18 only. These residues were then replaced by residues Ser, Pro, Phe, Arg, Ser, Val, and Gln respectively to mutate the aprotinin segment into that of the substrate analogues. After each replacement, a relatively unhindered conformation for the side chain chain atoms of each residue was determined. The structure in which all residues had been altered was energy minimized to yield the model used in these studies.

Peptide Synthesis: Peptides were synthesized on p-methylbenzhydrylamine resin by using standard techniques in solid phase synthesis. Synthetic peptides were characterized by amino acid analysis. Purity of the peptides was established by TLC and analytical HPLC. HPLC purifications were done on a Beckman ODS column (1X25 cm) with a gradient of 0-100% CH_3CN-0.2% CF_3COOH in H_2O-0.2% CF_3COOH over 20 min.

Results and Discussion

Conversion of a peptide inhibitor into a drug candidate involves size reduction and the elimination of moieties which may be labile under biologic conditions. In order to rationally eliminate non-essential residues in the peptide, quantitation of the interaction between the various residues and the target is necessary.

A systematic approach, in which all possible homologous peptides existing between any two residues in a peptide sequence are prepared and tested, is presented here. The number of non-trivial (>1 residue) substrate analogues is $\Sigma n - n$, where n is the number of amino acid residues in the synthetic sequence. For the kininogen sequence occurring between Ser[386] and Gln[392], n = 7 and the number of analogues is 21. The sequence of synthetic peptides and their inhibitory constants against β-PPK are shown in Table 1.

Table I. Inhibitory Constants and ΔG for Substrate Analogue Inhibitors

KKI-#	Sequence	K_i (μM)	ΔG (cal/mole)
1	Ac-Val-Gln-NH$_2$	NI[1]	-
2	Ac-Ser-Val-Gln-NH$_2$	NI[2]	-
3	Ac-Arg-Ser-Val-Gln-NH$_2$	950	-4287
4	Ac-Phe-Arg-Ser-Val-Gln-NH$_2$	230	-5161
5	Ac-Pro-Phe-Arg-Ser-Val-Gln-NH$_2$	167	-5358
6	Ac-Ser-Pro-Phe-Arg-Ser-Val-Gln-NH$_2$	101	-5668
9	Ac-Pro-Phe-Arg-Ser-Val-NH$_2$	266	-5071
19	Ac-Pro-Phe-Arg-Ser-NH$_2$	578	-4593
20	Ac-Pro-Phe-Arg-NH$_2$	NI[3]	-
21	Ac-Pro-Phe-NH$_2$	NI[4]	-
22	Ac-Phe-Arg-NH$_2$	NI[4]	-
23	Ac-Phe-Arg-Ser-NH$_2$	718	-4459
24	Ac-Ser-Pro-Phe-Arg-NH$_2$	2292	-3744
25	Ac-Ser-Pro-Phe-Arg-Ser-NH$_2$	223	-5180
26	Ac-Arg-Ser-NH$_2$	NI[3]	-
65	Ac-Ser-Val-NH$_2$	NI[3]	-
66	Ac-Ser-Pro-Phe-Arg-Ser-Val-NH$_2$	135	-5489
69	Ac-Phe-Arg-Ser-Val-NH$_2$	479	-4860
70	Ac-Arg-Ser-Val-NH$_2$	NI[3]	-
71	Ac-Ser-Pro-NH$_2$	NI[3]	-
72	Ac-Ser-Pro-Phe-NH$_2$	NI[3]	-

[1]NI: no inhibition (<5% > at 28 mM concentration of inhibitor.
[2]NI: no inhibition at 20 mM concentration of inhibitor.
[3]NI: no inhibition at 0.5 mM concentration of inhibitor.
[4]NI: no inhibition at 1 mM concentration of inhibitor.

The approach presented here makes it possible to evaluate the effect on K_i of addition of a residue K_i in n-3 cases for internal residues and n-2 cases for amino acid residues occurring at either terminus. Thus, addition of the N-terminal serine and C-terminal glutamine residues on K_i may potentially be evaluated in n-2 or 5 cases. Changes in K_i caused by addition of other residues may potentially be compared in n-3 or 4 cases.

Changes in the free energy of binding caused by addition of a single amino acid residue, $\Delta\Delta G$, may also be evaluated in quantitative terms by converting K_i values to ΔG (ΔG = -RTlnK_i) and then determining the effect of each residue on ΔG (Table II).

The values of $\Delta\Delta G$ obtained for addition of each amino acid residue appear to be reasonably consistent. The relatively similar changes in K_i caused by addition of a residue to a series of peptides, e.g. KKI-9 and KKI-5; and KKI-66 and KKI-6, indicate that for tissue kallikrein, inhibitors gain in affinity by filling discrete binding sites rather than by altering conformation of the inhibitors to open up new binding modes.

Table II. Calculation of $\Delta\Delta G$ for Amino Acid Residues in the Substrate Analogue Inhibitors.

Site	Residue	KKI-#	ΔG (cal/mole)	KKI-#	ΔG (cal/mole)	$\Delta\Delta G$ (cal/mole)
P_4	+Ser[386]	5	-5358	6	-5668	-310
		9	-5071	66	-5489	-418
		19	-4593	25	-5180	-587
		20	-	24	-3744	-
		21	-	72	-	-
						Average -438
P_3	+Pro[387]	4	-5161	5	-5358	-197
		69	-4860	9	-5071	-211
		23	-4459	19	-4593	-134
		22	-	20	-	-
						Average -181
P_2	+Phe[388]	3	-4287	4	-5161	-847
		70	-	69	-4860	-
		26	-	23	-4459	-
		71	-	72	-	-
P_1	+Arg[389]	2	-	3	-4287	-
		65	-	70	-	-
		72	-	24	-3744	-
		21	-	20	-	-
P_1'	+Ser[390]	1	-	2	-	-
		24	-3744	25	-5180	-1436
		20	-	19	-4593	-
		22	-	23	-4459	-
P_2'	+Val[391]	25	-5180	66	-5489	-309
		19	-4593	9	-5071	-478
		23	-4459	69	-4860	-401
		26	-	70	-	-
						Average -396
P_3'	+Gln[392]	66	-5489	6	-5668	-179
		9	-5071	5	-5358	-287
		69	-4860	4	-5161	-301
		70	-	3	-4287	-
		65	-	2	-	-
						Average -256

The effect of addition of the seryl residue at P_4 (serine) on K_i may potentially be evaluated in

5 cases (Table II). Comparison of the K_i value for KKI-5 (Ac-Pro-Phe-Arg-Ser-Val-Gln-NH$_2$, 167 μM) with that of KKI-6 (Ac-Ser-Pro-Phe-Arg-Ser-Val-Gln-NH$_2$, 101 μM) indicates that addition of the seryl residue to the substrate analogue sequence causes a measurable, though not marked, improvement in K_i . In two other cases a similar effect on K_i is also noted. These are: KKI-9 (266 μM) and KKI-66 (135 μM); KKI-19(578 μM) and KKI-25 (223 μM). In two remaining cases, (KKI-21 and KKI-72; KKI-20 and KKI-24), any change in affinity caused by addition of the seryl residue is undefined because at least one member of the pair does not have a measurable K_i. At S$_4$ Chen and Bode proposed 77that the naturally occuring glycyl residue of aprotinin does not interact with β-PPK. In the model77 used in which Gly^{12} is replaced with a seryl residue which does not appear to have any possible n77ew interactions with β-PPK that couls enhance binding. The value for $\Delta\Delta G$ at P$_4$ (-438 cal/mole) is consistent with lack of major interactions between the enzyme and the inhibitor.

Addition of the P$_3$ residue (proline) to the substrate analogues appears to have less effect on K_i than does addition of the seryl residue at P$_4$ (Table II). Changes in K_i may potentially be measured in 4 cases. Three of these are defined and show a slight improvement in K_i. One case is undefined. Both kininogen and aprotinin have a prolyl residue at P$_3$. At this position Chen and Bode propose that O of Pro^{13} in aprotinin H-bonds to N-H of Gly^{216} in the enzyme. In the model developed here, the O of Pro in KKI-5 and the N-H of Gly^{216} are 1.74 apart and the N-H-O angle is 175.4 , close to optimal for H-bond formation. This interaction would exist where the prolyl residue is replaced by an acetyl group. Loss of prolyl ring should not drastically alter the affinity of the inhibitor for the enzyme. The low value of $\Delta\Delta G$ (-181 cal/mole) is consistent with this observation.

The effect of the addition of the P$_2$ residue (phenylalanine) on K_i can potentially be evaluated in 4 cases. In three of these, at least one of the members of each pair has an undefined K_i. In the one case which is defined, KKI-4 *vs.* KKI-3, K_i is reduced approximately four fold by addition of the phenylalanyl residue. At the S$_2$ subsite the substrate analogues have a phenylalanyl residue while aprotinin has a cysteinyl residue that is part of a disulfide bridge that crosslinks the chain between positions 14 and 35. Chen an Bode hypothesize that the phenylalaninyl residue of kininogen fits into a wedge shape cavity formed between Trp^{215} and Tyr^{99} of β-PPK. The $\Delta\Delta G$ value (-847 cal/mole) for this residue is consistent with a moderate polar interaction at this position.

No inhibitor which lacks the arginyl residue measurably inhibits tissue kallikrein. Thus, while there are four potential ways to judge alterations in binding caused by addition of the arginyl residue, none yield useful information (Table III). $\Delta\Delta G$ values for the arginyl residues at P$_1$ cannot be calculated directly since analogues lacking this residue do not inhibit β-PPK in the assay employed here. Some idea of the importance of this residue can be obtained by comparing ΔG for the heptapeptide KKI-6 (-5668 cal/mole) with the sum of the contributions of the other individual residues shown in Table III. These calculations

[-5668 - (-438-181-847-1436-396-256)] give a value of -2114 cal/mole for the $\Delta\Delta G$ of the arginyl residue. The percentage contribution of each residue to the value of ΔG for KKI-6 may then be calculated as: Ser (8%), Pro (3%), Phe (15%), Arg (37%), Ser (25%), Val (7%), Gln (5%). Almost 80% of the total binding energy comes from the core sequence Phe-Arg-Ser. Summing the individual values of ΔG for each of the core residues (Table III) indicates that the tripeptide should have a ΔG of -4392 cal/mole (K_i, 800 μM) which compares well with the experimental value determined for KKI-23 (-4459 cal/mole; K_i, 718 μM).

The effect of addition of the seryl residue at $P_1{}'$ to the inhibitor sequence can potentially be evaluated in 4 cases. In only one of these (KKI-25 vs. KKI-24) are K_i values for both members defined. The effect of addition of the seryl-residue at this position is marked. The K_i value of the compound containing the seryl-residue at $P_1{}'$ is about one tenth of that of the homologous inhibitor lacking this residue. This strong effect may be contrasted with the relatively weak effect caused by addition of the same amino acid residue (serine) at P_4. At $S_1{}'$ the relatively large contribution of the serly residue to binding of the substrate analogues may also be explained by the model developed from the Chen-Bode coordinates. These authors propose that the side chain of the $P_1{}'$ residue in aprotinin (alanine) fits into a narrow channel formed between His^{57} and Cys^{42} of β-PPK. Replacement of Ala^{16} by a seryl residue indicates that the H-atom of side chain hydroxyl group is well placed to interact with either the O of the side chain amide of Gln^{41} or the O of His^{57}.

Addition of the $P_2{}'$ residue (valine) slightly improves the affinity of the inhibitors for β-PPK. Comparison of K_i values for KKI-25 and KKI-66, KKI-19 and KKI-9, KKI-23 and KKI-69, and KKI-26 and KKI-70 (Table III) indicates that addition of the valyl residue tends to increase binding somewhat. At S_2' no obvious explanation for the increase in $\Delta\Delta G$ is observed in the model. In the aprotinin — β-PPK complex S_2 is occupied by Arg^{27}. Chen and Bode suggested that energy gained by the binding of the arginyl residue permits the anomalous binding of kininogen so that the cleavage which releases lysyl-bradykinin occurs between the Met-Lys rather than, as expected, the Lys-Arg bond. Model building indicates that there is adequate room for the valyl residue in the S_2' pocket. In addition, the N-$\underline{H}$ of the valyl residue should be able to maintain the H-bond with O of Gln^{41} seen when the arginyl residue is in place.

Addition of glutamine at $P_3{}'$ improves binding of the inhibitors by a smaller amount than observed with the valyl residue at P_2'. The effect of this addition could be quantitated in two cases. Comparison of KKI-25 and KKI-6 (200 *vs*. 120 μM) and KKI-19 and KKI-1 (700 *vs*. 380 μM) indicates that affinity is almost doubled by addition of the glutaminyl residue at P_3'.

At S_3' the Ile[18] residue which occurs at P_3' of aprotinin forms two intramolecular hydrogen bonds in the Chen-Bode Model. As discussed previously these H-bonds are not possible with the kininogen substrate analogues which are missing the critical residues. Both the relatively large value for $\Delta\Delta G$ observed in these studies and the change in k_{cat}/K_m reported by Fiedler indicate that some type of interaction between the enzyme and the inhibitor does occur at this location.

References

1. Erdos, E. and Wilde A. In: Handbook of Experimental Pharmacology, Vol 25, Suppl. Erdos E. ed. Springer Verlag, New York, 1979.

2. Vavrek, R.J.; Stewart, J.M. Peptides, **1985**, 6, 161.

3. Deshpande, M.S.; Boylan, J.; Hamilton, J. A.; Burton, J. Int. J. Peptide Protein Res. **1991**, 37, 536.

4. Kettner,C.; Mirabelli, C.; Pierce, J.V.; Shaw, E. Arch. Biochem. Biophys. **1980**, 202, 420.

5. Okunishi, H.; Burton, J.; Spragg, H. Hypertension, **1986**, 8, I-114.

6. Fiedler, F. Eur. J. Biochem. **1987**, 163, 303.

7. Chen, Z.; Bode, W. J. J. Mol. Biol. **1983**, 164, 283.

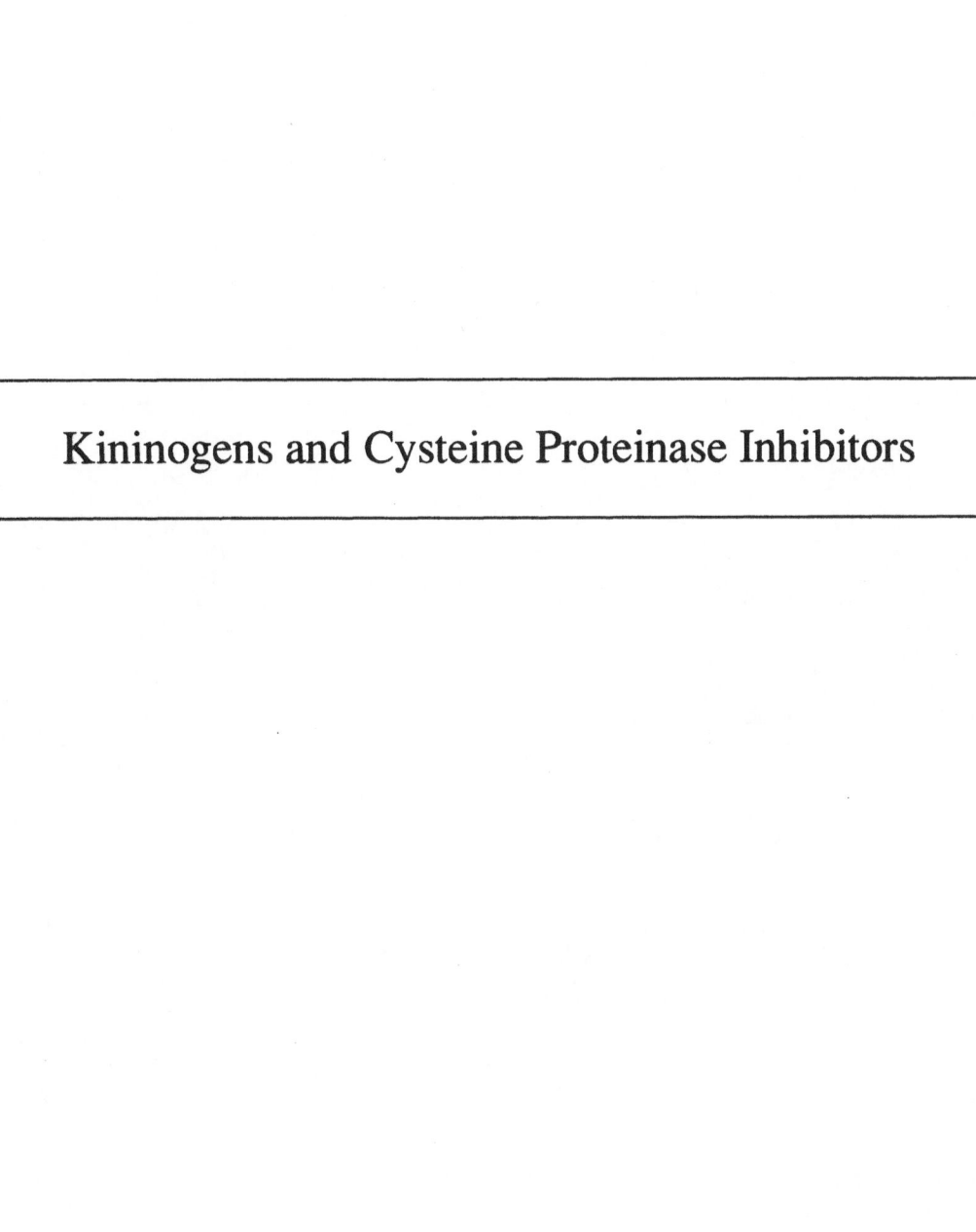

Kininogens and Cysteine Proteinase Inhibitors

HYDROXYLATED KININOGENS AND KININS

Hisao Kato and Kei-ichi Enjyoji

National Cardiovascular Center Research Institute,
Fujishirodai 5, Suita, Osaka 565, Japan

SUMMARY: Hydroxyprolyl-3-bradykinin was identified in the digest
of purified human high molecular weight (H) kininogen with plasma
kallikrein. Hydroxyproline was not detected in the heavy and
light chains portions of H kininogen, although they include three
possible sites for hydroxylation of proline by proline
hydroxylase. The content of hydroxyprolyl-3-bradykinin in H
kininogen from individual plasmas varied from 14 % to 64 % of
total kinin. The present results and our previous results
indicate that only kinin moity in H kininogen from human and
monkey plasmas has been partially hydroxylated post-
translationally by proline-4-hydroxylase.

INTRODUCTION

Hydroxyproline has been found in many proteins, including

collagen, elastin, C1q and osteocalcine. The mechanism of

hydroxylation of proline by proline hydroxylase has been

extensively studied on these proteins. Hydoxylated kinins have

been found in frog skin and wasp venom (1,2). McGee et al. found

that the third proline residue in synthetic kinin can be

hydroxylated by proline hydroxylase in 1971 (3). However, the

discovery of the hydroxylated kinin in mammalian kininogen was

made finally in 1988 by four independent groups (4, 7-9). It is

quite surprising that the presence of the kinin analogue in

kininogen was found after almost 30 years since the discovery of

bradykinin, despite the extensive studies on amino acid sequence and gene structure of kininogens. We found the hydroxylated kinins in human tumor ascites (4), human urine (5) and studied on the kinins in H kininogens from human and animal plasmas (6). We will describe the hydroxylated kinin in kininogen and discuss its possible function in the present paper.

MATERIALS AND METHODS

Human H kininogen was purified as described previously (6). Kinin-free protein was prepared by the digestion of H kininogen with plasma kallikrein. Heavy chain and light chain of the kinin-free protein was separated by gel-filtration after reduction and carboxymethylation. Reversed phase HPLC and amino acid and sequence analyses were performed as described previously (4). Synthetic hydroxyprolyl-3-bradykinin was prepared as described previously (4).

RESULTS AND DISCUSSION

The purified human H kininogen was incubated with plasma kallikrein and the digest was subjected to reversed phase HPLC. Two peaks of kinins were detected as shown in Fig. 1. These two kinins were determined to be bradykinin and hydroxyprolyl-3-bradykinin by the analyses of the amino acid composition and amino acid sequence and by the retention time of synthetic kinins. Therefore, it is clear that human H kininogen includes the hydroxylated kinin moiety, together with non-hydroxylated kinin moiety. The stereo form of the hydroxyproline in the hydroxylated bradykinin was determined to be trans-4-hydroxyproline, using isoforms of hydroxyproline (6), which

indicates that the third proline residue in bradykinin moiety was
post-translationally hydroxylated by proline-4-hydroxylase. The
result is consistent with the specificity of the hydroxylase,
-X-Pro-Gly-.

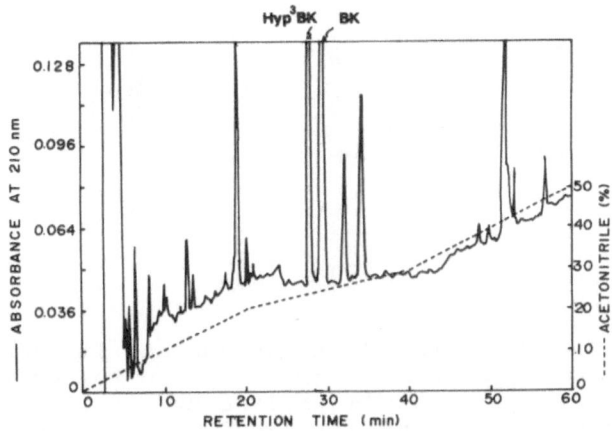

Figure 1. Separation of kinins from human H kininogen by HPLC

From the amino acid sequence of human H kininogen, we can find
one X-Pro-Gly sequence in the heavy chain portion and two in the
light chain portion as shown in Fig. 2. We isolated kinin-free
protein from human H kininogen and prepared its heavy chain and
light chain. The patterns of these derivatives on SDS-PAGE are
also shown in Fig.2. The amino terminal amino acid sequence study
on the light chain indicated that plasma kallikrein cleaved also
the peptide bonds between residue numbers 48 and 49 and between 68
and 69. The presence of hydroxyproline in the heavy chain and the
light chain was examined by the amino acid analyses after the
acid hydrolysis using Pico-Tag system. As shown in Fig. 3, no
significant amount of hydroxyproline was found in the both of
heavy and light chains. The result indicates that only kinin

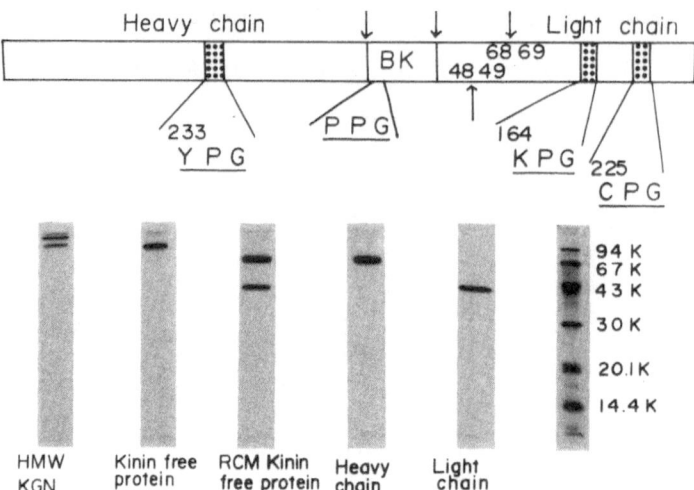

Figure. 2   SDS PAGE of human H kininogen and its derivatives.
The gross structure of human H kininogen and the position of the
possible hydroxylation sites by proline hydroxylase are shown at
the top of the figure. Number represents the residue number in
each heavy and light chain portions.

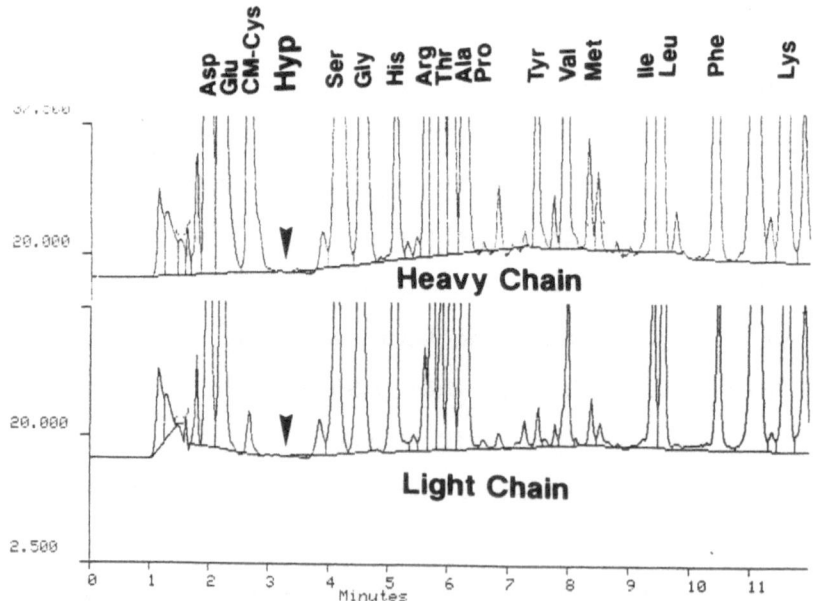

Figure.3   Amino acid analysis of heavy chain and light chain from
human H kininogen. Arrow indicates the elution position of
hydroxyproline.

moiety in human H kininogen has been hydroxylated by proline
hydroxylase.

We then examined the content of hydroxylated kinin in H kininogen
from individual plasma. Starting from 15 ml of individual plasma,
H kininogen was purified by Q-Sepharose column and zinc chelation
column. The liberated kinin from the kininogen by plasma
kallikrein was quantitated by reversed phase HPLC. As shown in
Table I, H kininogens from five individual plasma contained
various amounts of hydroxylated kinin. Similar experiments have
been reported by Maier et al.(7).

Table I Content of hydroxyprolyl-3-bradykinin in H kininogen from
individual plasma.

H kininogen	Hyp^3BK/BK mole ratio	$HypBK/(Hyp^3BK+BK)$ mole %
1	0.2/1	14
2	0.3/1	21
3	1.8/1	64
4	1.3/1	57
5	0.5/1	32

Hyp^3BK:hydroxyprolyl-3-bradykinin. BK:Bradykinin

We analyzed the liberation rate of bradykinin and
hydroxyprolyl-3-bradykinin from two H kininogens with different
hydroxylated kinin content using human plasma kallikrein.

The ratio of the initial velocity of the release of hydroxylated
kinin to non-hydroxylated kinin was comparable to the ratio of
the content of two kinins in kininogens. Although we did not make
kinetic analysis in these reactions, this result suggests that
hydroxylation of proline in bradykinin moiety does not change the

susceptibility of H kininogen to plasma kallikrein.

Using the enzyme immunoassay method, we measured the content of
hydroxylated kinin in human plasma and in animal plasmas (10) as
shown in Table II. This result clearly indicates that
hydroxylated kinin is present only in human and monkey plasmas,
but not in other animal plasmas.

We also prepared H kininogen from plasmas of monkey, guinea-pig,
rabbit and mouse and examined hydroxylated kinin by reversed
phase HPLC. We could confirm the hydroxylated kinin in monkey H
kininogen but not in H kininogen from other animals (6).

Table II Hydroxyprolyl-3-bradykinin content in human plasma and
animal plasmas (10).

Plasma	n	Hyp3BK (ng/ml)	Total kinin (ng/ml)
human	20	597	2300
monkey	10	955	1220
mouse	10	N.D.	5580
rat	10	N.D.	1160
dog	10	N.D.	4180
rabbit	10	N.D.	1070
guinea pig	10	N.D.	2180
bovine	9	N.D.	5273
pig	5	N.D.	1455

Plasma was treated with excess amounts of trypsin and the
hydroxylated kinin was measured using the monoclonal antibody
which recognized the amino terminal part of hydroxylated kinin.
Total kinin content was measured using the monoclonal antibody
which cross-reacts with the carboxy terminal part of kinin.
N.D.: Not detectable

By four independent groups, it has been demonstrated that
hydroxylated bradykinin or hydroxylated lysyl-bradykinin is
liberated from kininogen together with bradykinin or lysyl-
bradykinin. During these studies, the presence of other new

kinins, lysyl-alanyl-3-bradykinin (11) and desprolyl bradykinin
(12), has been reported. However, we now know that these new
kinins were mistakenly elucidated on hydroxylated kinins. It
should be emphasized that the identification of new kinin should
be completely consistent with all four criteria: (1), amino acid
composition, (2), complete amino acid sequence, (3), identical
retention time with synthetic new kinin on reversed phase HPLC or
other chromatographic techniques and (4), identical biological
activity with the synthetic new kinin. The lack of one of these
criteria will lead to a wrong structure of kinin.

As described in the present paper, only kinin mioety in H
kininogen is partially hydroxylated by proline hydroxylase after
the synthesis in liver microsome and secreted into blood stream.
Since heavy and light chain portions of H kininogen are
apparently not hydroxylated, cofactor activity or cysteine-
proteinase inhibitory activity of H kininogen may not be
influenced by the hydroxylation of kinin moiety. Susceptibility
of H kininogen to plasma kallikrein was also not significantly
influenced by the hydroxylation of kinin moiety. In our study,
hydroxylation of L kininogen was not examined. However, Maeir and
his colleagues domonstrated that the content of hydroxylated
kinin in L kininogen was very small (7). We have studied on the
degradation of hydroxylated kinin in plasma and could not find
any significant difference between hydroxylated and non-
hydroxylated kinins (13). A subunit of proline-4-hydroxylase is
identical with protein disulfide isomerase which catalyzes
disulfide exchange to make functionally active conformation after
the biosynthesis of proteins (14). Was the third proline residue

of bradykinin in H kininogen accidentally hydroxylated by the
action of these enzymes ? Or, is the hydroxylation necessary for
making the functionally active conformation of kininogen ? Why
are only human and monkey H kininogens hydroxylated by proline
hydroxylase, despite the presence of this enzyme in many other
animals ?

We have previously found that the content of hydroxylated kinin
in ascites from cancer patients is larger than that of non-
hydroxylated kinin (4). However, its mechanism and the
significance in tumor ascites await further investigation. One
more possible function of hydroxylated kinin which remains to be
established is the effect of biological activities of kinin. We
could expect some effect of hydroxylation on the interaction of
kinin with receptor.

REFERENCES

1. Kishimura H, Yasuhara T, Yoshida H. Chem Pharm Bull 1976;
   24:2896-2897.
2. Nakajima T, Yasuhara T, Faiconieri-Erspamer G. Experientia
   1979; 35: 1133.
3. McGee JO, Rhoads RF, Udenfriend S. Arch Biochem Biophys 1971;
   144: 343-351.
4. Maeda H, Matsumura Y, Kato H. J Biol Chem 1988; 263:16051-
   16054.
5. Kato H, Matsumura Y, Maeda H. FEBS lett 1988; 232: 252-254.
6. Enjyoji K, Kato H. FEBS lett 1988; 238: 1-4.
7. Maier M, Reissert G, Jerabek I, Lottspeich F, Binder BR. FEBS
   lett 1988; 232: 395-398.
8. Sasaguri M, Ikeda M, Ideishi M, Arakawa K. Biochem Biophys Res
   Commun 1988; 150: 511-516.
9. Mindroiu T, Carretero OA, Proud D, Walz D, Scicli AG. Biochem
   Biophys Res Commun 1988; 152: 519-526.
10. Kurooka S, Kaibe K, Ueyama H, Kido, K, Matumura Y, Maeda H,
    Kato H. J Immunol Methods 1989; 118: 147-149.
11. Mindroiu T, Scicli G, Perini F, Carretero OA, Scicli AG. J
    Biol Chem 1986; 261: 7407-7411.
12. Okuda M, Arakawa K. J Biochem 1982; 91: 633-641.
13. Matsumura Y, Maeda H, Kato H. Agents and Actions 1990; 29:
    172-180.
14. Koivu J, Myllyla R. J Biol Chem 1987; 262:6159-6164.

AAS 38/I
Recent Progress on Kinins
© 1992 Birkhäuser Verlag Basel

MAPPING OF THE H-KININOGEN BINDING SITE EXPOSED BY THE PREKALLIKREIN HEAVY CHAIN

H. Herwald, H. Hock*, W. Jahnen-Dechent, and Werner Müller-Esterl

Institute for Physiological Chemistry and Pathobiochemistry, Johannes-Gutenberg-University, Duesbergweg 6, D-6500 Mainz, Germany, and *Behringwerke AG, Postfach 1140, D-3550 Marburg, Germany

INTRODUCTION

H-kininogen, prekallikrein, factor XI and factor XII play a critical role in contact phase activation of the intrinsic blood coagulation. H-kininogen circulates in blood as a complex with either prekallikrein or factor XI. After vascular damage H-kininogen and factor XII bind to exposed negatively charged subendothelial surfaces. The local assembly of these factors allows the reciprocal activation of the zymogens prekallikrein and factor XII to the active factors, kallikrein and factor XIIa. Subsequently kallikrein cleaves H-kininogen thereby releasing the vasoactive peptide bradykinin; factor XIIa activates factor XI to factor XIa which triggers the intrinsic pathway of blood coagulation.

Six distinct domains have been identified in H-kininogen. The binding site for prekallikrein in H-kininogen has been mapped to the carboxyterminal domain D6 (1,2). Prekallikrein and factor XI are structurally closely related (3,4). Limited proteolysis of the proteins by FXIIa releases their corresponding heavy and light chains (Fig. 1). The heavy chains consists of 4 repeat units each ("apple domains" D1 to D4) of mutual sequence homology. This is followed by a short connecting region ("activation peptide") and the light chain region containing the catalytic triad of the serine proteinases ("catalytic domain").

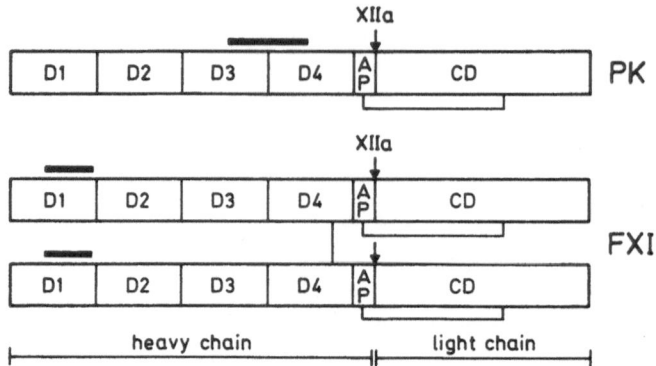

Figure 1. Domain structures of prekallikrein and factor XI.
Schematic representation of the prekallikrein (PK) and factor XI (FXI) molecules composed of four "apple" domains, D1 through D4, the connecting region, AP, and the
catalytic domain, CD [adapted from (10)]. Domains D1-D4 and AP constitute the heavy
chain; CD represents the corresponding light chain. H-kininogen binding sites mapped
for prekallikrein (7) and for factor XI (6) are indicated as solid bars above the gross
structures. The factor XIIa cleavage site generating the heavy and the light chain
portions of the molecules are given on top of the structures. Disulfide bridges linking the
chains are represented by thin lines. Note that factor XIa might use only one of the two
potential kininogen binding sites.

Prekallikrein and factor XI competitively bind to H-kininogen with similar
affinities (5) indicating that overlapping binding sites for the two factors exist in
H-kininogen. This in turn would suggest that the corresponding binding sites of
factor XI and prekallikrein are located on equivalent portions of these molecules.
The binding site for H-kininogen in factor XI has been mapped unequivocally to
apple domain 1 (6). The mutual sequence identity among the apple domains of
factor XI and prekallikrein is most pronounced for domain D1 (Table 1) as would
be expected for a common binding site. Therefore it seems likely that the H-
kininogen binding site of prekallikrein might be located in the corresponding
domain D1. Surprisingly Page and Colman (7) presented evidence for the localization of a H-kininogen binding site at the inter-domain junction of domains D3
and D4 of the prekallikrein heavy chain. In their experimental approach, monoclonal antibodies and synthetic peptides were used as probes to map the H-

kininogen binding site. Here we report on our preliminary experiments to identify the H-kininogen binding site on prekallikrein by an alternative approach, affinity cross-linking.

Table 1. Sequence identity among the apple domains D1 through D4 of factor XI and prekallikrein. Alignment of the sequences was done manually. The percentage of residues in identical positions is given.

prekallikrein		D1	D2	D3	D4
factor XI	D1	68%	34%	36%	32%
	D2	43%	63%	42%	34%
	D3	33%	52%	45%	36%
	D4	38%	36%	39%	59%

RESULTS AND DISCUSSION

Monoclonal antibody, PK6 raised against prekallikrein prevents the binding of H-kininogen to prekallikrein and is therefore likely to be directed against the H-kininogen binding site of prekallikrein (8). This antibody cross-reacts with factor XI indicating that PK6 recognizes an epitope which is well conserved among the two proteins (Fig. 2a). In a competition assay PK6 inhibited in a dose-dependent manner the binding of H-kininogen to immobilized factor XI (Fig. 2b). Furthermore a monoclonal antibody directed to the H-kininogen binding site of factor XI displaced PK6 in a concentration-dependent fashion (not shown). These results indicate that the H-kininogen binding site of factor XI identified by Baglia et al. (6) is immunologically and structurally similar to the corresponding binding site in prekallikrein.

Table 2. Primary structure of peptides HK31 (positions 565 to 595 human H-kininogen) and an aminoterminal version thereof, Tyr^0-HK31.

```
  S D D D W I P D I Q T D P N G L S F N P I S D F P D T T S P K
Y S D D D W I P D I Q T D P N G L S F N P I S D F P D T T S P K
```

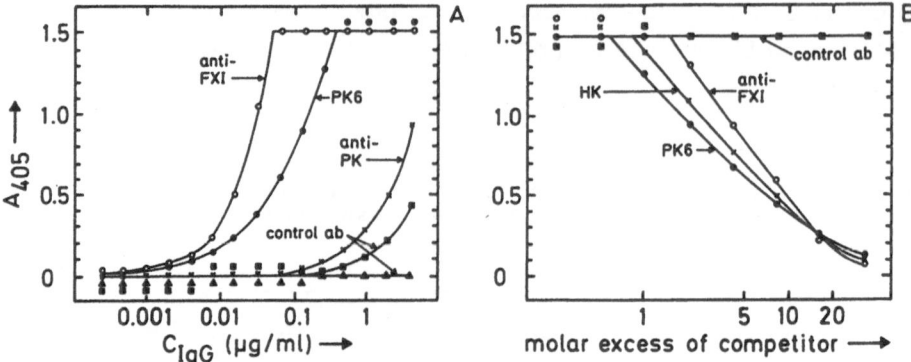

Figure 2. Cross-reactivity of monoclonal antibody PK6 with factor XI.
Panel A: For the indirect ELISA microtiter plates were coated with 0.5 μg/ml of factor XI. Serial dilutions (2^n) of antibodies against prekallikrein, i.e. monoclonal antibody PK6, affinity-purified polyclonal anti-prekallikrein IgG (anti-PK), monoclonal antibodies PK2 and PK4 were prepared (starting concentration 4 μg/ml) and delivered to the titer plate. For control, polyclonal anti-factor XI IgG (anti-FXI) was applied. Bound IgG was detected by peroxidase-coupled secondary antibodies using 2,2'-azino-di-(3-[ethylbenzthiazolin-sulfonat-(6)]) (ABTS) as the substrate.
Panel B: For the competitive ELISA, serial dilutions were prepared (2^n) of monoclonal antibody PK6, affinity-purified polyclonal anti-factor XI IgG, native H-kininogen and control antibody PK2. One hundred μl of each dilution was mixed with an equal volume of biotinylated H-kininogen (0.5 μg/ml), and applied to the wells of the plate previously coated with 0.5 μg/ml of factor XI. Bound H-kininogen was detected by the avidin-peroxidase complex and ABTS.

      To label the H-kininogen binding site in prekallikrein by affinity cross-linking we have synthesized peptides covering the prekallikrein binding site of H-kininogen (Table 2). The efficiency of cross-linkage of peptide HK31 (31mer) covering the entire prekallikrein binding site of H-kininogen was tested with monoclonal antibody HKL19 which specifically recognizes this peptide. Following complex formation between HK31 and HKL19, the homobifunctional crosslinker BS^3, bis(sulfosuccinimidyl) suberate was applied. The chemically linked antigen-antibody complex was subjected to SDS electrophoresis under reducing conditions, followed by immunoprint analysis using a specific poly-clonal antibody directed to HK31. Figure 3 illustrates that HK31 was cross-linked both to the heavy (50 kDa) and light (25 kDa) chains of HKL19 (Fig. 3, lanes 3, 4). Application of increasing concentration of the crosslinking reagent,

BS[3] resulted in the appearance of an additional band of 150 kDa (Fig. 3, lane 1,2) representing HKL19-HK31 complexes with extensive intra-molecular cross-linkage. Specificity of the cross-linking procedure was demonstrated by the application of an unrelated monoclonal antibody (raised against the nonapeptide bradykinin) which failed to give any cross-linkage with HK31 (Fig. 3, lane 5).

For the direct visualization of the HK31-prekallikrein conjugates a ^{125}I-labelled derivative of HK31 (^{125}I-Tyr[0]-HK31) was applied. Several chemical cross-linkers including BS[3], disuccinimidyl suberate (DSS), disuccinimidyl tratrate (DST), and difluorodinitrobenzene (DFDNB) were applied (Fig. 4). Among these, DST proved to be most suitable because it effectively crosslinked HK31 to prekallikrein without causing extensive intramolecular cross-linkage of prekallikrein as was observed with DSS (cf. Fig. 4, lanes 2 and 3).

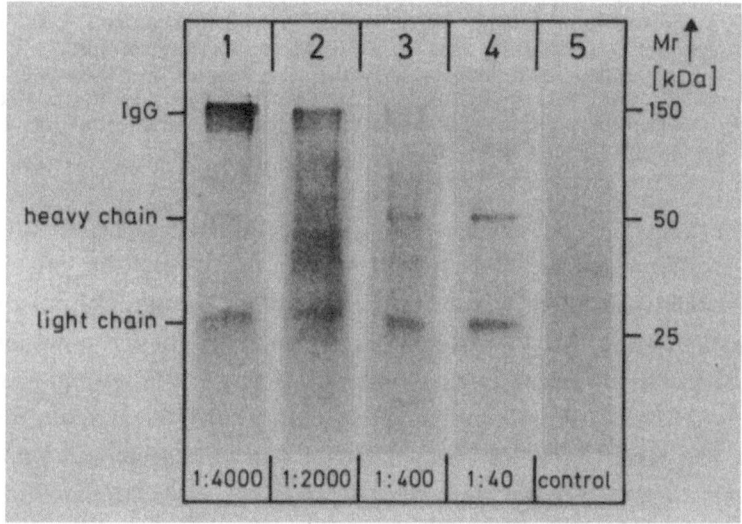

Figure 3. Specifity of cross-linking probed by monoclonal antibody HKL19 and peptide HK31.
The monoclonal antibody HKL19 directed to the prekallikrein binding site of H-kininogen was incubated with peptide HK31 (molar ratio of HKL19 to HK31 1:4) in presence of increasing concentration of crosslinker BS[3] (molar ratio of HKL19 to BS[3] is given below the lanes. The mixtures were separated by SDS polyacrylamide gel electrophoresis under reducing conditions, followed by Western blotting. The cross-linked peptide was detected by polyclonal anti-HK31 antibodies and a secondary peroxidase-labelled antibody. Note that the antigen binding sites of both immunoglobulin chains are labelled.

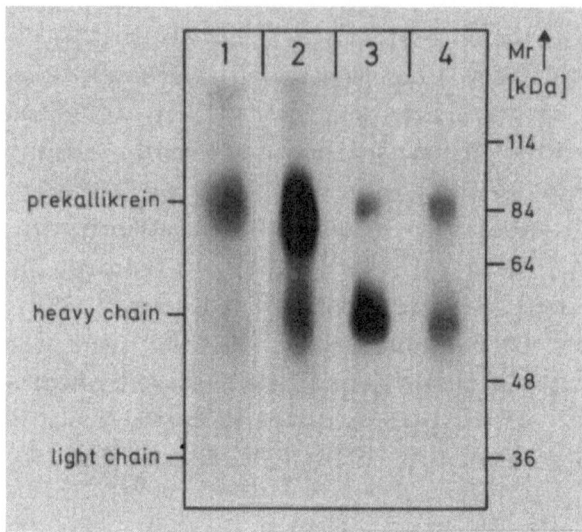

Figure 4. Affinity cross-linking of partially activated prekallikrein.
Prekallikrein was incubated with ^{125}I-Tyr^0-HK31 and various cross-linkers: lane 1, BS^3 [bis(sulfosuccinimidyl) suberate]; lane 2, DSS (disuccinimidyl suberate); lane 3, DST (disuccinimidyl tartarate), and lane 4, DFDNB (1,5-difluoro-2,4-dinitrobenzene). Note that DST (lane 3) cross-linked substantial amounts of the labelled peptide to the native prekallikrein and its heavy chain while intramolecular cross-linking was low compared to other cross-linkers (cf. lanes 1 and 2).

To further map the H-kininogen binding site, we have generated ^{125}I-labelled prekallikrein which was used as an internal marker. SDS electrophoresis and autoradiography (Fig. 5) revealed several distinct bands representing auto-catalytic degradation products of (pre)kallikrein (their relative molecular masses (9) are given in parenthesis): native prekallikrein (85/88 kDa), the heavy chain (52 kDa), the light chain (33/36 kDa), the carboxyterminal fragment of the heavy chain including apple domains D3 and D4 (28 kDa), and the aminoter-minal fragment of the heavy chain comprising apple domain D1 (18 kDa). Cross-linking of the labelled protein with peptide PK31 with DST resulted in an extra-band of M_r 58 kDa likely to represent an adduct of the heavy chain and HK31 of 3.5 kDa (cf. Fig. 5, lanes 1 and 2). Using unlabelled prekallikrein and ^{125}I-Tyr^0-HK31 extra bands of approximately 92 kDa, 58 kDa and 25 kDa were visible (not shown) suggesting that HK31 cross-linked to the parent molecule, its heavy chain and the 18 kDa fragment, respectively.

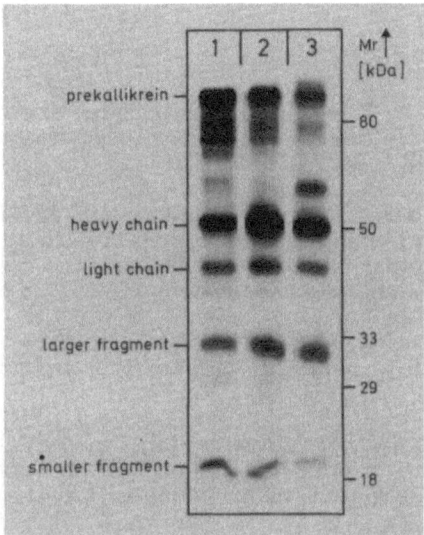

Figure 5. Affinity cross-linking of peptide HK31 and ^{125}I-prekallikrein.
Partially activated ^{125}I-prekallikrein (lane 1) which had been cross-linked in the absence (lane 2) or presence (lane 3) of peptide HK31 was resolved by SDS electrophoresis and visualized by autoradiography. Major fragments are identified on the left, and their apparent M_r are given on the right.

CONCLUSION

Together our results confirm that the H-kininogen binding site is located on the heavy chain of prekallikrein. Preliminary evidence suggests that the aminoterminal portion of the prekallikrein heavy chain might harbor relevant binding site(s) for H-kininogen. Refinement of the labelling and separation techniques should allow us to further narrow down the relevant binding segment of the molecule.

ACKNOWLEDGEMENTS

This work was supported by grants from the Deutsche Forschungsgemeinschaft and the Fonds der Chemischen Industrie (to WME). The secretarial help of S. Holz and the graphic work of E. Haas are gratefully appreciated.

REFERENCES

1. Tait JF, Fujikawa K Primary structure requirements for the binding of human high molecular weight kininogen to plasma prekallikrein and factor XI. J Biol Chem 1987; 262:11651.

2. Vogel R, Kaufmann J, Chung DW, Kellermann J, Müller-Esterl W Mapping of the prekallikrein binding site of human H-kininogen by ligand screening of lambda gt11 expression libraries. Mimicking of the predicted binding site by anti-idiotypic antibodies. J Biol Chem 1990; 265:12494.

3. Chung DW, Fujikawa K, McMullen BA, Davie EW. Human plasma prekallikrein, a zymogen to a serine protease that contains four tandem repeats. Biochemistry 1986; 25:2410.

4. Fujikawa K, Chung DW, Hendrickson LE, Davie EW. Amino acid sequence of human factor XI, a blood coagulation factor with four tandem repeats that are highly homologous with plasma prekallikrein. Biochemistry 1986; 25:2417.

5. Thompson RE, Mandle R, Kaplan AP. Studies of binding of prekallikrein and factor XI to high molecular weight kininogen and its light chain. Proc Natl Acad Sci USA 1979; 76:4862.

6. Baglia FA, Jameson BA, Walsh PN. Localization of the high molecular weight kininogen binding site in the heavy chain of human factor XI to amino acids phenylalanine 56 through serine 86. J Biol Chem 1990; 265:4149.

7. Page JD, Colman RW Localization of distinct functional domains on prekallikrein for interaction with both high molecular weight kininogen and activated factor XII in a 28-kDa fragment (amino acids 141-371). J Biol Chem 1991; 266:8143.

8. Hock J, Vogel R, Linke RP, Müller-Esterl W. High molecular weight kininogen-binding site of prekallikrein probed by monoclonal antibodies. J Biol Chem 1990; 265:12005.

9. Hojima Y, Pierce JV, Pisano JJ. Purification and characterization of multiple forms of human plasma prekallikrein. J Biol Chem 1985; 260:400.

10. McMullen BA, Fujikawa K, Davie, EW Location of the disulfide bonds in human plasma prekallikrein: the presence of four novel apple domains in the amino-terminal portion of the molecule. Biochemistry 1991; 30:2050.

AAS 38/I
Recent Progress on Kinins
© 1992 Birkhäuser Verlag Basel

CHARACTERIZATION OF CELL BINDING AND THROMBIN INHIBITORY REGIONS ON KININOGENS' HEAVY CHAIN

Y. P. Jiang and A. H. Schmaier

Thrombosis Research Center, Temple University School of Medicine, Philadelphia, PA 19140, and Division of Hematology and Oncology, Department of Internal Medicine, Simpson Memorial Research Institute, The University of Michigan Medical Center, Ann Arbor, MI 48109-0724 USA

This project was supported in part by a grant from the W.W. Smith Charitable Trust, and a grant (HL35553) from the National Institutes of Health. Dr. Schmaier is a recipient of a Research Career Development Award, HL01615.

SUMMARY: Investigations have been performed to determine the domain(s) on kininogens' heavy chain that binds to platelets and contains thrombin inhibitory region Domain 3, but not domains 1 or 2, completely inhibited ^{125}I-HK binding to platelets (K_i=24 nM $\pm$ 7, n=4). D3 binding to platelets was saturable with an apparent Kd of 39 nM $\pm$ 8 (n=4) and 1227 $\pm$ 404 binding sites/platelet. D3 inhibited ^{125}I-thrombin binding to platelets which prevented thrombin-induced platelet aggregation and secretion. These studies indicate that D3 on kininogens' heavy chain contains a cell binding region and another region which inhibits thrombin binding and activation of platelets.

INTRODUCTION

Although a single gene directs their synthesis, kininogens are present in the plasma in two different forms: high molecular weight kininogen (HK) with Mr = 120 kDa and low molecular weight kininogen (LK) with Mr = 66 kDa (1,2). There are numerous functions for the plasma kininogens. Firstly, the light chain of HK contains procoagulant activity which functions as a cofactor for the activation of the plasma zymogens including factor XII, prekallikrein, and factor XI (3-5). Secondly, both kininogens are the parent proteins for the nonapeptide bradykinin and the decapeptide lys-bradykinin. Thirdly, domains 2 and 3 of kininogens' heavy chains have cysteine protease inhibitory activity and contain a repeating amino acid sequence of glu-val-val-ala-gly which is highly conserved in cysteine proteases. Fourthly, domain 2 uniquely appears to be a good inhibitor of calpains, calcium-dependent tissue cysteine proteases (6). Fifthly, both HK and LK inhibit α-thrombin (IIa) binding to and activation of platelets (7,8). Lastly, studies also indicate that HK and LK directly bind to platelets and human endothelial cells (7-9). Since both HK and LK bind to platelets and inhibit thrombin binding to platelets, a cell binding site and a thrombin-inhibitory region must be contained on the heavy chain of kininogens. In this investigation the specific domain on the heavy chain of the plasma kininogens that contains the cell binding region to platelets and endothelial cells is identified. Further studies also show that this domain contains a region which has the ability to prevent thrombin binding to platelets.

MATERIALS AND METHODS

Plasmas, platelets, and human umbilical vein endothelial cells. Pooled normal plasma (lot N10) was purchased from George King Biomedical, Inc., Overland Park, KS. Total kininogen-deficient plasma, (i.e. deficient in both HK and LK), was donated by the late Mayme Williams of Philadelphia, PA. Fresh platelets were obtained from medication-free donors after obtaining their informed consent and blood was collected by venipuncture into 1/9 vol 3.8% sodium citrate. Platelet-rich plasma and gel filtered platelets were prepared according to the procedures described previously (7). Endothelial cells from human umbilical veins (HUVEC) which were grown to confluence on fibronectin-coated 96-well microtiter plates as described previously (9) were generously donated by Dr. Dougles B. Cines of the University of Pennsylvania, Philadelphia, PA.

Functional and immunochemical assays. HK procoagulant activity was measured by a one-stage activation assay (10) Purified HK and LK were quantitated by single radial immunodiffusion using antisera directed towards total human kininogen antigens. The concentration of these purified proteins was determined by reference to either purified HK or Fitzgerald plasma (plasma deficient in HK but containing 40% normal levels of LK) which had been previously assayed.

Purification of LK and its domains. LK was isolated from fresh human plasma by carboxyl-papain affinity chromatography followed by kaolin adsorption (11,12). Purified LK was then treated by limited digestion with trypsin (Ec 3,4,21,4 from bovine pancreas) according to the method of Salvesen et al. (13). the 20 kDa (domain 3) and 44 kDa peptides were separated by a Sephadex G75 gel filtration. The 44 kDa tryptic peptide was further digested for 20 min at 37°C with chymotrypsin at an enzyme to peptide weight ratio of 1:20 in 50 mM Tris-HCl buffer, pH 7.5. The reaction was stopped by addition of DFP (2 mM final concentration). The chymotrypsin-digested preparation was loaded on the CM-Papain-Sepharose column. The 23 kDa peptide of domain 2 bound to the column; a 17 kDa peptide which should be domain 1 did not bind to the column. The 23 and 17 kDa peptides were collected and concentrated and run on a Sephadex G75 gel filtration column to confirm their purity (11,12).

Iodination of proteins and binding experiments. Purified HK and domains of LK were radiolabeled with Na[125]I using Iodogen by the method of Fraker and Speck (14) under conditions previously described (7).

Expression and calculation of binding experiment data. Binding experiments were performed according to the procedures previously described (7). Nonspecific binding was measured in the presence of a 30-fold molar excess unlabeled domain 3 (D3) or 200-fold molar excess unlabeled HK.

Competition of ^{125}I-HK binding to HUVEC by unlabeled D3. HUVEC in microtiter plates (4 X 10^4 cells/per well) were cooled to 4°C and washed three times in Hepes-Tyrode's buffer containing 50 μM $ZnCl_2$. The cells were then incubated at 4°C for various periods of time with ^{125}I-HK (10 nM) in the absence or presence of unlabeled D3. After washing each well eight times with the Hepes-Tyrode's buffer, 50 ml of 1 N NaOH was added to each well to remove the cells from the plate. Total binding was determined by measuring the amount of ^{125}I-HK bound to the cells in the absence of any competitor and nonspecific binding was determined by the amount of ^{125}I-HK binding to HUVEC in the presence of 50-fold molar excess of unlabeled HK.

Platelet aggregation and secretion studies. Platelet aggregation and secretion studies were performed according to the methods described previously (7,12).

RESULTS

Indirect and direct binding of D3 to platelets. To determine the domain on kininogens' heavy chain that contained its binding site to platelets, washed platelets were incubated with ^{125}I-HK and increasing concentration of the purified, unlabeled domains (Figure 1). Specific ^{125}I-HK binding to platelets was completely inhibited by 25-fold molar excess domain 3, but not domain 1 or 2. D3 inhibited ^{125}I-HK binding to platelets with a mean IC_{50} of 50 nM from four experiments (Figure 1), which calculates to an apparent Ki of 24±7 nM. Further, unlabeled D3 inhibited ^{125}I-D3 binding to platelets with apparent Ki of 15±3 nM, n=3 (data not shown).

Time course studies of D3 binding to platelets and HUVEC. When washed platelets were incubated with ^{125}I-D3 , there was specific ^{125}I-D3 binding to platelets (Figure 2A). Both unlabeled D3 or HK were competitors to ^{125}I-D3 binding to platelets. Further studies were performed to determine if D3 would inhibit ^{125}I-HK binding to human umbilical vein endothelial cells (HUVEC). Binding of ^{125}I-HK to HUVEC was inhibited by unlabeled D3 (Figure 2B).

Reversibility and Saturability of D3 binding to platelets. The binding of ^{125}I-D3 to platelets was fully reversible (data not shown). When a 35-fold molar excess unlabeled D3 was added at 10, 30, and 50 min after binding of ^{125}I-D3 to platelets, the level of the bound radioligand decreased rapidly to the level of nonspecific binding. When increasing concentrations of ^{125}I-D3 were added to platelets in the absence or presence of a 35-fold molar excess unlabeled D3, a plateau of specific binding was observed between 30 and 40 nM added radioligand (data not shown). A single saturable binding site was found with a mean Kd of 39 nM ± 8 and 1227 ± 404 sites/platelet (n=4).

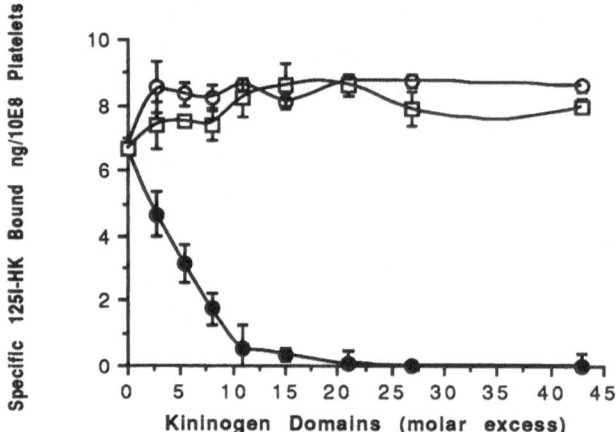

Figure 1.. **Competition of** ^{125}**I-HK binding to platelets by LK domains.** Gel-filtered platelets (2.0 x 10^8/ml) in Hepes-Tyrode's buffer were incubated for 20 min with 10 nM ^{125}I-HK in the presence of 50 μM Zn^{2+} and increasing concentration (10 to 430 nM) of unlabeled LK domains [D1(O), D2(□), and D3(●)]. Nonspecific binding was determined by adding a 50 molar excess of unlabeled HK. Specific binding was calculated by subtracting nonspecific binding from the total ^{125}I-HK binding. The figure presented is the mean ± SD of the data derived from four experiments.

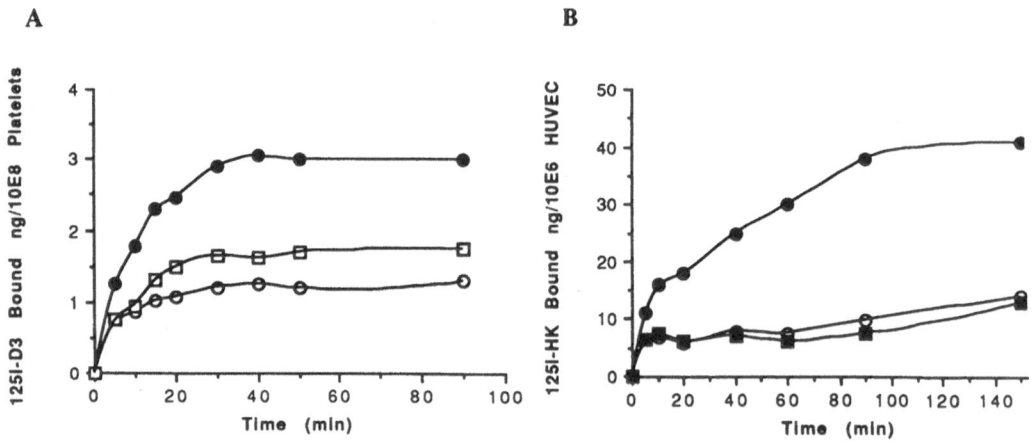

Figure 2. **(A).** **Time course of D3 binding to platelets.** Gel-filtered platelets (2.0 x 10^8/ml) in Hepes-Tyrode's buffer were incubated for 5 to 90 min at 37°C with ^{125}I-D3 (30 nM) without any competitor [●]. At each time point, samples were removed and the bound ^{125}I-D3 was separated from unbound. Nonspecific binding was measured concomitantly using replicate incubates containing a 35-fold molar excess of unlabeled D3 [O] or 200-fold molar excess HK [□]. The data plotted are the mean of 3 experiments. **(B). Competition of** ^{125}**I-HK binding to HUVEC by unlabeled D3.** Confluent monolayers of HUVEC in microtiter plates were

washed with Hepes-Tyrode's buffer, chilled on ice, and incubated with ^{125}I-HK (10 nM) in the absence (●)or presence of 30-fold molar excess of unlabeled D3 [■] for the indicated length of time. Nonspecific binding was determined by measuring the amount of ^{125}I-HK that binds to the cells in the presence of a 50-fold molar excess of unlabeled HK [○].

Effect of D3 on ^{125}I-thrombin binding to platelets and thrombin-induced platelet activation. Both HK or D3 were able to inhibit ^{125}I-thrombin binding to platelets (Figure 3A). Further studies were performed to determine if D3 binding to platelets, like HK and LK (10,11) could also influence platelet function (Figure 3B). Washed platelets activated with α–thrombin had an initial change in light transmittance of 50 Units/min. When purified HK was added, platelet aggregation was completely inhibited (5 Units/min), as previously reported (10). Similarly when purified D3 was added, platelet aggregation was also inhibited to a light transmittance value of less than 1 Unit/min (Figure 3B). D3 was also found to block thrombin-induced platelet secretion, independent of aggregation (Table I). D3, like HK and LK (10), decreased the ability of thrombin to induce secretion of a platelet-dense granule marker ([14C]5-hydroxytryptamine) in concentration-dependent fashion. The IC$_{50}$ for HK inhibition of thrombin-induced platelet secretion was between 30 to 50 nM versus an IC$_{50}$ between 125 to 200 nM for D3.

Table 1. HK and D3 inhibition of α-thrombin-induced platelet secretion

Dose	HK Treatment[*,+]	D3 Treatment[*,+]
μM	% secretion	
0	73	73
0.015	53	70
0.03	46	61
0.05	3	57
0.125	1	51
0.2	5	33
0.3	3	20
0.4	0.3	12
0.6	0	10

*Gel-filtered [14C]5-hydroxytryptamine radiolabeled platelets (2 x 10[8]/ml) were incubated in the absence or presence of each concentration of the HK or D3 indicated in the column under "Dose".

The reaction was initiated by the addition of 0.125 Unit/ml human α-thrombin. The data are the means of two full experiments on different samples of washed platelets with all of the concentrations of kininogen indicated.

+The numbers shown under the columns "HK" and "D3" represent percent secretion of [14C]5-hydroxytryptamine measured after the introduction of the thrombin.

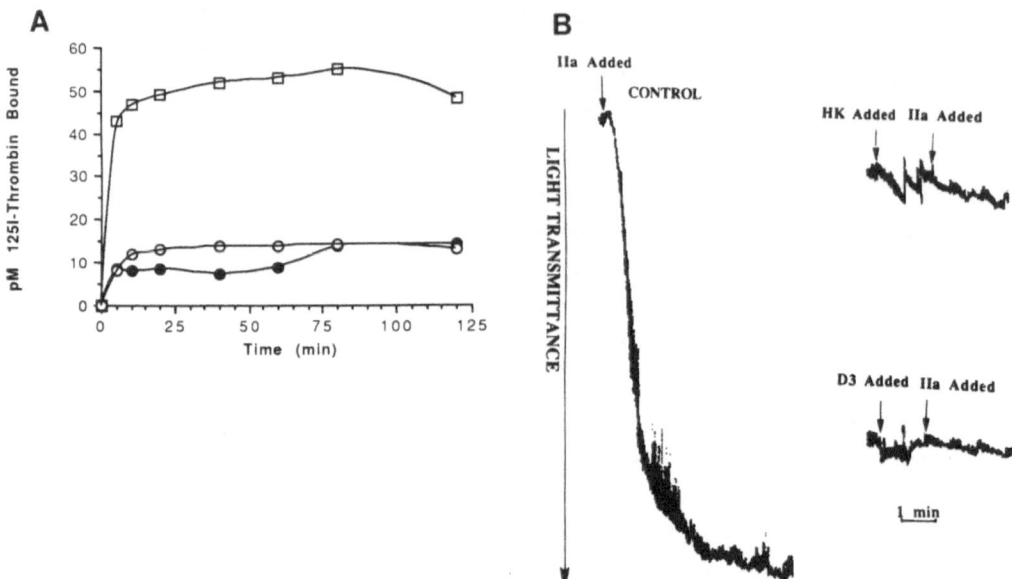

Figure 3. **D3 inhibition of thrombin-induced platelet activation by preventing thrombin binding.** (A). D3 inhibition of radiolabeled thrombin binding to platelets. Gel-filtered platelets (2×10^8/ml) in Hepes-Tyrode's buffer containing 50 μM $ZnCl_2$ and 2 mM $CaCl_2$ were incubated for 5-120 min at 37°C with 1 nM ^{125}I-thrombin alone [□] or in the presence of 200 nM HK [●] or 200 nM D3 [○]. The data plotted are the mean of two independent experiments. (B). HK and D3 inhibition of thrombin-induced platelet activation. Gel-filtered platelets (2.0×10^8/ml) in Hepes-Tyrode's buffer were treated with 1 μM HK or D3 for 1 min before the introduction of human thrombin (0.125 U/ml), indicated by the arrows. The platelet aggregation was measured for 5 min after the introduction of the agonist. **CONTROL** platelets received an identical volume of buffer. The figure is a representative experiment of three performed with different platelet donors and different batches of HK and D3 which were carefully dialyzed to remove any trace of proteolytic inhibitors added during their preparation.

DISCUSSION

The present studies were undertaken to further define the importance of kininogens' interaction with cells and to determine what domain on kininogens' heavy chain participates in these protein interactions. The current studies indicated that domain 3 of kininogens contained a cell binding region binding for platelets and HUVEC and a region to inhibit thrombin binding to platelets.

The importance of D3's ability to block ^{125}I-α-thrombin from binding to platelets was shown by further studies which indicate that D3 inhibited thrombin activation of platelets. D3, like HK and LK, has the ability to inhibit α–thrombin-induced platelet aggregation.and platelet secretion of [^{14}C] 5-hydroxytryptamine (7). However, D3 is a less efficient inhibitor of thrombin-induced platelet secretion than HK. The IC_{50} for HK's inhibition of secretion was between 30 to 50 nM but the IC_{50} for D3's inhibition was between 125 to 200 nM. These data are further confirmation that the kininogens are noncompetitive inhibitors of thrombin binding and activation of platelets. The larger, bulkier molecules of HK and LK serve as better noncompetitive inhibitors that the smaller D3. Alternatively, there is more than one binding site on HK that allows this larger molecule to function as a better inhibitor of thrombin-induced platelet secretion than D3. Studies from our laboratory indicate that there is a another region on the light chain of HK which also participates in its binding to platelets (15).

The finding that the kininogens and their cell binding domain inhibit thrombin binding to platelets suggest an antithrombotic function for this protein. The presence of HK in plasma requires higher concentrations of γ-thrombin to produce platelet aggregation (8). It is of interest that HK has the ability to decrease the heparin-induced enhancement of the rate of inactivation of α-thrombin by antithrombin (16). These direct anti-thrombotic effects are supported by further indirect influences of the kininogens on thrombosis. Bradykinin when liberated from the kininogens is a potent stimulator of prostacyclin production (17) and inducer of tissue-type plasminogen activator secretion from endothelial cells *in vivo* (18). It is as yet unclear whether these influences translate into a clinical increased risk for thrombosis in kininogen deficiency states.

REFERENCES

1. Vogel R, Asstolg-Machleidt I, Esterl A, Machleidt W, Muller-Esterl W. Proteinase-sensitive regions in the heavy chain of low molecular weight kininogen map to the inter-chain junctions. J Biol Chem 1988; 263:12661-12668.

2. Kitamara N, Kitagawa H, Fuknshima D, Takagaki Y, Miyata T, Nakanishi S. Structural organization of the human kininogen and a model for its evolution. J Biol Chem 1985; 260: 8610-8617.

3. Kerbiriou DM, Griffin JH. Human high molecular weight kininogen: studies of structure-function relationships and of proteolysis of the molecule occurring during contact activation of plasma. J Biol Chem 1979; 254:12020-12027.

4. Schiffman S, Mannhalter C, Tyner KD. Human high molecular weight kininogen. J Biol Chem 1980; 255:6433-6438.

5. Mandle R JR, Colman RW, and Kaplan AP. Identification of prekallikrein and high molecular weight kininogen as a complex in human plasma. Proc Natl Acad Sci 1976; 73:4179-4183.

6. Schmaier AH, Schutsky D, Farber A, Silver LD, Bradford HN, and Colman RW. Determination of the bifunctional properties of high molecular weight kininogen by studies with monoclonal antibodies directed to each of its chains. J Biol Chem 1987; 262:1405-1411.

7. Meloni FJ and Schmaier AH. Low molecular weight kininogen binds to platelets to modulate thrombin-induced platelet activation. J Biol Chem 1991; 266:6786-6794.

8. Puri R, Zhou F, Hu CJ, Colman RF, and Colman RW. High molecular weight kininogen inhibits thrombin-induced platelet aggregation and cleavage of aggregin by inhibiting binding of thrombin to platelets. Blood 1991; 77:500-507.

9. Schmaier AH, Kuo A, Lundberg D, Murray S, and Cines DB. Expression of high molecular weight kininogen on human umbilical vein endothelial cells. J Biol Chem 1988; 263:4689-4703.

10. Colman RW, Bagdasarian A, Talamo RC, Scott CF, Seavey M, Guimares JA, Pierce JV, and Kaplan AP. Williams trait: human kininogen deficiency with diminished levels of plasminogen proactivator and prekallikrein associated with abnormalities of the Hageman-dependent pathways. J Clin Invest 1975; 56:1650-1662.

11. Jiang YP, Kaufmann J, Meloni FJ, Muller-Esterl W, and Schmaier AH. Rapid purification of the domains of low molecular weight kininogen and their use in charactering monoclonal antibodies to kininogens. Thromb. Haemostas. 1991;65:1248.

12. Jiang YP, Muller-Esterl W, and Schmaier AH. Domain 3 of kininogens contains a cell-binding site and a site that modifies thrombin activation of platelets. J Biol Chem 1992; (in press).

13. Salvesen G, Parkes C, Abrahamson M, Grubb A, and Barrett A J. Human low-Mr kininogen contains three copies of a cystin sequence that are divergent in structure and in inhibitory activity for cysteine proteinases. Biochem. J. 1986; 234:429-434

14. Fraker PJ, and Speck SC, Jr. Protein and cell membrane iodinations with a spraingly soluble chloroamide, 1,3,4,6,-tetra-chloro-3 alpha, 6 alpha-diphenylglycoluril. Biochem. Biophys. Res. Commun. 1978; 80:849-857.

15. Meloni FJ, Gustafson EJ, and Schmaier AH. High molecular weight kininogen binds to platelets by its heavy and light chains and when bound has altered susceptibility to kallikrein cleavage. Blood 1992; (in press).

16. Bjork I, Olson ST, Sheffer RG, and Shore JD. Binding of heparin to human high molecular weight kininogen. Biochemistry 1989; 28:1213-1221.

17. Hong SL. Effect of bradykinin and thrombin on prostacyclin synthesis in endothelial cells from calf and pig aorta and human umbilical cord vein. Thromb Res 1980; 18:787-795.

18. Smith D, Gilbert M, and Owne WG. Tissue plasminogen activator release in vivo in response to vasoactive agent. Blood 1985; 66:835-839.

AAS 38/I
Recent Progress on Kinins
© 1992 Birkhäuser Verlag Basel

PARALLEL PROCOAGULANT AND ANTICOAGULANT PATHWAYS FOR HIGH MOLECULAR WEIGHT KININOGEN COAGULANT FUNCTION

S. T. Olson, R. Sheffer and J. D. Shore

Henry Ford Hospital, 2799 W. Grand Blvd., Detroit, MI 48202, USA

SUMMARY: High molecular weight kininogen (HK) or its procoagulant light-chain but not the heavy chain potentiated the heparin enhancement of antithrombin III inactivation of plasma kallikrein and factor XIa from 10-50-fold to ~1000-fold at I 0.15, pH 7.4, 25 °C. This potentiation resulted in antithrombin becoming a predominant inhibitor of kallikrein and factor XIa in heparinized normal but not HK-deficient plasmas. The heparin chain-length and salt dependence of this potentiation suggested an anticoagulant action of HK analogous to its procoagulant action.

INTRODUCTION

High molecular weight kininogen (HK) is a plasma glycoprotein with multiple functions. Besides being a precursor of the vasoactive nonapeptide, bradykinin, the protein additionally functions as a cofactor in the contact activation of the intrinsic blood coagulation pathway and as an inhibitor of cysteine proteinases. HK acts as a cofactor in the initiation of blood clotting by promoting the activation of two proenzymes, prekallikrein and factor XI, by their enzyme activator, factor XIIa, in the presence of a negatively charged surface (1). This function resides in two regions of the carboxy-terminal light chain of the kinin-free protein. One of these regions is histidine-rich and mediates the binding of the protein to a negatively charged surface whereas the other region is involved in forming tight complexes with prekallikrein and factor XI. The surface-dependent activation of the proenzymes is thus thought to result from HK mediating the binding of the proenzyme to the negatively charged surface where activation by surface-bound factor XIIa can rapidly occur (1, Fig. 1). Previous studies in our laboratory have shown that in addition to binding procoagulant surfaces, HK also binds to the anticoagulant glycosaminoglycan, heparin, which provides a catalytic surface for the rapid inactivation of blood coagulation enzymes by the protein inhibitor, antithrombin III (2). This observation in conjunction with the ability of HK to bind the enzymes, plasma kallikrein and factor XIa (1,3), led us to hypothesize that HK might function as an anticoagulant cofactor in a manner similar to its action as a procoagulant cofactor. Thus, it appeared that HK might promote the binding of these enzymes to the heparin surface where rapid

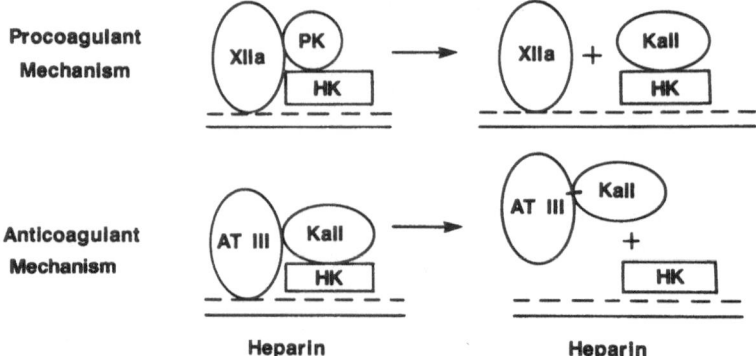

Figure 1. Hypothesized parallel procoagulant and anticoagulant modes of action of HK

inactivation by surface-bound antithrombin could occur (Fig. 1). In the present study we have confirmed this hypothesis by showing that HK greatly potentiates the heparin-dependent inactivation of kallikrein and factor XIa by antithrombin III by a mechanism which parallels the procoagulant mechanism of action of the cofactor protein. The significance of this potentiation is further demonstrated by showing that antithrombin is a predominant inhibitor of these enzymes when clinically relevant dosages of heparin are added to normal but not to antithrombin or HK-deficient plasmas.

MATERIALS AND METHODS

Proteins were purified from outdated plasma by published methods (1-4). A full-length heparin of reduced polydispersity (M_r ~8000) and with high-affinity for antithrombin was obtained by fractionation of commercial heparin (Diosynth), as described (4). A synthetic heparin penta-saccharide representing the antithrombin-binding sequence in high-affinity heparin was provided by Dr. Jean Choay of Sanofi Recherche. Concentrations of proteins were determined from the absorption at 280 nm along with published extinction coefficients or by active-site titration (2-4). Heparin concentrations were determined from the equivalence point of fluorescence titrations of antithrombin with the polysaccharide (4). The rates of enzyme inactivation by antithrombin were measured by discontinuous assays of residual enzyme activity as described (4) utilizing the tripeptide-p-nitroanilide substrates, S-2302 for kallikrein and S-2366 for factor XIa (Kabi). Experiments were performed at 25 °C in 0.1 M Hepes, 0.1 mM EDTA, 0.1% polyethylene glycol 8000, pH 7.4, containing 0.1 (I 0.15) or 0.25 (I 0.3) M NaCl. Enzyme inactivation in plasma was studied by addition of enzyme to 10-fold diluted normal or deficient plasmas and residual enzymatic activity measured discontinuously with the chromogenic substrate assay. Enzyme-inhibitor complexes formed in similar experiments were detected by SDS gel electrophoresis of plasma samples after complete (>97%) enzyme inactivation under nonreducing conditions. Kallikrein complexes were visualized by employing enzyme radiolabelled with NaI^{125} using Iodobeads (Pierce) to a specific radioactivity of 2.6 μCi/μg and performing autoradiography on dried gels. Factor XIa complexes were detected by Western blotting with polyclonal antibodies specific for C1-inhibitor, α_1-proteinase inhibitor and antithrombin III (The Binding Site). Quantitation of complexes was done by densitometry.

RESULTS

Figure 2A shows the results of kinetic studies of the inactivation of plasma kallikrein by antithrombin under pseudo-first order conditions in the absence and presence of either heparin or the cofactor protein, HK (kinin-free). The rate of kallikrein inactivation was found to be greatly stimulated by HK, but only in the presence of heparin. This stimulation was maximal at 200-400 nM HK, concentrations below those in plasma (~700 nM) and which were sufficient to bind all the kallikrein, given the previously measured dissociation constant of ~15 nM for this interaction (3). All reactions showed a simple exponential decay of kallikrein activity except when both heparin and the cofactor were present, in which case a biexponential decay of activity, with the final ~20% of the enzyme inhibited more slowly than the initial 80%, was observed. SDS gel electrophoresis revealed the presence of sufficient β-kallikrein in the α-kallikrein preparation to account for this slower phase, presumably due to the weaker affinity for HK of β-kallikrein than of α-kallikrein (5). Based on the second-order rate constants determined from an analysis of pseudo-first order inactivation rate constants as a function of the antithrombin or antithrombin-heparin complex concentration in the absence or presence of saturating HK in these and other experiments, HK was found to increase the heparin enhancement of the antithrombin-kallikrein reaction from 12-fold to a substantial 1200-fold (Table 1). Experiments with the heavy chain, i.e., kinin-free low molecular weight kininogen, and isolated light chain of HK showed that the potentiating effect of the cofactor resided in the light-chain, consistent with the region of HK mediating the procoagulant activity of the cofactor also mediating the anticoagulant effect.

Figure 2B shows the results of similar experiments performed with factor XIa. HK was found to also potentiate the inactivation of factor XIa by antithrombin, again only in the presence of the polysaccharide. In contrast to the cofactor effect on the heparin-accelerated antithrombin-kallikrein reaction, HK potentiated the heparin-accelerated antithrombin-factor XIa reaction for only about half of the reaction. This effect was not due to the failure to saturate factor XIa with the

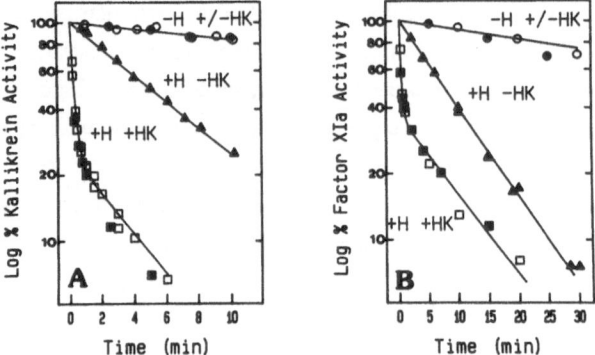

Figure 2. The effect of heparin (H) and HK on the rate of kallikrein (20 nM) or factor XIa (12 nM) inactivation by antithrombin (AT). A, 2 μM AT, 1 μM H, 0.2 (●,□) or 0.4 (■) μM HK; B, 0.5 μM AT, 0.1 μM H, 0.1 (□), 0.2 (■) or 1 (●) μM HK.

cofactor since the extent of the reaction potentiated was not altered when HK concentrations were increased from 100 to 200 nM. This incomplete potentiation was further shown to not be due to the well-characterized destruction of HK by XIa (6), since control experiments showed that such destruction occurred at a much slower rate at the XIa concentrations employed than that required to completely inactivate the enzyme. Moreover, 10-fold lower factor XIa concentrations did not alter the extent of the reaction potentiated. Autocatalytic degradation of factor XIa to an enzyme form not potentiated by the cofactor was also ruled out from the independence of the cofactor effect on preincubation of XIa prior to initiating the inactivation reaction. Together, such control experiments therefore suggested that HK was potentiating the inactivation of only one of the subunits of the dimeric factor XIa molecule. Again, the second-order rate constants determined for the fast phase in the presence of cofactor compared to those in the absence of cofactor indicated that HK potentiated the heparin-accelerated inactivation of one of the factor XIa subunits from ~50-fold to ~1000-fold.

To investigate whether the mechanism of HK potentiation of these heparin- accelerated antithrombin-proteinase reactions was similar to the procoagulant mechanism of action of the cofactor, further studies were done with kallikrein as the enzyme. The heparin chain-length requirements for cofactor potentiation were investigated by comparing a heparin pentasaccharide which constitutes the specific binding site for antithrombin with the full-length heparin used in the experiments of Fig. 2. The pentasaccharide was observed to accelerate kallikrein inactivation to the same extent as the full-length heparin, but was not potentiated by HK, suggesting that a heparin chain-length larger than that needed to bind the inhibitor was required for cofactor potentiation (Table 1). Moreover, pentasaccharide and full-length heparin accelerated reactions were unaffected by doubling the salt concentration in the absence of cofactor under conditions where these heparins were completely saturated with antithrombin, consistent with these accelerations not involving kallikrein binding to heparin (4). In contrast, the cofactor potentiation of the full-length heparin accelerated reaction was markedly dependent on salt under these same conditions, the rate enhancement decreasing from 1200 to 24-fold when the salt concentration was doubled (Table 1), despite the saturation of the enzyme with cofactor at both salt concentrations(3). Together, such experiments indicated that binding of HK-kallikrein complex to the heparin chain on which the inhibitor was bound was required for potentiation of the reaction.

Table 1. Second-order rate constants for antithrombin (AT) or antithrombin-heparin complex (AT-H) inhibition of kallikrein and kallikrein-HK complex

	Kallikrein $(M^{-1}s^{-1})$		Kallikrein-HK complex $(M^{-1}s^{-1})$	
	I 0.15	I 0.3	I 0.15	I 0.3
AT	180	180	180	ND[a]
AT-H5[b]	1900	2200	1900	ND
AT-H26[c]	2100	2100	210,000	4400

a ND, not determined
b Complex of antithrombin with the heparin pentasaccharide
c Complex of antithrombin with a ~26-saccharide heparin containing the pentasaccharide

To determine whether the cofactor-dependent enhancements of heparin-accelerated reaction rates were physiologically significant, the effect of heparin and HK on the inactivation of kallikein and factor XIa by other important plasma inhibitors of these enzymes was first investigated. The reactions of kallikrein and factor XIa with C1-Inhibitor, α_2-macroglobulin or α_1-proteinase inhibitor were not enhanced by HK either in the absence or presence of heparin. This observation together with the large cofactor-dependent enhancements of antithrombin inactivation of these enzymes in the presence of heparin suggested that the rate of inactivation of kallikrein and factor XIa in plasma should be enhanced by heparin. Both the rates of kallikrein and factor XIa inactivation as well as the enzyme-inhibitor complexes formed when these enzymes were added to normal plasma and plasmas deficient in antithrombin or HK were therefore investigated to test this prediction. Inhibitor-enzyme complexes were separated by SDS gel electrophoresis and visualized either by autoradiography of I^{125}-labelled enzyme in the case of kallikrein or by western blotting using inhibitor-specific antibodies in the case of factor XIa. These studies confirmed that heparin at a therapeutic dose of 0.5-1 unit/ml maximally accelerated kallikrein inactivation by 3.5-fold and factor XIa inactivation by 40-fold in plasma, consistent with a heparin-activatable inhibitor making greater than a 70% contribution to the inhibition of these enzymes. Indistinguishable results were obtained in factor XII-deficient and prekallikrein-deficient plasmas, indicating that no significant activation of the contact system enzymes by heparin was complicating these experiments. Examination of the inhibitor-enzyme complexes formed in the absence and presence of heparin on SDS gels confirmed that antithrombin made a minor contribution to the inhibition of these enzymes in the absence of heparin but accounted for more than half of the inhibition in the presence of heparin. Similar experiments in antithrombin-deficient and HK-deficient plasmas subtantiated the complete dependence of these effects on the presence of both antithrombin as well as the cofactor.

DISCUSSION

A high degree of homology between the histidine-rich surface-binding region of HK and a similar region in histidine-rich glycoprotein together with the demonstrated binding of the latter protein to the anticoagulant polysaccharide, heparin, led us to hypothesize that a similar interaction of HK with heparin might also occur (2). We were indeed able to demonstrate binding of HK to heparin from the retention of the cofactor by immobilized heparin and its elution from the matrix with ~0.25 M salt, as well as from the ability of HK to abolish the accelerating effect of heparin on the inactivation of thrombin by antithrombin (2). Heparin acceleration of the antithrombin-thrombin reaction is primarily due to the polysaccharide bridging specifically-bound antithrombin and nonspecifically-bound thrombin on the same polysaccharide chain (4). HK binding to heparin would thus be expected to antagonize the accelerating effect of heparin on this reaction by blocking the binding of the enzyme to heparin. However, in the case of the enzymes kallikrein and factor XIa, which form specific complexes with HK, we expected the cofactor to affect the heparin-accelerated reaction of antithrombin with these enzymes differently. In analogy to the procoagulant mode of action of the cofactor, we thus hypothesized that HK might promote rather than antagonize heparin's accelerating effect on the reaction of antithrombin with kallikrein and factor XIa by mediating the binding of these enzymes to the heparin surface where rapid inactivation by surface-bound antithrombin could occur (Fig. 1). Consistent with this prediction, HK or its procoagulant light chain was found to substantially stimulate the heparin-accelerated but not the unaccelerated reactions of antithrombin with kallikrein and factor XIa. With factor XIa, it appears that the potentiating effect of the cofactor involves only one of the subunits of this unique dimeric enzyme (1), suggesting the possibility that subunit-subunit interactions may play an important role in regulating this as well as other activities of this key clotting enzyme. Further studies are necessary to determine the molecular basis of this apparent half-of-the-sites reactivity.

In the case of kallikrein, evidence has been presented to show that the potentiating effect of the cofactor indeed results from HK promoting the binding of the enzyme to the heparin surface, analogous to the cofactor assisting the binding of the proenzyme to a procoagulant surface. Thus, the observations that 1) the cofactor enhances the acceleration of a full-length heparin but not a pentasaccharide heparin which specifically binds just antithrombin, despite the similar accelerations produced by these heparins, and 2) the cofactor-enhanced but not the unenhanced accelerations by these heparins are strongly dependent on salt even though the heparins are fully saturated with the inhibitor, together suggest that the cofactor potentiation requires the electrostatic binding of HK-kallikrein complex along with antithrombin to the heparin chain. The independence of heparin accelerations on the polysaccharide chain-length and salt observed in the absence of the cofactor indicate that such accelerations cannot involve kallikrein binding to the heparin chain and are likely due to the well-established conformational change induced in antithrombin when it specifically binds to the polysaccharide (4). The cofactor thus appears to be essential to allow the enzyme to bind to the heparin chain where it can react more rapidly with bound antithrombin.

HK was found to augment heparin rate enhancements of antithrombin reactions with kallikrein and factor XIa from modest values of 10-50-fold to a substantial ~1000-fold. Such polysaccharide rate enhancements are comparable to those observed for the reactions of antithrombin with its main target enzymes (4). No comparable effects of heparin or HK were found on the reactions of these enzymes with their major plasma inhibitors, namely, C1-Inhibitor and α_2-macroglobulin in the case of kallikrein (7), and α_1-proteinase inhibitor in the case of factor XIa (8). Such results suggested that antithrombin should be an important inhibitor of these enzymes when heparin is added to plasma. This prediction was confirmed by showing that the rates of kallikrein and factor XIa inactivation in plasma are significantly enhanced at therapeutic levels of heparin and that enzyme-complexes with antithrombin become predominant under such conditions. Such results were further completely dependent on the presence of both antithrombin and HK in the plasma as revealed by similar experiments in deficient-plasmas. These findings have implications for both the clinical use of heparin for the prophylaxis and treatment of venous thrombosis as well as for the in vivo regulation of kallikrein and factor XIa by endogenous heparin or anticoagulantly-active heparan sulfate glycosaminoglycans on the blood vessel wall. Thus, clinically administered or endogenous heparin or heparin-like molecules exposed to blood would be expected to increase the inhibitory potential of plasma with respect to these enzymes. Our data therefore provide a rational basis for early suggestions that heparin might be an effective treatment for patients with hereditary angioedema who are deficient in the primary kallikrein inhibitor in plasma, C1-Inhibitor (9). Our findings are also of interest with respect to the functional duality of the cofactor protein in both procoagulant and anticoagulant pathways. Such duality appears to be unique for HK since other nonhomologous cofactor proteins with similar function, such as factors Va and VIIIa, appear to act solely in a procoagulant manner (10). This duality can exist most likely because of the specificity of the surface. Thus, in the case of heparin, a specific pentasaccharide sequence which constitutes a "receptor" for antithrombin binding results in the polysaccharide acting in an anticoagulant fashion (4). Similarly, the probable procoagulant surfaces, namely platelets or endothelial cells, have been shown to expose specific receptors for HK binding upon activation which may direct a procoagulant mode of action (11). The appropriate action of HK may thus critically depend on the surfaces available for the cofactor to bind and their temporal presentation once vessel injury has occurred.

REFERENCES

1. Cochrane, CG, Griffin, JH. The biochemistry and pathophysiology of the contact system of plasma. Adv Immun 1982; 33:241-306.

2. Björk, I, Olson, ST, Sheffer, RG, Shore, JD. Binding of heparin to human high molecular weight kininogen. Biochemistry 1989; 28:1213-1221.

3. Bock, PE, Shore, JD, Tans, G, Griffin, JH. Protein-protein interactions in contact activation of blood coagulation. J Biol Chem 1985; 260:12434-12443.

4. Olson, ST, Björk, I, Sheffer, R, Craig, PA, Shore, JD, Choay, J. Role of the antithrombin-binding pentasaccharide in heparin acceleration of antithrombin-proteinase reactions. J Biol Chem 1992; in press.

5. Coleman, RW, Wachtfogel, YT, Kucich, U, Weinbaum, G, Hahn, S, Pixley, RA, Scott, CF, deAgostini, A, Burger, D, Schapira, M. Effect of cleavage of the heavy chain of human plasma kallikrein on its functional properties. Blood 1985; 65:311-318.

6. Scott, CF, Silver, LD, Purdon, AD, Colman, RW. Cleavage of human high molecular weight kininogen by factor XIa *in vitro*. J Biol Chem 1985; 260:10856-10863.

7. Schapira, M, Scott, CF, Colman, RW. Contribution of plasma protease inhibitors to the inactivation of kallikrein in plasma. J Clin Invest 1982; 69:462-468.

8. Scott, CF, Schapira, M, James, HL, Cohen, AB, Colman, RW. Inactivation of factor XIa by plasma proteinase inhibitors. J Clin Invest 1982; 69:844-852.

9. Colman, RW. Hereditary angioedema and heparin therapy. Ann Int Med 1976; 85:399.

10. Mann, KG, Jenny, RJ, Krishnaswamy, S. Cofactor proteins in the assembly and expression of blood clotting enzyme complexes. Ann Rev Biochem 1988; 57:915-956.

11. Greengard, JS, Griffin, JH. Receptors for high molecular weight kininogen on stimulated washed human platelets. Biochemistry 1984; 23:6863-6869.

AAS 38/I
Recent Progress on Kinins
© 1992 Birkhäuser Verlag Basel

PURIFICATION AND SOME PROPERTIES OF KININOGENS IN CANINE PLASMA

H. Mashiko and H. Takahashi

Meiji College of Pharmacy, 1-35-23 Nozawa, Setagaya-ku, Tokyo 154, JAPAN

SUMMARY: High molecular weight (HMW) and low molecular weight (LMW) kininogens were present in canine plasma, and its content ratio was 1:3. Both kininogens were purified by ion-exchange and affinity chromatographies. Purified HMW kininogen might be heterogeneous molecule. And two LMW kininogens were purified and properties of both LMW kininogens were almost the same.

INTRODUCTION

Kininogen, a precursor protein of vasoactive peptide, kinin, is a multifunctional glycoprotein, and composed of a single poly-peptide chain (1). It is well known that two types of kininogen, HMW and LMW kininogens, are present in mammalian plasmas. And third type of kininogen, a precursor of T-kinin (Ile-Ser-brady-kinin), was found in rat plasma (2). Thus, three types of kinin-ogen are discovered in mammalian plasmas.

Recently, it has been reported that HMW and LMW prekinin-ogen mRNAs are produced from a single gene a consequence of alternative RNA processing event. Both HMW and LMW kininogens consist of three domains: an amino-terminal heavy (H)-chain, bradykinin (BK) moiety and carboxyl-terminal light (L)-chain. So, H-chain, BK and amino-terminal 12 amino acid residues of L-chain of both kininogens are identical (3). Function of both H-chain is inhibition of cysteine proteinases (4), and function of L-chain of HMW kininogen is non-proteolytic co-factor in intrinsic blood coagulation system (5).

Both kininogens have been purified from various mammalian

plasmas. Though dog was used for bioassay of tissue kallikrein, the study of protein components related to plasma kallikrein-kinin system is very poor. So, we started to measure the amount of HMW and LMW kininogens. And both kininogens were purified and some properties of both kininogens were studied by comparison with those of other kininogens. This paper describes purification and some properties of HMW and LMW kininogens in canine plasma.

MATERIALS AND METHODS

Mongrel dog was anesthetized, and the blood was collected from the carotid artery with a polyethylene syringe. The blood was immediately mixed with 1/10 volume of 3.8% sodium citrate solution. Plasma was obtained by centrifugation at 3500 rpm for 30 min at room temperature, and storred at -80°C before use. Q-Sepharose Fast Flow, Chelating Sepharose 6B, S-Sepharose Fast Flow, Mono Q HR 5/5 and Sephacryl S-300 Superfine were products of Pharmacia LKB Biotechnology, Japan. The sources of other materials were as follows: Formyl-Cellulofine from Seikagaku Kogyo Co., Ltd., Japan; human HMW kininogen-deficient plasma from George King Bio-Medical, U.S.A.; Polybrene from Aldrich Chemicals Co., Inc., U.S.A.; benzamidine·HCl from Tokyo Kasei Kogyo Co., Ltd., Japan; soybean trypsin inhibitor (SBTI) and a kit of molecular weight markers (MW-SDS-200) from Sigma Chemical Co., U.S.A.; papain and ficin from Boehringer Mannheim, Germany; Pyr-Phe-Leu-p-nitroanilide (PNA) and synthetic BK from the Peptide Institute Inc., Japan; tosyl-phenylalanine chloromethyl-ketone (TPCK)-trypsin from Worthington Biochemicals Corp., U.S.A.; diisopropylfluorophosphate (DFP) from Katayama Kagaku Kogyo Co., Ltd., Japan; ε-aminocaproic acid (EACA) and phenyl-methylsulfonylfluoride (PMSF) from Nacalai Tesque Inc., Japan.

Differential assay for canine HMW and LMW kininogens was performed by the method of Uchida and Katori (6). Kinin liberation was estimated in terms of its ability to cause contraction of rat uterus, using synthetic BK as a standard (7).

Cysteine proteinase inhibitory (CPI) activity was measured by the method of Fillipova et al. (8), using Pyr-Phe-Leu-PNA and papain. The amount of p-nitroaniline released by papain was spectrophotometrically measured using a Hitachi model U-2000 spectrophotometer with absorbance at 410 nm.

Assay of HMW kininogen was carried out by a kaolin-activated partial thromboplastin time (APTT) method, using human HMW kinin-ogen-deficient plasma (9) with slight modification. One unit is defined as the amount of the activity which is present in 1.0 ml of the plasma.

Purified kininogen (0.2 ml), 0.2 ml of 1 M Tris-HCl buffer, pH 8.0, 0.1 ml of 30 mM o-phenanthroline and 0.1 ml of TPCK-trypsin solution (1 mg/ml) were incubated for 30 min at 37°C, and the reaction was terminated by addition of 25 μl of SBTI (40 mg/ml). The amount of kinin liberation was estimated by the method as described above.

Carboxymethylation of papain (100 mg) was performed by the method of Anastasi et al. (10). The carboxymethylated (Cm)-papain was coupled to Formyl-Cellulofine according to the instruction manual.

Polyacrylamide gel electrophoresis (PAGE) was carried out on 7% gels according to the method of Davis (11). Sodium dodecyl sulfate (SDS)-PAGE was performed on 10% gels according to the method of Laemmli (12).

Protein concentrations were determined by measurements of absorbance at 280 nm, assuming that an absorption value of 1.0 equals 1 mg/ml. When benzamidine was added in elution buffer, measurement of absorbance at 280 nm was carried out after removing benzamidine by dialysis.

RESULTS AND DISCUSSION

Evidence for presence of two kininogens in canine plasma

When the plasma was passed through a column (2.5 x 145 cm) of Sephacryl S-300 Superfine equilibrated with 0.02 M Tris-HCl

buffer, pH 8.0, containing 0.2 M NaCl, 3 mM EDTA-2Na and Polybrene (50 µg/ml), kinin activity released on incubation with
TPCK-trypsin was separated into two fractions. The former eluted
kininogen fraction showed the correction of the prolonged APTT
time of HMW kininogen-deficient plasma, however, the latter
eluted fraction did not show the correction of the plasma. These
results indicate that HMW kininogen is present in the former
eluted fraction, and LMW kininogen exists in the latter fraction.
The kininogen levels (µg BK equivalent/ml plasma) in canine
plasma were also determined by differential assay method (6) as
follows: total kininogen (4.13 ± 0.63); HMW kininogen (0.89 ±
0.13) and LMW kininogen (3.22 ± 0.38). Thus, two kininogens exist
in canine plasma, and we tried to purify simultaneously these
kininogens from canine plasma.

Purification and some properties of HMW and LMW kininogens from canine plasma

All purification procedures were performed in a cold room.
Various proteinase inhibitors were added to each elution buffer
or dialysed buffer during purification of HMW and LMW kininogens.
     The dialysed plasma (100 ml) was applied to a column (3.5 x
25 cm) of Q-Sepharose Fast Flow equilibrated with the dialysed
buffer. After washing the column with the equilibration buffer,
proteins were eluted by NaCl linear gradient in the equilibration buffer (each 2 liter). HMW and LMW kininogens adhered the
column, however, LMW kininogen fraction eluted prior to HMW
kininogen fraction. Each HMW or LMW kininogen fraction was
separately combined, and both fractions were used as starting
material for purification of these kininogens.
     The HMW kininogen fraction was applied to the zinc-Chelat-
ing Sepharose 6B column (4.5 x 24 cm). After washing the column
with the equilibration buffer, proteins were eluted by the
equilibration buffer containing EDTA-2Na. HMW kininogen was
eluted by the buffer containing EDTA-2Na, however, minor

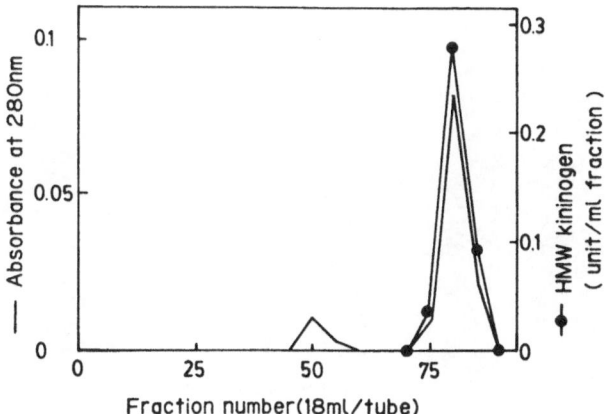

Figure 1. S-Sepharose Fast Flow column chromatography of HMW kininogen fraction

contaminating protein coexisted in the HMW kininogen fraction, judging from SDS-PAGE of the fraction.

After HMW kininogen fraction was dialysed, the dialysate was applied to an S-Sepharose Fast Flow column (3.6 x 13 cm) equilibrated with the dialysed buffer. The column was washed with the same buffer, and protein was eluted by NaCl linear gradient in the equilibration buffer (each 1 liter). As shown in Fig. 1, minor contaminating protein was separated from HMW kininogen.

When HMW kininogen preparation was subjected to PAGE at pH 8.3, the preparation gave two bands on the gels (Fig. 2). Such heterogeneity was also observed in HMW kininogen from bovine plasma (13). When the preparation was subjected to SDS-PAGE in the presence of 2-mercaptoethanol, the preparation gave a single band on the gel. And the kininogen was estimated to be about 135 Kd by comparison with those mobilities of marker proteins. The HMW kininogen, however, showed two bands on SDS-PAGE at non-reduced condition; the one was major with 205 Kd, and the other was minor with 130 Kd. Such heterogeneity was also appeared in HMW kininogen from human plasma (14). During the purification of the kininogen, we often obtained the cleaved form of the HMW kininogen. When such cleaved form of the kininogen was subjected to SDS-PAGE at non-reduced condition, the preparation

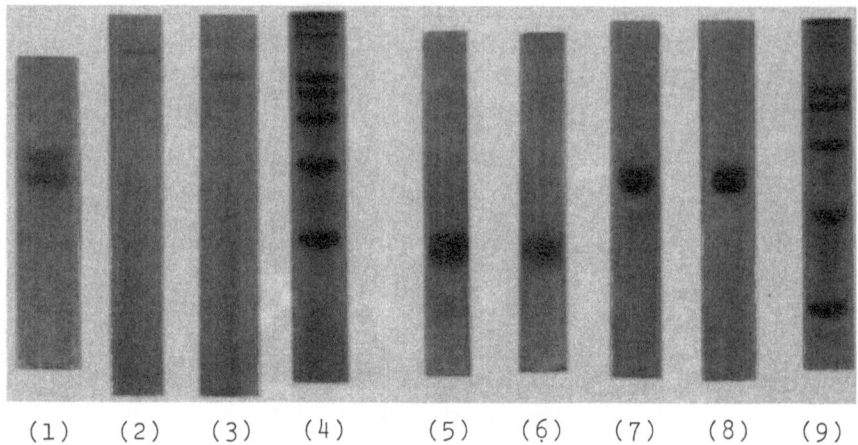

(1)   (2)   (3)   (4)   (5)   (6)   (7)   (8)   (9)

Figure 2. Polyacrylamide gel electrophoresis of canine HMW and
LMW kininogens in the presence or absence of SDS
(1) HMW kininogen (HMW-K) at pH 8.3; (2) non-reduced HMW-K; (3)
reduced HMW-K; (4) marker proteins; (5) LMW kininogen (LMW-K)-I
at pH 8.3; (6) LMW-K-II at pH 8.3; (7) non-reduced LMW-K-I; (8)
non-reduced LMW-K-II and (9) marker proteins. SDS-PAGE was (2)-
(4) and (7)-(9).

also gave two bands, but, the band of 205 Kd was minor and the
band of 130 Kd was major. So, the band of 205 Kd may correspond
to intact HMW kininogen in canine plasma, and the band of 130 Kd
may correspond to the cleaved form of the kininogen as like as
human HMW kininogen (14).

The HMW kininogen released kinin on incubation with trypsin,
and inhibited the activity of papain or ficin in proportion to
the amount of the preparation used.

LMW kininogen fraction obtained from Q-Sepharose Fast Flow
column chromatography was pooled. The fraction was applied on a
Cm-papain-Cellulofine column (1.5 x 10 cm). After washing the
column, proteins were eluted with the equilibration buffer
containing NaSCN. The LMW kininogen was eluted with NaSCN solution, and recovery of the kininogen was about 90% at this step.
The LMW kininogen fraction was pooled and dialysed.

Dialysate was chromatographed on a Mono Q column (1.5 x 5

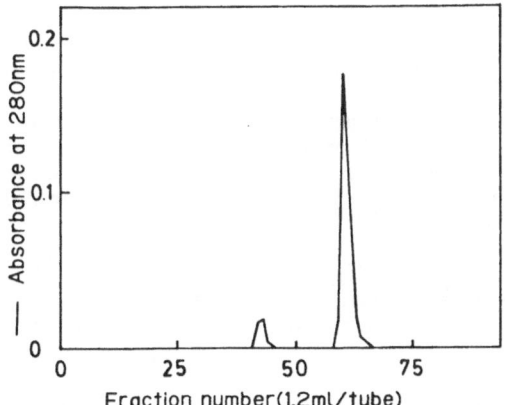

Figure 3. Mono Q column chromatography of LMW kininogen fraction

cm) equilibrated with the dialysed buffer. As shown in Fig. 3, LMW kininogen was separated into two fractions, and both fractions showed a potent CPI activity. The former eluted kininogen was named LMW kininogen-I, and the latter eluted kininogen was named LMW kininogen-II, tentatively. The recovery ratio of these kininogens, however, was varied by every lot of canine plasma.

These preparations were subjected to PAGE at pH 8.3, and SDS-PAGE in the absence of 2-mercaptoethanol. As shown in Fig. 2, there was no significant difference between LMW kininogen-I and -II. And their molecular weights were estimated to be about 60 Kd. And also they inhibited the activity of papain or ficin, and the ability of inhibition of these proteinases showed no significant difference between LMW kininogen-I and -II. Moreover, both kininogens released kinin on incubation with trypsin. The difference of these kininogens will be studied in near future.

REFERENCES

1. Müller-Esterl W, Iwanaga S, Nakanishi S. Kininogens revisited. TIBS 1986; 11: 336.

2. Okamoto H, Greenbaum LM. Isolation and structure of T-kinin. Biochem Biophys Res Commun 1983; 112: 701.

3. Takagaki Y, Kitamura N, Nakanishi S. Cloning and sequence analysis of cDNAs for human high molecular weight and low molecular weight prekininogens. J Biol Chem 1985; 260: 8601.

4. Sueyoshi T, Enjyoji K, Shimada T, Kato H, Iwanaga S, Bando Y, Kominami E, Katsunuma N. A new function of kininogens as thiol-proteinase inhibitors: Inhibition of papain and cathepsins B, H and L by bovine, rat and human plasma kininogens. FEBS Lett 1985; 182: 193.

5. Griffin JH, Cochrane CG. Mechanisms for the involvement of high molecular weight kininogen in surface-dependent reaction of Hageman factor. Proc Natl Acad Sci USA 1976; 73: 2554.

6. Uchida Y, Katori M. Differential assay method for high molecular weight and low molecular weight kininogens. Thromb Res 1979; 15: 127.

7. Kato H, Nagasawa S, Iwanaga S. HMW and LMW kininogens. In: Methods in Enzymology; Vol. 80, Lorand L. editor. New York: Academic Press, 1981: 172-198.

8. Fillipova Y, Lysogorskaya EN, Oksenoit ES, Rudenskaya GN, Stepanov VM. L-Pyroglutamyl-L-phenylalanyl leucine-p-nitroanilide. A chromogenic substrate for thiol proteinase assay. Anal Biochem 1984; 143: 293.

9. Hayashi I, Ito T, Kato H, Iwanaga S, Nakano T, Oh-ishi S. Demonstration of the third kininogen in high and low molecular weight kininogens-deficient Brown Norway Katholiek rat. Thromb Res 1984; 36: 509.

10. Anastasi A, Brown MA, Kembhavi AA, Nicklin MJH, Sayers CA, Sunter DC, Barrett AJ. Cystatin, a potent inhibitor of cysteine proteinases. Improved purification from egg white, characterization, and detection in chicken serum. Biochem J 1983; 211: 129.

11. Davis BJ. Disc electrophoresis II. Method and application to human serum protein. Ann N Y Acad Sci 1964; 121: 404.

12. Laemmli UK. Cleavage of structural proteins during the assembly of the head of bacteriophage T4. Nature 1970; 227: 680.

13. Komiya M, Kato H, Suzuki T. Bovine plasma kininogens I. Further purification of high molecular weight kininogen and its physicochemical properties. J Biochem (Tokyo) 1974; 76: 811.

14. Higashiyama S, Ohkubo I, Ishiguro H, Kunimatsu M, Sawai K, Sasaki M. Human high molecular weight kininogen as a thiol proteinase inhibitor: Presence of the entire inhibition capacity in the native form of heavy chain. Biochemistry 1986; 25: 1669.

AAS 38/I
Recent Progress on Kinins
© 1992 Birkhäuser Verlag Basel

DETERMINATION OF HUMAN LOW MOLECUIAR WEIGHT KININOGEN

BY IMMUNOASSAY

I. Jerabek, Z. Stetina, R. Furtner, B.R. Binder and M. Maier

Lab. Clin. Exp. Physiology, Dept. Med. Physiology, Univ. Vienna
Schwarzspanierstr. 17, A-1090 Vienna, Austria

SUMMARY: It was the aim of the present investigation to develop a convenient method for determination of human kininogens. Using mono- and polyclonal antibody preparations an ELISA-system for specific determination of LMWK could be developed. In addition, the specificity of the monoclonal antibody suggests that their epitope in HMWK and its heavy chain is different to that in LMWK.

INTRODUCTION

Two types of kininogens - the multifunctional proteins which release kinin upon cleavage by kallikrein - exist in human plasma (1,2). High molecular weight kininogen (HMWK) with a mass of about 120 kD and low molecular weight kininogen (LMWK) with a mass of 68 kD. Both forms have identical heavy chains with a mass of 62 kD, whereas their light chains are different (1). The light chain of HMWK has a mass of 62 kD and contains the binding sites for prekallikrein, factor XI and for negatively charged surfaces (1,3). In contrast, the light chain of LMWK has a molecular mass of only 4 kD and its physiological function -if any- is unknown (4). Antibodies generated against the entire LMWK-molecule reportedly cross react with HMWK due to identical heavy chain sequences (5). It was therefore postulated that antibodies must be directed against the small light chain of LMWK to restrict specificity for this molecule (5). In our effort to learn more about synthesis and metabolism of kininogens and for measurement of their concentrations in biological samples, antibodies against single chain intact LMWK were raised in rabbits and mice and characterized. Based on their specificity an ELISA system could be developed for specific measurement of LMWK.

MATERIALS AND METHODS

In brief native, functionally active human LMWK was purified by a six- step procedure as described earlier (6). Rabbits and mice were immunized according to a
standard protocol and polyclonal as well as monoclonal antibodies, respectively, were
isolated (7). The antibodies were characterized by means of SDS-electrophoresis,
subclass determination (Clonotyping System III, Southern Biotechnology Associates
Inc., USA), immunoblotting and functional inhibition studies. Antibodies were blotted
against human plasma and against purified LMWK and HMWK both in their native
and kinin free forms (2,8). Samples of purified rat (unpublished) and bovine kininogens
(9) were added as controls.

The following sandwich ELISA-protocol was used: After overnight coating of ELISA-
plates (Greiner, Austria) with the monoclonal mouse antibody (2LMWK11) at 4°C,
purified human LMWK standard (0.1ml, 1μg-1ng/ml) and unknown samples were incubated for 1h at 37°C. After washing the plates three times with phosphate buffer
(10, pH=7.4) containing 0.5% Tween (Merck, Germany) incubation was continued after
addition of the polyclonal rabbit antibodies for 1h at 37°C. The plates were again
washed and incubated with a peroxidase-linked anti-rabbit IgG antibody (Amersham,
UK)for another hour at 37°C. The developed color reaction was quantified by means
of an ELISA-assay reader (Anthos 2001, Labtech Instruments, Austria).

The values obtained in the ELISA were compared to those from functional studies
carried out with the rat-uterus bioassay. Purified kininogens alone (0.1-2.0μg/ml) or
kininogens added to plasma samples were incubated with 80ng of purified human
urinary kallikrein (11) for 5 minutes and released kinin was determined by measuring
the magnitude of the smooth muscle contractile response (7). Values for kininogens
were expressed as ng of bradykinin released per 5 minutes.

Using the newly established ELISA system, LMWK was determined in a variety of
body fluids. Samples of normal human plasma (n>30), urine (n=6), saliva (n=6), amniotic fluid (n=20), ascitic fluid (n=12), pleura effusion (n=12), synovial fluid (n=6), liquor
(n=1) and aqueous humor (n=1) were obtained. Further, supernatants from a variety of
human cell cultures were also screened for their content of LMWK. These included
the following primary and established cell lines of both normal and malignant tissues:
Liver (Chang Liver, Hep G2 and primary human liver cell culture), kidney (TCL 598
and primary cultures TU 4 - TU 35), prostate gland (PC-3, DU 145, LNCaP and
primary cultures), melanoma cell lines (Bowes, GUBSB, MJZJ, G-361, RA, GeJ, C'G
and primary cultures), osteosarcomas (CRL 1422, HTB 166, HTB 86, EW2, EW11, SIM,
KAL), primary amnion cell line cultures (n=8), colon carcinoma cell lines (SW620,

SW480, WiDr), lymphoma (U-937, H33HJ-JA1), leukemia (HL-60, K-562, MOLT-4), cervix- (HeLa, HeLa S3, HTB 35), mamma- (BT-20, MCF 7) and ovary carcinomas (Caov-3, Caov-5, PA-1, HEY 28, HOC) a rabdomyosarcoma (A673), human foreskin fibroblasts (HF), human pulmonal artery smooth muscle cells (HPASMC) and epithelial cells (HPAEC) and finally human umbilical vein epithelial cells (HUVEC). All samples were measured in duplicate.

RESULTS

Characterization by immunoblotting of the rabbit antiserum revealed that these poly-clonal antibodies recognize single chain HMW- and LMW-kininogens and their kinin-free forms only (Fig.1). These antibodies recognized neither the isolated HMWK-heavy chain nor the SH-reduced forms of both kininogens. Further, they did not cross-react with rat and bovine kininogens. In contrast, the monoclonal antibody 2LMWK11 (IgG2a kappa) bound to LMWK and its kinin-free form only, but also recognized the HMWK-heavy chain after reduction of the purified cleaved HMWK. However, the single chain, kinin containing form of HMWK was recognized only in a tenfold molar excess over LMWK.

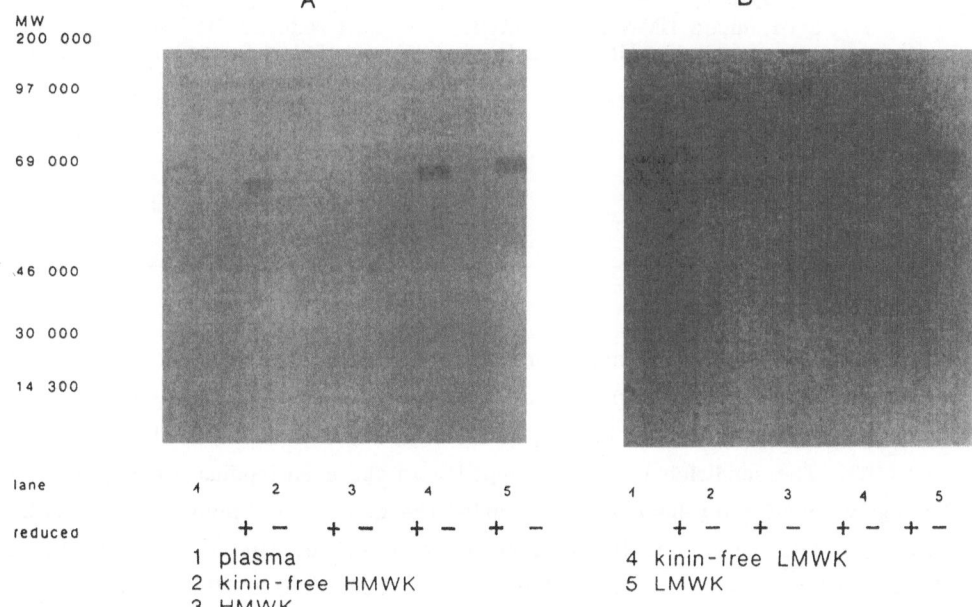

Figure 1. Characterization of the monoclonal (A) and polyclonal (B) antibodies by immunoblotting

Like the polyclonal rabbit antibodies, 2LMWK11 interacted neither with SH-reduced forms of human LMWK and HMWK nor with the kininogens from other species. In functional studies carried out in the bioassay, preincubation of purified LMWK with purified 2LMWK11 had no influence on the amount of kinin released upon subsequent incubation with purified human urinary kallikrein. The characteristics of the rabbit and mouse antibodies are summarized in Table 1.

Table 1. Characteristics of the polyclonal and monoclonal antibodies (AB) as revealed by SDS-PAGE, immunoblotting and functional studies.

	RABBIT AB	MONOCLONAL AB
	IgG	IgG 2a, kappa
recognizes:	single chain LMWK single chain HMWK	single chain LMWK HMWK-heavy chain
does not recognize:	HMWK-heavy chain SH-reduced HMWK and LMWK rat and bovine HMWK and LMWK	single chain HMWK SH-reduced HMWK and LMWK degraded forms of HMWK and LMWK rat and bovine HMWK and LMWK
additional characterisation:		no inhibition of LMWK-cleavage by kallikrein

These data suggest that the monoclonal antibody 2LMWK11 is directed against an epitope localized on the common heavy chain of kininogens; however, while this epitope is easily recognized in LMWK, it is not easily available for binding on single chain HMWK. The sandwich ELISA developed with these antibodies proved, therefore, to be highly specific for human LMWK under the conditions employed. The calibration curve of the assay was linear between amounts of 1ng and 1μg of purified LMWK/ml and addition of purified HMWK (up to 500ng/ml) to the LMWK standards did not influence the calibration curve. The lower detection limit of the assay was 1ng/ml. Recovery of known amounts of LMWK added to plasma was higher than 91%.

The inter- and intraassay variations for identical samples were less than 6% and less than 4%, respectively.

Comparison of values determined in the ELISA with those obtained in the bioassay revealed an excellent correlation (r=0.98) for both purified LMWK alone and purified LMWK added to plasma. When these experiments were done with either purified HMWK or HMWK added to plasma, a much higher concentration of HMWK (approximately twenty times more) was necessary for detection in the ELISA, while kinin release measured in the bioassay was comparable with LMWK. Therefore, despite a good correlation of the two assays for measurement of HMWK, the slope of the regression line was very steep (Fig. 2).

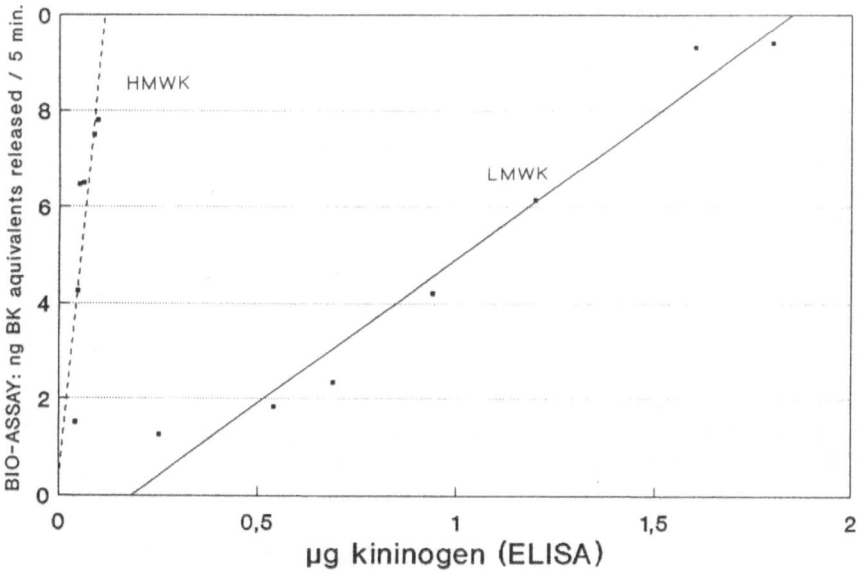

Figure 2. Relationship between measurements for purified HMWK and purified LMWK performed with the rat uterus bioassay and with the newly developed ELISA

Serial dilutions of samples from plasma, ascitic fluid, amniotic fluid and pleural effusion were parallel to the standard curve (Fig. 3) indicating that the assay can be employed to specifically measure LMWK in these samples. Quantitative determination of LMWK was therefore performed in a number of biological samples, the results of which are given in Table 2. No LMWK could be detected in saliva. The results obtained upon measurement of LMWK in a variety of cell culture supernatants are given in Table 3. The highest values were measured in the human hepatoma cell line Hep G2.

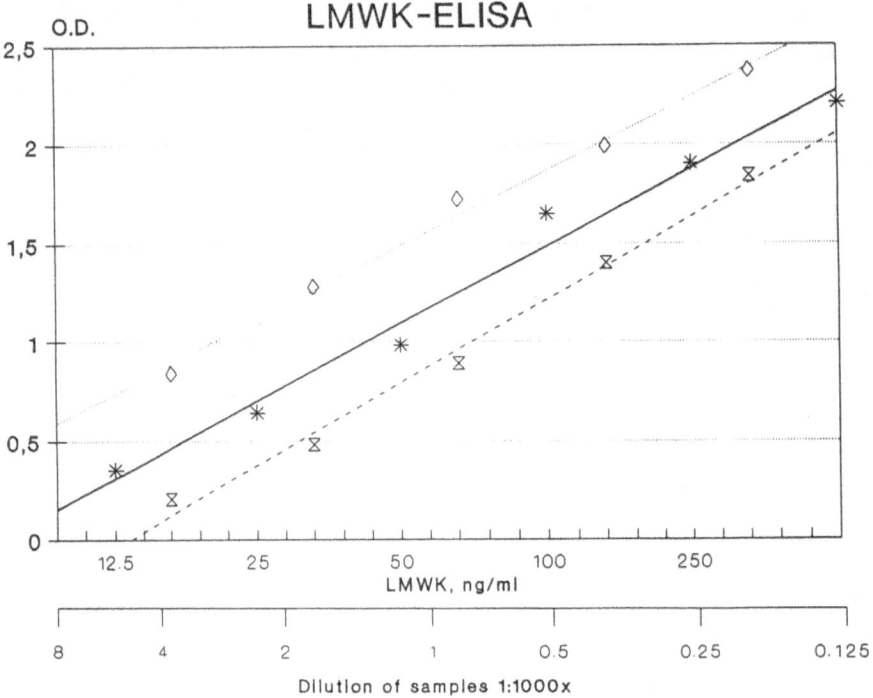

Figure 3. Serial dilutions of ascitic fluid ····· and pleural effusion --- were parallel to the standard curve —

Table 2.   LMWK concentration

Plasma	40-100μg/ml	n>30
Amniotic fluid	20- 70μg/ml	n=20
Pleura effusion	20-100μg/ml	n=12
Ascitic fluid	20-500μg/ml	n=12
Synovial fluid	10-300μg/ml	n= 6
Urine	100-200ng/ml	n= 6
Liquor	150ng/ml	n= 1
Aqueous humor	300ng/ml	n= 1

Table 3. Cell culture supernatants   LMWK, ng/24h/10^6 cells

Hep G2	29.31	SW620	1.10
Chang liver	0.92	WiDr	0.44
G-361	0.77	A673	0.24
HL-60	1.02	Caov-3	0.36
U-937	0.57	Caov-5	0.74
H33HJ-JA1	0.40	PA-1	0.32
HeLa	0.77	PC-3	0.38
BT-20	0.30	DU 145	0.29
MCF7	1.00	LNCaP	0.48

DISCUSSION

The monoclonal antibody 2LMWK11 was capable of binding to intact LMWK and to the isolated heavy chain of HMWK (Fig 1., Tab. 1). However, since the rabbit polyclonal antibodies did not bind to the isolated heavy chain of HMWK but only to both intact LMWK and HMWK and since the latter in turn was not bound to the monoclonal antibody, the sandwich ELISA developed is specific for LMWK (Fig 2.). A reliable method for determination of human LMWK in a variety of biological samples was established (Fig. 3). The values obtained for plasma samples were similar to those found by other authors using different assay methods (12). Rather high concentrations were measured in samples of ascites obtained from patients suffering from liver cirrhosis. Since kininogens are produced in the liver (13) one might expect rather reduced concentrations and low amounts of kininogen accompanying this desease. However, the high values of LMWK might be due to reduced protease activity or due to diminished clearance from plasma (prolonged half life) in these patients. LMWK measured in pleural effusions of patients with both malignant and non-malignant disease showed no difference between these two groups. In saliva no kininogen was found, suggesting that it is not synthesized at all or that it is immediately degraded. In contrast, kininogen concentrations found in urine were high. Because of the presence of kallikrein in the urine (11,14) LMWK from this source might, at least in part, be kinin-free. A similar conclusion was reached by other investigators (15). As evident from Figure 1, it was not possible to distinguish between the active and the kinin-free form with our determination method.

Binding of 2LMWK11 to only the isolated heavy chain of the HMWK-molecule indicates that the structures of intact HMWK (and its heavy chain within the intact molecule) and of the kinin-free molecule, respectively are somewhat different from those of the isolated heavy chain and from those of intact LMWK. Because of the known homology of kininogens in their amino-terminal heavy chain region (13) the epitope in LMWK recognized by the antibody might therefore have a different structure or might be covered by the larger C-terminal chain in HMWK. Neither antibody was able to bind to SH-reduced LMWK, again indicating the fundamental importance of the intact structures provided by the inter- and intrachain disulfide bridges (16). In our effort to characterize the epitope further the antibodies were used in functional studies. The results show that in the bioassay the monoclonal antibodies were not able to interfere with kinin release by human urinary kallikrein (Table 1). This result suggests that they were not competing with purified human urinary kallikrein for its binding site on both HMWK and LMWK.

Our ELISA-system is a reliable and accurate method for screening biological samples for their content of LMWK and will be a valuable tool in the field of further kininogen research.

REFERENCES

1. Müller-Esterl W.: Kininogens, Kinins and Kinships. Thromb. Haemostas. 1989; 61: 2-6.

2. Maier M., Austen K. F. and Spragg J.: Kinetic analysis of the interaction of human tissue kallikrein with single-chain human high and low molecular weight kininogens. Proc. Natl. Acad. Sci. USA 1983; 80: 3928-3932.

3. Tait J. F. and Fujikawa K.: Identification of the Binding Site for Plasma Prekallikrein in Human High Molecular Weight Kininogen. J. Biol. Chem. 1986; 261: 15396-15401.

4. Lottspeich F., Kellermann J., Henschen a., Rauth G. and Müller-Esterl W. Human low-molecular-mass kininogen. Eur. J. Biochem. 1984; 142: 227-232.

5. Proud D., Perkins M., Pierce J.V., Yates K.N., Highet P.F., Herring P.L., Mang kornkanok/Mark M., Bahu R., Carone F and Pisano J.J. Characterization and Localization of Human Renal Kininogen. J. Biol. Chem. 1981; 256: 10634-10639.

6. Maier M., Austen F.K. and Spragg J.: Purification of Single-Chain Human Low-Molecular-Weight Kininogen and Demonstration of Its Cleavage by Human Urinary Kallikrein. Analyt. Biochem. 1983; 134:336-346.

7. Maier M., Jerabek I., Reissert G., Höltzl E. and Binder B.R.: Correlation of two different assays for urinary kallikrein in normotensive and hypertensive subjects. Clinica Chimica Acta 1988; 178: 127-140.

8. Maier M., Austen K. F. and Spragg J.: Characterization of the Procoagulant Chain Derived From Human High Molecular Weight Kininogen (Fitzgerald Factor) by Human Tissue Kallikrein. Blood 1983; 62: 457-463.

9. Maier M., Zhegu Z and Binder B.R. Hemodynamics of the isolated perfused rat kidney in the absence and presence of kallikrein substrate. in: Kinins IV, Lowell M. Margolius (ed.), Plenum Publishing Corporation, 1986; 173-180.

10. Muellbacher W., Maier M and Binder B.R. Regulation of plasminogen activation in isolated perfused rat kidney. Am. J. Physiol. 1989; 256: F787-F793.

11. Ole-MoiYoi O., Spragg J. and Austen K.F. Structural studies of human urinary kallikrein (urokallikrein). Proc. Natl. Acad. Sci. USA 1979; 76: 3121-3125.

12. Adam A., Albert A., Calay G., Closset J., Damas J. and Franchimont P. Human Kininogens of Low and High Molecular Mass: Quantification by Radioimmuno assay and Determination of Reference Values. Clin. Chem. 1985; 31: 423-426.

13. Takagaki Y., Kitamura N. and Nakanishi S. Cloning and Sequence Analysis of cDNAs for Human High Molecular Weight and Low Molecular Weight Prekininogens. J. Biol. Chem. 1985; 260: 8601-8609.

14. Scicli A.G. and Carretero O.A. Renal kallikrein-kinin system. Kidney Int. 1986; 29: 120-130.

15. Weinberg M.S., Azar P., Trebbin W.M., Solomon R.J. The role of urinary kininogen in the regulation of kinin generation. Kidney Int. 1985; 28: 975-981.

16. Kellermann J., Thelen C., Lottspeich F., Henschen A., Vogel R. and Müller-
    Esterl.Arrangement of the disulphide bridges in human low-Mr kininogen.
    Biochem. J. 1987; 247: 15-21.

AAS 38/I
Recent Progress on Kinins
© 1992 Birkhäuser Verlag Basel

KININOGENS AS INHIBITORS OF CALPAINS: CHARACTERISTICS AND

BIOLOGICAL IMPLICATIONS OF THE REACTION

M. Sasaki, I. Ohkubo* and M. Kunimatsu

Department of Biochemistry, Nagoya City University Medical
School, Mizuho-ku, Nagoya 467, Japan

INTRODUCTION

Kininogens are multifunctional proteins, which participate in the
inflammatory process by liberating kinins (1) and in the
regulation of cysteine proteinases including calpains I and II
(2) and cathepsins B, H and L (3). High molecular weight
kininogen additionally serves as a cofactor in the initial phase
of blood coagulation (4). Calpains are also multifunctional
proteins consisting of two subunits: a large subunit, which
contains a papain-like cysteine proteinase domain, a calmodulin-
like calcium binding domain (5) and a chemotactic factor
releasing domain (6); and a small subunit, which includes a
calmodulin-like calcium binding domain (5) and a chemotactic
factor releasing domain (7). Interaction of the two
multifunctional proteins is therefore not a simple reaction
between a protease and an inhibitor, but results in concomitant
reactions including degradation of kininogens and liberation of
kinin (8). Several characteristics and possible biological
implications of the reaction are described.

---

*Present address: Department of Medical Biochemistry, Shiga
 University of Medical Science, Ohtsu 520-21, Japan

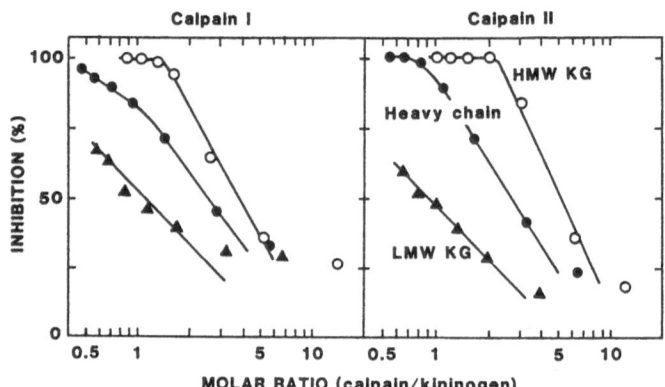

Figure 1. Inhibition of caseinolytic activity of calpains by HMW and LMW kininogens and the heavy chain (2).

BINDING CAPACITY OF KININOGENS

In the presence of the calcium ion, calpains I and II are inhibited by high molecular weight (HMW) and low molecular weight (LMW) kininogens and their heavy chain. Although the reactive sites of kininogens and the heavy chain with cysteine proteinases are known to be localized in domains 2 and 3 of the heavy chain and are identical to each other (9, 10), inhibition patterns of HMW and LMW kininogens and the heavy chain are considerably different. As shown in Fig. 1, calpain II is completely inhibited by HMW kininogen at a molar ratio of 2 : 1, whereas it is almost totally inhibited by the heavy chain at a molar ratio of 1 : 1. However, LMW kininogen cannot completely inhibit calpain II (2). Likewise, similar but weaker inhibitions are

Table 1. Molar ratios of calpain to kininogen and papain to kininogen which give maximum inhibition

	Calpain I	Calpain II	Papain
HMW-KG	1.4	2.0	1.4
LMW-KG	<0.5	<0.5	1.4
heavy chain	0.7	0.8	2.0

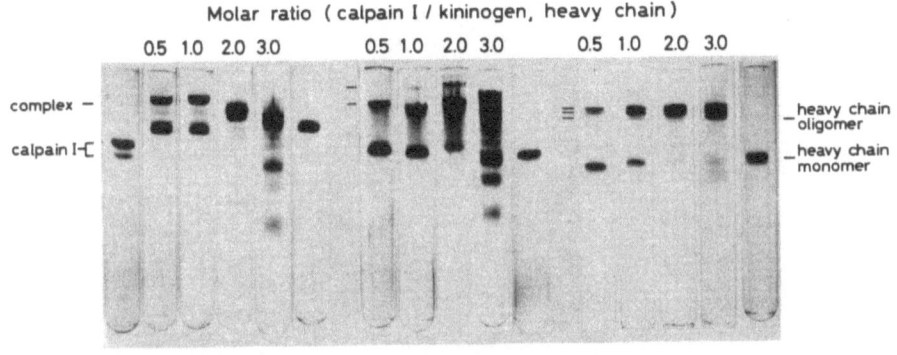

Figure 2. Disc gel electrophoretic analysis of complex formation between calpain I and HMW and LMW kininogen or heavy chain (2).

observed with calpain I. Details of the mechanism resulting in such a large difference in inhibition by the two kininogens and the heavy chain are not clear, but it could be due to the effect of size and charge differences in the two light chains of HMW and LMW kininogens. In Table 1, the data are summarized and compared to results of papain inhibition (11). In the case of papain, the reaction occurs without the calcium ion and full inhibition at a 2 : 1 molar ratio is obtained only with the heavy chain. The effect of light chains on inhibitory activity is almost identical for both HMW and LMW kininogens at a molar ratio of 1.4.

In order to characterize the interaction of calpains with kininogens and the heavy chain, various amounts of calpain I were incubated with a constant amount (7.5×10^{-11} mol) of kininogen or heavy chain and complex formation was analyzed by disc gel electrophoresis (Fig. 2)(2). Gel 1 was loaded with calpain I, gel 6 with HMW kininogen, gel 11 with LMW kininogen, gel 16 with the heavy chain, and the other gels were loaded with mixtures of calpain 1 and HMW kininogen (gels 2-5), LMW kininogen (gels 7-10) and the heavy chain (gels 12-15). Molar ratios are shown above the panels. At molar ratios of 0.5 and 1.0 (gels 2 and 3), HMW kininogen is still detectable, whereas at a molar ratio of 2.0,

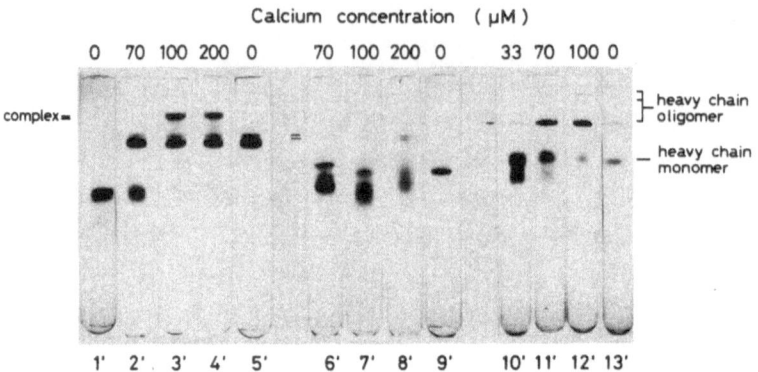

Figure 3. Disc gel electrophoretic analysis of complex formation
between calpain II and kininogens or heavy chain (2).

both calpain I and HMW kininogen almost disappear, forming
colmplexes. In a molar ratio of 3.0, some degradation products
appear, indicating that the 2 to 1 mixture is optimal for the
reaction. Likewise, with the heavy chain, at a molar ratio of
2 : 1, both calpain and the heavy chain almost disappear.
However, with LMW kininogen, even at a molar ratio of 2 : 1,
calpain and/or kininogen can sitll be detected. These results
are compatible with the inhibition data, suggesting loose
association of the complex with LMW kininogen. Since the calcium
ion seems to play an important role in the reaction between
kininogen and calpain, the effect of the calcium ion on complex
formation was examined (Fig. 3) (2). Gel 1' was loaded with
calpain II, gel 5' with HMW kininogen, gel 9' with LMW kininogen,
and gel 13' with the heavy chain. To the other gels, 1 : 1
mixtures of calpain II and kininogens or heavy chain were applied
at various calcium concentrations from 0 to 100 µM or to 200 µM.
The complex appears at a calcium concentration of 100 µM with HMW
kininogen and from 70 µM with the heavy chain, although calpain
II requires mM levels of calcium ion for activation, suggesting
that the calcium ion required for complex formation is not
related to the activation of calpains. This was more clearly
demonstrated by experiments using several other divalent cations.

REQUIREMENT OF DIVALENT CATIONS FOR COMPLEX FORMATION

Figure 4 shows complex formation involving several divalent
cations at two concentrations (2): 100 µM and 10 mM. The upper
two panels show complex formation between calpain I and the heavy
chain, and the bottom two panels show calpain II and the heavy
chain.

At a cation concentration of 100 µM, calpains I and II
formed complexes in the presence of only calcium ions, but at a
concentration of 10 mM, other cations, Mn^{2+}, Sr^{2+} and Ba^{2+} also
participated in complex formation. The results are summarized in
Table 2 referring to the data with the activation of calpains
(2). For complex formation, four cations, Mn^{2+}, Ca^{2+}, Sr^{2+} and
Ba^{2+} are effective. For activation of calpain I, Ca^{2+}, Sr^{2+} and

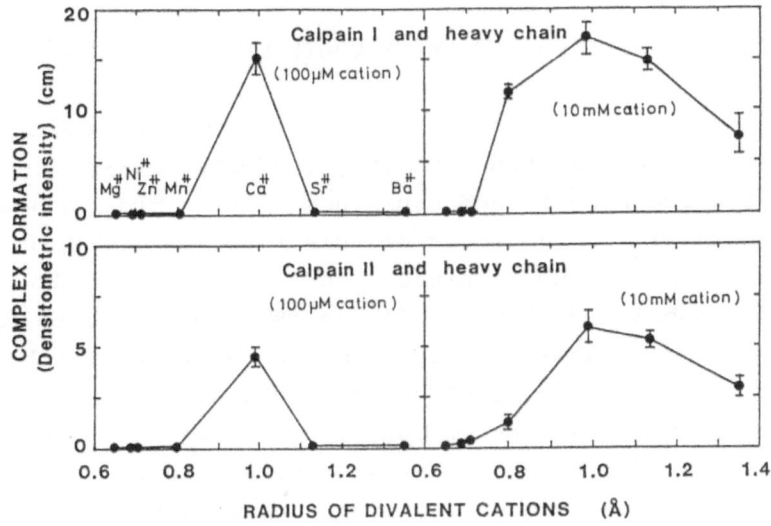

Figure 4. Effects of various divalent cations on complex
formation between calpains and the heavy chain.
After a 15-min incubation of calpain I or II with the heavy
chain, aliquots were subjected to polyacrylamide disc gel
electrophoresis. The gels were stained with Coomassie brilliant
blue R-250 and subjected to densitometric analysis. The
absorption peaks (height) of the band(s) for the complex(es) were
plotted against ionic radii of divalent cations (2).

Table 2. Roles of divalent cations in activation of calpains
and complex formation with the heavy chain of kininogen

Cations	Calpain I			Calpain II		
	Activation		Complex formation	Activation		Complex formation
	5 (mM)	10 (mM)		5 (mM)	10 (mM)	
Ca^{2+}	100	–	+	100	100	+
Mg^{2+}	0	0	–	3.8	7.6	–
Ni^{2+}	9.6	9.7	–	7.6	11.0	–
Zn^{2+}	0	0	–	0	0	–
Mn^{2+}	3.4	4.9	+	0	3.8	+
Sr^{2+}	103.2	105.1	+	0	3.8	+
Ba^{2+}	44.4	91.9	+	3.8	7.6	+

Ba^{2+} are effective, whereas for calpain II, Ca^{2+} alone is
effective, indicating that the divalent cations acting in complex
formation and those acting in calpain activation are different.

CALCIUM BINDING SITE ON THE HEAVY CHAIN OF KININOGEN

Calcium binding sites capable of inducing conformational changes
of kininogen were searched employing conformation-specific
antibodies which bind to HMW kininogen only in the presence of
calcium ion (12). An antibody of this type was isolated from the
IgG fraction of anti-HMW kininogen antiserum using a HMW
kininogen-immobilized column. The antibody was able to bind to
the CB-1 fragment (domain 1 region of the heavy chain) but not to
domains 2 and 3 and the light chain of HMW kininogen. Therefore,
a sequence search was carried out, and a calmodulin-like sequence
was revealed at the N-terminal region of domain 1. Figure 5
shows the N-terminal sequence of human kininogens in comparison
with other amino acid sequences of the E-F hand structures (12).
In the 28 N-terminal sequence of kininogen, the E-F hand-like
structure of the 12 amino acid sequence stretch is involved.
This sequence has considerably high sequence homology with the
E-F hand structure of the sarcoplasmic Ca^{2+}-binding protein
(SCP), whereas it has rather low homology with those of
calmodulin and calpains. Conformational changes of the CB-1

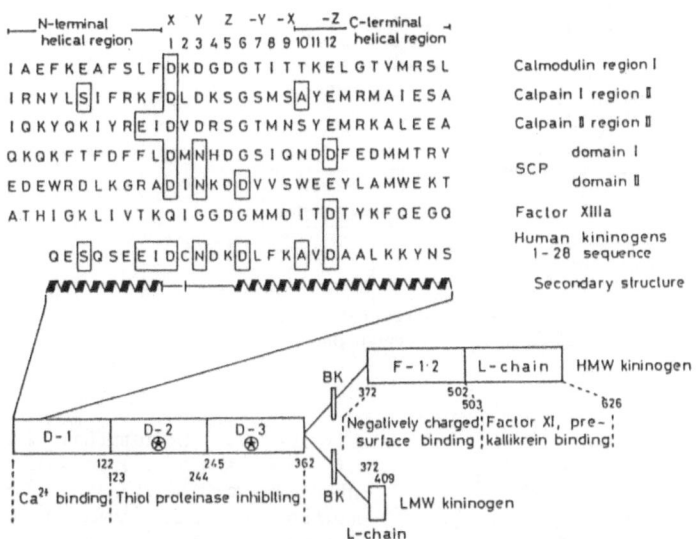

Figure 5. Comparison of the amino acid sequence of the amino-terminal 28 residues of kininogens with the EF hand site sequences of Ca^{2+}-binding proteins and linear model of kininogen domain structure and functions (12).

fragment and the heavy chain induced by divalent cations, including the calcium ion, was demonstrated in circular dichroism spectra (12).

KININ RELEASE

Another interesting observation of the interaction of kininogen with calpain is the liberation of kinin (Lys-bradykinin)(8). Kinin release occurred over a limited range of calpain I to kininogen molar ratios of 2 : 1 to 8 : 1. The maximum level of kinin release is 25% where calpain I is inhibited approximately 30% by each kininogen. Likewise, kinin release by calpain II also takes place over a limited range of calpain to kininogen molar ratios, and the maximum levels of kinin release from HMW and LMW kininogens are 6% and 20%, respectively.

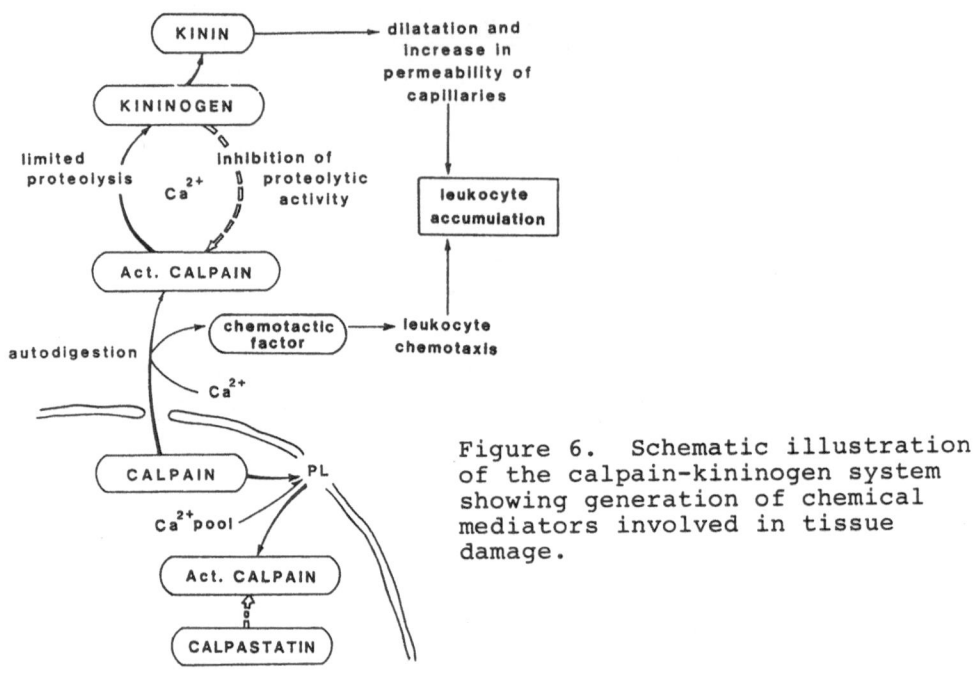

Figure 6. Schematic illustration of the calpain-kininogen system showing generation of chemical mediators involved in tissue damage.

BIOLOGICAL IMPLICATIONS OF THE REACTION

The kininogen-calpain interaction in vivo may occur when calpains are released from cells (13). In the case of tissue injury, calpains might be released into the interstitial connective tissues, where they may be activated with an excess amount of Ca^{2+} and autodigested, liberating leukocyte chemotactic factors (6, 7). Activated calpains are trapped with kininogens in tissue fluids with simultaneous generation of kinin (8). Kinin may act on the capillary wall inducing dilatation and increasing capillary permeability. This increase may cooperatively facilitate migration and accumulation of neutrophils (Fig. 6). Thus, the interaction of kininogens with calpains can be summerized as follows.

1. Characteristic binding stoichiometry: a high binding ratio and highly efficient inhibition of calpains by HMW kininogen. a low binding ratio and poor inhibition by LMW kininogen.

2. Requirement of the calcium ion not only for activating calpains but also for complex formation.
3. Degradation of kininogens and simultaneous liberation of kinin.
4. Possible participation in inflammation caused by tissue damage.

REFERENCES

1. Ryan GB, Majno G. Acute inflammation. Amer J Pathol 1977; 86:185-276.

2. Ishiguro H, Higashiyama S, Namikawa C, Kunimatsu M, Takano E, Tanaka K, Ohkubo I, Murachi T, Sasaki M. Interaction of human calpains I and II with high molecular weight and low molecular weight kininogens and their heavy chain: mechanism of interaction and the role of divalent cations. Biochemistry 1987; 26:2863-2870.

3. Sueyoshi T, Enjyoji K, Shimada T, Kato H, Iwanaga S, Bando Y, Kominami E, Katunuma N. A new function of kininogens as thiol proteinase inhibitors: inhibition of papain and cathepsins B, H and L by bovine, rat and human plasma kininogens. FEBS Lett 1985; 182:193-195.

4. Jackson CM, Nemerson Y. Blood coagulation. Ann Rev Biochem 1980; 49:765-811.

5. Suzuki K. Calcium activated neutral protease: domain structure and activity regulation. Trend Biochem Sci 1987; 12:103-105.

6. Kunimatsu M, Higashiyama S, Sato K, Ohkubo I, Sasaki M. Calcium dependent cysteine proteinase is a precursor of a chemotactic factor for neutrophils. Biochem Biophys Res Comm 1989; 164:875-882.

7. Kunimatsu M, Ma XJ, Nishimura J, Baba S, Hamada Y, Shioiri T, Sasaki M. Neutrophil chemotactic activity of N-terminal peptides from the calpain small subunit. Biochem Biophys Res Comm 1990; 169:1242-1247.

8. Higashiyama S, Ishiguro H, Ohkubo I, Fujimoto S, Matsuda T, Sasaki M. Kinin release from kininogens by calpains. Life Sci 1986; 39:1639-1644.

9. Ohkubo I, Kurachi K, Takasawa T, Shiokawa H, Sasaki M.
   Isolation of a human cDNA for α_2-thiol proteinase inhibitor
   and its identity with low molecular weight kininogen.
   Biochemistry 1984; 28:5691-5697.

10. Salvesen G, Parkes C, Abrahamson M, Grubb A, Barrett A.
    Human low-Mr kininogen contains three copies of a cystatin
    sequence that are divergent in structure and in inhibitory
    activity for cysteine proteinases. Biochem J 1986; 234:429-
    434.

11. Higashiyama S, Ohkubo I, Ishiguro H, Kunimatsu M, Sawaki K,
    Sasaki M. Human high molecular weight kininogen as a thiol
    proteinase inhibitor: presence of the entire inhibition
    capacity in the native form of heavy chain. Biochemistry
    1986; 25:1669-1675.

12. Higashiyama S, Ohkubo I, Ishiguro H, Sasaki M. Heavy chain
    of human high molecular weight and low molecular weihgt
    kininogens binds calcium ion. Biochemistry 1987; 26:7450-
    7458.

13. Sasaki M, Kunimatsu M, Tada T, Nishimura J, Ma XJ, Ohkubo I.
    Calpain and kininogen mediated Inflammation. Biomed Biochim
    Acta 1991; 50:499-508.

AAS 38/I
Recent Progress on Kinins
© 1992 Birkhäuser Verlag Basel

KININOGEN DEFICIENCY IN THE RAT

S. Oh-ishi, I. Hayashi, K. Yamaki, and I. Utsunomiya

Department of Pharmacology, School of Pharmac. Sci., Kitasato Univ., Shirokane, Minato-ku, Tokyo, Japan

SUMMARY: The Brown Norway Katholiek (B/N-Ka) strain rat is the only animal strain that demonstrates deficiency in plasma HMW- and LMW-kininogens with a low level of prekallikrein. We developed an RIA for rat HMW-kininogen, LMW-kininogen, and T-kininogen, and using them measured these proteins in B/N-Ka and normal strain (B/N-Ki) rats. Plasma level of immunoreactive as well as kinin-releasing HMW-kininogen and LMW-kininogen in B/N-Ka rats was either around 3 % of their levels in the normal B/N-Ki rats.

The cause of the plasma deficiency of kininogens in the B/N-Ka strain was examined by ^{35}S-methionine uptake of primary cultures of hepatocytes from the B/N-Ki and B/N-Ka strains. The results indicated that the kininogens were synthesized in the B/N-Ka liver but not secreted into the medium. Northern blot analysis of poly A(+)RNA extracted from the livers of both strains demonstrated that the band corresponding to mRNA of HMW-kininogen was present in the mRNA from B/N-Ka liver as well as in that from the B/N-Ki one. The band was similar in size and intensity in both cases. This result confirmed the data that immunoreactive HMW-kininogen was found in the liver of B/N-Ka rats (12). Thus, the cause of plasma deficiency of HMW-kininogen in the mutant appears to be secretry defect in nature.

The B/N-Ka rats showed less reactivity to the inflammatory stimulus, such as carrageenin or kaolin, but the strain expressed almost the same response as normal rats to phorbol ester (PMA) or zymosan for pleurisy induction. These results indicate that kinin may play an important role in exudation in carrageenin- and kaolin-induced edema but not in that induced by PMA or zymosan. The deficient rat strain could be useful for differentiation of the inflammatory model which shows involvement of the kinin system.

INTRODUCTION

The rat strain, Brown Norway mai f, has been kept in the animal

laboratory of Katholiek University, Liege, and was discovered by

J.Damas as a mutant strain having a defective plasma kallikrein-kinin system (1). The same strain kept in Kitasato University was found to be normal and was named B/N-Kitasato (B/N-Ki), whereas the deficient strain was termed B/N-Katholiek (B/N-Ka). The origin of B/N rats is historically described in a book (2), which indicates the B/N strain was developed in the Wistar Institute and originated from the same wild rats from which the Wistar rats had been derived. As shown in Fig. 1, B/N rats in Katholiek University had been transferred there from National Institutes of Health, Bethesda, while the same strain kept at the NIH was normal (3). The reason for the mutation is not known.

Both normal and mutant strains have been extensively studied, and the B/N-Ka strain has been confirmed to have a congenital plasma kininogen deficiency with a low level of plasma pre-kallikrein (4-6). The deficiency is very similar to the human kininogen deficiency, which has previously been reported (5-8). B/N-Ka rats has been used to evaluate the role of the kallikrein-kinin system in the response to various stimuli, and these rats have been shown to be low responders to some inflammatory stimuli (9-11). In this paper we describe and summarize the nature of the deficiency of this strain and reactivity of the body defense system of these animals to various stimuli, and then discuss some genetic features of the deficiency.

MATERIALS AND METHODS

Animals: Sprague-Dawley (SD) rats were purchased (SLC, Hamamatsu). Brown Norway Kitasato (B/N-Ki) and Brown Norway Katholiek (B/N-Ka) rats were kept and bred in the animal labora-

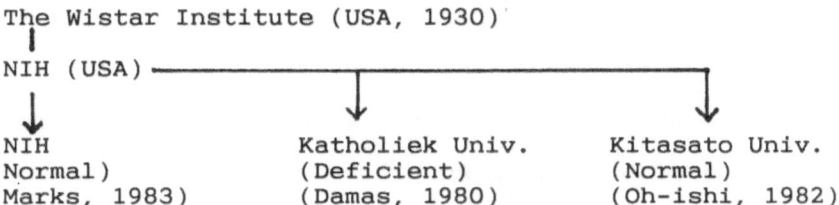

ORIGIN OF THE BROWN NORWAY RAT (B/N Mai pfd f)

The Wistar Institute (USA, 1930)

NIH (USA)

NIH	Katholiek Univ.	Kitasato Univ.
(Normal)	(Deficient)	(Normal)
(Marks, 1983)	(Damas, 1980)	(Oh-ishi, 1982)

Figure 1.   Origin of the Brown Norway rat.

The ancestor of laboratory rats were bred at the Wistar Institute from wild rats and used to establish colonies of rat strains
(2).   One of them, the Brown Norway, was received by the National
Institutes of Health, USA, and later transfered to laboratories
world-wide, including those at Katholiek University, Belgium, and
the National Institute of Health, Japan.

Figure 2.   Kininogen contents
of human plasma and rat plasma

HMW-kininogen (H) and LMW-
kininogen (L) in human plasma
were measured by bradykinin
released when the plasma was
incubated with kaolin or with
snake venom kininogenase as
described in the method.   H
and L, and T-kininogen (T) in
rat plasma were assayed by
radioimmunoassay and also in
terms of bradykinin released
when incubated with rat kallikrein. Numbers above columns
indicate numbers of samples
used, and bars standard er-
rors.

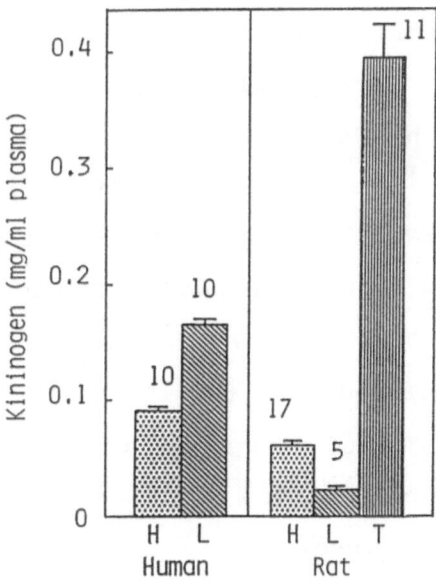

tory of Kitaso University, School of Pharmaceutical Sciences.

Kininogens and their antibodies: HMW-, LMW- and T-kininogens were purified as previously reported (13,14); and RIA was performed as previously (15,16), using antiserum to the light chain of HMW-kininogen and mouse monoclonals to HMW-kininogen or T-kininogen.

Assays of components: Measurement of kinins by a bioassay based on rat uterus contraction was made as previously reported (6), and that by an enzyme immunoassay (Markit-BK, a kind gift from Dainippon Pharmaceutical Co., Osaka) was also carried out as described earlier (17).

Plasma prekallikrein was measured in termes of amidase activity toward a synthetic substrate, carbobenzoxyl-L-phenylalanyl-L-arginyl-4-methylcoumaryl-7-amide (Peptide Institute, Minoh) after activation with kaolin-activated Factor XII as described previously (18).

Western blot analysis was made as previously reported (12), with rabbit antisera to the light chain of HMW-kininogen.

Northern blot analysis was carried out with a probe of rat HMW-kininogen mRNA (kind gift from Dr. N.Kitamura, Kansai Univ.). The probe used was a 618 base-pair of cDNA from number 1242 to 1859 of the HMW-kininogen gene (19). Poly A(+) RNA (10 µg) was isolated from the livers of B/N-Ki (Ki) and B/N-Ka (Ka) rats, subjected to agarose gel electrophoresis, and transferred to a nylon membrane followed by hybridization with the ^{32}P-labeled cDNA probe.

Primary culture of hepatocytes: The livers were perfused with physiological buffer after exsanguination, and then the buffer was replaced with collagenase-containing buffer as described previously (12). Isolated hepatocytes were incubated in a plastic plates (35 mm, Corning) in the presence or absence of ^{35}S-methionine (Amersham Japan). Kininogens in the medium or cell fraction were assayed by RIA. Alternatively immunoreactive kininogen was precipitated by monoclonal antibodies to each kininogen and then autoradiography was performed as described (20).

Procedure for induction of pleurisy in rats: Male B/N-Ki and B/N-Ka rats were injected under light ether anesthesia with 0.1 ml saline solution or a suspension of one of the following inducers, as previously reported : 2% carrageenin (9), 1% kaolin (21), 1 µM PMA (22,) or 2% Zymosan (23). At the indicated times after the intrapleural injection, rats were intravenously injected with 50 mg/kg pontamine sky blue saline solution; and then 20 min later they were exsanguinated. Plasma and pleural exudates were collected immediately, and examined.

Collection of urine: Urine was collected from the ureter of B/N-Ki and B/N-Ka rats into tubes containing kininase inhibitors, and subjected to gel chromatography as previously reported (17). Kinin in each fraction was measured by bradykinin EIA as described above.

RESULTS

First of all, kininogen contents in rat plasma were measured in comparison with those in human plasma. As shown in Fig. 2, kininogen contents in human plasma were measured by bioassay of

the released kinin according to the classical method described by
Jacobsen (24).   That is, bradykinin can be released from HMW-
kininogen when plasma is activated with kaolin in the presence of
kininase-inhibitors: and bradykinin can also be released from
HMW- and LMW-kininogen when plasma is incubated with partially
purified snake venom kininogenase (6).   The released kinins were
assayed by rat uterus contraction or bradykinin-EIA kit.   We
measured rat kininogens in normal rat (male SD) plasma in the
same way as for HMW-kininogen and LMW-kininogen in human plasma
as shown in Fig. 2.   HMW-kininogen content was also measured by
an RIA for rat HMW-kininogen using antibody to the light chain.
Estimates by bioassay and RIA agreed well, indicating both measurements to be reliable.   The T-kininogen level was measured by
an RIA using monoclonals to rat T-kininogen (15).   Then using
these methods we measured kininogen contents of plasma samples of
male B/N-Ki and B/N-Ka rats (20-40 week-old), as shown in Fig. 3.
Contents of HMW- and LMW-kininogens in B/N-Ka plasma were around
3% of the normal level, while T-kininogen levels were almost the
same between B/N-Ki and B/N-Ka rats.

As shown in Fig. 4, the kininogen content of medium condi-
tioned by liver cells in primary culture reflected the findings
in plasma; i.e., whereas T-kininogen was detected at the same
level and with the same kinetics in the medium from both normal
and mutant cells, only the normal cells also secreted HMW- and
LMW-kininogens.   As it is possible that the B/N-Ka liver may
synthesize these kininogens but not secrete them, we pulse-
labeled the liver cells for 3 hr with ^{35}S-methionine, and then

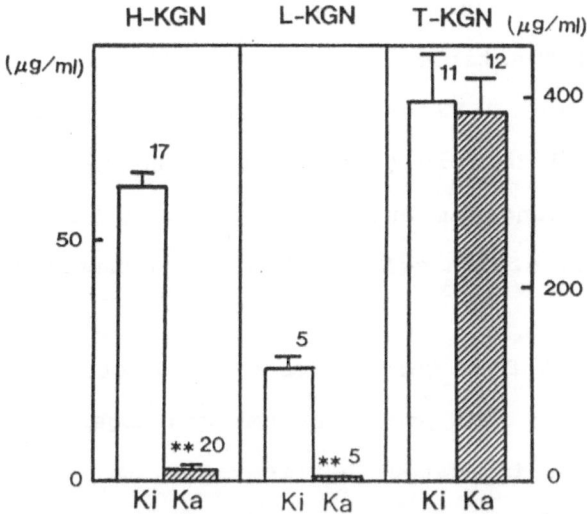

Figure 3.   Contents of kininogens in B/N-ka and B/N-Ki rat plasma

HMW-kininogen (H-KGN) and T-kininogen (T-KGN) were measure by
RIA, and LMW-kininogen (L-KGN) was assayed by kinin-release with
rat glandular kallikrein.   Numbers above columns indicate numbers
of rats used.

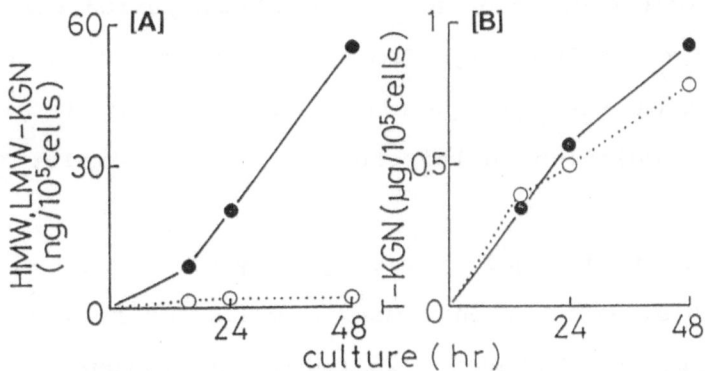

Figure 4. Synthesis and release of kininogens in rat hepatocyte
primary cultures

HMW- and LMW-kininogens released into the medium were measured
bu RIA using heavy chain-specific antibody [A], and T-kininogen
was measured by RIA [B].   -●-, B/N-Ki; -o-, B/N-Ka

examined both cells and medium for the presence of radioactivity precipitable with antibody specific for the heavy chain of HMW- and LMW-kininogens. Figure 5 indicates that the B/N-Ka liver cells did indeed contain (and hence synthesize) radio-labeled HMW- and LMW-kininogens but were unable to release them. In contrast, normal strain cells (B/N-Ki) synthesized and secreted the kininogens.

Poly A(+) RNA from the livers of both strains was examined with a ^{32}P-labeled cDNA probe for HMW-kininogen as shown in Fig. 6; and the result indicated that the mRNA for HMW-kininogen from both strains is almost the same size (2.3 kb) and amount.

The time course of development of carrageenin pleurisy was compared between B/N-Ki and B/N-ka rats and is illustrated in Fig. 7. Accumulation of pleural exudate [C] was significantly less in B/N-Ka strain rats. The exudation rate [B], which was expressed as volume of exudated over a 20-min period starting at the indicated times, was significantly less at 3 to 5 hr after the injection of the carrageenin. The time course of total leukocyte accummulation in the exudate [A] was similar in both strains.

Fig. 8 illustrates gel chromatography of urinary kinin excreted by both strains. When urine was collected from the ureter and fractionated by Sephadex G-25 column chromatography, there two immunoreactive kinin fractions, protein fraction (MW > 50,000) and kinin fraction (MW = ca. 1,000), were obtained. While in B/N-Ka urine there was no immunoreactive material in the kinin fraction, therewas some positive material in the > 50,000 MW protein fraction (17).

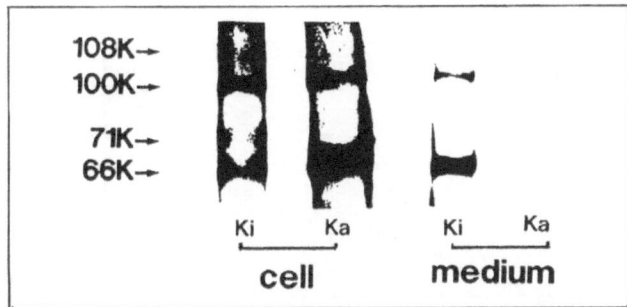

Figure 5. Autoradiography of immunoreactive ^{35}S-labeled kinino-gens produced in primary cultures of hepatocytes.

Hepatocytes from normal (Ki) and mutant (Ka) B/N rats were pulse-labeled with ^{35}S-methionine as described in Materials and Methods, and immunoprecipitation of cell lysates and medium was done with antibody specific for the H-chain of HMW- and LMW-kininogens. Following electrophoresis of the immunoprecipitates autoradiography was performed.

Figure 6. Northern blot analysis of HMW-kininogen mRNA from the livers of B/N-Ki and B/N-Ka

Isolated poly A(+) RNA (10 ug) from the liver of B/N-Ki (Ki) and B/N-Ka (Ka) rats was subjected to agarose gel electrophoresis and trans-ferred to a nylon membrane followed by hybridization with a ^{32}P-labeled cDNA probe for rat HMW-kininogen.

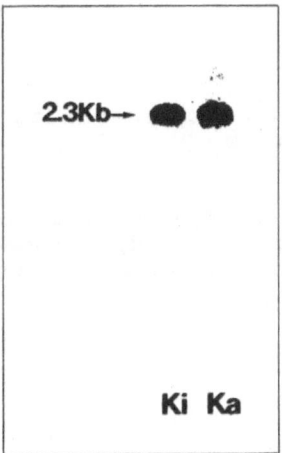

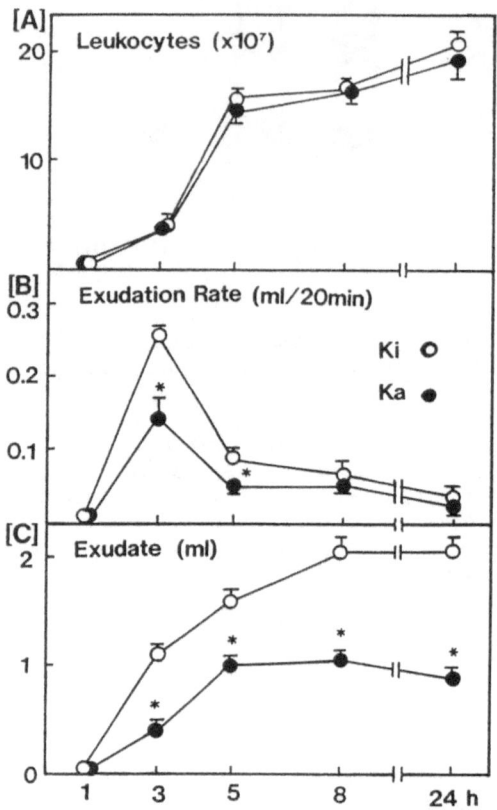

Figure 7.   Time course of carrageenin-induced pleurisy in B/N-Ki and B/N-Ka rats

[A] Total leukocytes in the exudate, [B] Exudation rate for 20 min is expressed as dye exudation, [C] Exudate volume.   Details are described in Materials and Methods.

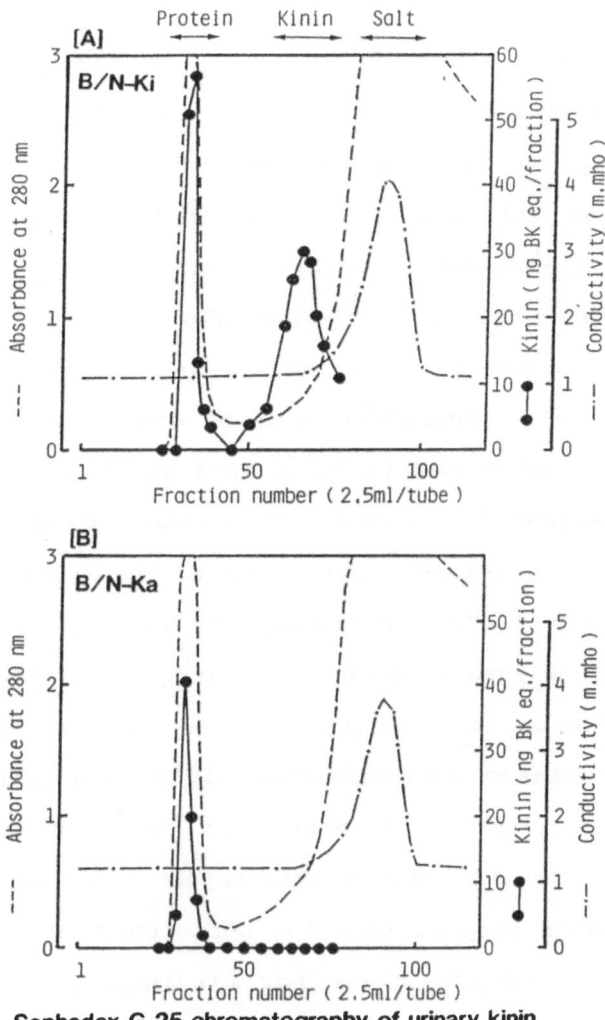

Sephadex G-25 chromatography of urinary kinin

Figure 8. Gel chromatographic patterns of urinary kinin of B/N-Ki (A) and B/N-Ka (B)

Kinin in each fraction was assayed by the bradykinin EIA as described in Materials and Methods.

DISCUSSION

Before discussing kininogen deficiency, we will first consider the contents of kininogens in normal rat plasma and human plasma. As shown in Fig. 2, human plasma contains about twice as much LMW-kininogen as HMW-kininogen, while in rat plasma the reverse applies. Rat plasma additionally contains T-kininogen, whose amount is several-fold over that of HMW-kininogen even in the normal condition; and it increases up on inflammatory or infectious stimulation. Therefore in this study the estimates for kininogens were measured in rats that were kept in strictly controled SPF animal laboratory. This basal data gives rise to several important questions pertaining to the role(s) of kininogens in the body. For instance, why is the amount of LMW-kininogen in rat plasma is so small in comparison with that of T-kininogen ?, What is the specific role of LMW-kininogen ?, etc.

B/N-Ka rat plasma contains about 3% of the normal level of HMW- and LMW-kininogens. We found that the liver cells of B/N-Ka could synthesize HMW- and LMW-kininogens but could not release them. These facts suggest that the deficiency is caused by some secretory defect of the liver for kininogens. As shown in Fig.4, hepatocytes of B/N-Ka could synthesize and secrete T-kininogen just as B/N-Ki. Furthermore the amount of T-kininogen in their plasma is similar to that of B/N-Ki or SD rats. Therefore the defect is focussed specifically on the release of HMW- and LMW-kininogen proteins. The HMW-kininogen synthesized in the livers of both strains seems to be almost the same size as judged from the ^{35}S-methionine experiment (Fig. 5). This puzzule should be clarified in future.

Susceptibity to inflammatory stimuli was examined by induction of pleurisy. The time course of development of carrageenin pleurisy (Fig. 7) indicates that HMW- and/or LMW-kininogen may have some role in exudation but no role in leukocyte migration. The lesser exudation rate of B/N-Ka at 3-5 hr indicates that for the exudation in the initial phase kininogen may play a major role, whereas at the later stage it might not be so important, since there was no significant difference between the two strains later in the time course.

In addition to carrageenin pleurisy, B/N-Ka rats showed significantly less exudation in kaolin-induced pleurisy. On the contrary, exudate volumes of PMA-induced or zymosan-induced pleurisy were not significantly different in both strains. The results indicate that involvement of the kinin system could be minor in the latter types of pleurisy. The B/N-Ka rats are useful for differentiation of the type of inflammation, i.e., kininogen dependent vs independent.

B/N-Ka rats did not release a detectable amount of kinin into their urine (Fig. 8), suggesting that urinary kinin may be derived fron plasma kininogens.

ACKNOWLEDGEMENTS

The authors express their thanks to Dr. Takeshi Nakano, Emeritus Professor of Kitasato University, and to Dr. Tatsuo Suzuki, Kitasato Institute, for their kind suggestions and technical help in the breeding of the rats. This work was supported in part by a Grant-in-Aid for Scientific Research (62480424, 01771989) from the Ministry of Education, Science, and Culture of Japan.

REFERENCES

(1) DAMAS,J. and ADAM,A. Congenital deficiency in plasma kallik-
     rein and kininogens in the brown Norway rat. Experientia
     36, 586-587, 1980
(2) LINDSEY,J.R. Historical foundations. In The Laboratory rat
     vol. I, Biology and Diseases. Eds. BAKER,H.J., LINDSEY,J.R.
     and WEISBROTH,S.H., pp 1-36, 1979, Academic Press, New York
(3) MARKS,E, ALVING,B. and PISANO,J.J. The kallikrein-kinin
     system in the Brown Norway rat. Thrombosis Res., 31, 653-
     656, 1983
(4) OH-ISHI,S., SATOH,K., HAYASHI,I., YAMAZAKI,K. and NAKANO,T.
     Differences in prekallikrein and high molecular weight
     kininogen levels in two strains of Brown Norway rat (Kitasa-
     to strain and Katholiek strain). Thrombosis Res., 28, 143-
     147, 1982
(5) OH-ISHI,S., HAYASHI,I., SATOH,K. and NAKANO,T. Prolonged
     activated thromboplastin time and deficiency of high molecu-
     lar weight kininogen in Brown Norway rat mutant (Katholiek
     strain). Thrombosis Res., 33, 317-377, 1984
(6) HAYASHI,I., INO,T., KATO,H., IWANAGA,S., NAKANO,T. and
     OH-ISHI,S. Demonstration of the third kininogen in high and
     low molecular weight kininogens-deficient Brown Norway
     Katholiek rat. Thrombosis Res., 36, 509-516, 1984
(5) WUEPPER,K.D., MILLER,D.R., Lacombe,M.J. Flaujeac trait.
     Deficiency of human plasma kininogen. J.Clin.Invest., 56,
     1663-1672, 1975
(6) SAITO,H., RATNOFF,O.D., WALDMANN,R. and ABRAHAM,J.P. Fitz-
     gerald trait. Deficiency of a hitherto unrecognized agent,
     Fitzgerald factor, participating in surface-mediated reac-
     tions of clotting, fibrinolysis, generation of kinins, and
     the property of diluted plasma enhancing vascular permeabil-
     ity (PF/Dil). J.Clin.Invest., 55, 1082-1089, 1975
(7) COLMAN,P.W., BAGDASARIAN,A., TALAMO,R.C., SCOTT,C.F., SEAVY,
     M., GUIMARAEES,J.A., PIERCE,J. and Kaplan,A.P. Williams
     trait. Human kininogen deficiency with diminished level of
     plasminogen proactivator and prekallikrein associated with
     abnormalities of the Hageman factor-deficient pathways.
     J.Clin.Invest., 56, 1650-1662, 1976
(8) OH-ISHI,S., UENO,A., UCHIDA,Y., KATORI,M., HAYASHI,H., KOYA,
     H., KITAJIMA,K. and KIMURA,I. Abnormalities in the contact
     activation through Factor XII in Fujiwara trait: a deficien-
     cyin both high molecular weight and low molecular weight
     kininogens with low level of prekallikrein. Tohoku J.exp.
     Med., 133, 67-80, 1981
(9) OH-ISHI,S., HAYASHI,I., HAYASHI,M., YAMAKI,K., YAMSU,A.,
     NAKANO, T., UTSUNOMIYA,I. and NAGASHIMA,Y. Evidence for a
     role of the plasma kallikrein-kinin system in acute inflam-
     mation: Reduced exudation during carrageenin- and kaolin-
     pleurisies in kininogen-deficient rats. Agents Actions 18,
     450-454, 1986
(10) OH-ISHI,S., HAYASHI,I., UTSUNOMIYA,I., HAYASHI,M., YAMAZAKI,
     K., YAMASU,A. and NAKANO,T. Roles of the kallikrein-kinin
     system in acute inflammation: Studies on high- and low-
     molecular weight kininogens deficient rats (B/N-Katholiek
     strain). Agents Actions 21, 384-386, 1987

(11) DAMAS,J. and REMACLE-VOLON,G. Some acute inflammatory reactions in a strain of Brown-Norway rats which are deficient in kallikrein-kinin system. Arch.int.Pharmacodyn., **260**, 274-276, 1982

(12) HAYASHI,I., MARUHASHI,J. and OH-ISHI,S. Functionally active high molecular weight-kininogen was found in the liver, but not in the plasma of Brown Norway Katholiek rat. Thrombosis Res., **56**, 179-189, 1989

(13) HAYASHI,I., KATO,H., IWANAGA,S. and OH-ISHI,S. Rat plasma high-molecular weight kininogen: A simple method for purification and its characterization. J.Biol.Chem., **260**, 6115-6123, 1985

(14) ENJYOJI,K., KATO,H., HAYASHI,I., OH-ISHI,S. and IWANAGA,S. Purification and characterization of two kinds of low molecular weight kininogens from rat (non-inflamed) plasma: One resistant and the second sensitive to rat glandular kallikreins. J.Biol.Chem., **263**, 965-972, 1988

(15) UTSUNOMIYA,I., OH-ISHI,S., HAYASHI,I., MARUHASHI,J., TSUJI, N., YAMAMOTO,N. and YAMASHINA,S. Monoclonal antibodies against rat T-kininogen: Application to radioimmunoassay and immunohistochemistry. J.Biochem.,**103**, 225-230, 1988

(16) HAYASHI,I., OH-ISHI,S., ENJYOJI,K., KATO,H. and IWANAGA,S. A radioimmunoassay for rat T-kininogen as an acute phase reactant. Chem.Pharm.Bull., **34**, 3502-3505, 1986

(17) YAMSU,A., OH-ISHI,S., HAYASHI,I., HAYASHI,M., YAMAKI,K., NAKANO,T. and SUNAHARA,N. Differentiation of kinin fractions in ureter urine and bladder urine of normal and kininogen-deficient rats. J.Pharnaco-Dyn., **12,** 287-292, 1989

(18) OH-ISHI,S. and KATORI,M. Fluorometric assay for plasma pre kallikrein using peptidylcoumarinylamide as a substrate. Thrombosis Res.,**14**, 551-559, 1979

(19) FRUTO-KATO,S., MATSUMOTO,A., KITAMURA,N. and NAKANISHI,S. Primary structures of the mRNAs encoding the rat precursors for bradykinin and T-kinin. J.Biol.Chem.,**260,** 12054-12059, 1985

(20) HAYASHI,I. and OH-ISHI,S. Demonstration of biosynthesis of kininogens in the liver of Brown Norway Katholiek rat (a deficient strain of HMW- and LMW-kininogens in the plasma). Japan.J.Pharmacol.,**52** Suppl., 89P, 1990

(21) KAWAMURA,K. and OH-ISHI,S. Rat pleurisy induced by kaolin or croton oil: Time course of fluid accumulation, exudation rate and white cell migration, and the effect of some pretreatments. Int.J.Tissue Reactions **7,** 381-386, 1985

(22) KIKUCHI,M. and OH-ISHI,S. Involvement of histamine in vascular permeability increase of rat pleurisy induced by phorbol myristate acetate. Japan.J.Pharmacol., **39,** 467-473, 1985

(23) IMAI,Y., HAYASHI,M. and OH-ISHI,S. Key role of complement activation and platelet-activating factor in exudate formation in zymosan-induced rat pleurisy. Japan.J.Pharmacol.,**57,** 225-232, 1991

(24) JACOBSEN,S. Substrates for plasma kinin forming enzymes in human, dog and rabbit plasmas. Brit.J.Pharmacol., **26,** 403-411, 1966

AAS 38/I
Recent Progress on Kinins
© 1992 Birkhäuser Verlag Basel

THE STRUCTURE AND EXPRESSION OF THE GENES FOR
T-KININOGEN IN THE RAT

T. J. Cole[1] and G. Schreiber

The Russell Grimwade School of Biochemistry, University of Melbourne, Parkville,
Victoria, 3052, Australia.

[1] Institute for Cell and Tumor Biology, German Cancer Research Center, Im
Neuenheimer Feld 280, D-6900 Heidelberg 1, Germany.

SUMMARY: T-kininogen plays an important role in the acute phase response to
trauma in the rat as a possible source of kinins and as a cysteine proteinase
inhibitor.   Two T-kininogens are expressed by rat liver from two separate genes.
T-kininogen expression in liver during the acute phase response is regulated at
the level of transcription.   The similarity in T- and K-kininogen gene structure
suggests divergent evolution from a common gene ancestor.

INTRODUCTION

Kininogens are the precursor proteins for the vasoactive kinins (1).   There are
two forms of kininogens synthesized by the liver, the high molecular weight
(HMW) and the low molecular weight (LMW) kininogens.   HMW and LMW
kininogen mRNAs are generated from a single gene by alternate RNA splicing (2).
In the rat two closely related LMW kininogens have been characterized and have
been termed K-kininogen and T-kininogen.   T-kininogen was first described as
one of the most prominent rat acute phase proteins (3, then called major acute
phase α_1 protein or MAP).   Its concentration in plasma increased 16 fold 48 hours
after experimentally induced inflammation, due to an increase in synthesis rate
by the liver (3, 4).   This protein was also characterized as an additional kininogen
in rat plasma and called T-kininogen (5).   It contains the vasoactive kinin-like
peptide, Ile-Ser-Bradykinin, called T-kinin and on induction of an acute
inflammation limited release of T-kinin has been detected *in vivo* (6, 7).   The
cDNAs for T-kininogen mRNAs were subsequently cloned from liver cDNA
libraries (8, 9, 10).   Two T-kininogen cDNAs were isolated which were 96%
identical at the nucleotide level.   Also cloned from liver was a rat LMW K-
kininogen cDNA which was approximately 90% homologous in nucleotide

sequence to T-kininogen (9). Kininogens have recently been shown to also function as cysteine proteinase inhibitors (11). T-kininogen is a strong inhibitor of cysteine proteinases such as papain and the lysosomal cathepsins and for this reason has also been given the name thiostatin (12, 13, 14). In this paper we describe the structure of the T-kininogen genes and their regulation during the acute phase response.

MATERIALS AND METHODS

All materials and methods are as described in the quoted original references.

RESULTS

Rat kininogen and related genes have been isolated by a number of groups (13, 15, 16). We have isolated two different T-kininogen genes, one K-kininogen gene and one structurally related pseudogene from a Buffalo rat genomic library (13). These are shown schematically in Fig. 1.

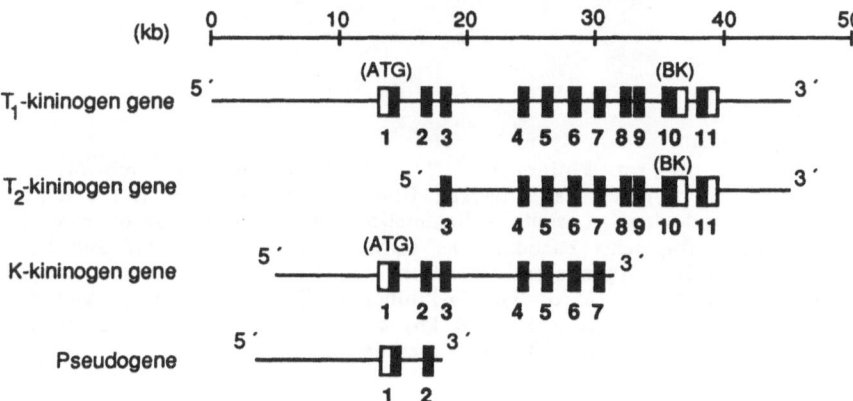

Figure 1. The rat kininogen genes. Four genes termed T_1-kininogen, T_2-kininogen, K-kininogen, and a pseudogene are depicted. Coding exons are represented by filled boxes and non-coding parts of exons by open boxes. Introns and flanking regions are shown by thick lines. ATG; codon initiating translation, BK; bradykinin sequence. From Fung and Schreiber (13), with permission.

The T$_1$-kininogen gene was isolated in full and spans 24 kb. It is composed of
11 exons, has a similar genomic organization to the previously isolated bovine
kininogen gene (2), and also encodes the HMW and LMW specific sequences on the
separate and adjacent exons 10 and 11.   Exon 10 of both T-kininogen genes code for
the T-kinin sequence and also sequences similar to the light chain region of HMW
K-kininogen.   Analysis of the rat T-kininogen and the K-kininogen genes
indicate that their genomic organization is very similar (Fig. 1).   Nucleotide
sequence analysis of the T-kininogen and K-kininogen genes show a high
similarity of approximately 90%, and it is clear that these genes share an
evolutionary origin.   The expression of the T-kininogen and the K-kininogen
genes in the liver, before and after induction of the acute phase response, has
been analysed by Northern blots (13).   This is shown in Fig. 2.

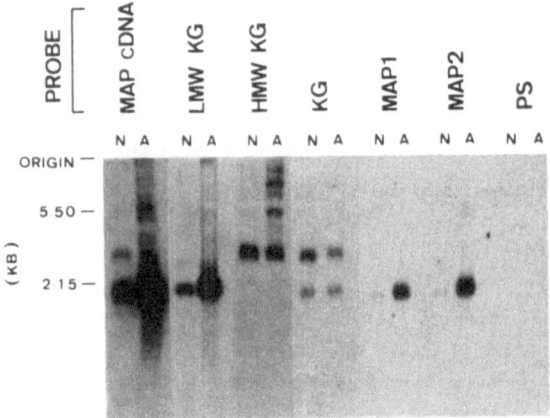

Figure 2.   Analysis of rat kininogen RNA by Northern blot hybridization.
Polyadenylated RNA (3 ug/lane) was analysed from normal rat liver (N) and from
liver 24 hours after inducing an acute inflammation (A).   Probes used were T$_1$-
kininogen cDNA, DNA fragments encoding the carboxyl termini of LMW and HMW
kininogen, and synthetic oligonucleotides with sequences specific for the K-
kininogen (KG), T$_1$-kininogen (MAP 1), T$_2$-kininogen (MAP 2), and pseudo (PS)
genes.   Size markers were the rat 28S (5.50 kb) and 18S (2.15 kb) ribosomal RNA
bands.   From Fung and Schreiber (13), with permission.

Using a full length T$_1$-kininogen cDNA as a probe, mRNAs of approximately
3.0 and 1.6 kb are detected and correspond to both T-kininogen and K-kininogen
mRNAs.   An oligonucleotide probe specific for the K-kininogen gene detects both
LMW and HMW K-kininogen mRNAs (KG, Fig. 2) and their levels of expression is
unaffected by induction of the acute phase response.   Only the specific T$_1$- and T$_2$-

kininogen mRNAs of 1.6 kb are inducible, but no HMW-mRNA form of either T-kininogen is detectable. The T-kininogen genes only express a LMW mRNA form. This indicates differences in RNA splicing between the highly similar T-kininogen and K-kininogen genes. The molecular basis of this has been studied in detail and results from several mutational changes in the HMW-specifying regions of both T-kininogen genes (13, 15). These mutations to the T-kininogen genes include a nucleotide substitution in the putative polyadenylation signal site for its HMW mRNA and also the presence of repetative DNA insertions in the HMW-specifying region of exon 10 (15). There is also a single nucleotide deletion in exon 10 of the T_2-kininogen gene resulting in a frame shift leading to premature termination of translation. The increase in the synthesis rates of T-kininogen in liver during the acute phase response is paralleled by an increase in their mRNA levels. This is shown in Fig. 3 for both T-kininogen genes using specific oligonucleotide probes.

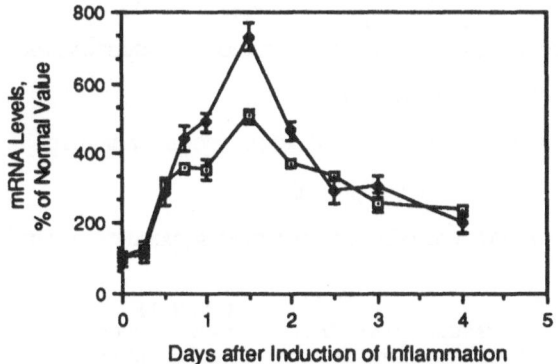

Figure 3. Level of T_1- (open boxes) and T_2-kininogen (closed circles) mRNA in rat liver after turpentine induced acute inflammation (in days). Cytoplasmic extracts were prepared from livers at various times after induction of inflammation, spotted onto nitrocellulose membranes, and hybridized with ^{32}P-labelled T_1- and T_2-kininogen specific oligonucleotides (13). Messenger RNA levels were calculated as a percentage of the value for normal liver. Each point is the mean $\pm$ S. E. (standard error; indicated by bars for each time point) for eight rats.

T-kininogen mRNA levels increase 5-8 fold 36 hours after turpentine induced inflammation. This was also demonstrated by S1-nuclease analysis after lipopolysaccharide induced inflammation (17). Changes in mRNA levels can result from regulation at the level of transcription, mRNA stability, or mRNA degradation. The transcription rate of the T-kininogen genes was measured during the acute phase response and found to increase dramatically paralleling the increase in mRNA levels (18). This indicates that the T-kininogen genes are primarily regulated at the level of transcription. A comparison of the 5′ flanking regions of the T-kininogen genes and the K-kininogen gene is shown in Fig. 4.

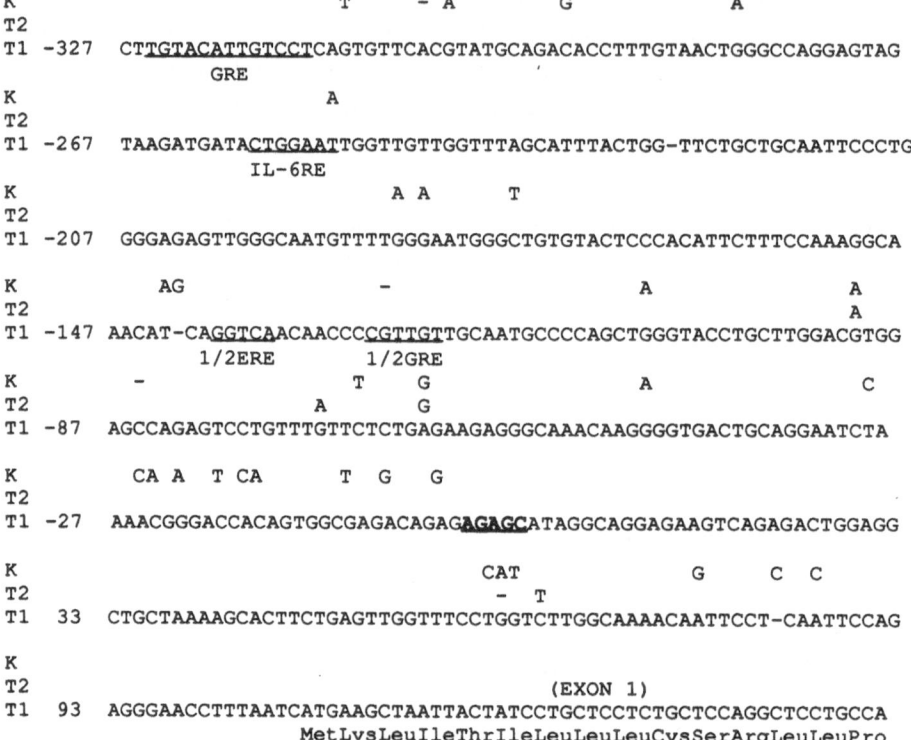

Figure 4. Nucleotide sequences of the 5′ flanking regions of the rat T_1-kininogen (T1), T_2-kininogen (T2) and K-kininogen (K) genes. Nucleotide differences for the T2 and K genes are displayed above the nucleotide sequence of the T_1-kininogen gene. The deduced amino acid sequence for part of exon 1 of the T_1-kininogen gene is displayed below the nucleotide sequence. Start sites of transcription (spread over 5 nucleotides) are in bold and underlined. Putative half or full consensus sites for glucocorticoid response elements (GRE), estrogen response elements (ERE), and IL-6 response elements (IL-6RE), are underlined and labelled. Modified from Fung and Schreiber (13), with permission.

They are very similar up to 1 kilobase upstream of the proposed transcriptional start site (13). Transfection experiments using deletion constructs of the 5′ region of the T_1-kininogen gene, showed that a 321 base pair fragment was sufficient to confer responsiveness to the cytokine interleukin-6 (19).

Analysis of this fragment revealed the presence of an IL-6-like response element (CTGGAAT) about 230 base pairs upstream of the transcription start site (Fig. 4). This sequence could, in part, be responsible for mediating the effects of IL-6 on T-kininogen expression during the acute phase response.

DISCUSSION

The rat has a K-kininogen gene similar to the kininogen gene found in other mammals and also two T-kininogen genes.   The K-kininogen gene generates two mRNAs encoding LMW and HMW kininogen through the differential splicing of its two 3′ terminal exons, 10 and 11, while only LMW T-kininogen mRNA has been detected for both T-kininogen genes.   A model explaining this difference in splicing has been suggested (20) and proposes that stretches of naturally occurring repeated sequences exist in exon 10 of the K-kininogen gene which modifies normal splicing function.   The HMW-specific sequences of exon 10 are not always spliced out and allows formation of a HMW K-kininogen mRNA.   For the T-kininogen genes, mutations in exon 10 disrupt this process and therefore a processive spliceosome efficiently splices the pre-mRNA into LMW T-kininogen mRNA.

Cytokines released from activated macrophages and monocytes following inflammation are responsible for induction of acute phase protein synthesis (21). These cytokines include interleukin-6 (IL-6) and interleukin-1 (IL-1).   IL-6 is now recognized as responsible for the induction of the majority of acute phase proteins, including T-kininogen, in the liver.   IL-6 exerts its effect by binding to a cell surface IL-6 receptor and induces the interaction of a transcription factor called IL-6 DNA binding protein to specific IL-6 response elements (IL-6REs) upstream of acute phase protein gene promoters (22).   This results in an increase in the rate of transcription.   T-kininogen expression is also regulated by steroid hormones.   Dexamethasone was shown to be required for induction of T-kininogen by IL-6 in hepatoma cells (23) and acted synergistically with IL-6 to induce T-kininogen expression in transfection experiments (19).   Furthermore administration of dexamethasone after induction of an acute inflammation will down regulate the expression of both T-kininogen genes in the liver (24). Analysis of the 5′ flanking sequences of the T-kininogen genes reveals a number of consensus sequences to the previously described glucocorticoid (GRE) and estrogen (ERE) response elements (25).   Some of these elements are boxed and marked in Fig. 4.   The similarity in structure between the K- and T- kininogen genes suggest they have evolved from a common ancestor. A T-kininogen homologue has not been detected in mouse and indicates that an initial gene duplication from an ancestoral kininogen gene occurred after divergence of rat and mouse. The next important change was the introduction of an inducible promoter bringing expression under the control of the acute phase response. A second gene duplication occurred followed by additional structural mutations to produce the two T-kininogen genes as they occur today. By gene duplication and gene conversion the rat has evolved a kininogen multigene family.

ACKNOWLEDGMENTS

This work was supported by grants from the National Health and Medical Research Council of Australia and the Australian Research Council.

REFERENCES

1. Kato H, Nagasawa S, Iwanaga S. HMW and LMW kininogens. Methods Enzymol 1981; 80: 172-198.

2. Kitamura N, Takagaki Y, Furuto S, Tanaka T, Nawa H, Nakanishi S. A single gene for bovine high molecular weight and low molecular weight kininogen. Nature 1983; 305: 545-549.

3. Urban J, Chan D, Schreiber G. A rat serum glycoprotein whose synthesis rate increases greatly during inflammation. J Biol Chem 1979; 254: 10565-8.

4. Schreiber G, Tsykin A, Aldred AR, Thomas T, Fung WP, Dickson PW, Cole T, Birch H, De Jong FA, Milland J. The acute phase response in the rodent. Ann N Y Acad Sci 1989; 557: 61-85.

5. Barlas A, Okamoto H, Greenbaum LM. T-kininogen - the major plasma kininogen in rat adjuvant arthritis. Biochem Biophys Res Commun 1985; 129: 280-286.

6. Okamoto H, Greenbaum LM. Kininogen substrates for trypsin and cathepsin D in human, rabbit, and rat plasmas. Life Sci 1983; 32: 2007-2013.

7. Barlas A, Okamoto H, Greenbaum LM. Release of T-kinin and bradykinin in carrageenin-induced inflammation in the rat. FEBS Lett 1985; 190: 268-270.

8. Cole T, Inglis AJ, Roxburgh CM, Howlett GJ, Schreiber G. Major acute phase α_1-protein of the rat is homologous to bovine kininogen and contains the sequence for bradykinin: its synthesis is regulated at the mRNA level. FEBS Lett 1985; 182: 57-61.

9. Furuto-Kato S, Matsumoto A, Kitamura N, Nakanishi S. Primary structures of the mRNAs encoding the rat precursors for bradykinin and T-Kinin. J Biol Chem 1985; 260: 12054-9.

10. Anderson KP, Heath EC. The relationship between rat major acute phase protein and the kininogens. J Biol Chem 1985; 260: 12065-12071.

11. Müller-Esterl W, Iwanaga S, Nakanishi S. Kininogens revisited. Trends Biochem Sci 1986; 11: 336-9.

12. Moreau T, Gutman N, El Moujahed A, Esnard F, Gauthier F. Relationship between the cysteine-proteinase-inhibitory function of rat T-kininogen and the release of immunoreactive kinin upon trypsin treatment. Eur J Biochem 1986; 159: 341-6.

13. Fung WP, Schreiber G. Structure and expression of the genes for major acute phase α_1- protein (thiostatin) and kininogen in the rat. J Biol Chem 1987; 262: 9298-9308.

14. Cole T, Schreiber G. Synthesis of thiostatins (major acute-phase α_1 proteins) in different strains of *Rattus Norvegicus*. Comp Biochem Physiol 1989; 93B: 813-6.

15. Kitagawa H, Kitamura N, Nayashida H, Miyata T, Nakanishi S. Differing expression patterns and evolution of the rat kininogen gene family. J Biol Chem 1987; 262: 2190-8.

16. Anderson KP, Croyle ML, Lingrel JB. Primary structure of a gene encoding rat T-kininogen. Gene 1989; 81: 119-128.

17. Kageyama R, Kitamura N, Ohkubo H, Nakanishi S. Differential expression of the multiple forms of rat prekininogen mRNAs after acute inflammation. J Biol Chem 1985; 260: 12060-4.

18. Birch HE, Schreiber G. Transcriptional regulation of plasma protein synthesis during inflammation. J Biol Chem 1986; 261: 8077-8080.

19. Chen HM, Considine KB, Liao WSL. Interleukin-6 responsiveness and cell-specific expression of the rat kininogen gene. J Biol Chem 1991; 266: 2946-2952.

20. Kakizuka A, Ingi T, Murai T, Nakanishi S. A set of U1 snRNA - complementary sequences involved in governing alternative RNA splicing of the kininogen genes. J Biol Chem 1990; 265: 10102-8.

21. Heinrich PC, Castell JV, Andus T. Interleukin-6 and the acute phase response. Biochem J 1990; 265: 621-636.

22. Poli V, Cortese R. Interleukin 6 induces a liver-specific nuclear protein that binds to the promoter of acute-phase genes. Proc Natl Acad Sci USA 1989; 86: 8202-8306.

23. Baumann H, Richards C, Gauldie J. Interaction among hepatocyte-stimulating factors, interleukin 1, and glucocorticoids for regulation of acute phase plasma proteins in human hepatoma (HepG2) cells. J Immunol 1987; 139: 4122-8.

24. Howard EF, Thompson YG, Lapp CA, Greenbaum LM. Reduction of T-kininogen messenger RNA levels by dexamethasone in the adjuvant-treated rat. Life Sci 1990; 46: 411-7.

25. Anderson KP, Lingrel JB. Glucocorticoid and estrogen regulation of a rat T-kininogen gene. Nucleic Acids Res 1989; 17: 2835-2848.

AAS 38/I
Recent Progress on Kinins
© 1992 Birkhäuser Verlag Basel

T-KININOGEN, PROCESSING AND FUNCTIONS

L. M. Greenbaum, E. Howard, U. Albus, C. Lapp and XX. Gao

Departments of Pharmacology and Biochemistry and School of Graduate Studies, Medical College of Georgia, Augusta, GA 30912, USA.

SUMMARY

Studies are presented which indicate that T-kininogen, the acute phase kininogen of the rat, could be a healing protein because of its properties as a cysteine protease inhibitor. Evidence is also presented that mRNA of T-kininogen synthesis may be a function of interleukin 6 production. A regulatory mechanism is postulated by which SH cofactors could determine if T-kinin is released or whether the T-kininogen molecule would remain intact. Evidence is also presented that T-kinin acts through kinin B_2 receptors. No specific binding of bradykinin or T-kinin could be detected in rat heart preparations.

INTRODUCTION

The discovery of T-kininogen and T-kinin (Ile-Ser-Bradykinin) by Okamoto and Greenbaum in the rat in 1983 (1) has opened a Pandora's box of questions which we are still struggling to find answers for. The reason for the questions is that T-kininogen, unlike high and low molecular weight kininogens, is an acute phase protein which is synthesized in the rat liver in very great quantities a short time after challenges such as LPS, carrageenin, adjuvant arthritis, or surgery etc. Why does the rat expend so much energy on synthesis of these proteins (T-kininogens I and II)? There are two possibilities; one is that T-kinin released from T-kininogen supports the imposed inflammation because of its properties which resemble bradykinin; the second is that the properties of T-kininogen supports "healing".

Background information on T-kininogen - The discovery of T-kininogen as a unique rat kininogen could have been predicted by the work of Fasciola and Halvorsen who showed that the blood of rats was kallikrein resistant but not trypsin resistant in releasing kinin-like material (2). Okamoto in our laboratory made the cardinal finding that Ile-Ser-bradykinin which we named T-kinin, was not released from its precursor protein, T-kininogen by kallikrein but by large quantities of trypsin (thus the name T for trypsin) (3). Subsequently, the term K kininogens and T-kininogens was adopted for the kininogens which are kallikrein-sensitive and T-kinin releasers following trypsin activity respectively. The partial sequences of rat T and K kininogens are as follows:

-Val-Ser-Ile-Arg-*Arg-Pro-Pro-Gly-Phe-Ser-Pro-Phe-Arg*-Ala- (K)

-Met-Met-*Ile-Ser-ArgPro-Pro-Gly-Phe-Ser-Pro-Phe-Arg*-Leu- (T)

Trypsin cleaves both T-kininogen and K-kininogens to release the italicized products. Kallikreins release bradykinin only from the K kininogens.

Table 1. **Concentration of kininogens in normal plasmas**
(µg bradykinin equivalents)

Species	Total KGN	T-KGN	HMW-KGN	LMW-KGN
Rat	10.44	8.82	1.01	0.61
Mouse	6.68	None	0.98	5.71
Rabbit	2.26	None	0.08	2.19
Guinea-pig	4.06	None	0.27	3.80

Table 1 demonstrates that T-kininogen makes up about 88% of the total kininogen content of blood in the rat. No T-kininogen has been found in species other than the rat so far although Fasciola and Halvorsen's experiments also indicated that kinin release by kallikrein in the guinea pig is quite low as it is in the rat.

RESULTS AND DISCUSSION

T-kininogen as an acute phase protein - A number of laboratories have observed a dramatic increase in the kininogen content of plasma in rats following the administration of inflammatory agents such as Freund's adjuvant, croton oil, acetic acid, and turpentine, etc. However, until the early part of the 1980s, the lack of HPLC technology prevented the identification of which kininogen(s) were involved. Furthermore, the discovery of T-kininogen in 1983, and our ability to identify it in plasma, provided Barlas in our laboratory with the necessary technology to identify which of the kininogens was synthesized following the inflammatory response. He clearly showed (Fig. 1) that T-kininogen was expressed into the blood as an "acute phase protein". The K kininogens did not respond at all to the inflammatory challenge (4).

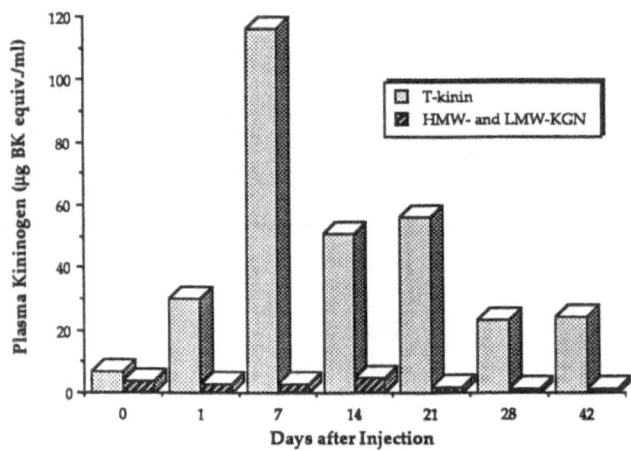

Fig. 1. Response of plasma kininogens after injection of adjuvant

The results were rapidly confirmed by Nakanishi et al. (5) who showed that the mRNA of T-kininogens but not K-kininogens followed the same pattern as we had shown in blood levels. Nakanishi's group also showed that while K kininogens are coded by one gene, two separate genes code for mRNAs of T-kininogen I and II.

T-kininogen, dexamethasone, and interleukin 6 - Howard in our laboratory has clearly demonstrated that the anti-inflammatory steroid, dexamethasone, sharply and dramatically reduces the expression of messenger RNA of T-kininogen following the challenge by adjuvant arthritis (6). This confirms the original observation made by our laboratory that dexamethasone reduces the plasma levels of T-kininogen ususally seen following an inflammatory challenge such as adjuvant arthritis or carrageenin (3). Howard further pursued his observation to determine whether dexamethasone acted directly on the T-kininogen gene or some intermediary cytokine. His findings point to the actions of dexamethasone as reducing interleukin synthesis, particularly interleukin 6. Thus, our working hypothesis is that T-kininogen synthesis involves activaiton of the gene expression of T-kininogen by interleuklin 6. Dexamethasone, however, reduces the gene expression of interleukin 6 mRNA thus reducing this important interleukin for activating T-kininogen mRNA synthesis. Support for this hypothesis comes from the efforts of Lapp in our laboratory who has shown that in cell culture, dexamethasone actually enhances T-kiningoen synthesis as opposed to the *in vivo* effect (7).

Factors influencing transcription of T-kininogen mRNA - T-kininogen is a very dynamic protein. Transcription of mRNA is enhanced by hormones such as estrogen, prolactin, and tryroid hormone (7,8). Inflammatory agents such as LPS, carrageenin, Freund's adjuvant and surgery itself have been shown to cause remarkable elevations of both T-kininogen I and II. Lactating mothers, probably because of prolactin, and newborns have 2-3 times normal levels of T-kininogen in the blood. Normal levels are about 200 µg/ml for the male and about 600 µg/ml for the female rat.

"Healing" properties of T-kininogen - Evidence has accumulated that while very significant synthesis of T-kininogen occurs following a variety of challenges as described above, only one report, which comes from our laboratory, has shown that T-kinin is released in large quantities. It is evident that under most conditions, T-kininogen itself is an inhibitor of cysteine proteases such as cathepsin B (Fig. 2). In fact, a polypeptide in humans which is a cysteine protease inhibitor, cystatin, is a conserved T-kininogen sequence. Thus, there is a significant possibility that T-kininogen's function is to reduce the degradative actions of cathepsin-like enzyme and to ameliorate or reduce the inflammatory response, i.e., to act as a "healing" protein.

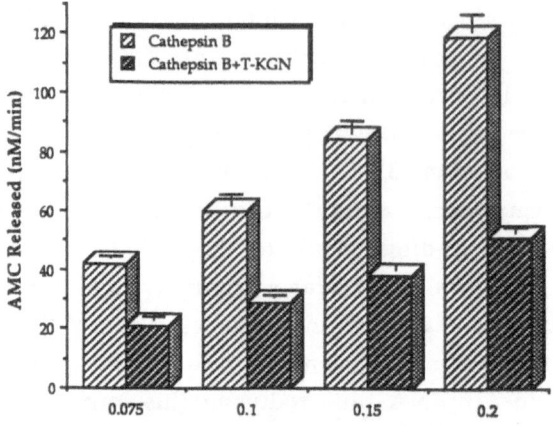

Fig. 2. Inhibiton of cathepsin B by T-kininogen

Regulation of T-kinin release from T-kininogen - T-kininogen is substrate for T-kininogenase which catalyzes the release of T-kinin (10). T-kininogenase has been found in salivary glands. T-kininogenase releases T-kinin, but needs SH cofactors for its actions. The enzymes has a neutral pH optima and has been purified by Barlas in our laboratory. There has been some reports of "look-alike" enzymes; but there is some question if they differ from T-kininogenase. The fact that SH factors activate T-kininogenase, provides a real possibility of this mechanism as a regulatory factor as is described in Fig. 3.

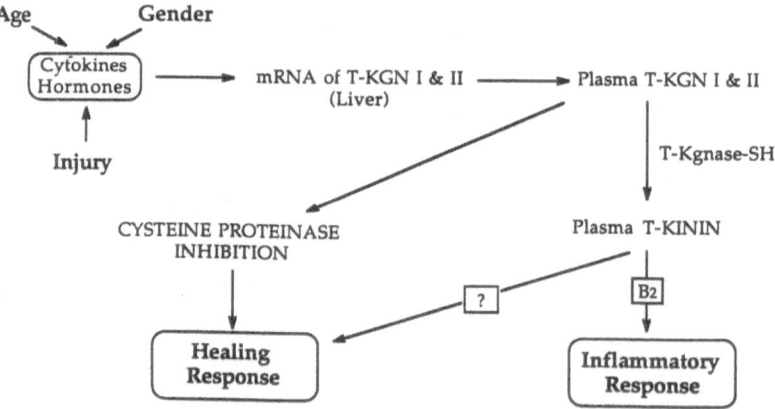

Fig 3. The T-kinin, T-kininogen system in the rat and its regulation.

Receptor properties of T-kinin - T-kinin has now been shown by Gao (11, 12) to act on kinin B_2 receptors present in the isolated rat uterus and in rat myometrium membrane preparations. Albus in our laboratory investigated kinin binding in the rat left ventricle. By the techniques he used, he could not identify any specific binding for kinins including T-kinin in his preparations (13).

CONCLUSION

The T-kininogen - T-kinin system is one of the most dynamic systems in the rat. T-kininogen, as an acute phase protein, represents a potential healing agent because of its anti-proteinase properties. Its relationship to cytokines and proteinases such as T-kininogenases are just beginning to be understood including regulation of the system by SH factors. The role of T-kinin needs further clarification although we now know that it acts through kinin B_2 receptors.

REFERENCES

1. Okamoto H and Greenbaum LM, Kininogen substrates for trypsin and cathepsin D in human, rabbit and rat plasmas. Life Sciences 1983; 32: 2007-2013.

2. Fasciola JC, Halvorsen K, Sosa HO, and Carrizo A, Specificity of mammalian kallidinogen, Am J Physiol 1964; 207: 901-905.

3. Okamoto H and Greenbaum LM, Isolation and structure of T-kinin. Biochem Biophys Res Commun 1983; 112(2): 701-708.

4. Barlas A, Gao X, and Greenbaum LM, Isolation of a thiol-activated T-kininogenase from the rat submandibular gland. FEBS 1987; 218(2): 266-270.

5. Kagayama R, Kitamura N, Ohkubo H, and Nakanishi S, Differential expression of the multiple forms of rat prekininogen mRNAs after acute inflammation. J Biol Chem 1985; 260: 12060-12064.

6. Howard EF, Thompson YG, Lapp CA, and Greenbaum LM, Reduction of T-kininogen messenger RNA levels by dexamethasone in the adjuvant-treated rat. Life Sci 1990; 46(6): 411 -417.

7. Lapp AL, Howard EF, and Greenbaum LM, Modulation of hepatocyte secretion of the acute phase protein T-kininogen by prolactin. Progress in NeuroEndocrinImmunology 1991; 4(4): 248-257.

8. Oh-ishi S, Hayashi I, Kusunoki A, Nagashima Y, Hayadi M, Yamaki K, Utsunomiya I, and Yamasu A, Developmental and sexual differences of T-kininogen levels in rat plasma and liver. Biochem Biophys Res Commun 1988; 150, 1069-1076.

9. Bouhnik J, Savoie F, Baussant T, Michard A, Alhenc-Gelas F, and Corvol P, Effect of thyroidectomy on rat T-kininogen. Am J Physiol 1988; 255(4) Pt1): E411-415.

10. Barlas A, Okamoto H, and Greenbaum LM, T-kininogen - the major plasma kininogen in rat adjuvant arthritis. Biochem Biophys Res Commun 1983; 129, 280-286.

11. Gao X, Regoli D, Stewart JM, Vavrek RJ, and Greenbaum LM, Studies on T-kinin receptors, The Pharmacologist 1989; 31:3.

12. Gao XX, Stewart JM, Vavrek RJ, and Greenbaum LM, Characterization of receptor-mediated action of T-kinin and [D-Ile[1]]-T-kinin, indicating the existence of a subtype of bradykinin B_2 receptors, (This volume)

13. Albus, U, Gao, XX, and Greenbaum, LM, Lack of specific binding of bradykinin and D-Arg[Hyp[3],Thi[5], D-Tic, Oic[8]]Bradykinin in membranes from the heart. Abst. PS 3.11, Kinin '91 Munich, International Congress.

AAS 38/I
Recent Progress on Kinins
© 1992 Birkhäuser Verlag Basel

INCREASED UPTAKE OF T-KININOGEN BY THE LIVER IN INFLAMMATORY CONDITIONS

M. Takano, K. Yayama, Y. Miyawaki, N. Itoh and H. Okamoto

Department of Pharmacology, Faculty of Pharmaceutical Sciences, Kobe-Gakuin University, Ikawadani-cho, Nishi-ku, Kobe 651-21, Japan

SUMMARY: The distribution of [^{125}I]T-kininogen in the liver of rats was found to be increased by laparotomy-, turpentine- or lipopolysaccharide-induced inflammation, whereas no such increase was observed in other organs or when ^{125}I-labeled carboxymethylated T-kininogen, which does not inhibit cysteine proteinase, was used. These results suggest that the liver plays an important role in clearing T-kininogen from the circulation during inflammation.

INTRODUCTION

Kininogens, including rat T-kininogen (T-Kgn), have been shown to be cysteine proteinase inhibitors (1). T-Kgn has also been identified as an acute-phase protein; its concentration in plasma increases several-fold after induction of inflammation (2,3). Although these properties of T-Kgn suggest that this plasma protein may play a role in inflammation, there is no evidence to support this.

In order to clarify the function of T-Kgn in inflammation, we investigated the tissue distribution of [^{125}I]T-Kgn in normal rats and those with induced inflammation.

MATERIALS AND METHODS

Rat T-Kgn was purified as described previously (4). S-Carboxymethylated T-Kgn was prepared by reduction of T-Kgn with dithiothreitol and subsequent alkylation with iodoacetate (5). T-Kgn was radioiodinated with [^{125}I]Bolton-Hunter reagent and purified by Sephadex G-50 chromatography. Male Sprague-Dawley rats, weighing 140-150 g, were used. Acute inflammation was induced by injection of turpentine (1 ml/100 g, s.c.) or lipopolysaccharide (LPS;

50 µg/100 g, i.p.). Tissue injury was induced by making a bilateral flank incision through the skin, muscle mass and peritoneum under pentobarbital anesthesia. The animals were anesthetized with pentobarbital sodium and received via a femoral vein a single bolus injection of [^{125}I]T-Kgn (1 x 10^6 cpm/20 ng) in 200 µl of 0.2 M sodium phosphate, pH 7.4, containing 1% bovine serum albumin. Two hours or 30 min after the injection of [^{125}I]T-Kgn, the peritoneal aorta was cannulated under pentobarbital anesthesia, and total exsangination was carried out by infusion of about 100 ml of cold phosphate-buffered saline for 5 min. The liver, kidneys, heart, brain, lung and testis were removed, weighed, and their radioactivity counted using a gamma-counter. Radioactivity was calculated per unit of whole tissue, and data were expressed as percentages of total injected radioactivity.

RESULTS

The tissue distribution of radioactivity in normal rats 2 h after a single bolus i.v. injection of [^{125}I]T-Kgn was, in descending order: liver 1.7%, testis 1.6%, kidneys 1.1%, lung 0.2%, heart 0.2% and brain 0.1% (Fig. 1). When plasma samples collected 2 h after injection of [^{125}I]T-Kgn were analyzed by SDS-PAGE followed by autoradiography, a single radioactive band corresponding to the molecular mass of native T-Kgn was observed (data not shown). In order to clarify whether tissue injury influenced the distribution of [^{125}I]T-Kgn, rats were laparotomized 90 min before injection of [^{125}I]T-Kgn. As shown in Fig. 1, about a 3-fold increase in the distribution of radioactivity was found in the liver, but not in other organs.

To determine whether the laparotomy-induced increase in T-Kgn distribution to liver is a response associated with inflammation, the distribution of radioactivity in the liver and kidneys 30 min after injection of [^{125}I]T-Kgn was determined in rats after induction of inflammation by injection of turpentine or LPS. As shown in Fig. 2, the distribution of radioactivity in the liver was significantly higher in rats treated with turpentine or LPS than in normal rats, whereas no significant differences were observed in the distribution to kidneys between turpentine- or LPS-treated rats and normal rats. Similar results were obtained in rats treated by laparotomy (Fig. 2). When turpentine was injected at different times before injection of [^{125}I]T-Kgn, a significantly higher distribution of radioactivity in the liver was found in the rats which had been treated with turpentine 0.5 - 2 h before injection of [^{125}I]T-Kgn, but not in the rats treated 4 and 8 h before injection of [^{125}I]T-Kgn (Fig. 3).

In order to clarify whether the inflammation-induced increase in T-Kgn distribution to the liver was associated with the function of T-Kgn as a cysteine proteinase inhibitor, the disulfide bonds of T-Kgn were reduced and carboxymethylated with iodoacetate prior to radioiodination. The characteristic properties of T-Kgn as a cysteine proteinase inhibitor, such as binding activity to papain-agarose or inhibition of the amidolytic activity of papain, were completely lost after carboxymethylation. As shown in Fig. 4, no significant increase in T-Kgn distribution in the liver was observed in turpentine-treated rats, when carboxymethylated T-Kgn was used   as a radiolabeled protein.

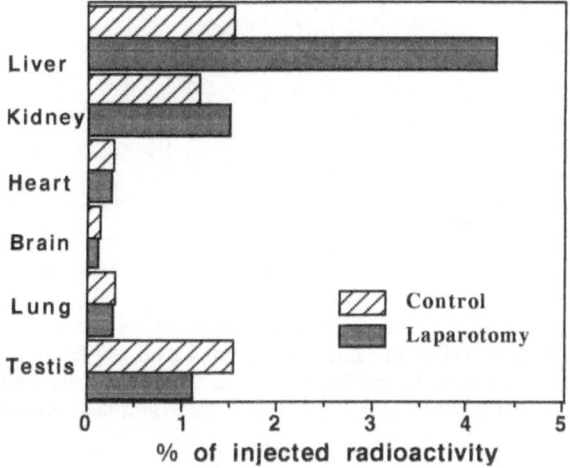

Figure 1. Tissue distribution of radioactivity in rats following injection of [^{125}I]T-kininogen ([^{125}I]T-Kgn).   [^{125}I]T-Kgn was injected i.v., and then tissues were removed 2 h later. Laparotomy was carried out 90 min before injection of [^{125}I]T-Kgn.   Data represent mean values from two animals, and are expressed as percentages of total injected radioactivity.

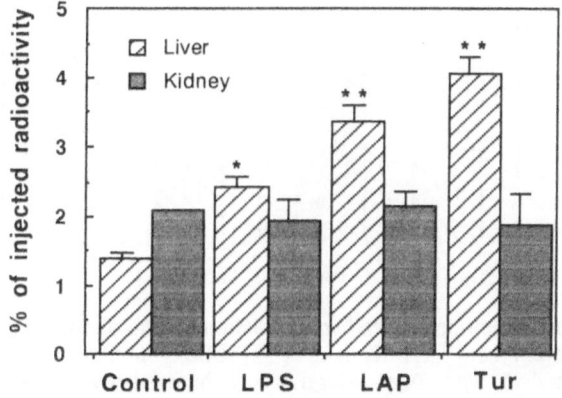

Figure 2. Distribution of radioactivity to the liver and kidney of rats with induced inflammation following injection of [^{125}I]T-Kgn.   The rats were laparotomized (LAP) or injected with lipopolysaccharide (LPS) i.p. or turpentine (TUR) s.c. 1 h before injection of [^{125}I]T-Kgn, and then the liver and kidneys were removed 30 min later. Data represent mean values ± S.D. from four animals. Significantly different from control (*P<0.05, **P<0.001).

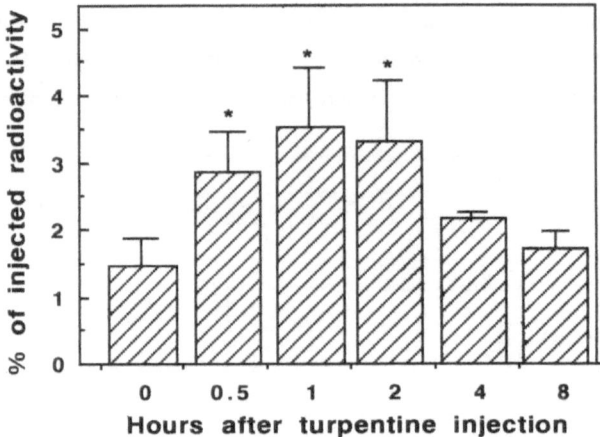

Figure 3. Effect of turpentine-induced inflammation on the distribution of radioactivity to the liver following injection of [^{125}I]T-Kgn. Rats were treated with turpentine at different times before injection of [^{125}I]T-Kgn, as shown in the figure. The liver was removed 30 min after injection of [^{125}I]T-Kgn. Data represent mean values ± S.D. from three animals. Significantly different from control (*P<0.05).

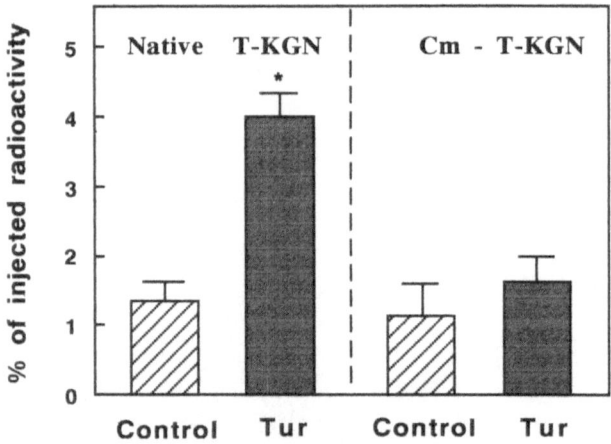

Figure 4. Effect of turpentine-induced inflammation on the distribution of radioactivity to the liver following injection of [^{125}I]T-Kgn or [^{125}I]carboxymethylated T-Kgn. [^{125}I]T-Kgn or [^{125}I]carboxymethylated T-Kgn (Cm-T-Kgn) was injected i.v. into normal or turpentine (TUR)-pretreated rats, and then the liver was removed 30 min later. Turpentine was injected 30 min before injection of radiolabelled protein. Data represent mean values ± S.D. from four animals. Significantly different from control (*P<0.001).

DISCUSSION

In the present study, we found that the distribution of radioactivity in the liver after injection of [^{125}I]T-Kgn was increased in rats which had been exposed to inflammatory stimuli, such as laparotomy, and injection of turpentine or LPS. Since no degradation products of [^{125}I]T-Kgn were found in plasma 2 h after injection, it seems likely that the level of radioactivity measured in organs reflects the amount of T-Kgn taken up by these organs. Interestingly, the distribution of [^{125}I]T-Kgn in organs besides the liver was not influenced by inflammation. These results suggest that T-Kgn uptake into the liver occurs through a mechanism different from that in other organs.

When the distribution of [^{125}I]T-Kgn in liver was measured at different times after injection of turpentine, increased uptake of radioactivity was observed even 30 min after injection, but not at 4 and 8 h, indicating that uptake of T-Kgn into the liver is increased during the early phase of inflammation. Furthermore, the inflammation-induced increase in T-Kgn uptake by the liver was not observed after T-Kgn had been inactivated by carboxymethylation, suggesting that the function of T-Kgn as a cysteine proteinase inhibitor is involved in inflammation-induced T-Kgn uptake.

Taken together, it is likely that the liver plays an important role in clearing T-Kgn from the circulation during inflammation. Like α_2-macroglobulin (6), there is a possibility that T-Kgn functions under inflammatory conditions by trapping cysteine proteinases, which leak from site of inflammation, to form complexes that are cleared efficiently from the circulation by the liver. Further studies will be needed in order to demonstrate this hypothesis.

REFERENCES

1. Müller-Esterl W, Iwanaga S, and Nakanishi S, *Kininogens revisited.* Trends Biochem Sci *11*, 336-339 (1986).
2. Barlas A, Okamoto H, and Greenbaum LM, *T-Kininogen, the major plasma kininogen in rat adjuvant arthritis.* Biochem Biophys Res Commun *129*, 280-286 (1985).
3. Kageyama R, Kitamura N, Ohkubo H, and Nakanishi S, *Differential expression of the multiple forms of rat prekininogen mRNA after acute inflammation.* J Biol Chem *260*, 12060-12064 (1985).
4. Greenbaum LM and Okamoto H, *T-Kinin and T-kininogen.* Methods Enzymol *163*, 272-282 (1988).
5. Crestfield AM, Moore S, and Stein WH, *The preparation and enzymatic hydrolysis of reduced and S-carboxymethylated proteins.* J Biol Chem *238*, 622-627 (1963).
6. Moestrup SK and Gliemann J, *Purification of the rat hepatic α_2-macroglobulin receptor as an approximately 440-kDa single chain protein.* J Biol Chem *264*, 15574-15577 (1989).

AAS 38/I
Recent Progress on Kinins
© 1992 Birkhäuser Verlag Basel

THE ROLE OF THE KININOGENS AS CYSTEINE PROTEINASE INHIBITORS IN LOCAL AND SYSTEMIC INFLAMMATION

I. Assfalg-Machleidt[a], A. Billing[b], D. Fröhlich[b], D. Nast-Kolb[c], Th. Joka[d], M. Jochum[e] and W. Machleidt[a]

[a]Institut für Physiologische Chemie, Physikalische Biochemie und Zellbiologie der Universität München, Goethestrasse 33, D-8000 München 2, Germany; [b]Chirurgische Klinik und Poliklinik der Universität München, Klinikum Großhadern; [c]Chirurgische Klinik Innenstadt der Universität München; [d]Chirurgische Universitätskliniken D-4300 Essen; [e]Abteilung für Klinische Chemie und Klinische Biochemie in der Chirurgischen Klinik Innenstadt der Universität München

SUMMARY: The contribution of the kininogens and cystatin C to the functional inhibitory capacity for cysteine proteinases of blood plasma and inflammatory secretions was estimated from *ex vivo* experiments. 98.5 % of the inhibitory capacity of blood plasma for cathepsin L (4-5 μM) is provided by the kininogens ensuring a complete control of this enzyme even at a lowered kininogen concentration. Control of cathepsin B activity by the kininogens is incomplete and depends critically on the active concentration of cystatin C (70 nM in normal plasma), which is reduced in blood plasma of polytraumatized and septic patients and very low in epithelial lining fluid of the shock lung.

INTRODUCTION

A major portion of the lysosomal proteinases responsible for intracellular degradation of phagocytized proteins are cysteine proteinases (cathepsins B, H, L and S). Increased cysteine proteinase activity has been found in blood plasma of polytraumatized and septic patients as well as in local inflammatory secretions like epithelial lining fluid (ELF) of the shock lung and peritonitis exudate indicating that these proteinases are discharged from the phagocytes (1,2). In several clinical studies we have verified the release of E-64 sensitive peptidase activity in correlation to the severity of inflammation and have shown that the released enzymatic activity is mainly due to cathepsin B dissociating from its complexes with endogenous protein inhibitors (1,2). Cathepsin L, if discharged simultaneously with cathepsin B, would not be detectable as active enzyme because it is very tightly bound to the protein inhibitors (3).

According to their inhibition constants and their immunologically determined concentrations, the kininogens and the low-M_r protein inhibitor cystatin C have been predicted to be the biologically most significant cysteine proteinase inhibitors of the extracellular space (3,4). However, no data are vailable on the inhibitory capacity of blood plasma and secretions for the lysosomal cysteine proteinases, and the functional share of the individual inhibitors. The aim of this work was to determine from *ex vivo* experiments the inhibitory capacity of the kininogens and the low-M_r cystatins under normal and various inflammatory conditions.

MATERIALS AND METHODS

Papain (Type III from Sigma), human cathepsin B, cystatin C (Medor, D-8036 Herrsching), LMW- and HMW-kininogen (Novabiochem, D-6902 Sandhausen) were used without further purification.

Samples from patients were obtained as published in detail elsewhere (5-7). Activity of cysteine proteinases was measured with the fluorogenic peptide substrates Z-Phe-Arg-NH-Mec and Bz-Arg-NH-Mec (Bachem, Heidelberg) using the instrumentation described previously (1). The assay buffer was 0.3 M sodium acetate buffer pH 5.5 containing 1 mM dithiothreitol, 2 mM EDTA, and 0.015 % Brij 35.

The inhibitory capacity for papain of the *ex vivo* samples was determined by titration of E-64-standardized papain as described previoulsly (2). The capacity of ELF was obtained by multiplication of the BALF value by 8.3 correcting for dilution of the epithelial lining fluid during the bronchoalevolar lavage procedure (8).

Plasma and peritonitis exudate samples were separated on a Superose 12 FPLC column (HR 10/30), Pharmacia) eluted with the assay buffer devoid of dithiothreitol (0.2 ml/min) at room temperature. Fractions of 0.4 ml (2 min) were collected. The fractions (and aliquots of the samples applied to the column) were tested for inhibition of papain (0.2-10 nM) and cathepsin B (0.090 nM) in stopped assays with the substrates Z-Phe-Arg-NH-Mec (5 μM for papain after dilution of the formed enzyme-inhibitor complex, 10 μM for cathepsin B) and Bz-Arg-NH-Mec (50 μM for papain). After 15-60 min incubation at 30 °C, the reactions were stopped with sodium monochloroacetate (50 mM final concentration). Properly diluted samples were used for the determination of the inhibitory capacity of individual fractions.

Effective K_i values of plasma, exudate and BALF for cathepsin B inhibition were estimated by dilution experiments essentially as described (2). The K_i was calculated from the equation for classical inhibition, $v_i/v_o = 1/(1+I_t/K_i)$, (v_i, reaction rate at enzyme-inhibitor equilibrium; v_o, reaction rate in the absence of inhibitor; I_t, active concentration of inhibitor) by nonlinear regression analysis (see Fig. 3 for experimental details).

RESULTS

Inhibitory capacity of blood plasma and secretions

The inhibitory capacity for cysteine proteinases was determined by titration of E-64-standardized papain with increasing amounts of samples. Equivalence was assumed when a constant papain activity was reached due to α_2-macroglobulin-bound papain which is still able to catalyze the cleavage of the small substrate (2). The results obtained with this method are summarized in Table 1. The normal inhibitory capacity of blood plasma, around 5 μM, was found to be significantly reduced in patients after multiple injury and was lower in peritonitis exudates compared to non-purulent exudates. Very low inhibitory capacity was found in bronchoalveolar lavage fluid (BALF) of patients suffering from an adult respiratory distress syndrome (ARDS).

Table 1. Inhibitory capacity for cysteine proteinases

Sample	Inhibitory capacity [μM] Mean	Range
Blood plasma		
Healthy persons (n=2)	4.9	4.2 - 5.6
Polytrauma patients (n=11)	3.4	1.35 - 5.2
Peritoneal exudate		
Clear exudate (n=2)	2.4	2.4 - 2.4
Peritonitis (n=3)	1.2	0.6 - 1.6
Bronchoalveolar lavage fluid		
Respiratory distress		
syndrome (n=2)	0.0035	0.0015 - 0.0055

Contribution of kininogens and low-M_r cystatins

The inhibitory fractions of blood plasma of a healthy person were separated by fast gel chromatography on a Superose 12 column (Fig. 1A) calibrated by isolated HMW- and LMW-kininogen and cystatin C as standards (Fig. 1B). The major portion of papain inhibition (Fig. 1C) was found in the elution position of LMW-kininogen (M_r = 68,000) and only 1/70 of this capacity in the position of cystatin C (M_r = 13,300). In blood plasma, a separate peak of inhibition corresponding to HMW-kininogen was not resolved, though HMW-kininogen separated from LMW-kininogen in the standard chromatogram.

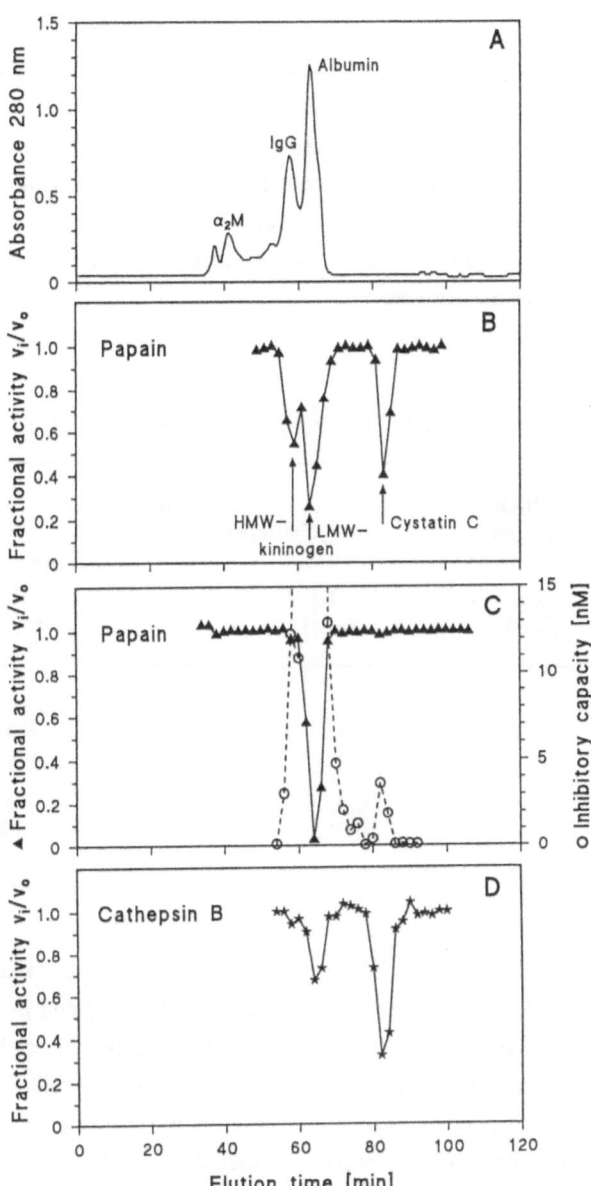

Figure 1. Cysteine proteinase inhibitors of normal blood plasma. A, Separation of blood plasma (0.1 ml diluted 1:1) on a Superose 12 column; B, Papain inhibition by a mixture of isolated HMW-kininogen (0.12 nmol), LMW-kininogen (0.23 nmol), and cystatin C (0.12 nmol) separated on the same column; C, Elution profile of papain inhibition and inhibitory capacity for papain obtained with the plasma sample shown in A; D, elution profile of cathepsin B inhibition in the same experiment.

In contrast to papain inhibition, inhibition of cathepsin B (Fig. 1D) was lower in the kininogen than in the cystatin C fraction, reflecting the low affinity of cathepsin B for kininogen. The *ex vivo* inhibition constants calculated from this experiment were 356 nM for the LMW-kininogen fraction and 1.6 nM for the low-M_r cystatin fraction (Table 2). The inhibition constants for the interaction of isolated human LMW-kininogen with isolated human cathepsin B reported in the literature vary between 600 nM (our laboratory, 3) and 30 nM (4). As the result of a carefully designed redetermination, we obtained a K_i of 390 nM which is quite close to the value of 356 nM estimated from the *ex vivo* experiment.

Table 2. Cysteine proteinase inhibition by normal blood plasma and isolated proteins

| Fraction | Inhibitory capacity | Inhibition of | | | |
| | | Cathepsin L | | Cathepsin B | |
	I_t [nM]	K_i [nM]	I_t/K_i	K_i [nM]	I_t/K_i
Kininogen					
ex vivo	4435	n.d.		356	13
LMW-Kininogen		0.012	4.0×10^5	390	11
Low-M_r cystatins					
ex vivo	65	n.d.		1.6	41
Cystatin C		<0.005	1.3×10^4	0.8	81

Two inhibitory fractions corresponding to the kininogens and low-M_r cystatins, respectively, were also found in blood plasma of polytraumatized patients (Fig. 2) and in peritonitis exudate (not shown). Dilution of samples results in the dissociation of the cathepsin B-inhibitor complexes (Fig. 3). From the dilution curves and the total functional inhibitor concentration, I_t, determined by titration, an effective K_i of cathepsin B inhibition can be calculated for the *ex vivo* samples. Assuming that two inhibitory fractions with very different K_i values for cathepsin B are present, the "global" I_t/K_i ratio, which determines the degree of inhibition, is the sum of the two individual ratios, $I_t/K_i = I_1/K_{i1} + I_2/K_{i2}$, and $I_t = I_1 + I_2$. On the basis of a K_{i1} of 390 nM (see above) for LMW-kininogen and a K_{i2} of 0.8 nM for cystatin C (determined in our laboratory), the functional concentrations of the two inhibitor fractions, I_1 and I_2, were calculated.

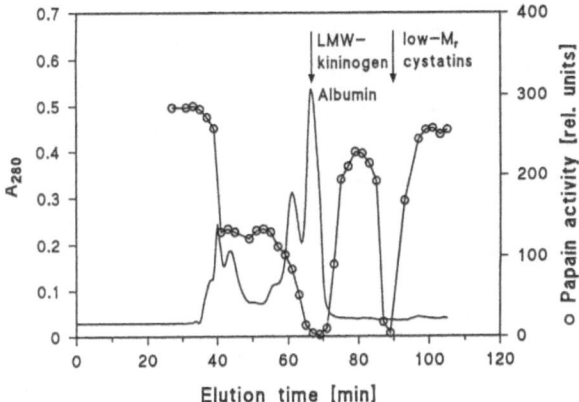

Figure 2. Cysteine proteinase inhibitors in blood plasma of a polytraumatized patient (9th day after accident). 0.1 ml of 1:4 diluted plasma were separated on a Superose 12 column as in Fig. 1. Inhibition of papain (0.2 nM) by 1/5 of each fraction was determined in a stopped assay with the fluorogenic substrate Z-Phe-Arg-NH-Mec. Under these conditions, papain inhibition is not linear with inhibitor concentration.

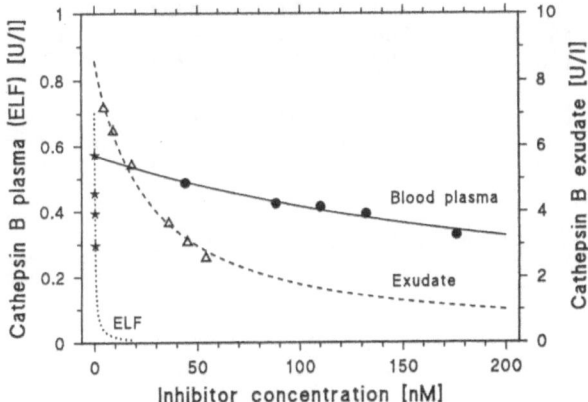

Figure 3. Determination of the effective inhibition constant (K_i) for cathepsin B by dilution analyis of *ex vivo* samples. Blood plasma of a polytraumatized patient, peritoneal exudate of a peritonitis patient, and bronchoalveolar lavage fluid of a patient with shock lung, of known inhibitor concentration (determined by papain titration), were diluted to the concentrations shown on the abscissa. Cathepsin B activity was determined as the E-64-sensitive peptidase activity with the fluorogenic substrate Z-Phe-Arg-NH-Mec obtained after dissociation of the complexes (60 min). Activity in the epithelial lining fluid (ELF) was calculated for the BALF samples (see Methods). See (2) for a discussion of the specificity of the assay for cathepsin B activity.

Preliminary data obtained with this approach are summarized in Table 3. Even when the total inhibitory capacity for papain was not significantly diminished, a reduced contribution of the low-M_r cystatin (cystatin C) fraction was observed in blood plasma of polytraumatized and septic patients. The active cystatin concentration in the exudate of a peritonitis patient was close to the normal plasma value. In the epithelial lining fluid of the lung the total inhibitor concentration was very low; the inhibitory capacity for cathepsin B was almost exclusively due to the low-M_r cystatin fraction.

Table 3. Inhibition of cathepsin B by kininogen and low-M_r cystatins

Sample	Total		Kininogen		Low-M_r-cystatins	
	I_t [nM]	I_t/K_i	I_1 [nM]	I_1/K_{i1}	I_2 [nM]	I_2/K_{i2}
Blood plasma						
healthy person*	4500	94	4434	11	66	83
Sepsis pat. 431	4300	33	4282	11	18	22
Polytrauma pat. 43	4200	30	4185	11	15	19
Polytrauma pat. 116	3300	16	3294	8	6	8
Exudate						
Peritonitis pat. 75	1350	65	1301	3	49	62
ELF lung						
Shock lung (ARDS)	18	13	8	0.02	10	13

*from the results of FPLC separation (see Fig. 1 and Table 2)

DISCUSSION

In this study, the functional inhibitory capacity of blood plasma and secretions for lysosomal cysteine proteinases was determined by titration of papain, a plant cysteine proteinase with very high affinity for kininogen (K_i = 0.012 nM) and cystatin C (K_i = < 0.005 nM). The determined inhibitory capacity, 4-5 μM in normal plasma, should be also available for the inhibition of cathepsin L which is very similar to papain in its affinity for the protein inhibitors (3). Most of the inhibitory potential (98.5%) of blood plasma is due to the kininogens, only 1-2 % are provided by low-M_r cystatins like cystatin C. These functional data agree well with previously published antigen concentrations of total kininogen, 3.6 μM (9), and cystatin C, 0.1 μM (4), in blood plasma and ensure a complete control of cathepsin L released into the circulation $(I_t/K_i > 10^5)$.

In contrast, due to its low affinity, the activity of cathepsin B discharged into the blood plasma is not sufficiently controlled by the kininogens $(I_t/K_i < 15)$. Therefore the control of cathepsin B activity critically depends on the functional concentration of low-M_r cystatins, presumably cystatin C. In normal blood plasma, the control of cathepsin B by cystatin C seems to be sufficient $(I_t/K_i>80)$. However, the inhibitory capacity of the cystatin fraction was found to be significantly reduced in blood plasma of polytraumatized and septic patients, whereas the kininogen fraction was low in peritonitis exudate. A diminished functional capacity of cystatin C may be due to N-terminal truncation and partial inactivation by released PMN elastase (10). Dissociation of active cathepsin B from its inhibitor complexes may well occur *in vivo* wherever the local concentrations of kininogens and/or cystatin C are reduced at sites of inflammation.

It has been suggested that cystatin C plays a major role in the control of cysteine proteinase activity in the bronchoalveolar fluid into which it is secreted by epithelial cells and alveolar macrophages (11,12). This is consistent with our results that the epithelial lining fluid (ELF) of the shock lung has a low active inhibitor concentration (10-50 nM) for cysteine proteinases half of which is due to low-M_r cystatins. The same samples contained appreciable amounts of proteolytically active PMN elastase (13) which might be responsible for the inactivation of cystatin C. As alveolar macrophages harbour cathepsin L (14), a very low functional cystatin C concentration would allow released cathepsin L to cleave elastin at local sites of inflammation, and, furthermore, to cleave and inactivate α_1-proteinase inhibitor (15). The mutual enhancement of proteolyis by PMN elastase and cathepsin L by inactivation of the protein inhibitors may contribute to irreversible tissue destruction in the shock lung.

CONCLUSIONS

The functional inhibitory capacity of blood plasma for cysteine proteinases is due to the kininogens and to the low-M_r cystatins, mainly cystatin C. The kininogens provide an excessive inhibitory potential for the control of cathepsin L activity which is bound quasi-irreversibly. Inhibition of cathepsin B by the kininogens, however, remains incomplete enabling the dissocation of free enzyme from the complexes whenever the inhibitory capacity is lowered. Therefore the control of cathepsin B activity in local and systemic inflammation should depend critically on the functional capacity of cystatin C which is present in much lower concentrations but is a 500-fold better inhibitor of cathepsin B.

ACKNOWLEDGEMENTS

The expert technical assistance of Gerda Behrens and Rita Zauner is greatly appreciated. We wish to thank Prof. Hans Fritz, München, for generous support. The investigations were supported by the Sonderforschungsbereich 207 of the University of Munich (grants G1 to W.M. and A.B, and G5 to M.J.)

REFERENCES

1. Assfalg-Machleidt I, Jochum M, Klaubert W, Inthorn D, Machleidt W. Enzymatically active cathepsin B dissociating from its inhibitor complexes is elevated in blood plasma of patients with septic shock and some malignant tumors. Biol Chem Hoppe-Seyler 1988; 369 Suppl:263-269.

2. Assfalg-Machleidt I, Jochum M, Nast-Kolb D, Siebeck M, Billing A, Joka Th, Rothe G, Valet G, Zauner R, Scheuber H-P, Machleidt W. Cathepsin B - Indicator for the release of lysosomal cysteine proteinases in severe trauma and inflammation. Biol Chem Hoppe-Seyler 1990; 371 Suppl:211-222.

3. Machleidt W, Ritonja A, Popovic T, Kotnik M, Brzin J, Turk V, Machleidt I, Müller-Esterl W. Human cathepsins B, H and L: Characterization by amino acid sequences and some kinetics of inhibition by the kininogens. In: Cysteine proteinases and their inhibitors. Turk V, editor. Berlin: Walter de Gruyter, 1986:3-18.

4. Abrahamson M, Barrett AJ, Salvesen G, Grubb A. Isolation of six cysteine proteinase inhibitors from human urine. J Biol Chem 1986; 261:11282-11289.

5. Nast-Kolb D, Waydhas C, Jochum M, Duswald K-H, Machleidt W, Spannagl M, Schramm W, Fritz H, Schweiberer L. Biochemische Faktoren als objektive Parameter zur Prognoseabschätzung beim Polytrauma. Unfallchirurg 1992; 95:59-66.

6. Billing A, Fröhlich D, Assfalg-Machleidt I, Machleidt W, Jochum M. Proteolysis of defensive proteins in peritonitis exudate: Pathobiochemical aspects and therapeutical approach. Biomed Biochim Acta 1991; 50:399-402.

7. Kreuzfelder E, Joka, Th, Keinecke H-O, Obertacke U, Schmit-Neuerburg K-P, Nakhosteen JA, Paar D, Scheiermann N. Adult respiratory distress syndrome as a specific manifestation of a general permeability defect in trauma patients. Am Rev Respir Dis 1988; 137:95

8. Holter JF, Weiland JE, Pacht ER, Gadek JE, Davis WB. Protein permeability in the adult respiratory distress syndrome. J Clin Invest 1986; 78:1513-1522.

9. Müller-Esterl W, Just I, Fritz H. Quantitation and differentiation of human kininogens by enzyme-linked immunosorbent assays (ELISA). Fresenius Z Anal Chem 1984; 317:733-734.

10. Abrahamson M, Mason RW, Hansson H, Buttle DJ, Grubb A, Ohlsson K. Human cystatin C. Role of the N-terminal segment in the inhibition of human cysteine proteinases and its inactivation by leucocyte elastases. Biochem J 1991; 273:621-626.

11. Chapman HA jr, Reilly JJ jr, Yee R, Grubb A. Identification of cystatin C, a cysteine proteinase inhibitor, as a major secretory product of human alveolar macrophages in vitro. Am Rev Respir Dis 1990; 141:698-705.

12. Warfel AH, Cardozo Ch, Yoo OH, Zucker-Franklin D. Cystatin C and cathepsin B production by alveolar macrophages from smokers and nonsmokers. J Leucocyte Biol 1991; 49:41-47.

13. Jochum M, Machleidt W, Fritz H. Phagocyte proteinases in multiple trauma and sepsis: Pathomechanisms and related therapeutic approaches. In: Molecular aspects of inflammation. 42. Colloquium Mosbach 1991. Sies H, Flohé L, Zimmer G, editors. Berlin: Springer-Verlag, 1991:73-92.

14. Reilly JJ jr, Mason RW, Chen P, Joseph LJ, Sukhatme VP, Yee R, Chapman HA jr. Synthesis and processing of cathepsin L, an elastase, by human alveolar macrophages.

15. Johnson DA, Barrett AJ, Mason RW (1986) Cathepsin L inactivates α_1-proteinase inhibitor by cleavage in the reactive site region. J Biol Chem 1986; 261:14748-14751.

AAS 38/I
Recent Progress on Kinins
© 1992 Birkhäuser Verlag Basel

CAIMAN KININOGEN-LIKE CYSTEINE PROTEINASE INHIBITOR

M.S. Araujo MS, Andreotti* R, Chudzinski** AM, Sampaio CAM and
Sampaio MU

Departamento de Bioquimica, Escola Paulista de Medicina. 04034
S.Paulo, SP; *EMBRAPA Centro de Pesquisa Agropecuaria do
Pantanal, 79300 Corumba, MS; **Laboratorio de Fisiopatologia,
Instituto Butantan, 05503 São Paulo, SP, Brazil

SUMMARY

Kininogens are the major mammalian plasma cysteine proteinase
inhibitors; a kininogen-like protein was also found in the
snake Bothrops jararaca plasma. This communication describes a
kininogen-like protein in plasma of Caiman crocodilus yacare.
Caiman crude plasma, unlike snake plasma, contains a detectable
cysteine proteinase inhibitor. The inhibitor was purified by
DEAE-Sephadex ion-exchange chromatography and chromatography on
carboxy-methylated-papain-Sepharose. The estimated molecular
weight of Caiman cysteine proteinase inhibitor is 70,000. Caiman
plasma also hydrolyzes plasma kallikrein synthetic substrates
and inhibits trypsin. Reptilian kininogen may lack the site for
interaction with plasma prokallikrein, and the sequence of the
released kinin may be distinct from bradykinin. The poor
effectiveness of bradykinin on reptile smooth muscle shows that
the reptile kinin receptors may be adapted to a specific kinin.

INTRODUCTION

Mammalian plasma contains at least two types of kininogens, high and low molecular weight kininogens. The same gene directs the biosynthesis of both kininogens. Although they share the heavy chains and the consecutive kinin moiety, they differ in the structural properties of the C-terminus sequences where the light-chains are located (1).

Mammalian kininogens are now also known as the main plasma cysteine proteinase inhibitors, being this inhibitory activity associated with the heavy chain of high and low molecular weight kininogens. Both kininogens contain three repeating domains in the heavy chains, with high homology to the cystatins, and two of these domains can inhibit cysteine proteinases (2).

High-molecular-weight kininogen is associated with the initiation of the blood clotting cascade, participating in the activation of plasma prokallikrein and Factor XII. Only the light chain of high- molecular-weight kininogen fits the prokallikrein binding site, distal to bradykinin and proximal to the C-terminus region of the molecule (1).

Studies on the presence of kininogen in snake plasma have been approached by the estimation of released kinin, upon incubation with kininogenases. Contrary to what is seen in mammalian plasma, kinin was not demonstrated in Bothrops jararaca plasma, on isolated preparations such as guinea pig ileum or rat uterus (3). Snake plasma was reported to lack kininogen, or alternatively, the absence of detectable amounts of kinins was attributed to a rapid and potent inactivation of the released kinin by kininases (4).

B. jararaca plasma was shown to release a polypeptide active
on snake smooth muscle (5) and also to contain a cysteine
proteinase inhibitor able to yield a polypeptide active on snake
smooth muscle (6). A kininogen-related protein was found in
chicken and turtle plasma, and both released kinins are
different from bradykinin (7,8). The aim of the present study
is to describe in Caiman crocodilus yacare plasma the presence
of a kininogen-type protein that inhibits cysteine proteinases.

MATERIAL AND METHODS

Caiman crocodilus yacare plasma was collected from male and
female adults (15 kg average weight). Blood was drawn from the
heart into plastic tubes containing 0.4% sodium citrate (final
concentration). Plasma separated by centrifugation was frozen in
liquid nitrogen and stored at -70°C

Papain was from Boehringer; bromelain, bovine trypsin,
phenylmethylsulfonyl-fluoride (PMSF), L-trans-epoxysuccinyl-L-
leucyl-amido-(4-guanidino)-butane (E-64), DL-dithiothreitol
(DTT), were from Sigma; bovine thrombin was from Roche; human
plasma kallikrein was purified by a described procedure (10).
DEAE-Sephadex A 50 was a Pharmacia product. Carboxy-methylated-
papain-Sepharose was made by reacting the active thiol group of
the enzyme with iodoacetamide, and subsequently coupling to
CNBr-activated Sepharose (9).

Tosyl-L-arginine methyl ester (TAME) was from Merck, and the
chromogenic substrate N-acetyl-L-phenylalanine-L-arginine p-
nitroanilide (Ac-Phe-Arg-Nan) was a kind gift of Dr. L. Juliano,
Departamento de Biofísica, Escola Paulista de Medicina.
Hexadimetrine bromide (Polybrene) was from EGA-Chemie, and
Nembutal was from Abbott.

Papain activity was measured by the hydrolysis of 1.0 mM Ac-Phe-Arg-pNA, in 10 mM sodium phosphate buffer, 1.0 mM EDTA, pH 6.8, after activation of the enzyme with 2.0 mM DTT, for 15 min, at 37°C, as described elsewhere (10). Papain inhibition was followed by incubation of increasing concentrations of the inhibitor (from 0.5 to 4 ug) with 12.0 ng E-64-titrated papain (11).

DEAE-Sephadex A 50 was equilibrated with 0.05 M tris-HCl, pH 8.0 buffer, containing 1 mM EDTA, 1 mM PMSF, 100 mg/L polybrene, 0.01 % timerosal and 0.03 M NaCl. Following sample application (10 ml Caiman plasma dyalized against the equilibrium buffer), the column was extensively washed with equilibrium buffer until absorbance at 280 nm (A280) was lower than 0.05, and subsequently with increasing NaCl concentrations (0.3 M and 0.5 M) in the same buffer system.

Gel filtration was performed in a Fast Protein Liquid Chromatography equipament from Pharmacia, using a Superose 12 column equilibrated with 0.1 M tris-HCl buffer, pH 8.0, and developed at 0.25 mL/min flow rate.

CM-papain-Sepharose (2 mL) was equilibrated with 0.1 M tris-HCl buffer, pH 7.0. The resin was extensively washed with the same buffer, following sample (10 mL Caiman plasma diluted to 20 mL with equilibrium buffer) application, until the absorbance at 280nm was lower than 0.05. Elution of bound material was carried out with 0.05 M NaOH, pH 11.0, in 2.0 mL fractions which were immediately neutralized with 60 uL 1.0 M tris-HCl, pH 8.0 buffer. Protein elution was monitored at 280 nm.

Polyacrylamide gel eletrophoresis was performed on 5-15 % or 10-20% gradient slab gels, under the conditions described by Laemmli (12), and stained with Coomassie Blue or silver nitrate(13).

Kininogen biological activity was assayed on isolated guinea-pig ileum preparations, bathed with 10 mL Tyrode solution, and standardized with synthetic bradykinin; variable amounts of the purified Caiman plasma inhibitor were assayed in the presence of an excess of trypsin (50 to 500 ug); bradykinin elicited contractions were recorded for 1 min, and contractions elicited by trypsin direct incubation were recorded for about 3 min (14). Biological activity was also analyzed on isolated C.c.yacare intestine bathed with a Ringer solution for reptile at 22°C, bradykinin-like activity was measured as in guinea-pig ileum.

RESULTS

Papain inhibition was detected directly in Caiman plasma and it was separated after chromatography on a DEAE-Sephadex column, the cysteine proteinase inhibitor was found in the effluent eluted by 0.2 M NaCl (figure 1).

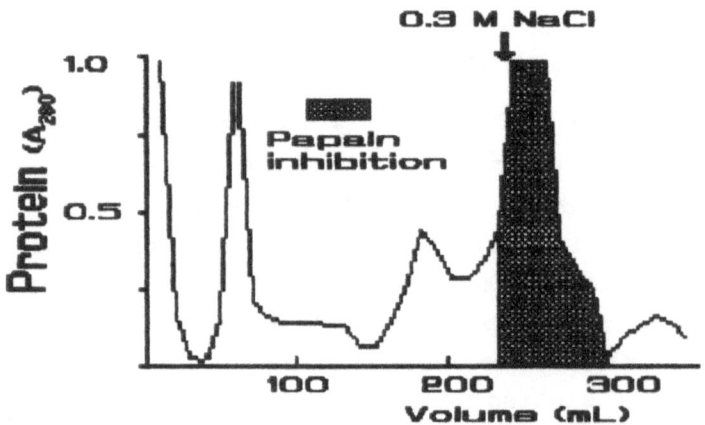

Figure 1. DEAE-Sephadex chromatography. Column (22.5 x 1 cm) equilibrated with 0.05 M tris-HCl buffer, pH 8.0, and eluted with 0.3 and 0.5 M NaCl in the same buffer. Sample: C.c.yacare plasma (10 mL) in tris-HCl equilibrium buffer.

The pooled active fractions were subjected to a gel filtration in Superose 12 yielding two peaks active upon papain, being the first eluted peak pool a correspondent to Mr 70,000 (Figure 2).

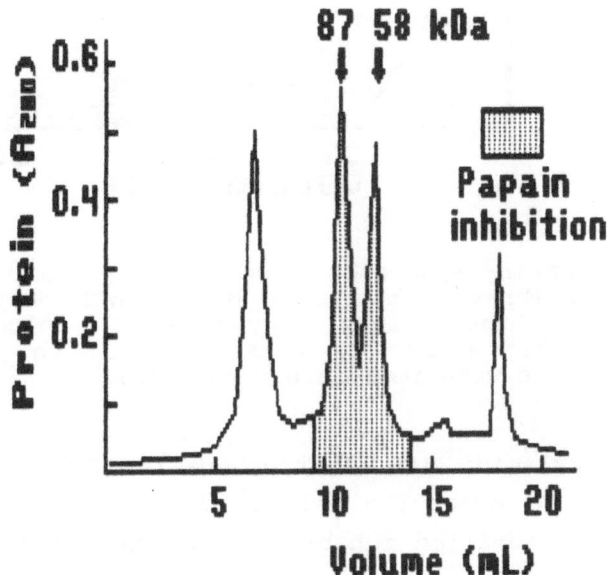

Figure 2. Chromatography in a Pharmacia FPLC system (Superose 12 column) with resin equilibrated with 0.1 M tris-HCl, 0.1 M NaCl, pH 8.0 buffer, flow rate 0.25 mL/min. Sample: active pool from DEAE-Sephadex chromatography.

Cysteine proteinase inhibitor activity was bound to CM-papain-Sepharose, under the conditions used, and eluted by alkalinization, and immediate neutralization of the collected fractions. A single peak of a material which presents a kininogen-like activity after incubation with excess trypsin (100 ug/mL) was obtained (figure 3).

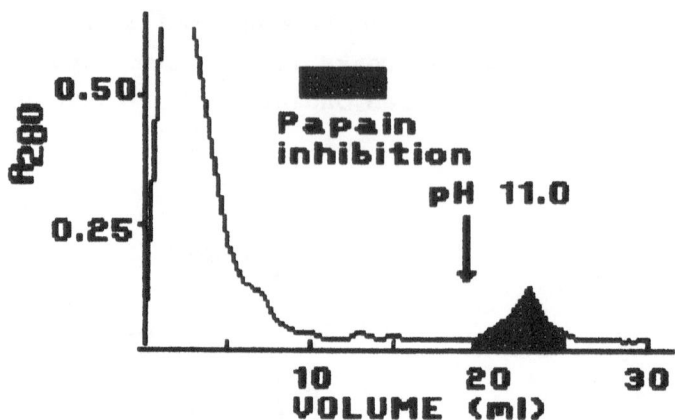

Figure 3. CM-papain-Sepharose chromatography. Column (4.0 ml) with resin equilibrated in 0.1 M tris-HCl buffer, pH 7.0. Sample: inhibitor eluted from Superose 12 column (pool a). Bound inhibitor was eluted by alkalinization to pH 11.0, and collected fractions were immediately neutralized.

SDS-polyacrylamide gel electrophoresis (9) showed a single major band with a molecular weight of 70,000. Dithiothreitol reduction of the purified inhibitor indicated that the material is mainly a single-chain polypeptide (not shown).

The inhibition of papain by the Caiman kininogen is concentration dependent (Figure 4), with an apparent Ki value 3.27 nM, calculated as for Bothrops kininogen (7). Trypsin was poorly inhibited by Caiman plasma (Ki = 0.22 uM).

A bradykinin like activity released by trypsin was detected both in plasma and the purified cysteine proteinase inhibitor eluted from DEAE-Sephadex, either on the guinea-pig ileum or Caiman isolated intestine preparation.

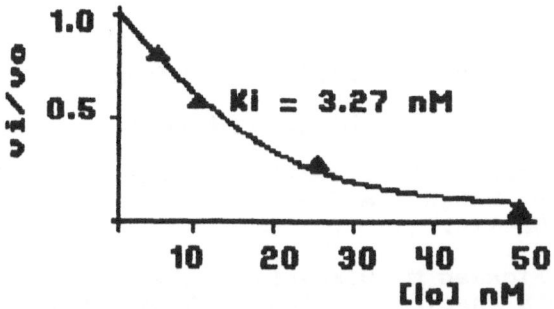

Figure 4. Inactivation of papain by _C.c.vacare_ cysteine proteinase inhibitor. Papain (1.2 nM) was incubated with the inhibitor (10 to 50 nM) in 10 mM sodium phosphate buffer, pH 6.8, containing 1 mM EDTA, for 15 min at 37°C. Residual papain activity was determined by measuring the hydrolysis of 1.0 mM Ac-Phe-Arg-pNA (7). Data are reported as percent activity in the absence of inhibitor.

DISCUSSION

The presence of a kininogen-like protein in _Caiman crocodilus vacare_ plasma confirms the presence of the kininogen gene in reptiles. Structural data are not yet available, and the biological activity of the tryptic hydrolysates on the isolated guinea pig ileum is very weak. However, these data suggest that a peptide is released, as plausibly explained by the presence of a structural domain related to the kinin-yielding moiety in the molecule. A low activity on non-homologous organs would be expected, as seen for the chicken kininogen (7) and turtle kininogen (8).

REFERENCES

1. Müller-Esterl W (1987). Sem.Thromb. Hemost. 13:115-126.

2.Barret AJ (1986). Biomed. Biochem. Acta 45:1363-1374.

3.Lavras AAC, Fichman M, Hiraichi E, Boucault M, Tobo T, Schmuziger P, Nahas L and Picarelli ZP (1979). Ciência e Cultura 31:168-174.

4.Lavras AAC., Fichman M, Hiraichi E, Todo, T and Boucault, MA (1980) Acta Physiol. Latinoam. 30:269-274 .

5.Prezoto BC, Hiraichi E, Abdalla FMF, Picarelli ZP and Lavras AAC (1987). Kinin 87 Tokyo International Congress Abstracts, 146.

6.Chudzinski, AM, Oliva ML, Sampaio MU and Sampaio CAM (1989) Braz. J. Med Biol. Res. 22: 945-94

7.Kimura M, Sueyoshi T, Takada T, Tanaka K, Morita T and Iwanaga S (1987). Eur. J. Biochem. 168: 493-501

8.Colon JM, Hicks, JW and Smith, DD (1990) Endocrinology 126: 985-991.

9.Anastasi A, Brown MA, Kembhavi AA, Nicklin MJH, Sayers CA, Sunter DC and Barret AJ (1983). Biochem. J. 211:129-138.

10.Oliva MLV, Sampaio MU and Sampaio CAM (1988). Biol. Chem. Hoppe-Seyler 369:229-232.

11.Zucker S, Buttle DJ, Nicklin MJ and Barret AJ (1985). Biochim. Biophys. Acta 828:196-204.

12.Laemmli UK (1970). Nature, 227:680-685.

13.Morrissey JH (1981). Anal. Biochem., 117:307-312 .

14.Sampaio CAM, Nunes ST, Mazzacoratti, MGN and Prado JL (1976). Biochem. Pharmacol. 25:2391-2396 .

AAS 38/I
Recent Progress on Kinins
© 1992 Birkhäuser Verlag Basel

ISOLATION AND CHARACTERISATION OF CHICKEN L- AND H- KININOGENS AND THEIR INTERACTION WITH CHICKEN CYSTEINE PROTEINASES AND PAPAIN

Janko Kos, Marko Dolinar and Vito Turk

Department of Biochemistry, J. Stefan Institute, Jamova 39,
61000 Ljubljana, Slovenia

SUMMARY

We have isolated L- and H-kininogens from chicken egg white and plasma using affinity chromatography on CM-papain Sepharose, Con-A Sepharose, gel filtration and ion exchange chromatography, in pure form. In chicken plasma mostly HK was present, whereas in chicken egg white both LK and HK were identified. The determined Mr of LK and HK were 69000 and about 96000, respectively. They occured in multiple forms with pI 4.3 - 5.2. The inhibitory activity of chicken HK was tested against cysteine proteinases cathepsins B and L, isolated from chicken liver, and papain. The obtained Ki values demonstrated that chicken H-kininogen is a strong inhibitor of chicken cathepsin L and papain, but much weaker inhibitor of chicken cathepsin B.

INTRODUCTION

During the last few years much attention has been paid to cystatins, the protein inhibitors of cysteine proteinases. They were isolated from different animal tissues and characterized (1). On the basis of their primary structures they were divided into three families: the stefin and the cystatin family, both composed of low-Mr proteins of Mr about 11000 - 13000, and the kininogen family with Mr of about 65000 and higher (2).

Kininogens are further divided into three types: H-kininogens, L-kininogens and T-kininogens (3). All three types share the heavy chain, located at the N-terminus and the kinin fragment, but they differ in their light chains at the C-terminus. The heavy chain contains three domains homologous to chicken cystatin, a representative of the inhibitors of cysteine proteinases, isolated from chicken egg white (4). Domain 1 from the N-terminus is inhibitory inactive, domain 2 inhibits calpain, papain and cathepsin L , whereas domain 3 strongly inhibits only papain and cathepsin L (5).

In mammals, the structure and function of the kininogens have been extensively studied, but in contrast, the knowledge of the nonmammalian kininogens is very limited.

In the present work we have isolated L- and H-kininogens from chicken egg white and plasma using the procedure, developed for the isolation of chicken cystatin (6). Here we report some of the biochemical characteristics of these two inhibitors of cysteine proteinases, as well as kinetic data for interactions of H-kininogen with papain and previously isolated chicken cathepsins B and L.

MATERIALS

Chicken eggs were purchased from the chicken farm Jata, Ljubljana. Chicken plasma was prepared at the Biotechnical faculty, University of Ljubljana. CNBr-activated Sepharose 4B, Sephadex G-75 and Sephacryl S-200 were from Pharmacia, Sweden. Ampholines were from Serva, FRG, as well as benzoyl-D,L-arginine-2-naphtyl amide (BANA) and L-cysteine. Papain (twice crystallized) was from Sigma, USA. CM-papain-Sepharose 4B was prepared in our laboratory as described previously (7). Ep-475 was a gift of K. Hanada (Japan). Z-Phe-ArgNMec and Z-Arg-ArgNMec were from Bachem, Switzerland. All the other reagents were of analytical grade.

METHODS

Isolation of the L-kininogen from egg white. We started our preparation from 3600 fresh chicken eggs. The first purification steps, including affinity chromatography on CM-papain-Sepharose, were done according to Anastasi et al. (8). The inhibitory active fractions, eluted from affinity resin, were pooled, concentrated and applied to the gel filtration column (Sephadex G75, 6 x 90 cm), equilibrated with 2 mM solution of ammonia. Four protein peaks were eluted at a flow rate of 54 ml/h. Fractions of the second peak, containing kininogen, were further rechromatographed on CM-papain-Sepharose 4B and then applied to the Sephacryl S-200 column (2.4 x 115 cm), equilibrated and eluted with 0.05 M TRIS/HCl buffer, pH 8.0, containing 0.5 M NaCl at a flow rate of 18 ml/h.

After the gel filtration active material was dialysed against 0.02 M TRIS/HCl buffer, containing 0.5 M NaCl (starting buffer), and applied to the Con-A Sepharose column (3.5 x 4 cm). The unbound protein was washed off by the starting buffer. For the elution of glycosilated proteins a linear gradient of methylglucoside (0 - 0.5 M) was used. Fractions of 6 ml were collected at a flow rate of 30 ml/hr and assayed for inhibitory activity.

Isolation of H-kininogen from chicken serum. 100 ml of chicken plasma, containing 20 mM phosphate buffer + 0.5 M NaCl, pH 6.5 were applied to the column (4 x 2.5 cm) of Cm-papain Sepharose 4B. After washing the column with equilibrating buffer, bound proteins were eluted by 0.1 M Na_3PO_4, pH 11.5. Inhibitory active fractions were pooled, concentrated, dialysed against 40 mM

TRIS/HCl buffer, pH 7.9 and applied to the MONO Q column (FPLC), equilibrated with the same buffer. Proteins were eluted by a linear gradient of NaCl from 0 to 0.5 M. The final purification step was affinity chromatography on Con-A Sepharose under the same conditions as for chicken egg white L-kininogen.

Inhibitor assay. The inhibitory activity was assayed on papain using BANA as a substrate, according to Barrett (7). One inhibitory unit (IU) corresponds to the inhibition of 1 μg of active papain previously titrated by Ep-475.

Gel electrophoresis. Polyacrylamide gel electrophoresis was performed as described previously (9) on Pharmacia gradient gels. The protein standards used for Mr determination were: phosphorylase B (94000), bovine serum albumin (67000), ovalbumin (43000), carbonic anhydrase (29000), soya-bean trypsin inhibitor (21000) and lactalbumin (14000).

Isoelectric focusing. Analytical gel electrofocusing was carried out on 1 mm thick 5% polyacrylamide gel plates with carrier ampholines (pH 3-10) as described (8), using a Desaga apparatus.

Protein determination. Protein concentration was determined by the method of Lowry et al. (10).

N-terminal amino acid sequence determination. Amino acid sequences were determined by automated solid-phase Edman degradation according to ref. (11).

Preparation of the enzymes. Chicken cathepsins B and L were isolated from chicken liver according to the procedures, described for human cathepsins B (12) and L (13).
Papain (Sigma, 2x crystallized) was repurified by affinity chromatography on papain inhibitor Gly-Gly-Tyr(Bzl)-Arg as described (14). All enzymes were titrated by Ep-475 to determine their active concentration.

Determination of kinetic constants. The rate constants (kass, kdiss) for the inactivation of papain and chicken cathepsins B and L by H-kininogen were determined by continous rate assays according to Morrisson (15). Progress curves for the inhibition of proteinases were monitored on spectrofluorimeter (Perkin-Elmer LS 3). Fluorescence was continuously measured, digitized and stored in IBM XT microcomputer using FLUSYS (16) software package, and further analysed by non-linear regression method.

Before starting the reaction, the enzyme (50 ul) was added to fluorimetric cuvette, containing 2.9 ml of assay buffer (20 mM Na acetate buffer, pH 6.0, 2 mM dithiotreitol, 1 mM EDTA and 0.05 % Brij 35). After 5 min of activation (at 25°C) 50 ul of the mixture of substrate and inhibitor was added.

For papain, 2.5×10^{-10} M final concentration of activatable enzyme was used, with inhibitor ranging from 1.5 to 7.5×10^{-9} M and Z-Phe-ArgNMec as substrate at 10 μM final concentration.

For chicken cathepsin L 1×10^{-10} M final concentration was used with inhibitor ranging from 1 to 6×10^{-9} M and 5 μM Z-Phe-ArgNMec as substrate. For cathepsin B 2×10^{-8} M final concentration was used with inhibitor ranging from 0.8 to 1.8×10^{-7} M and Z-Phe-ArgNMec as substrate at 10 μM final concentration.

In all experiments the substrate consumption was less than 3%.

RESULTS AND DISSCUSION

Chicken kininogen has already been isolated and sequenced from chicken plasma and the name ornitho-kininogen was proposed for it (17). While it has an apparent molecular weight of 74 kDa, determined on Ferguson plot, it migrates as a 95 kDa component on SDS-PAGE. The HMW inhibitor of cysteine proteinases that we isolated from chicken plasma, has similar mobility on SDS-PAGE gel - 96 kDa. Considering also the same N-terminal amino acid sequence (T P L P F E F) our protein is very probably identical to ornitho-kininogen (17).

In the absence of 2-mercaptoethanol H-kininogen gave a single band on SDS-PAGE at Mr of 96 kDa (Fig. 1, samples a,b), whereas under reducing conditions additional slight bands occured at Mr 63 kDa and 54 kDa, respectively, probably corresponding to the kinin-free protein (Fig. 1, sample c). On isoelectric focusing H-kininogen shows two bands at pI 4.3 and 4.6 (results not shown). We estimated the concentration of H-kininogen in chicken plasma to be about 120 μg/ml (Table 1).

HMW inhibitor of cysteine proteinases isolated from chicken egg white is in contrast similar to L-kininogens. On SDS-PAGE under reducing conditions it shows two bands with Mr of 63000 and 69000. The first one corresponds to the heavy chain and the second to the full length molecule (Fig. 2, sample a). Additionally a slight band appears at Mr of 96000 indicating also the presence of low amounts of H- kininogen in egg white. On isoelectric focusing L-kininogen shows several multiple forms in the pH range 4.9 - 5.2 (Fig. 3). The estimated concentration of L-kininogen in egg white is 3 to 7 μg/ml (Table 1), that is 20 fold lower than the concentration of H-kininogen in blood plasma. Considering that the concentration of chicken cystatin in egg white is at least 80 μg/ml (6,8) the role of L-kininogen as inhibitor in egg white is negligible.

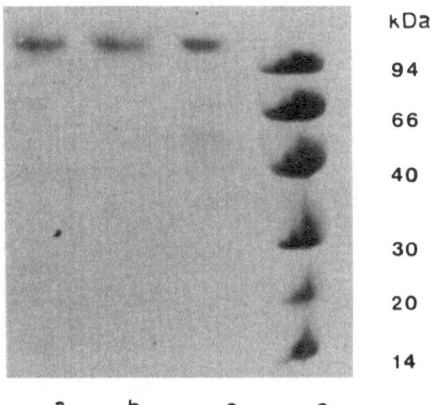

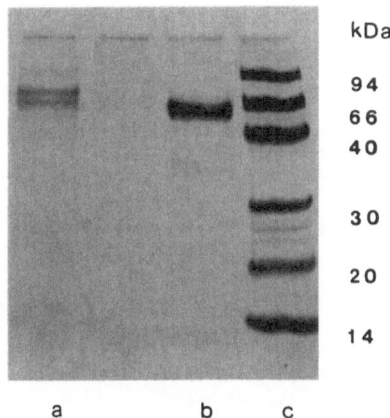

Figure 1: SDS-PAGE
a, b - chicken H-kininogen, isolated from blood
plasma,without 2-mercaptoethanol, c - chicken
H-kininogen with 2-mercaptoethanol, s - standards

Figure 2: SDS-PAGE under reductive conditions
a - chicken egg white L-kininogen, b - human
   L-kininogen, c - standards

Table 1:Purification of L- and H- kininogens from chicken egg white and chicken blood plasma.
O Data comprise cystatin and kininogen activity

Steps	Protein (g)	Total activity (IU x 10^3)	Specif. activity (IU/mg)	Yield (%)
Egg white	1800	3600	2	100
Eluate after aff. chromatography	8.7	1800	135.6	50
Gel filtration on Sephadex G75	1.8	120	83.3	3.3
Rechromatography on CM-papain Sepharose 4B	0.15	82	446	2.2
Gel filtration on Sephacryl S200	0.06	57	950	1.55
Con-A Sepharose	0.025	32	1240	0.90
O chicken plasma	7.5	30	4	100
ion exchange chromatography	0.01	16	1600	53
Con-A Sepharose	0.004	10	2500	33.3

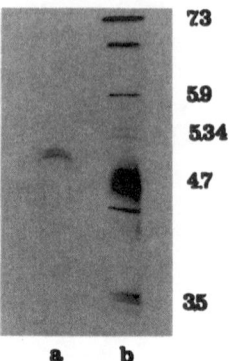

Figure 3: Analytical isoelectric focusing
a - L-kininogen from chicken egg white
b - standards

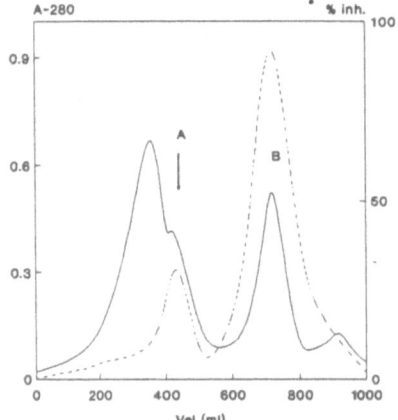

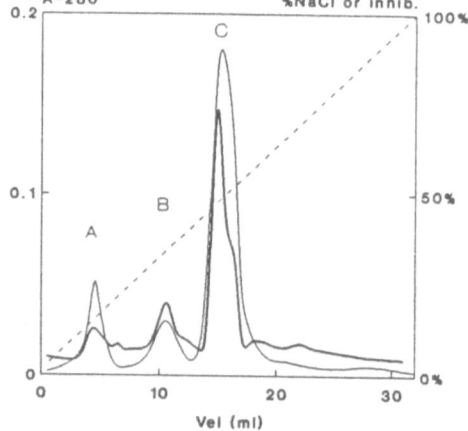

Figure 4: Gel filtration on Sephadex G-75 column
Isolation of L-kininogen from chicken egg white.
A - Inhibitory fractions corr. to kininogen,
B - Inhibitory fractions corr. to cystatin.
____ A280 - protein concentration,
- - - - % of inhibition of papain.

Figure 5:   Ion exchange chromatography on
MONO Q (FPLC) column.
Isolation of chicken H-kininogen from plasma
A, B - chicken cystatin, C - kininogen
____ A280 - protein conc., - - - % of inhibition
of papain, NaCl concentration

The isolation procedure from egg white includes more steps than that from chicken plasma. In both
cases the affinity chromatography on CM-papain Sepharose was used as the initial step, resulting in
high (700-fold) increase of specific activity. From elution profile on Fig. 4 it is evident that chicken
cystatin contributes much more to the total inhibitory activity of egg white than kininogen, whereas in
blood plasma the concentration of cystatin is lower (1) and inhibitory activity is mainly due to
kininogen (Fig. 5).

Like other kininogens, chicken LK and HK are glycosilated and they can be bound to Con-A Sepharose. This fact was used for the final separation of kininogens from higher molecular weight aggregates of chicken cystatin (Fig. 6).

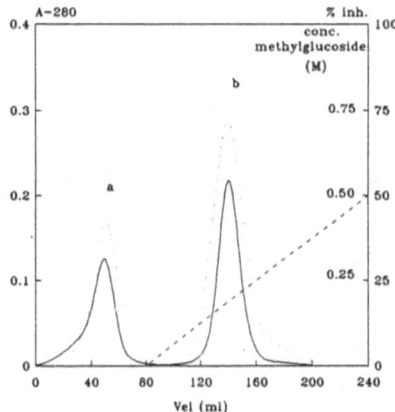

Figure 6: Affinity chromatography on Concavalin-A Sepharose
Final purification step for chicken L- and H- kininogens.
- - - - A280 - protein concentration, _____ gradient of
methyl-glucoside, ... % of inhibition of papain

Rate and equilibrium constants, describing interactions between H-kininogen and papain, cathepsin B and L are presented in Table 2.

Table 2: Inhibition constants and rate constants for the interactions between chicken H-kininogen and papain. chicken cathepsin L and chicken cathepsin B

	K_i (nM)	k_{ass} ($M^{-1}s^{-1}$)	k_{diss} (s^{-1})
papain	0.016	5.4×10^6	0.9×10^{-4}
cathepsin L	0.025	1.4×10^7	3.6×10^{-4}
cathepsin B	44	$1.1. \times 10^4$	4.9×10^{-4}

Progress curves of the inhibitor-enzyme interactions were fitted to the equation (15)

$$P = v_s t (v_o - v_s) (1-e^{-kt})/k$$

by non-linear least-squares analysis to obtain the best estimates for v_0, v_s and k. Rate constants k_{ass} and k_{diss} were calculated using following equations:

$$k = k_{ass} I_0 / (1+S_0/K_m) + k_{diss}$$
$$k_{diss} = k \ v_s/v_0$$
$$K_i = k_{diss}/k_{ass}$$

The K_m values for chicken cathepsins B (23 μM) and L (3.5 μM) were calculated by non-linear least-squares analysis from initial velocities, measured at six to eight different substrate concentrations. For papain and Z-PheArgNMec as substrate K_m was published to be 65 μM (18).

From kinetic data it is evident that chicken H-kininogen is a potent inhibitor of papain and chicken cathepsin L (K_i 10^{-11}), whereas for chicken cathepsin B the inhibition is 1000 fold weaker (K_i 10^{-8}M).

AKNOWLEDGEMENTS

This work was supported by Slovene Ministry of science and technolology. We thank Dr. Dušan Benčina for providing chicken blood plasma and Dr. Marina Drobnič Košorok for amino acid sequence determination.

REFERENCES

1. Barrett, A.J., Rawlings, N.D., Davies, M.E., Machleidt, M., Salvesen, G. and Turk, V. (1986) in: Proteinases inhibitors (Barrett, A.J. and Salvesen, G. eds.) Elsevier, Amsterdam, New York, 515-569.

2. Barrett, A.J., Fritz, H., Grubb, A., Isemura, S., Jarvinen, M., Katunuma, N., Machleidt, W., Sasaki, M., Turk, V. (1986) Biochem. J. 238, 236-312.

3. Barrett, A.J. (1987) TIBS 12, 193-196.

4. Okhubo, I., Kurachi, K., Takasawa, T., Shiokawa, H., Sasaki, M. (1984) Biochemistry 23, 5691-5697.

5. Salvesen, G., Parkes, C., Abrahamson, M., Grubb, A., Barrett, A.J. (1986) Biochem. J. 234, 429-434.

6. Kos, J., Dolinar, M., Turk, V. (1986) in: Cysteine proteinases and their inhibitors (Turk, V. ed.) Walter de Gruyter Berlin, New York, 583-591.

7. Barrett, A.J. (1981) Methods Enzymol. 80, 771-778 .

8. Anastasi, A., Brown, M.A., Kembhavi, A.A., Nicklin, M.J.H., Sayers, C.A., Sunter, D.C., Barrett, A.J. (1983) Biochem. J. 211, 129-138.

9. Laemmli, U.K. (1970) Nature 227, 680-685.

10. Lowry, O.H., Roseborough, N.J., Farr, A.L., Randall, R.J. (1951) J. Biol. Chem. 193, 265-275.

11. Ritonja, A., Popović, T., Turk, V., Wiedenmann, K. and Machleidt, W. (1985) FEBS Lett. 181, 169-172.

12. Popović, T., Brzin, J., Kos, J., Lenarčič, B., Machleidt, W., Ritonja, A., Hanada, K. and Turk, V. (1988) Biol. Chem. Hoppe-Seyler 371, Suppl., 175-183.

13. Kotnik, M., Popović, T., Turk, V. (1986) in: Cysteine proteinases and their inhibitors (Turk, V. ed.) Walter de Gruyter Berlin, New York, 583-591.

14. Blumberg, S., Schechter, I. and Berger, A. (1970) Eur. J. Biochem. 15, 97-102 .

15. Morrisson, J.F. (1982) TIBS 7, 102-105.

16. Rawlings, N.D., Barrett, A.J. (1990) CABIOS 6, 118-119.

17. Kimura, M., Sueyoshi, T., Takada, K., Tanaka, K., Morita, T., Iwanaga, S. (1987) Eur. J. Biochem. 168, 493-501.

18. Zucker, S., Buttle, D.J., Nicklin, M.J.H. and Barrett, A.J. (1985) Biochem. Biophys. Acta 828, 196-204.

CHARACTERIZATION OF TWO MEMBERS(CST4 and CST5) OF THE CYSTATIN GENE FAMILY

AND MOLECULAR EVOLUTION OF CYSTATIN GENES

Eiichi Saitoh, Satoko Isemura, Kazuo Sanada and Koji Ohnishi*

Department of Oral Biochemistry, Nippon Dental University at Niigata,
1-8 Hamaura-cho, Niigata 951, JAPAN and *Department of Biology, Faculty of
Science, Niigata University, Ikarashi-2, Niigata 950-21, JAPAN

SUMMARY: Two members(CST4 and CST5) of the cystatin gene family have been characterized partially by DNA analysis. The CST4 clone contained the gene coding
for the precursor form(141 amino acids) of cystatin S, and its exon-intron
organization is the same as that of other members(the cystatin SN gene at the
CST1 locus, the cystatin SA gene at the CST2 locus, the cystatin C gene at the
CST3 locus and a cystatin pseudogene at the CSTP1 locus). The second cystatin
pseudogene was elucidated in the clone, CST5, and it was assigned to the CSTP2
locus. Alignment of DNA sequences of cystatin genes with other genes suggested
that the genes for cystatins, kininogens, and Bowman-Birk type inhibitors have
evolved from an ancient ribonuclease-like gene.

INTRODUCTION

Endogenous cysteine proteinase inhibitors belonging to the cystatin superfamily
are found in various body fluids and tissues of animals. They are divided into
at least three families: I(the stefin family), II(the cystatin family) and III
(the kininogen family)(1). The members of the cystatin superfamily are proposed to be derived from a common ancestor(2) and they are considered to
regulate intracellular protein catabolisms or to protect the cells from attacks
by foreign proteinases. Human cystatins of family II are secretory proteins
with two disulfide bonds and molecular weights about 15,000. Four molecular
species of this class, salivary(S-type) cystatins(cystatins S, SA, and SN), and
cystatin C, have been isolated from human body fluids(3-7).

We have already shown that cystatins S, SA, SN, and C are determined by a
multigene family(seven members) on human chromosome 20-the cystatin gene family
(8-11). Six out of seven cystatin loci(CST1, CST2, CST3, CST4, CSTP1 and CST5)
have been cloned(8-10), and four genes were assigned to the corresponding loci:
the cystatin SN gene to the CST1, the cystatin SA gene to the CST2, the
cystatin C gene to the CST3, and a cystatin pseudogene to the CSTP1(8-10).

Hin dIII

AAGCTTGGGAGCACTGGGGAAGAGAGGCATGGCTCAGGGAGGTCGCAGTGAGGACTGGAGTGGGGAGGAGGGGGAGATGGAGGAGGAGGCCTGGGAGGGG

CAGGGGGAACTTAGGCAGGGAGGGAGCTTGTAGTGGTGGGGGAGTGAAAAGAGAGATGGAGAAAGAGGGGATGGGCTGAAAGAGGAGGAGGAGTCAGGGG

CAGGGCATGGAGGTGGGTGGGGCTGGGCTGCCAAAGCAGGATAAATGCACACCTGCCTGCTGGTCTGGGCTCCCTGCCTCAGGCTCTCACCCTCCTCTCC

Exon 1

TGCAGCTCCAGCTCTGTGCTCTGCCTCTGAGGAGACCATGGCCCGGCCTCTGTGTACCCTGCTACTCCTGATGGCTACCCTGGCTGGGGCTCTGGCCTCG
                                        M A R P L C T L L L L M A T L A G A L A S

Sac I   -20   -1 +1
AGCTCCAAGGAGGAGAATAGGATAATCCCAGGTGGCATCTATGATGCAGACCTCAATGATGAGTGGGTACAGCGTGCCCTTCACTTCGCCATCAGCGAGT
 S S K E E N R I I P G G I Y D A D L N D E W V Q R A L H F A I S E Y

                                                              ▼
ACAACAAGGCCACCGAAGATGAGTACTACAGACGCCCGCTGCAGGTGCTGCGAGCCAGGGAGCAGGTGGGTGCTGCCTCCACCCCAGGGGTCCTNAGCCC
 N K A T E D E Y Y R R P L Q V L R A R E Q
                                                              56

TAGCCTGGTTTGTTGCCGG--------- Intron 1 ----------TCTGCAACTGTAAGAGACACCTAAGGTGTGCTGCTGACTTGAGAAATGTA

TCTTGAACCTCACACTTGAAATGGTGGCATCTGGGCGGCCCCATTGACCCAAAATATCTGTGTGTGTGAAGCATCTCATTTCCTACTCTAAGTGAAGTAA

TAAATCTAGGTTAAATGGAGGGAATAAGATTTTCGTGAGTTAGGTGAAATTTTGTCATCAGACAGCCTTCCTAGAAAAGAGTCAGTGTTCCCTCGCCCCT

              EcoRI
GAGCCACAGGCAGCAGAATTCAATGAATCCTCTTACCCAGCACAGAGAAAACGATGTTTAAGAGCGGGCATGAGGCTCAGCACCCTGCCAGCTGACAGGA

AGAGGGGGCTTGTGTGCCTTGTGTTGACATGTGGGCAGCTCACGAAGCCCCCAAGCAAGTCCAGTGACTCAGCCACAGTGAAGTGCCTGTGAGTGCATGA

                                        Exon 2
ACTGATGGGGGCGCTGTCCGTGCTTCCTGTTTTCTCCTGTGTGCAGACCTTTGGGGGGGTGAATTACTTCTTCGACGTAGAGGTGGGCCGCACCATATGT
                                        T F G G V N Y F F D V E V G R T I C
                                        57
                                                              ▼   Sma I
ACCAAGTCCCAGCCCAACTTGGACACCTGTGCCTTCATGAACAGCCAGAACTGCAGAAGGTACGTTCCTGATGCGGGTCCCGGGCCAGTCATGCATGCA
 T K S Q P N L D T C A F H E Q P E L Q K
                                                         94

CTGCAGAGGGGTGCGTATGTGTCAGCCTCTGTGCCTACCCATGTTTGGACGGTGTGTGTGTGTGCAGGTGGGTATGTGGGGAGCCGTGTATGCATGGATGTGT

ACGTGTTCATGTACTTATGGGGGGGTGTGTGCATTTAGGTGTGCATGTGGAAAAGGTGCACGTGTGTGTACACACATGTGCCAGTGTGTGCGGGTAGGTGTATGG

AAGCATGTGTGCCTGTGTGTGTGGGTGTGTG---------- Intron 2 ----------GGTGGGGTCCCAATGCCACCTGGTGACTTGGAGCCTTGGG

AGGGGTAATGGTACAGTCACTACTCATTCTAGTTCAGTGCTCTGGGACTCAGCAGGGGTGGGTGAGGGTGCAGTGTCTCACCTCCATCCTCCTCACCCAG

                                                              Exon 3
GCTCTGACATCTCATGCCTGGGCATCTTCCCCTTTAACTGTAACCCACACTGATTGGCCCTCTCTCTCTTCCCTTTCACAGAAACAGTTGTGCTCTTTCGAG
                                                              K Q L C S F E
Bgl II   EcoRI   95
ATCTACGAAGTTCCCTGGGAGGACAGAATGTCCCTGGTGAATTCCAGGTGTCAAGAAGCCTAGGGGTCTGTGCCAGGCCAGTCACACCGACCACCACCCA
 I Y E V P W E D R M S L V N S R C Q E A *
                                                     121
CTCCCACCCCCTGTAGTGCTCCCACCCCTGGACTGGTGGCCCCCACCCTGCGGGAGGCCTCCCCATGTGCCTGTGCCAAGACACAGACAGAGAAGGCTGC

AGGAGTCCTTTGTTGCTCAGCAGGGCGCTCTGCCCTCCCTCCTTCCTTCTTGCTTCTAATAGACCTGGTACACACACCCCCACCTCCTGCAATTAAACAG

TAGCATCGCC

Fig. 1

In this communication, we analyze the clones, CST4 and CST5, and assign the cystatin S gene to the CST4 locus and a cystatin pseudogene elucidated in the CST5 clone to the CSTP2 locus. In addition, we describe a homology relationship among kininogens, cystatins, Bowman-Birk type inhibitors and ribonucleases.

MATERIALS AND METHODS

The clones, CST4 and CST5, were previously isolated from a bacteriophage Charon 35 library containing HindIII digests of human genomic DNA(8-10). The cloned DNAs were digested with HindIII, and the excised fragments were subcloned into the pUC 118 plasmid vector. Plasmid DNA was purified from selected clones by the alkaline lysis method. Exonuclease III(Promega Biotec.) was used to gene-rate a set of overlapping deleted fragments from each subclone. The nucleotide sequences were determined by the method of Sanger(12) using $[^{35}S-\alpha]dATP(1,000-1,500$ Ci/mmol)(Dupont), the 17-mers universal and reverse primers (Toyobo) and modified T7 DNA polymerase(U.S. Biochemical Corp.).

Homology levels between every pair of aligned gene sequences were evaluated by $P_{nuc}(m,n)$, which denotes probability by chance for m-base matches in an n-base alignment, as described before(13). Gaps were ignored for calculation.

RESULTS AND DISCUSSION

In a series of our previous study on the cystatin gene family, we have demon-strated the isolation of seven clones(CST1,CST2,CST2B,CST3,CST4,CSTP1 and CST5) from a human genomic library and characterized four of them (CST1,CST2,CST3 and CSTP1)(8-11). To clarify the proteins encoded by all the member genes and determine the corresponding loci, we further analyzed gene sequences in the clones, CST4 and CST5. The restriction maps and exon-intron organization of the genes contained in the two clones were previously reported(10).

We first characterized the CST4 clone. The nucleotide sequence is shown in Fig. 1 together with the deduced amino acid sequence. Three exons and two

Fig. 1. Nucleotide sequence of the CST4 gene. Splicing sites are indicated by downward arrowheads. Possible CAT and ATA boxes, the Kozak initiation consensus (ACCATGG) and the poly(A) addition signal(AATTAAA) are underlined. The deduced amino acid sequence is indicated under the nucleotide sequence. Numbering of the amino acid sequence is based on the published sequence of cystatin S(3,14). Asterisk denotes a termination codon.

introns were assigned by comparison to the amino acid sequence of cystatins reported previously(3-5,14). The DNA sequences of two RNA splicing donor and acceptor sites are all in agreement with the consensus sequences described by Mount(15). The sequence of three exons indicates that this clone carries the gene coding for the precursor form of cystatin S consisting of 141 amino acids. The first 20 amino acids, rich in hydrophobic residues, encoded by the open reading frame,is considered to be a secretory signal sequence, since the Ala-X-Ala, here Ala-Leu-Ala, is the most frequent sequence preceding the signal peptidase cleavage site(16). The mature form(121 amino acids) thus excised is identical in size to the published sequence of cystatin S(3,14). The Kozak initiation consensus (ACCATGG) abuts the ATG initiation codon as well as other human cystatin genes(8,9,17,18). A possible ATA-box sequence(ATAAA), which is common to many eukaryotic promoters, is present 96 base pairs(bp) upstream to the ATG codon. A putative CAT-box sequence(CAT) is found 34 bp upstream from the ATA-box. About 230 bp downstream to the ATG termination codon, there is the heptanucleotide (AATTAAA) common to the S-type cystatin genes(8), a variant of the polyadenylation signal(AATAAA). The 5'-flanking region from the CAT-box, is remarkable for its high content of purine (80 % A + G). The CST4 gene does not have any typical features of a pseudogene. Therefore, the third S-type cystatin genes is now to be determined, in addition to the cystatin SN gene(CST1) and the cystatin SA gene(CST2).

Subsequently, we sequenced three regions in the CST5 clone that hybridized to the three DNA probes(the exon 1, exon 2 and exon 3 probes from the CST1 gene) (8-10). Three exons and two introns were assigned by homology. We describe below that the gene in the CST5 clone is a cystatin pseudogene, which we urge to call "CSTP2" according to the nomenclature proposed by us(8).

The first exon in the CSTP2 gene is 85% identical to that of CST4 gene. Two frame shift deletions were found in the exon 1(data not shown). A possible CAT-box sequence (CAT) and a putative ATA-box sequence were found in the 5'-flanking region. The second exon of CSTP2, located approximately 1800 bp downstream from exon 1, shares 73% sequence identity with the second exon of CST4. A premature termination codon (TAA) occurs in this exon. The third exon of CSTP2, located approximately 1500 bp downstream from the second exon, shows 86% sequence identity with the third exon of CST4. A mutation occurs at the acceptor splicing site of the third exon(a mutation from consensus AG to GG). Taking these observations into consideration, it can be concluded that CSTP2 is a cystatin pseudogene, and this can be assigned to the sixth cystatin locus. Several structural features of the CSTP2 are given in Table 1.

Table 1. Summary of structures of seven members from the human cystatin gene family

Locus	Gene Product	5'-Flanking Region	Sequence of Donor Site	Sequence of Acceptor Site	3'-Flanking Region
CST1	Cystatin SN (121 Residues)	CAT-box(CAT) ATA-box(ATAAA)	Exon 1-GTAGGTGCTCCCTCC Exon 2-GTACGTTCCTGATGC	GTTTTCTCCTGTGTGCAG-Exon 2 CTCTCTTCCCTTCACAG-Exon 3	Poly(A)-addition Signal (AATTAAA)
CST2	Cystatin SA (121 Residues)	CAT-box(CAT) ATA-box(ATAAA)	Exon 1-GTGGGTGCTGCCTCC Exon 2-GTACGTTCCTGATGT	GTTTTCTCATGTGTTGCAG-Exon 2 CTCTCTTCCCTTCACAG-Exon 3	Poly(A)-addition Signal (AATTAAA)
CST3	Cystatin C (120 Residues)	GC-box(GGGCGG) ATA-box(ATAAA)	Exon 1-GTGCGTGCCGCCCCC Exon 2-GTATGTGCCTTATAT	GCTCTTTCACATGTGTAG-Exon 2 CTCTGTTTCCTTTCACAG-Exon 3	Poly(A)-addition Signal (AATAAA)
CST4	Cystatin S (121 Residues)	CAT-box(CAT) ATA-box(ATAAA)	Exon 1-GTGGGTGCTGCCTCC Exon 2-GTACGTTCCTGATGC	GTTTTCTCCTGTGTGCAG-Exon 2 CTCTCTTCCCTTCACAG-Exon 3	Poly(A)-addition Signal (AATTAAA)
(CST4)	Cystatin D (Not isolated)	GC-box(GGGCGG) ATA-box(ATAAA)	Exon 1-GTGCGTGCTACCACC Exon 2-GTATGTGCCTGATGT	GCTCTTCCACGCGTGTAG-Exon 2 ATCTCTTTCTTTTCACAG-Exon 3	Poly(A)-addition Signal (AATTAAA)
CSTP1	Pseudogene	CAT-box(CAT)	Exon 1-GTGGGTGATGCCACC Exon 2-GTATGTGACTGATGT	GCTCTTTCGTGCTTGTAG-Exon 2 CTCTCTTTCCTTTCACAG-Exon 3	Poly(A)-addition Signal (AATTAAA)
CSTP2 (CST5)	Pseudogene	CAT-box(CAT) ATA-box(ATAAA)	Exon 1-GTGGGTGCTGCCACC Exon 2-GTGTGTGCATGATGT	GCTCTTTCACGTGAGTAG-Exon 2 CTCTCTTTCCTTTCACGG-Exon 3	N.D.

Notes:The nucleotide sequence sources are as follows;The CST1,CST2 and CSTP1 genes(ref.8),The CST3 gene(refs.9,17, 18),The cystatin D gene(ref.19),The CST4 gene for cystatin S(ref.10 and present study),The CSTP2 gene(present study). The consensus sequences(GT and AG) at the splicing donor and acceptor sites are shadowed. N.D.= not determined.

Recently Freije and co-workers have cloned a human gene and assigned three exons to its gene(19) by comparison of DNA sequence identity with cystatin genes hitherto sequenced. Since the deduced amino acid sequence from this gene is 51 - 55 % identical to human cystatins of family II, a name "cystatin D" was introduced tentatively for the gene product. In addition, it is reported that the cystatin D mRNA was expressed only in human parotid gland with high level, although the corresponding protein has not been elucidated yet. The cystatin D gene is considered to fill up the seventh locus of the cystatin gene family. The cystatin D gene was assigned to the CST4 locus by chance, however, we assigned the cystatin S gene to the CST4 locus(ref.10 and this study). The subject on the gene assignment to this locus will be discussed elsewhere. Table 1 compares several features of the cystatin D gene with those of other six members from the cystatin gene family identified by us.

Cystatin genes are composed of three exons encoding 76 or 81(exon 1),38(exon 2), and 27(exon 3) amino acids(8-11). The 5'-nine exons of kininogen genes are known to have evolved by triplication of an ancestral three-exon DNA segment closely homologous to the cystatin genes(3,11). We have reported that cystatins and kininogens are evolutionary related to Bowman-Birk type serine proteinase inhibitors(10).

On the other hand, it is known that E. coli ribonuclease (RNase) P is composed of M1 RNA(a ribozyme) and a protein encoded by rnpA gene(20). Recent observation of the sequence homology between rnpA gene and M1 RNA strongly suggests that the rnpA protein is a candidate for a member of most primitive proteins in early life(21).

The DNA sequences encoding these proteinase inhibitors were further compared with the E. coli rnpA and rnh genes (22), the latter coding for RNase H. The resulting alignment is shown in Fig. 2. In the CST4(cystatin S gene), the exon

Fig. 2. Alignment of cystatin-related proteinase inhibitor genes with ribo-nuclease genes. Nucleotide and deduced amino acid sequences are aligned. Lower case letters indicate intron and 3'-untranslated sequences. "< " and " >" show exon-intron boundaries. ## denotes continuity of sequence. Base matches to CST4-exon 2 region are underlined. Other base matches are indicated in the figure. CST4, human cystatin S gene; cyst.D, human cystatin D gene(19); C-II, soybean inhibitor C-II; TI-II, tomato leaf inhibitor II; rnh, RNase H gene(21); rnpA, gene for the protein moiety of RNase P(20). Note:See references cited in ref.(10) for other sequence sources.

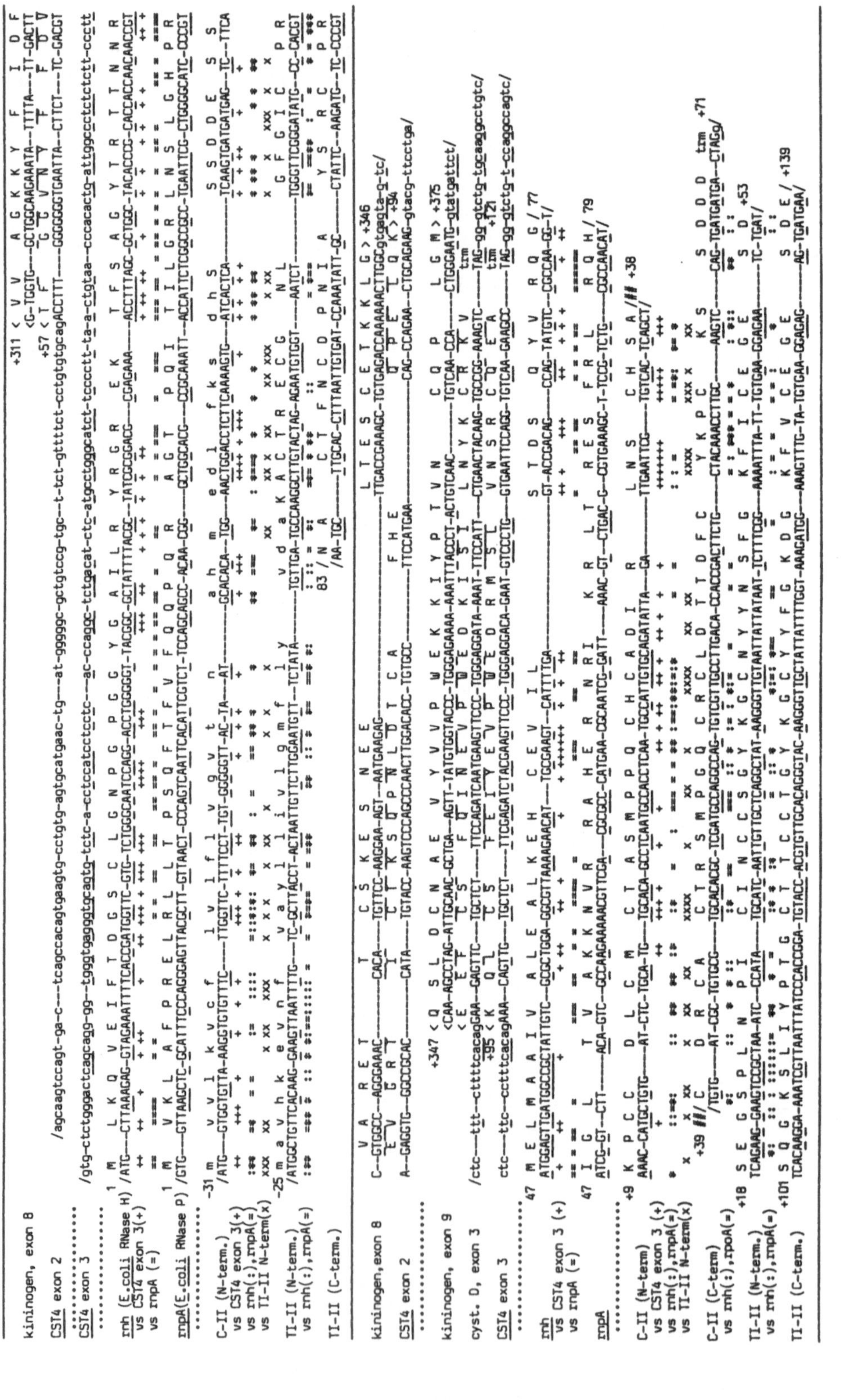

kininogen, exon 8

CST4 exon 2

CST4 exon 3

rrn (E.coli RNase H)
vs CST4 exon 3(+)
vs rrnpA (=)

rrnpA(E.coli RNase P)

C-II (N-term.)
vs CST4 exon 3(+)
vs rrnh(±),rrnpA(=)
vs TI-II N-term(x)

TI-II (N-term.)
vs rrnh(±),rrnpA(=)

TI-II (C-term.)

kininogen, exon 8

CST4 exon 2

kininogen, exon 9

cyst. D, exon 3

CST4 exon 3

rrn
vs CST4 exon 3 (+)
vs rrnpA

rrnpA

C-II (N-term.)
vs CST4 exon 3 (+)
vs rrnh(±),rrnpA(+)
vs TI-II N-term(x)

C-II (C-term.)
vs rrnh(±),rpoA(=)

TI-II (N-term.)
vs rrnh(±),rrnpA(=)

TI-II (C-term.)

Fig. 2

2 regions (including its 5'- and 3'-flanks) showed an evident homology [48.3% base match, $P_{nuc}(97,201) = 1.0 \times 10^{-13}$] to the CST4-exon 3 and its flanks. The C-II(a Bowman-Birk type inhibitor from soybean) gene segment encoding its amino (N-) terminal region (amino acids from -31 to +38) is weakly homologous to the CST4-exon 3 and its flanks giving a 42.8% base match [$P_{nuc}(80,187) = 0.84 \times 10^{-7}$]. On the other hand, an rnh gene segment encoding the N-terminal 77 amino acids of RNase H is not only markedly homologous to the rnpA gene[50.7%, $P_{nuc}(105,207) = 0.18 \times 10^{-14}$], but also to the CST4-exon 2 and its 5'-flank [49.5%, $P_{nuc}(91,184) = 0.84 \times 10^{-12}$], and to the CST4-exon 3 and its 5'-flank [45.0%, $P_{nuc}(91,202) = 0.49 \times 10^{-9}$]. These results and the alignment in Fig. 2 permit us to conclude that the second and third exons(including their flanks) of the cystatin genes and of three cystatin gene-like domains in the kininogen genes have evolved from a very ancient gene encoding a primitive RNase-like protein. Further details will be published elsewhere.

ACKNOWLEDGMENTS

This study was supported in part by a Grant-in-Aid for Scientific Research(C) (No.2670842 to ES), a Grant-in-Aid for Scientific Research(C) (No. 04671140 to ES and SI) and a Grant-in-Aid for Scientific Research on Priority Areas (No.319 to KO) from the Ministry of Education, Science and Culture of Japan.

REFERENCES

1. Barrett AJ, Fritz H, Grubb A, Isemura S, Järvinen M, Katunuma N, Machleidt W, Müller-Esterl W, Sasaki M, Turk V. Nomenclature and classification of the proteins homologous with the cysteine proteinase inhibitor chicken cystatin. Biochem J 1986; 236:213.
2. Müller-Esterl W, Iwanaga S, Nakanishi S. Kininogens revisited. Trend Biochem Sci 1986; 11:336-339.
3. Isemura S, Saitoh E, Sanada K. Isolation and amino acid sequence of SAP-1, an acidic protein of human whole saliva, and sequence homology with γ-trace. J Biochem 1984; 96:489-498.
4. Isemura S, Saitoh E, Sanada K. Characterization of a new cysteine proteinase inhibitor of human saliva, cystatin SN, which is immunologically related to cystatin S. FEBS Lett 1986; 198:145-149.
5. Isemura S, Saitoh,E, Sanada K. Characterization and amino acid sequence of a new acidic cysteine proteinase inhibitor (cystatin SA) structurally closely related to cystatin S, from human whole saliva. J Biochem 1987; 102:693-704.
6. Isemura S, Saitoh E, Sanada K, Isemura M, Ito S. Cystatin S and the related cysteine proteinase inhibitors in human saliva.In:Cysteine Proteinases and their Inhibitors. Turk V, editor. Berlin and New York: Walter de Gruyter & Co,1986:497-505.

7. Grubb A, Löfberg H. Human γ-trace, a basic microprotein: Amino acid se-
    quence and presence in the adenohypophysis. Proc Natl Acad Sci USA 1982;
    79:3024-3027.
8. Saitoh E, Kim H-S, Smithies O, Maeda N. Human cysteine proteinase inhibi-
    tors: Nucleotide sequence analysis of three members of the cystatin gene
    family. Gene 1987;61:329-338.
9. Saitoh E, Sabatini LM, Eddy RL, Shows TB, Azen AE, Isemura S, Sanada K.
    The human cystatin C gene(CST3) is a member of the cystatin gene family on
    chromosome 20. Biochem Biophys Res Commun 1989;162:1324-1331.
10. Saitoh E, Isemura S, Sanada K, Ohnishi K. The human cystatin gene family:
    Cloning of three members and evolutionary relationship between cystatins
    and Bowman-Birk type proteinase inhibitors. Biomed Biochim Acta 1991; 50:
    599-605.
11. Saitoh E, Isemura S, Sanada K, Kim H-S, Maeda N, Smithies O. Cystatin
    superfamily: Evidence that family II cystatin genes are evolutionarily
    related to family III cystatin genes. Biol Chem Hoppe-Seyler 1988; 369
    Suppl:191-197.
12. Sanger F, Nicklen S, Coulson AR. DNA sequencing with chain terminating
    inhibitors. Proc Natl Acad Sci USA 1977;74:5463-5467.
13. Ohnishi K. Domain structures and molecular evolution of class I and class
    II major histocompatibility gene complex(HMC) products deduced from amino
    acid and nucleotide sequence homologies.Origins Life 1984;14:707-715.
14. Isemura S, Saitoh E, Sanada K, Minakata K. Identification of full-sized
    forms of salivary (S-type) cystatins (cystatin SN, cystatin SA, cystatin S
    and two phosphorylated forms of cystatin S) in human whole saliva and de-
    termination of phosphorylation sites of cystatin S. J Biochem 1991;110:
    648-654.
15. Mount S. A catalogue of splice junction sequence. Nucl Acids Res 1982; 10:
    459-472.
16. Perlman D, Halvorson HO. A putative signal peptidase recognition site and
    sequence in eukaryotic and prokaryotic signal peptides. J Mol Biol 1983;
    167:391-409.
17. Levy E, Lópetz-Otín C, Ghiso J, Geltner D, Frangione B.Stroke in Icelandic
    patients with hereditary amyloid angiopathy is related to a mutation in
    the cystatin C gene, an inhibitor of cysteine proteinases. J Exp Med 1989;
    169:1771-1778.
18. Abrahamson M, Olafsson I, Palsdottir A, Ulvsbäck M, Lundwall Å, Jensson O,
    Grubb A. Structure and expression of the human cystatin C gene. Biochem J
    1990;268:287-294.
19. Freije JP, Abrahamson M, Olafsson I, Velasco G, Grubb A, Lópetz-Otín C.
    Structure and expression of the gene encoding cystatin D, a novel Human
    cysteine proteinase inhibitor. J Biol Chem 1991; 266: 20538-20543.
20. Hansen FG, Hansen EB, Atlung T. Physical mapping and nucleotide sequence
    of the rnpA gene that encodes the protein component of ribonuclease P in
    E. coli. Gene 1985;38: 85-93.
21. Ohnishi K. Possible evolutionary origin of primitive protein encoding
    mRNAs as avirusoid-like ribo-organism. Nucl Acids Res Symp Ser 1990; 22:
    39-40.
22. Kanaya S, Crouch RJ. DNA sequence of the gene coding for Escherichia coli
    ribonuclease H. J Biol Chem 1983; 258:1276-1281.

Kininases and Kininase Inhibitors

THE ANGIOTENSIN I-CONVERTING ENZYME (KININASE II) : MOLECULAR AND REGULATORY ASPECTS

E. Jaspard, O. Costerousse, L. Wei, P. Corvol and F. Alhenc-Gelas

INSERM U367 and U36, Paris, FRANCE

The angiotensin I-converting enzyme or kininase II (dipeptidyl peptidase A, EC 3.4.15.1, ACE) is an important enzyme in vascular tone and blood pressure regulation, that may have also other function related to the processing of peptides in the central nervous system and in adsorptive epithelium. The two best known substrates of ACE are angiotensin I and bradykinin. (1-3) Angiotensin I is converted into the vasopressor and aldosterone stimulating peptide angiotensin II by removal of the carboxyterminal dipeptide. Angiotensin II is not further cleaved by ACE. Because of these specificities and of the wide distribution of ACE in the circulation, both as an ectoenzyme on the surface on the endothelial cells and as a soluble enzyme in plasma, ACE is responsible for most if not all of angiotensin II formation in the circulation. The best substrate known so far for ACE, i.e. the substrate with the most favorable kinetic parameters, is bradykinin (BK). ACE cleaves sequencially two carboxyterminal dipeptides from bradykinin and analogues, suppressing the biological effects of this peptide. There are increasing evidences to suggest that kinin can be involved in the control of vascular tone and blood flow in certain circulations, for exemple the renal circulation, and that ACE may also regulates vascular tone through bradykinin metabolism. Furthermore ACE cleaves at least in vitro substance P and has a peculiar specificity here, as it cleaves a protected carboxyterminal dipeptide or a tripeptide. ACE is indeed able to act, depending on the substrate, either as an ectopeptidase or as an endopeptidase cleaving protected dipeptides or tripeptides on the carboxyterminal side (substance P) or even the aminoterminal side of the peptide, such as in the luteinizing hormone releasing hormone. The concept that ACE was somehow a borderline enzyme between endo and exopeptidases resulted from these observations and suggested that it may be an interesting enzyme to study and compare to other peptidases for understanding the evolution of this class of enzymes. (3) Moreover ACE is a target for the inhibition of the renin angiotensin system in hypertension and cardiac insufficiency. (4) It was of interest to try to precise the molecular mechanism of action of the therapeutically active ACE inhibitors which have been designed largely on the basis of a theoretical model of the active site and proved to be very effective, even if they appear to be perhaps incomplete blockers of the formation of angiotensin II in vivo (5) . Finally the regulation of ACE expression in tissues remained largely unknown specially in humans and was of interest to consider with regard to cardiovascular regulation and susceptibility to hypertension.

Recently the primary structure of ACE has been disclosed by protein sequencing and cDNA cloning and these experiments followed by expression of recombinant enzyme and site-directed mutagenesis, allowed to discover that ACE was composed of two homologous domains, each possessing a functionnal active site. These active sites are certainly highly homologous in their structure, but display differences in substrate specificity and sensitivity to regulatory factors, that suggest structural and functionnal differences between them, currently being investigated.

Concerning the regulation of ACE expression, an other unexpected and potentially important result has been obtained : The observation has been made that the large interindividual variability in ACE levels in man was for a part genetically determined, and this observation has been subsequently linked to a polymorphism of the gene coding for ACE.

Structure and processing of ACE

The primary structure of ACE was revealed by protein sequencing of human kidney ACE followed by cDNA cloning in endothelial cells libraries (6). The sequence of the mouse enzyme has been also determined and found to display a high overall homology with human ACE (7). ACE is encoded by a 4.3 Kb mRNA species in human endothelial cells and in other somatic tissues. The coding sequences comprises 1306 residues including a signal peptide of 29 amino-acids. ACE is mostly a membrane bound enzyme and has been identified as an ectoenzyme of the vascular endothelial cells or the absorptive epithelial cells of the intestinal or renal brush borders. Protein sequencing of the mature kidney enzyme has indicated that the signal peptide was cleaved off during the processing, and therefore the enzyme could not remain anchored to the membrane by this peptide. However there was in the sequence another hydrophobic sequence located 47 amino-acids upstream the carboxyterminal extremity and constituted by a segment of 17 amino-acids highly hydrophobic and having the characteristics of a transmembrane domain (6). Anchorage through a C terminal transmembrane domain was also consistent with previous solubilization experiments (8). However to establish definitively the anchorage mechanism of ACE, recombinant enzyme has been expressed in CHO cells. A mutant where the first amino-acid of the putative transmembrane domain was replaced by a codon, and therefore lacking these putative transmembrane domain and intracellular region, was also expressed (9). The wild type recombinant ACE was expressed mostly as a membrane bound ectoenzyme. Experiments with an antibody directed against a synthetic peptide corresponding to the last 20 amino-acids of the endothelial ACE sequence (i.e. to the putative intracellular domain) and recognizing the ACE molecule showed that ACE was indeed orientated in a C in, N out direction. By contrast the mutant lacking the C-terminal part was not incorporated into the membrane but secreted into the culture medium. (9) These experiments also allowed to understand the mechanism of ACE secretion by the cell. Indeed, beside the membrane bound form of ACE there is also a soluble form circulating in plasma and present in several other body fluids (3,10). The plasma enzyme is believed to originate from endothelial cells .

Purification of plasma ACE and experiments with the anti C-terminal sequence antibody allowed to establish that the plasma enzyme was truncated in the carboxyterminal region (9). This result excluded the possibility that the plasma ACE was simply produced by leakage of the ectoenzyme. The other possibilities for ACE secretion included translation of the soluble form from a different mRNA that did not encode for the transmembrane domain, but a single mRNA was detected in human tissues. (6) The soluble form also could have been produced by a post-translationnal cleavage of the membrane anchor. Experiments in CHO cells allowed to establish that this last mechanism was most likely the mechanism involved in ACE secretion. Indeed the cells transfected with the wild type recombinant enzyme were able not only to express ACE as an ectoenzyme but also to secrete it in the culture medium. The secreted form did not react with the anticarboxyterminal antibody. These results indicated that in CHO cells and presumably in endothelial cells as well the soluble form is produced by a post-translational proteolytic cleavage of the carboxyterminal region of the membrane bound form. (9) It is not known at the present time where the cleavage site is located and whether the cleavage takes place intracellularly or on the membrane. However the enzyme cleaving ACE is certainly a cellular enzyme rather than a circulating enzyme as ACE secretion was observed in serum free medium. Similar findings have been obtained by transfection of the human testicular ACE CDNA. (11) The putative ACE processing enzyme may be interesting to characterize further because many other ectoproteins are similarly anchored near their carboxyterminal extremity, and several of them have a soluble counterpart that may be generated by a proteolytic cleavage. Alteration in this mechanism may occur in disease and has been proposed has a possible mechanism for deposit of the amyloïd precursor protein in Alzeihmer's disease.

Demonstration of the presence of two active sites. Is ACE a bifunctional enzyme ?

An unexpected observation made after the cloning was that the ACE molecule probably resulted from an ancestral gene duplication and was organized in two large homologous domains, surrounded by short non homologous regions (6,7). These latter included the signal peptide and the carboxyterminal anchor and intracellular domain. Each of these two homologous domains comprised short sequences homologous to the zinc binding sequences of other metallopeptidases (thermolysine, endopeptidase 24-11, collagenase), and therefore beared a putative active site. It was not possible to predict by sequence analysis wether only one or both of these putative active sites was functionnal. However all the previous experiments suggested that only one of these sites was functionnal. For exemple a single zinc atom was found to be bound to the ACE molecule. Moreover several studies using competitive ACE inhibitors were in favor of a single high affinity binding site on ACE (12-14). Finally it was known that a peculiar form of ACE was expressed in the testis, equally active toward angiotensin I but translated as a shorter molecular species of 80 Kd instead of 140 Kd in somatic tissues (15). The testicular enzyme was indeed encoded by a shorter mRNA, transcribed from the same gene as the somatic enzyme, but having a size of 3 Kb instead of of 4.3 Kd in endothelial cells (6). When the cDNA for the testicular enzyme was cloned and sequenced it was observed that it corresponded to the 3' part of the endothelial transcript and encoded only for the second domain (i.e. the domain located in the carboxyterminal half of the molecule) followed by the transmembrane and intracellular regions and preceeded by a short testicular specific region of 65 aminoacids, rich in serine and threonine and probably glycosylated (16-18).

These results suggested that the testicular transcript corresponded to the ancestral form of the gene. (16) They also suggested that the endothelial and the testicular forms of ACE mRNA were from different transcription initiation sites under the influence of different promoters. (16). This was later established after analysis and sequencing of the ACE gene and of its promoters (19-21). As the structure of testicular ACE corresponded only to the second of the two homologous domains of endothelial ACE this domain at least, beared a functionnal active site. All these data taken together suggested that the aminoterminal domain perhaps did not contain a functionnal active site despite its homology to the carboxyterminal domain. However this turned out to be untrue and ACE is indeed a two active sites enzyme. The expression of ACE mutants either truncated, or mutated on putative zinc binding or catalytic residues of each of the two putative active sites allowed indeed to establish that both domains were in fact enzymatically active (22).

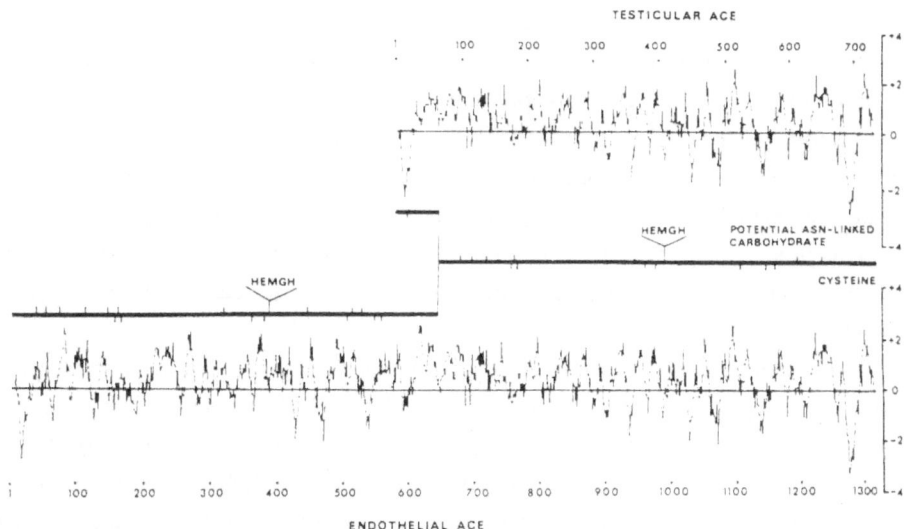

Fig.1. Schematic representation of testicular and endothelial ACE. (Middle) Diagram showing cysteine positions, potential asparagine-linked glycosylation sites, and positions of putative residues of active site of the two enzymes (HEMGH). Beyond the point of divergence, the testicular enzyme is shown on the upper line and the endothelial enzyme on the lower line. (Top, bottom) Hydropathy plots of the predicted testicular (top) and endothelial [5] (bottom) amino acid sequences by the method of kyte and Doolittle with a window size of 10 residues [18]. Negative values indicate increasing hydrophobicity. Amino acid numbering presented above and below the hydropathy plots. Reproduced from reference 16.

The two active sites of endothelial ACE (called here the N and C active sites) hydrolyze angiotensin I and bradykinin and seem to function independantly and additively. However they display differences in catalytic parameters and chloride activation profile (chloride is a known activator of ACE) that suggest physiologically relevant structural differences between them. For exemple, as expected, the carboxyterminal domain hydrolyzes well Hip-His-Leu and angiotensin I and has a chloride activation profile that it is similar to that described for the testicular or endothelial ACE. However the aminoterminal domain hydrolyzes ten times less (Kcat/Km) Hip-His-Leu at 300 mM Nacl. Both domains convert angiotensin I with kinetic parameters in the same order of magnitude but the N domain appears less chloride dependent. Finally the two domain display differences in sensitivity to competitive ACE inhibitors (22).

Reappraisal of the zinc content and inhibitor stocheiometry of ACE allowed to confirm these observations by showing that in fact there was two zinc atoms bound per molecule of ACE and (23) two high affinities inhibitor binding sites, although, like for susbstrates , they display chloride related differences in sensitivity to these inhibitors (22,23). Previous results for zinc and inhibitors were probably explained by difficulties in assessing the correct molecular weight of ACE prior to the knowledge of the sequence and by the poor stability of the enzyme in some experimental conditions. In summary it is now established that ACE possesses in fact two active sites, highly homologous in their structure, but not completely identical (22).

The question then arises of wether ACE is a bifunctionnal enzyme. These enzymes usually have two actives sites also resulting form an ancestral gene duplication but these active sites display less structural homology and a clear difference in substrate specificity. Several arguments suggest that the N active site of ACE may hydrolyse different substrates than the carboxyterminal active site, although a specific substrate has not yet been identified. These arguments are the differences in catalytic parameters for at least one substrate (Hip-His-Leu) and the different chloride and inhibitors sensitivity profiles. Preliminary results indicate that both active sites are able to make the endoproteolytic cleavage of substance P, although there may be differences in the cleavage of another in vitro ACE substrate LHRH, that undergo a peculiar aminoterminal endoproteolytic cleavage. (24) A recent report suggests that the endothelial but not the testicular enzyme is able to perform this cleavage and therefore that the N active site may be specifically involved in this reaction (23). Concerning bradykinin preliminary results indicate that both active site hydrolyse well bradykinin and BK is also the substrate possessing the best kinetic parameters for each active site (25). Like there are two angiotensin I-converting enzymes in the angiotensin I-converting enzyme molecule, there seems to be two kininase II as well... Further studies are in progress to characterize the substrate specificity of each active site, and to try to find out what can be the specific function of the aminoterminal domain of ACE. One can only speculate at the present time that this domain might play a specific and important function because it appeared more recently and was conserved during evolution.

Genetic determinism of angiotensin I converting enzyme levels in man

As mentionned earlier a soluble form of ACE circulates in plasma at the relatively high concentration of 10^{-9} M, although the plasma enzyme is probably physiologically less important for blood pressure regulation than the membrane bound endothelial enzyme. (3,10)

However ACE levels are monitored in certain diseases, such as adult respiratory distress syndrome, were they are decreased as a results of pulmonary circulation damage, or in granulomatous diseases such as sarcoidosis were activated macrophages secrete large amount of the enzyme. ACE levels are also increased in diabetes and may be linked to vascular complications. The interindividual variability of plasma ACE levels in healtly subjects is very large as those levels can range from 1 to 6. However when measured repeteadly in a given subject plasma ACE levels remain remarkably constant (10,26). No association with candidate hormonal on environmental parameters was found to explain this variability. We performed a study of plasma ACE levels in nuclear families to test the hypothesis that this interindividual variability was geneticaly determined. Indeed intra familial correlations between geneticaly related members were found and the genetic analysis suggested that a major gene affected the phenotype and was responsible for a significant part of the interindividual variability in plasma ACE levels. (27) This was later confirmed and extendent after the cloning of ACE cDNA where an insertion/deletion polymorphism, located is an intron of the ACE gene, was discovered and when it was recognized that this polyphormism was associated with differences in the concentration of ACE in plasma (28). Subjects homozygotes for the insertion have lower levels that those homozygote for the deletion, heterozygotes having intermediate levels.

There are several possible developments to these observations. First it is necessary to precise the mechanism linking the insertion-deletion polymorphism to the synthesis of ACE. Most likely the genetic control is excerted at the transcriptional level but its exact mechanism remain to determine. Preliminary results indicate that ACE is expressed in circulating mononuclear cells, mainly lymphocytes and that the genetic polymorphism of ACE is linked also to differences in the level of membrane bound ACE in these cells (29). These results also suggest that in the many cell type where ACE is expressed the level of the enzyme is genetically determined. Then the physiological consequences, if any, of these observations for peptide metabolism and blood pressure regulation have to be investigated. There are evidences to suggest that ACE is a rate limiting step in angiotensin II formation, for exemple in the kidney (30,31), and differences in the level ACE expression may be physiologicaly relevant. Finally it is now possible to define more appropriate reference intervals for normal values by establishing these normal values per genotype. This will allow to compare putative pathological values to more appropriate reference intervals and presumably to increase the specificity and the sensitivity of plasma ACE measurements in disease.

REFERENCES

1. Skeggs LTD Jr., Kahn JR, Shumway NP. The preparation and function of the hypertensive-converting enzyme. J Exp Med 1956 ; 103 : 295-299.

2. Erdös EG, Yang HYT. An enzyme in microsomal fraction of the kidney that inactivates bradykinin. Life Sci 1967 ; 6 : 569-574.

3. Erdös EG . Angiotensin I converting enzyme and the changes in our concept through the years Lewis K. Dahl Memorial Lecture. Hypertension.1990 ; 16 : 363-370.

4. Cushman DW, Ondetti MA. Inhibitors of angiotensin-converting enzyme. Prog Med Chem 1980 ; 17 : 42-104.

5. Juillerat L, Nussberger J, Menard J, Moeser V, Christen Y, Waeber B, Graf P and Brunner H.R. Determinants of angiotensin II generation during converting enzyme inhibition. Hypertension 1990 ; 16 : 564-572.

6. Soubrier F, Alhenc-Gelas F, Hubert C , Allegrini J, John M, Treager J, Corvol P. Two putative active centers in human angiotensin I-converting enzyme revealed by molecular cloning. Proc Natl Acad Sci USA. 1988 ; 85 : 9360-90.

7. Bernstein KE, Martin BM, Edwards AS, Bernstein EA. Mouse angiotensin-converting enzyme is a protein composed of two homologous domains. J Biol Chem 1989 ; 264 : 11945-11951.

8. Hooper NM, Ken J, Pappin DJ, Turner AJ. Pig kidney angiotensin-converting enzyme : purification and characterization of amphipatic and hydrophilic forms of the enzyme establishes C-terminal anchorage to the plasma membrane. Biochem J 1987 ; 247 : 85-93.

9. Wei L, Alhenc-Gelas F, Soubrier F, Michaud A, Corvol P, Clauser E. Expression and characterization of recombinant human angiotensin I-converting enzyme. J Biol Chem 1991 ; 266 : 5540-5546.

10. Alhenc-Gelas F, Weare JA, Johnson RL, Erdös EG. Measurement of human converting enzyme level by direct radioimmunoassay. J Lab Med 1983 ; 101 : 83-96.

11. Ehlers W, Chen YNP, Riordan JF. Spontaneous solubilization of membrane-bound human testis angiotensin-converting enzyme expressed in chinese hamster ovary cells. Proc Natl Acad Sci 1991, 88 : 1009-1013.

12. Strittmatter SM, Snyder SH, Characterization of angiotensin converting enzyme by (3H) captopril binding. Mol Pharmacol 1986 ; 29 : 142-8.

13. Bull HG, Thornberry NA, Cordes MHJ, Patchett AA, Cordes EH. Inhibition of rabbit lung angiotensin-converting enzyme by N^{α} [(S)- carboxy-3 phenylpropyl] L-alanyl-L-proline and N^{α} [(S)- carboxy-3 phenylpropyl] L-Lysyl-L-proline. J Biol Chem 1985 ; 260 : 2952-2962.

14. Cumin F, Vellaud V, Corvol P, Alhenc-Gelas F. Evidence for a single active site in the human angiotensin I-converting enzyme from inhibitor binding studies with [^{3}H] RU 44 403 : Role of chloride. Biochem Biophys Res Comm 1989 ; 163 : 718-725.

15. El Dorry H, Pickett CB, Mac Gregor JS, Soffer RL. Tissue specific expression of mRNAs for dypeptidyl carboxypeptidase isoenzymes. Proc Natl Acad Sci 1982 ; 79 : 4295-4297.

16. Lattion AL, Soubrier F, Allegrini J, Hubert C, Corvol P, Alhenc-Gelas F. The testicular transcript of angiotensin I-converting enzyme encodes for the ancestral, non-duplicated form of the enzyme. FEBS Lett 1989 ; 252 : 99-104.

17. Kumar RS, Kusari J, Roy SN, Soffer RL, Sen GC. Structure of testicular angiotensin-converting enzyme. A segmental mosaic isozyme. J Biol Chem 1989 ; 264 : 16754-16578.

18. Ehlers MRW, Fox EA, Strydom DJ, Riordan JF. Molecular cloning of human testicular angiotensin-converting enzyme : the testis isozyme is identical to the C-Terminal half of endothelial angiotensin-converting enzyme. Proc Natl Acad Sci 1989 ; 86 : 7741-7745.

19. Howard TE, Shai SY, Langford KG, Martin BM, Bernstein KE. Transcription of testicular angiotensin-converting enzyme (ACE) is initiated within the 12th intron of somatic ACE gene. Mol Cell Biol 1990 ; 10 : 4294-4302.

20. Kumar RS, Tekkimkara TJ, Sen GC. The mRNAs encoding the two angiotensin-converting isozymes are transcribed from the same gene by a tissue-specific choice of alternative transcriptiion sites. J Biol Invest 1990 ; 85 : 1328-1332.

21 Hubert C, Houot AM, Corvol P, Soubrier F. Structure of the angiotensin I-converting enzyme gene. Two alternate promoters correspond to evolutionary steps of a duplicated gene.J Biol Chem 1991 ; 266 : 15377-15383.

22. Wei L, Alhenc-Gelas F, Corvol P, Clauser E. The two homologous domains of human angiotensin I-converting enzyme are both catalytically active. J Biol Chem 1991 ; 266 : 9002-9008.

23. Ehlers MRW, Riordan JF. Angiotensin-converting enzyme : Zinc-and inhibitor-binding stoichiometries of the somatic ans testis isozymes. Biochem 1991 ; 30, 7118-7126.

24. Skidgel RA, Defendini R, Erdös EG. Angiotensin I converting enzyme and its role in neuropeptide metabolism, in Turner AJ, ed. Neuropeptides and their peptidases. Chishester, England, Ellis-Horwood, 1987, pp 165-182.

25. Jaspard E, Wei L, Clauser E, Corvol P, Alhenc-Gelas F. Hydrolysis of bradykinin by angiotensin I-converting enzyme (kininase II) and mutants possessing only one functionnal active site. Abstract kinin 91, Munich 1992 p 323.

26. Alhenc-Gelas F, Richard J, Courbon D, Warnet JM, Corvol P. Distribution of plasma angiotensin I-Converting enzyme in healthy men. Relationship to environmental and hormonal parameters. J Lab Clin Mad 1191 ; 117 : 33-39.

27. Cambien F, Alhenc Gelas F, Herbeth B, André JL, Rakotovao R, Gonzalez MF, Allegrini J, Block JC. Familial resemblance of plasma angiotensin-converting enzyme level : the Nancy study. Am. J Hum Genet 1988 ; 43 : 774-80.

28. Rigat B, Hubert C, Alhenc-Gelas F, Cambien F, Corvol P, Soubrier F. An insertion/deletion polymorphism of the angiotensin I-converting enzyme gene accounting for half the variance of serum enzyme levels. J Clin Invest 1990; 86 : 1343-1346.

29. Costerousse O, Allegrini J, Lopez M, Corvol P, Alhenc-Gelas F. Expression of angiotensin I-converting enzyme (kininase II) in human mononuclear cells. Abstract kinin 91, Munich 1992 p 324.

30. Marchetti J, Roseau S, Alhenc-Gelas F. Angiotensin I converting enzyme and kinin hydrolyzing enzymes along the ravbbit nephron. Kidney Int 1987 ; 31 : 744-751.

31. Semple PF. Angiotensin I and II in renal vein blood. Kidney Int 1979 ; 15 : 276-282.

32. Alhenc-Gelas F, Soubrier F, Hubert C, Allegrini J, Lattion AL, Corvol P. The angiotensin I-converting enzyme (kininase II) : progress in molecular and genetic structure. J Cardiovasc Pharmacol 1990 ; 15, suppl 6, 525-528.

AAS 38/I
Recent Progress on Kinins
© 1992 Birkhäuser Verlag Basel

STRUCTURAL FEATURES OF TWO KININASE I-TYPE ENZYMES
REVEALED BY MOLECULAR CLONING

Randal A. Skidgel and Fulong Tan

Laboratory of Peptide Research and Departments of Pharmacology and Anesthesiology
University of Illinois College of Medicine at Chicago
835 S. Wolcott (M/C 868)
Chicago, Illinois, USA 60612

SUMMARY: Kininase I-type carboxypeptidases remove a single C-terminal Arg residue from kinins. The circulating kininase I (carboxypeptidase N) contains two types of subunits: a 50 kDa catalytic subunit and an 83kDa carrier subunit which protects the active subunit in blood. The 83 kDa subunit contains 12 leucine-rich tandem repeats, similar in sequence to other proteins with binding functions. Human carboxypeptidase M is a widely distributed "tissue kininase I" bound to plasma membranes. It has 41% sequence identity with the 50 kDa subunit of carboxypeptidase N and may regulate the activity of kinins and other peptides at the cell surface.

INTRODUCTION

In the early 60's, studies by Erdös and co-workers on bradykinin metabolism in plasma led to the discovery of kininase I (carboxypeptidase N) which inactivates bradykinin by removal of the C-terminal Arg (1). Further studies led to the discovery of another kininase (II) in plasma which was later proved to be identical with the angiotensin I converting enzyme (2,3).

Although scattered reports (2,4) indicated the possible existence of a "tissue" kininase I, it was not clear whether this activity was a different form of plasma carboxypeptidase N or pancreatic carboxypeptidase B or might represent a different enzyme. After purifying a carboxypeptidase-type kininase from human urine, which differs in structural and enzymatic characteristics from plasma carboxypeptidase N (5), we began investigations into the possible existence of a membrane bound carboxypeptidase in kidney and other tissues. We discovered a membrane-bound carboxypeptidase B-type enzyme which is present in a variety of tissues including kidney, lung, placenta and blood vessels, and in cultured endothelial cells and fibroblasts (6,7). The enzyme was purified to homogeneity from human placenta and analysis of its enzymatic and structural characteristics proved it is a unique enzyme (8). We named it carboxypeptidase "M" to denote the fact that it is membrane bound.

RESULTS AND DISCUSSION

Primary Structure of Carboxypeptidase M. In order to unequivocally prove that the membrane bound carboxypeptidase we purified is distinct from other known carboxypeptidases, the cDNA coding for the enzyme was cloned from a human placental cDNA library and sequenced (9). The cDNA codes for a mature protein of 426 amino acids (after removal of the signal peptide) whose N-terminal sequence (31 amino acids) matches that of the sequence determined for the purified protein (9). Because carboxypeptidase M is membrane bound, hydropathic analysis of the sequence was carried out in order to identify potential membrane spanning regions. Only a single candidate sequence was found at the extreme C-terminus (Fig. 1). However, the sequence is unlikely to function as a true transmembrane spanning region as it is too short (15 amino acids) to cross the

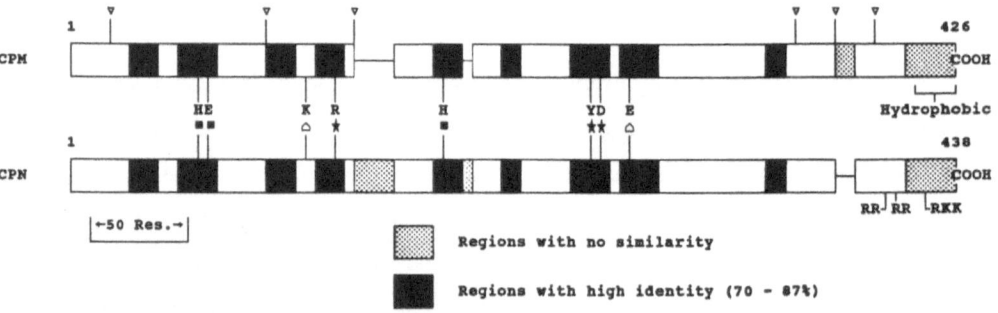

Figure 1. Schematic diagram comparing the primary structures of human carboxypeptidase M (CPM) and the 50 kDa active subunit of human carboxypeptidase N (CPN). Regions of high identity (70-87%) are denoted by solid boxes and regions with no similarity by stippled boxes. Gaps of 3 or more amino acids are indicated by a single connecting line. Potential Asn-linked glycosylation sites are marked with triangles (▽). Potential active site residues are shown in single letter amino acid code and include zinc binding residues (■), substrate binding residues (★) and amino acids involved in catalysis (△).

lipid bilayer as an α-helix and the cytoplasmic domain would consist of only a single lysine residue (9). The C-terminal hydrophobic domain is similar to those found on proteins attached to membranes via a phosphatidylinositol-glycan anchor where the C-terminus acts as a temporary anchor for the newly synthesized protein in the Golgi membrane (10). The hydrophobic region is then removed and the new C-terminal residue simultaneously attached to the ethanolamine of a preformed phosphatidylinositol-glycan anchor (10). The release of carboxypeptidase M from membrane fractions with bacterial phosphatidylinositol-specific phospholipase C and radiolabeling of the enzyme in Madin Darby canine kidney cells with [^{3}H]ethanolamine, in addition to other experiments, proved that carboxypeptidase M is indeed attached to plasma membranes by a phosphatidylinositol-glycan anchor (11,12).

The sequence of carboxypeptidase M proved that it is not identical with any other known protein. However, as expected, it does exhibit sequence similarity with other known carboxypeptidases. In the case of the bovine pancreatic carboxypeptidases A and B, the sequence identity is only 15% with human carboxypeptidase M (9), but all of the zinc binding residues and most of the amino acids involved in substrate binding and catalysis have been conserved (Fig. 1). Carboxypeptidase M has a higher degree of identity (41%) with either the active 50 kDa subunit of human carboxypeptidase N or bovine secretory granule carboxypeptidase H (9), indicating all three of these regulatory carboxypeptidases are more closely related to each other than they are to the pancreatic carboxypeptidases.

Comparison of Carboxypeptidase M with Carboxypeptidase N. There are some obvious differences between carboxypeptidases M and N; carboxypeptidase M is a single chain membrane bound enzyme whereas carboxypeptidase N is a tetrameric soluble plasma enzyme. In addition, carboxypeptidase M preferentially cleaves substrates with C-terminal Arg while carboxypeptidase N prefers C-terminal Lys (2,6,8,12). Nevertheless, there are also some similarities. For instance, both are zinc metalloenzymes which can be activated by replacing zinc with cobalt in the active site and both are inhibited by the same inhibitors (e.g., chelating agents, DL-2-mercaptomethyl-3-guanidinoethylthiopropanoic acid and guanidinoethylmercaptosuccinic acid) (2,8,13). Carboxypeptidase M and N also cleave only C-terminal basic amino acid residues and have maximal activity in the neutral pH range (2,8,13). As might be expected from similarities in their enzymatic properties, molecular cloning of the carboxypeptidase N 50 kDa subunit (14) and carboxypeptidase M (9) revealed similarities in their primary sequences.   Although the overall sequence identity is 41%, nine regions comprising 146 residues (out of 426 or 438 residues for carboxypeptidase M or N) are highly conserved with 70 - 87% sequence identity (Fig. 1).   Most of these regions contain putative active site residues (Fig. 1) as determined by comparing the sequences with those of carboxypeptidases A and B (9).   These include the zinc binding residues (His, Glu, His), substrate binding residues (Arg, Tyr, Asp) and amino acids involved in the catalytic step (Lys, Glu) (Fig. 1).   Comparison of the sequences also reveals some striking differences.   In order to align the sequences, significant gaps (of 3 or more amino acids) had to be introduced in two regions of carboxypeptidase M and one in the carboxypeptidase N 50 kDa subunit sequence (Fig. 1).   Moreover, the C-terminal 26 amino acids of each enzyme have no similarity.   As mentioned above, this region contains the C-terminal hydrophobic signal for phosphatidylinositol-glycan attachment in carboxypeptidase M whereas in carboxypeptidase N, the C-terminal 33 amino acids of the 50 kDa subunit contain four potential proteolytic cleavage sites, comprised of dibasic residues, which are not present in carboxypeptidase M (Fig. 1).   This is consistent with previous findings that the active subunit of carboxypeptidase N is very sensitive to serine proteases and can be rapidly converted to forms of slightly lower molecular weight (2,15-17).   The other major difference between the two enzymes is the presence of 6 potential glycosylation sites in carboxypeptidase M and the lack of any glycosylation sites in the active subunit of carboxypeptidase N (Fig. 1).   This confirms previous biochemical studies showing the lack of carbohydrate in the 50 kDa subunit of carboxypeptidase N (15,16) and the high carbohydrate content (23% by weight) of carboxypeptidase M (8).

Molecular Cloning of the 83 kDa Subunit of Carboxypeptidase N.   Owing to its small size, lack of carbohydrate and relative instability at 37°C (15), the 50 kDa subunit of carboxypeptidase N would not be expected to survive by itself in the circulation for very long. Intact carboxypeptidase N contains an additional 83 kDa subunit which fulfills the role of carrying and protecting the 50 kDa subunit in the blood.   In order to explore the nature of the 83 kDa subunit (which has no intrinsic activity of its own) we cloned and sequenced the cDNA coding for this protein from a human liver cDNA library (18).   The deduced protein sequence contains 536 amino acids (calculated Mr = 58,762) and has no similarity to the 50 kDa active subunit or any other carboxypeptidases (18).   As expected from its high carbohydrate content (27% by weight), the sequence contains 7 potential Asn-linked glycosylation sites and, in addition, a region rich in threonine and serine which may contain O-linked carbohydrate (18).

The 83 kDa Subunit Contains Leucine-Rich Tandem Repeats. The most notable feature of the deduced sequence is a domain comprising about 54% of the protein which contains 12 leucine-rich tandem repeats of 24 amino acids each (18). This repeating pattern was first discovered in the leucine-rich α_2-glycoprotein (19) and has since been found in at least 20 other proteins (Fig. 2). The consensus repeated sequence in the 83 kDa subunit contains conserved residues in 10 positions out of 24 the amino acids in each repeat, primarily consisting of leucine in 6 positions, leucine and other hydrophobic amino acids in the 4th and 5th positions, proline in the first position and asparagine in the 19th position (Fig. 2). The consensus sequence is strikingly similar to those found in a variety of other mammalian proteins including platelet

PROTEIN	# of REPEATS	CONSENSUS REPEATED SEQUENCE
CPN 83 kDa SUBUNIT	12	P - - α F - - L - - L - - L - L - - N - L - - L
Leu-RICH α₂-GLYCOPROTEIN	8	P - - L L - - - - - L - - L - L - - N - L - - L
PLATELET GPIbα	7	P - G L L - - L P - L - - L - L S - N - L T T L
PROTEOGLYCAN I	12	P - - - F - - L - - L - - L - L - - N - I - - V
RNASE INHIBITOR	8 (A)	- C - - L - - - L - 5 L E - L - L - - C - L T - -
	7 (B)	G α - - L - - α L - 4 L - E L - L - - N - L G D -
LH-CG RECEPTOR	14	P S - A F - - L - - α - 2 L - L - - - - L - - α
PLATELET GP V	>6	P - - - F - - L - - L - - L - L - - N - L - - L
OLIGODENDROCYTE/MYELIN GP	7	P - - - L - - - - - L - - L - L S - N - L - - L
U2 snRNP-A'	5	- - - - - - - L - - L - - L - α - - N - α - - L

Figure 2. Comparison of consensus sequences in selected mammalian proteins with leucine-rich tandem repeats. Consensus sequences are derived from published data. The repeats are 24 amino acids long except in the case of the RNAse inhibitor (two types of repeats of 28 or 29 residues) and the LH-CG receptor (25 residues). Residues conserved among the consensus sequences of different proteins are boxed. α = aliphatic amino acids (I, L, V). - = any amino acid. Abbreviations: GP, glycoprotein; CPN, carboxypeptidase N; LH-CG, luteinizing hormone-choriogonadotropin; snRNP, small nuclear ribonucleoprotein.

GPIb$_\alpha$, GP V and GP IX, proteoglycans, RNAse inhibitor, luteinizing hormone receptor, oligodendrocyte/myelin glycoprotein and U2 snRNP-A' (Fig. 2). This type of structure is even found in *Drosophila*, yeast, bacterial and viral proteins. These data would indicate that the leucine-rich repeat region forms an important structural or functional element which is critical for the functioning of these proteins, especially considering that in some cases nearly the entire protein ($\approx 90\%$) consists of leucine-rich repeats. Our data regarding the 83 kDa subunit would support this hypothesis. For example, predicted chain flexibility analysis of the deduced protein sequence shows that the leucine-rich repeat region has the lowest overall flexibility, indicating it may form a more rigid structural domain. In addition, when we isolated tryptic peptides from the 83 kDa subunit for sequencing, we found they came from either the N- or C-terminal regions but not the leucine-rich repeat domain (18), indicating it may form a structure relatively inaccessible to proteases. Secondary structure predictions do not give an unambiguous answer as to the nature of the structure in this region of the 83 kDa subunit. Computer analyses of the sequences of a few other leucine-rich proteins indicate the repeats may form α-helices although recent evidence, obtained by studying the structure of a synthetic peptide corresponding to a single repeat in the *Drosophila* protein chaoptin, supports an amphipathic ß-sheet structure for this region (20).

Interaction of the 50 kDa and 83 kDa Subunits of Carboxypeptidase N. The precise role of the leucine-rich tandem repeats has not been clearly defined in any protein to date. The only common feature among this diverse group of proteins is their participation in some sort of binding function (e.g., protein-protein or protein-membrane interactions). We therefore propose that the leucine-rich repeat region in the 83 kDa subunit may mediate its interaction with the 50 kDa active subunit to form a heterodimer (Fig. 3). This interaction probably involves a combination of hydrophobic and ionic interactions as chaotropic agents such as 3 M guanidine or ionized detergents can dissociate them (15,16). If this is the case, then it is likely that the N- and C-terminal domains of the 83 kDa subunit are responsible for association of the two heterodimers to form the tetramer. This could involve ionic interactions of the N-terminus of one 83 kDa subunit (which contains many acidic residues) with the C-terminus of the other 83 kDa subunit (which contains numerous basic residues) (Fig. 3). This proposal is consistent with our preliminary findings that plasmin converts the tetrameric carboxypeptidase N into an active heterodimer by removal of a 13 kDa fragment from the 83 kDa subunit (17).

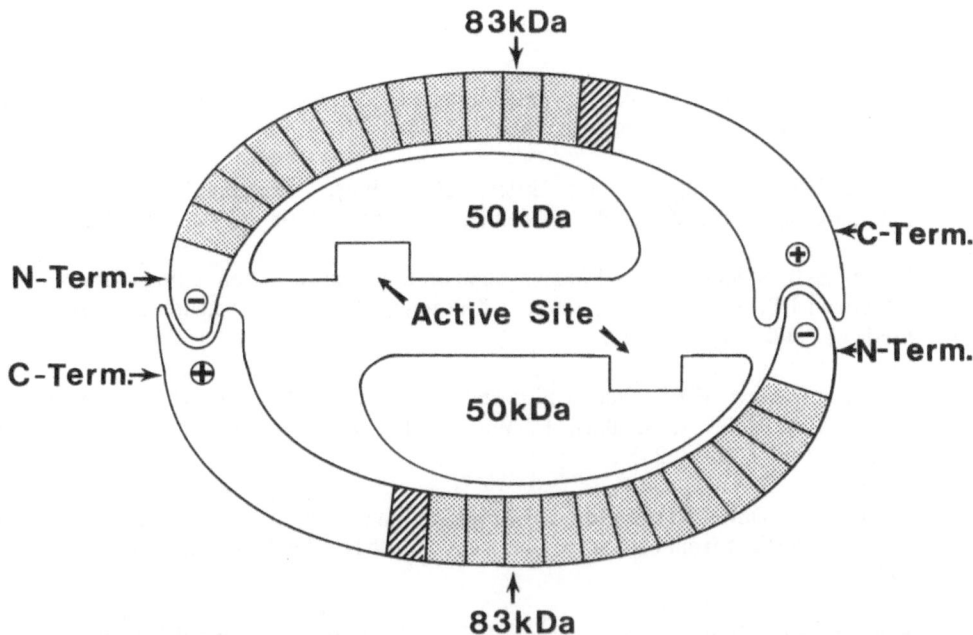

Figure 3. *Hypothetical model illustrating possible subunit interactions in carboxypeptidase N.* The leucine-rich repeat region in the 83 kDa subunit (stippled boxes) may mediate its interaction with the 50 kDa catalytic subunit. The association of the heterodimers to form the tetramer may be due to the interaction of the negatively charged N-terminal domain (N-Term.) of one 83 kDa subunit with the positively charged C-terminal domain (C-Term.) of the other. Hatched bars indicate the threonine/serine-rich region.

Elucidation of the exact structure and function of the leucine-rich repeat motif in the 83 kDa subunit and other proteins will require further studies using X-ray crystallography, NMR, site-directed mutagenesis and other biochemical techniques.

ACKNOWLEDGEMENTS

These studies were supported by NIH grants DK 41431, HL 36743 and HL 36082. We thank Dr. Ervin G. Erdös for encouragement and support.

REFERENCES

1. Erdös, EG, Sloane, EM. An enzyme in human blood plasma that inactivates bradykinin and kallidins. Biochem. Pharmacol. 1962; 11:585-92.

2. Erdös, EG. Kininases. In: Erdös, EG, editor. Handbook of Experimental Pharmacology, Vol. 25 Suppl. Heidelberg: Springer-Verlag, 1979:427-448.

3. Erdös, EG, Skidgel RA. Biochemistry of angiotensin I converting enzyme. In: Robertson JIS, Nicholls, MG, editors. The renin angiotensin system. London: Gower Medical Publishing, in press.

4. Erdös, EG, Yang, HYT. Inactivation and potentiation of the effects of bradykinin. In: Erdös, EG, Back, N, Sicuteri, F, Wilde, AF. Hypotensive peptides. New York: Springer-Verlag, 1966:235-250.

5. Skidgel, RA, Davis, RM, Erdös, EG. Purification of a human urinary carboxypeptidase (kininase) distinct from carboxypeptidases A, B, or N. Anal. Biochem. 1984; 140:520-31.

6. Skidgel, RA, Johnson, AR, Erdös EG. Hydrolysis of opioid hexapeptides by carboxypeptidase N. Presence of carboxypeptidase in cell membranes. Biochem. Pharmacol. 1984; 33:3471-8.

7. Johnson, AR, Skidgel, RA, Gafford, JT, Erdös, EG. Enzymes in placental microvilli: Angiotensin I converting enzyme, angiotensinase A, carboxypeptidase, and neutral endopeptidase ("enkephalinase"). Peptides 1984; 5:789-96.

8. Skidgel, RA, Davis, RM, Tan, F. Human carboxypeptidase M. Purification and characterization of a membrane-bound carboxypeptidase that cleaves peptide hormones. J. Biol. Chem. 1989; 264:2236-41.

9. Tan, F, Chan, SJ, Steiner, DF, Schilling, JW, Skidgel, RA. Molecular cloning and sequencing of the cDNA for human membrane-bound carboxypeptidase M. J. Biol. Chem. 1989; 264:13165-70.

10. Low, MG. Glycosyl-phosphatidylinositol: a versatile anchor for cell surface proteins. FASEB J. 1989; 3:1600-8.

11. Deddish, PA, Skidgel, RA, Kriho, VB, Becker, RP, Li, X-Y, Erdös, EG. Carboxypeptidase M in cultured Madin-Darby canine kidney cells. Evidence that carboxypeptidase M has a phosphatidylinositol glycan anchor. J. Biol. Chem. 1990; 265:15083-9.

12. Skidgel, RA, Tan, F, Deddish, PA, Li, X-Y. Structure, function and membrane anchoring of carboxypeptidase M. Biomed. Biochim. Acta 1991; 50:815-20.

13. Skidgel, RA. Basic carboxypeptidases: regulators of peptide hormone activity. Trends Pharmacol. Sci. 1988; 9:299-304.

14. Gebhard, W, Schube, M, Eulitz, M. cDNA cloning and complete primary structure of the small, active subunit of human carboxypeptidase N (kininase 1). Eur. J. Biochem. 1989; 178:603-7.

15. Levin, Y, Skidgel, RA, Erdös, EG. Isolation and characterization of the subunits of human plasma carboxypeptidase N (kininase I). Proc. Natl. Acad. Sci. USA 1982; 79:4618-22.

16. Plummer, TH Jr, Hurwitz, MY. Human plasma carboxypeptidase N. Isolation and characterization. J. Biol. Chem. 1978; 253:3907-12.

17. Skidgel, RA, Weerasinghe, DK, Erdös, EG. Structure of human carboxypeptidase N (kininase I). Adv. Exp. Med. Biol. 1989; 247A:325-9.

18. Tan, F, Weerasinghe, DK, Skidgel, RA, Tamei, H, Kaul, RK, Roninson, I, Schilling, JW, Erdös, EG. The deduced protein sequence of the human carboxypeptidase N high molecular weight subunit reveals the presence of leucine-rich tandem repeats. J. Biol. Chem. 1990; 265:13-19.

19. Takahashi, N, Takahashi, Y, Putnam, FW. Periodicity of leucine and tandem repetition of a 24-amino acid segment in the primary structure of leucine-rich α_2-glycoprotein of human serum. Proc. Natl. Acad. Sci. USA 1985; 82:1906-10.

20. Krantz, DD, Zidovetzki, R, Kagan, BL, Zipursky, SL. Amphipathic ß structure of a leucine-rich repeat peptide. J. Biol. Chem. 1991; 266:16081-7.

AAS 38/I
Recent Progress on Kinins
© 1992 Birkhäuser Verlag Basel

COMPARATIVE MOLECULAR MODELING OF THE ACTIVE SUBUNIT OF HUMAN KININASE I

Dirk Hendriks[1], Martin Vingron[2], Gerrit Vriend[2] , Wei Wang[1], Dominique Nalis[2], and Simon Scharpé[1]

[1]Department of Pharmaceutical Sciences, Laboratory of Medical Biochemistry, University of Antwerp, Universiteitsplein 1, 2610, Wilrijk, Belgium and [2]European Molecular Biology Laboratory, Meyerhofstrasse 1, 6900 Heidelberg, Germany

ABSTRACT

The structure of the enzymatically active subunit of human plasma carboxypeptidase N was determined by computer aided model building by homology using the structural coordinates from carboxypeptidase A. The active site of carboxypeptidase N has been well conserved in comparison with carboxypeptidase A. Differences in substrate specificity can be explained by the comparison of energetically favorable binding sites for different atomic probe groups.

INTRODUCTION

The human plasma carboxypeptidase N (CPN, kininase I, arginine carboxypeptidase, anaphylatoxin inactivator, EC 3.4.17.3) is a Zn^{2+} containing exopeptidase which catalyzes the release of the basic amino acids lysine and arginine from the C-termini of peptides and proteins. Its most important physiological substrates are bradykinin and kallidin [1] and the anaphylatoxins C3a, C4a and C5a [2-3]. Also the fibrinopeptides 6A and 6D [4], the hexapeptide enkephalins [5] and the creatine kinase MM-isoenzyme [6,7] can be cleaved by carboxypeptidase N.

The enzyme is synthesized in the liver [1] and circulates as a 280 000 M_r tetrameric complex, composed of two identical high molecular weight subunits (M_r 83 000) which are heavily glycosylated and lack enzymatic activity, and two identical low molecular weight subunits (M_r 55 000) which lack carbohydrate but contain the active center. The subunits are held together by non-covalent bonds as they can be dissociated with guanidine or with an ionizing detergent such as SDS. The high molecular weight subunit functions to stabilize the active subunit at body temperature and keep it in the circulation [8,9].

Gebhard *et al.* recently isolated a cDNA clone containing the entire coding sequence of the small subunit of carboxypeptidase N from a human liver cDNA library. This cDNA clone encodes a signal sequence of 20 amino acids and the 438 amino acids of the mature subunit .

There is a strong primary structure similarity to bovine carboxypeptidase H (enkephalin convertase) and human carboxypeptidase M, and a more distant relationship to bovine pancreatic carboxypeptidases A (CPA) and B (CPB) [10].

In order to understand the difference in substrate specificity between CPN and CPA, a three-dimensional model of CPN was built. To do so we exploited the homology of the CPN enzymatically active subunit with other carboxypeptidases.

MATERIALS AND METHODS

Sequence alignments

Sequences were extracted from the EMBL/Swissprot [11] database and aligned using combined information from several approaches. The methods applied were intended to delineate reliable information about location and extent of sequence similarity. The Sensitive Sequence Comparison Method [12, 13] was used to calculate dotplots between carboxypeptidase N and the other sequences. Given the low overall similarity in this family of proteins, the sequences still had to be compared as a set. This was done using a newly developed approach based on the consistent occurence of similarities in the entire set of pairwise comparisons [14]. This method not only calculates a multiple alignment but at the same time highlights those parts of the alignment which may be trusted in a structural sense.

Model building procedure

The atomic model of carboxypeptidase N was built using the structure of carboxypeptidase A [15] and replacing its sequence by the CPN sequence in a way similar to that described by Eijsink et al. [16], using the automated homology building module of the program WHAT IF [17] with subsequent energy minimization and molecular dynamics to overcome the problem of local minima. Several surface loops for which no related loop was present in the CPA structure were not modeled. Atomic coordinates were obtained from the PDB Protein Data Bank [18]. Energy minimization and molecular dynamics were carried out with GROMOS [19]. The molecular display system consisted of an Evans and Sutherland PS390 system attached to a VAX-cluster.

Determination of energetically favorable binding sites

Binding energies for the different atomic probe groups in the active sites of the carboxypeptidase A structure and the carboxypeptidase N model were computed using the program GRID [20]. Contour surfaces at appropriate energy levels are calculated for each atomic probe group and displayed using the GRID interface module of the WHAT IF program.

RESULTS AND DISCUSSION

From a sequence database search, the following sequences were retained to be used in the alignment study: carboxypeptidases A (bovine) [15], A (rat) [21], A (human mast cell) [22], B (bovine) [23], M (human) [24], H (bovine) [25] and N (human plasma) [10]. Figure 1 shows the alignment between the seven carboxypeptidases. Only the part of the sequences that can be aligned with CPA are shown. This means that the carboxyterminal part of CPN is not aligned and therefore not modeled. The alignment between carboxypeptidase N and A reveals an overall homology of only 18 %, which is very near to the downlimit where model building by homology is still useful. Indeed, parts of the model of CPN cannot be modeled with any degree of confidence. However, the sequence alignment techniques used allow us to determine an alignment for exactly those regions where the result is likely to be correct. Fortunately, the sequence spans around the active site could be aligned that way. Taking into consideration only those residues within 8 angstrom of the Gly-Lys dipeptide docked into the active site of the CPN, we find that 16 out of 37 (43%) residues are identical, which allows us to built the active site with great confidence. It is therefore safe to assume that around the active site the CPN model is good enough to permit qualitative analysis of its atomic constellation.

Zones of good homology between CPA and CPN include the area around the three conserved zinc binding ligands (His-69, Glu-72, His-196), around the substrate binding region (conserved Asn-144, Arg-145, Asn-146), and around the active site (conserved Tyr-248 and Glu-270, Leu-271). Because of low homology in certain regions and the presence of a 12 amino acid insertion (CPN 208-219), two external loops (CPN 146-169 and 208-219) have not been built. These loops however are situated far away from the active center, and are unlikely to interfere with substrate binding or enzymatic activity.

Plausible candidates for nucleophylic attack at the scissile carbonyl of the substrate in the hydrolysis reaction are either Zn-hydroxyl (the general base mechanism) or Glu-270 (the acyl-mechanism) [26,27]. The active site zinc is coordinated to His-69, Glu-72 and His-196. Zn,

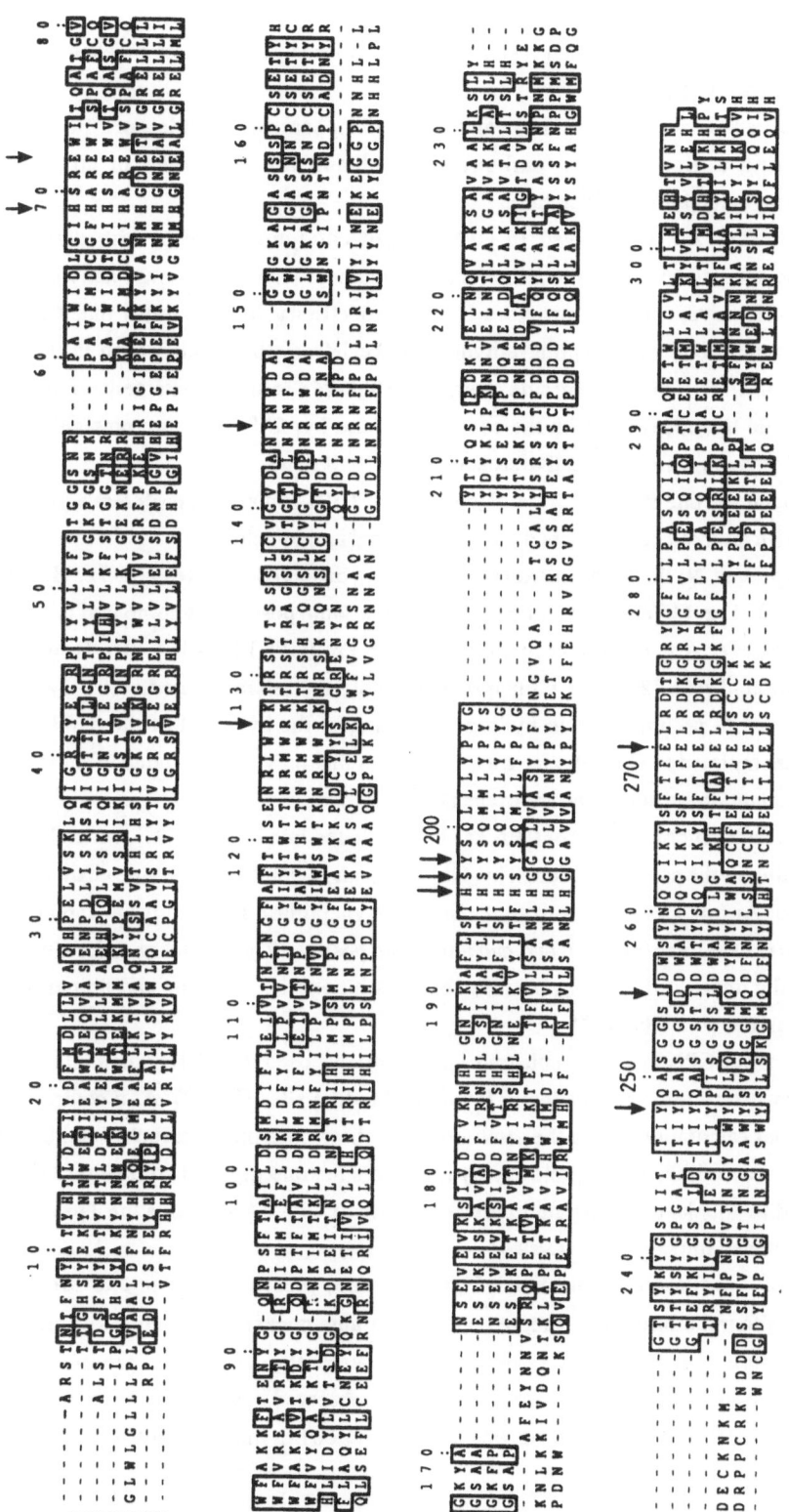

Fig. 1. Similarity of the small unit of human carboxypeptidase N (7) to carboxypeptidase A from bovine (1), from rat (3), from human mast cell (4), bovine carboxypeptidase B (2), human carboxypeptidase M (5) and bovine carboxypeptidase H (6). Residues identical (and conservative changes) in at least four proteins are boxed. Arrows mark important residues thought to be involved in the enzymatic mechanism.

Glu-270 and Arg-127 are three crucial residues in the proposed general-base mechanism for CPA-catalyzed hydrolysis [27].

Arg-145 (positively charged), Asn-144, and Tyr-248 appear to provide specificity for substrates bearing a free terminal carboxylate [28] and are conserved in all of the carboxypeptidases taken into consideration.

The function of Tyr-248 (conserved in CPN) is not catalytic, since by site-directed mutagenesis the Tyr was mutated into a Phe, and normal peptidase and esterase activity was observed [29]. However Tyr-248 provides binding specificity for substrates that have a penultimate peptide bond by accepting a hydrogen bond from the amide group in the P1 position of the substrate. The phenolic side chain of the Tyr-248 is in the characteristic "down" position for bound ligands [25]. With the exception of the Tyr-248, there are no significant conformational deviations from the native structure at the active site.

Ile-255 is a crucial residue in the hydrophobic pocket of CPA and allows preference of CPA for substrates with aromatic and branched chain C-terminal amino-acids [30].

In carboxypeptidase N, the mechanistically important conserved residues Glu-72, His-69, His-196, Glu-270, Arg-145 and Tyr-24 are exactly in the same position as compared to CPA. In our model however Arg-127 has been changed into a Pro (CPN) (Lys in CPE). However, the alignment around Arg-127 in the CPN model was not very reliable. The Ser197-Tyr198, which are believed to be important in hydrogen bonding of the hydroxyl of the tetrahydral intermediate, are mutated to Gly-Gly. Because of the fact that only the backbone of these two residues is important, these mutations are irrelevant.

Ile-255 in the hydrophobic pocket of CPA has been mutated into a Gln (CPN), which has its sidechain pointing in the same direction. This Gln forms an H-bond with the side chain of the carboxyterminal Arg or Lys of the substrate. In carboxypeptidase B, there is an Asp at this position, which is negatively charged and can attract the positively charged Arg or Lys, which might explain the increased K_{cat}/K_m on the substrates hippuryl-L-arginine and hippuryl-L-lysine in comparison with CPN [31].

In order to test our CPN model on substrate specificity, we used the GRID potential energy method [23] for determining energetically favorable binding sites (Fig. 2). As a control, we performed similar calculations using the same atomic probe groups on the carboxypeptidase A coordinates. The coordinates of the slowly hydrolyzed substrate glycyl-L-tyrosine [32] for CPA were used to "dock" the substrate in the active site of CPN. Afterwards the Tyr of this inhibitor was mutated into an Arg or Lys.

Using the NH_3^+ -probe group and $=NH_2^+$ probe group, present in lysine and arginine respectively, we found a bifurcated energetically favourable pocket in the active site cleft of CPN in a position that coincides with the place were the guanidine group of the carboxyterminal arginine fits (Fig. 2). This pocket is not observed in CPA. Histidine, which is positively charged at the pH where the enzyme is active, doesn't fit into the active site cleft.

Using an aromatic carbon as a probe group, CPA shows a wide energetically favourable pocket where an aromatic ring can fit, whereas with CPN a narrow pocket is available which is not wide enough to contain a phenyl ring (Fig. 2).

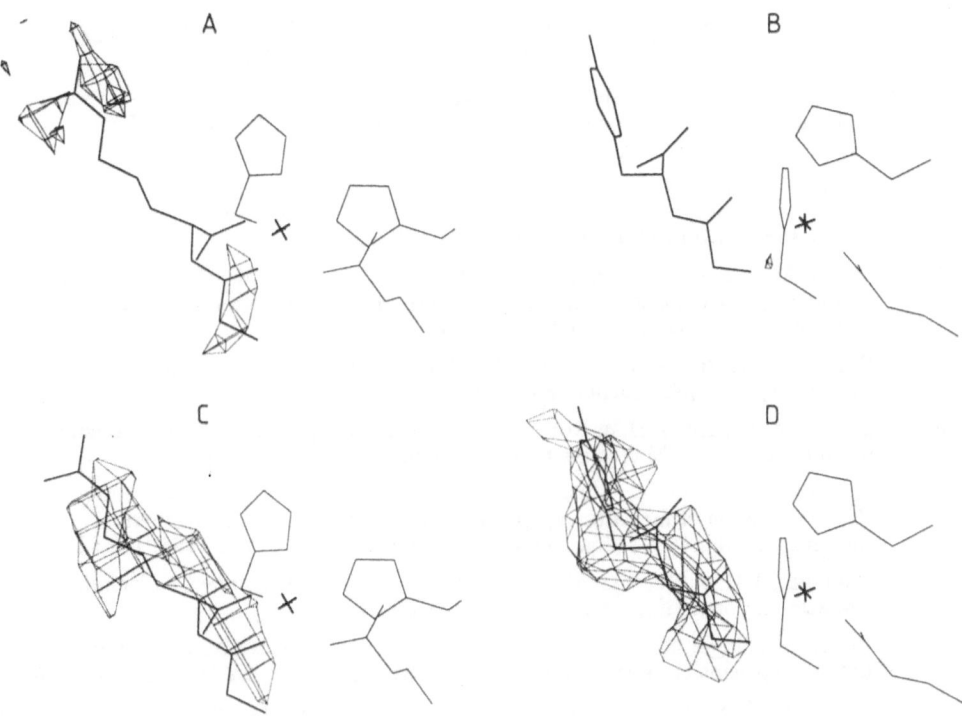

Fig. 2. Contour plots of the energetically favorable binding sites in the substrate binding cleft of carboxypeptidase N and A.
Contours are plotted for a sp3 positively charged amino-group for CPN at -15 kcal/mol (A) and for CPA at -15 kcal/mol (B), for a methylene group for CPN at -3 kcal/mol (C) and for an aromatic carbon atom for CPA at -2 kcal/mol (D). In A and C the dipeptide Gly-Arg is shown with thick solid lines. In B and D the inhibitor Gly-Tyr is shown.

Both for CPN and CPA, energetically favourable places for a methylene probe group coincide with the alpha-carbon chain part of the chain of the substrate. It seems therefore likely that substrates containing a C-terminal residue with an aliphatic sidechain shorter than Arg or Lys (leucine, isoleucine) could be cleaved by CPN (as is the case with CPA), although presumably at a rate which is lower than the hydrolysis of basic residues.

Proteolysis of the active subunit of carboxypeptidase N by serine proteases (trypsin, plasmin) yields two fragments of 27 kDa and 21 kDa [8,9]. This could be explained by a cleavage of the Arg-218/Arg-219 peptide bond situated in an external loop.

REFERENCES

1. Erdös, E.G. In: Bradykinin, Kallidin and Kallikrein, Handbook of Experimental Pharmacology (Erdös, E.G., ed) 1979; Vol 25 (Suppl), 427-487.

2. Bokish, V.A. & Müller-Eberhard, H.J. Anaphylatoxin inactivator of human plasma : its isolation and characterization as a carboxypeptidase. J Clin Invest 1970; 49: 2427-2436.

3. Hugli, T., Gerard, C., Kawahara, M., Scheetz, M., Barton, R., Bruggs, S., Koppel, G. & Russell, S. Isolation of three separate anaphylatoxins from complement-activated human serum. Mol Cell Biochem 1981; 41 : 59-66.

4. Belew, M., Gerdin, B., Lindeberg, G., Porath, J, & Wallin, R. Structural-activity relationships of vasoactive peptides derived from fibrin or fibriongen degraded by plasmin. Biochim Biophys Acta 1980; 621: 169-178.

5. Skidgel, R.A., Johnson, A.R. & Erdös, E.G. Hydrolysis of opioid peptides by carboxypeptidase N. Biochem Pharmacol 1984; 33: 3471-3478.

6. Perryman, M., Knell, D. & Roberts, R. Molecular mechanism for the production of multiple forms of MM creatine kinase. Experientia 1984; 40 : 1275-1277.

7. Hendriks, D., Soons, J., Scharpé, S., Wevers, R., van Sande, M. & Holmquist, B. Identification of the carboxypeptidase responsible for the post-synthetic modification of creatine kinase in human serum. Clin Chim Acta 1988; 172 : 253-260.

8. Plummer, T.H. & Hurwitz, M.Y. Human plasma carboxypeptidase N: isolation and characterization. J Biol Chem 1978; 253 : 3907-3912.

9. Levin, J., Skidgel, R.A. & Erdös, E.G. Isolation and characterization of the subunits of human plasma carboxypeptidase N. Proc Nat Acad Sci USA 1982; 79 : 4618-4622.

10. Gebhard, W., Schube, M. & Eulitz, M. cDNA cloning and complete primary structure of the small, active subunit of human carboxypeptidase N. 1989; Eur J Biochem; 178: 603-607.

11. SWISS-PROT Protein Sequence Database. EMBL Data Library, D-6900 Heidelberg, FRG & Amos Bairoch, Departement de Biochimie Medicale, Centre Medicale Universitaire, 1211 Geneva 4, Switzerland.

12. Argos, P. A sensitive procedure to compare amino acid sequences. J Mol Biol 1987; 193 : 385-396.

13. Rechid, R., Vingron, M. & Argos, P. A new interactive protein sequence alignement program and comparison of its results with widely used algorithms. Comp Appl Biosc 1989; 5 : 107-113.

14. Vingron, M. & Argos, P. Determination of reliable regions in protein sequence alignements. Protein Engineering 1990 ; 3 : 565-569.

15. Rees, D.C., Lewis, M. & Lipscomb, W.N. Refined crystal structure of carboxypeptidase A at 1.54 Å resolution. J Mol Biol 1983; 168 : 367-387.

16. Eijsink, V.G., Vriend, G., Van Den Burg, B., Venema, G., & Stulp, B.K. Contribution of the C-terminal amino acid to the stability of Bacillus subtilis neutral protease. Protein Engineering 1990 ; 4 : 99-104.

17.   Vriend, G. WHAT IF : a molecular modeling and drug design program. J Mol Graphics 1990; 8 : 52-56.

18.   Bernstein, F.C., Koetzle, T.F., Williams, G.J.B., Meyer, E.F., Brice, M.D., Rodgers, J.R., Kennard, O., Shimanouchi, T., Tasumi, M. The Protein Databank: a computer-based archival file for macromolecular structures. J Mol Biol 1977; 112 : 535-542.

19.   Van Gunsteren, W.F. & Berendsen, H.J. (1987) BIOMOS, Biomolecular Software, Laboratory of Physical Chemistry, University of Groningen, Groningen, The Netherlands.

20.   Goodford, P.J. A computational procedure for determining energetically favorable binding sites on biologically important macromolecules.J Med Chem 1985; 28 : 849-857.

21.   Quinto, C., Quiroga, M., Swain, W.F., Nikovits, W.C., Standring, D.N., Pictet, R.L., Valenzuela, P., Rutter, W.J. Rat preprocarboxypeptidase A : cDNA sequence and preliminary characterization of the gene. Proc Natl Acad Sci USA, 1982; 79:31-35.

22.   Cole, K.R., Kumar, S., Trong, H.L., Woodbury, R.G., Walsh, K.A., Neurath, H. Rat mast cell carboxypeptidase : amino acid sequence and evidence of enzyme activity within mast cell granules. Biochemistry 1991; 30 : 648-655.

23.   Titani, K., Ericsson, L.H., Walsh, K.A., Neurath, H. Amino acid sequence of bovine carboxypeptidase B. Proc Natl Acad Sci USA 1975; 72: 1666-1670.

24.   Tan, F., Chan, S.J., Steiner, D.F., Schilling, J.W., Skidgel, R.A. Molecular cloning and sequencing of the cDNA for human membrane bound carboxypeptidase M. J Biol Chem 1989; 264 : 13165-13170.

25.   Fricker, L.D., Evans, C.J., Esch, F.S., Herbert, E. Cloning and sequence analysis of cDNA for bovine carboxypeptidase E. Nature 1986 ; 323 : 461-464.

26.   Christianson, D.W., David, P.R. & Lipscomb, W.N. Mechanism of carboxypeptidase A: hydration of a ketonic substrate analogue. Proc Natl Acad Sci USA 1987; 84 : 1512-1515.

27.   Kim, H. & Lipscomb, W.N. Crystal structure of the complex of carboxypeptidase A with a strongly bound phosphonate in a new crystalline form: comparison with structures of other complexes. Biochemistry 1990; 29 : 5546-5555.

28.   Christianson, D.W. & Lipscomb, W.N. Comparison of carboxypeptidase A and thermolysin : inhibition by phosphonamidates. J Am Chem Soc 1988; 110: 5560-5565.

29.   Gardell, S.J., Craik, C.S., Hilvert, D., Urdea, M.S. & Rutter, W.J. Site directed mutagenesis shows that tyrosine 248 of carboxypeptidase A does not play a crucial role in catalysis. Nature 1985; 317 : 551-555.

30.   Hanson, J.E., Kaplan, A.P., Bartlett, P.A. Phosphonate analogues of carboxypeptidase A substrates are potent transition-state analogue inhibitors. Biochemistry 1989; 28 : 6294-6305.

31.   McKay, T., Phelan, A., Plummer, T. Comparative studies on human carboxypeptidases B and N. Arch Biochem Biophys 1979; 197 : 487-492.

32.   Christianson, D.W. & Lipscomb, W.N. X-ray crystallographic investigation of substrate binding to carboxypeptidase A at subzero temperatures. Proc Natl Acad Sci 1986; 83 : 7568-7572.

AAS 38/I
Recent Progress on Kinins
© 1992 Birkhäuser Verlag Basel

TISSUE SPECIFIC EXPRESSION OF ANGIOTENSIN CONVERTING ENZYME

K.E. Bernstein, T.E. Howard, S-Y. Shai, K.G. Langford and R. Balogh

Department of Pathology and Laboratory Medicine, Emory University, Atlanta, Georgia, USA 30322

SUMMARY: Angiotensin converting enzyme (ACE) is a component of the renin-angiotensin system and is critical in the homeostatic control of systemic blood pressure. There are two isozymes of ACE that result from two distinct promoter regions with the single ACE gene. In this article, we discuss the biochemistry of tissue specific promoter recognition as exemplified by the ACE gene.

INTRODUCTION

The renin-angiotensin system is central to the control of blood pressure. Angiotensin II (ang II) is the final product of this system and leads to volume expansion and vasoconstriction, mechanisms that combine to raise blood pressure. Ang II is synthesized in two discrete steps. The precursor protein angiotensinogen is cleaved by renin to produce angiotensin I. This is rapidly converted to ang II by angiotensin converting enzyme (ACE). ACE is rather non-specific in substrate specificity, and many small peptides including bradykinin are also hydrolyzed by this enzyme. Thus the actions of ACE are to produce the vasoconstrictor ang II and to eliminate bradykinin, a potent vasodilator. Over the last 5 years, our laboratory has investigated the regulated expression of the ACE gene within the mouse and human genomes. Though encoded by a single gene, there are two isozymes of angiotensin converting enzyme. One isozyme is produced by several tissue types including endothelial cells, areas of the gut, and renal proximal tubular epithelium. This form of ACE is referred to as somatic ACE; it is the isozyme produced by all somatic tissues expressing this enzyme. It has a molecular weight of approximately 160 kDa. The second isozyme is only expressed by developing spermatozoa and is referred to as testis ACE. Testis ACE is smaller than somatic ACE, with a molecular weight of approximately 95 kDa.

Thus all cells can be categorized into three patterns of ACE expression. Those tissues such as the kidney or vascular endothelium that make somatic ACE, developing spermatozoa which express testis ACE, and many tissues such as hepatocytes that produce no ACE.

RESULTS

In order to study the regulated expression of the angiotensin converting enzyme gene, we cloned cDNA encoding somatic ACE. To do this, mouse kidney ACE was purified to homogeneity using affinity chromatography.[1] Partial amino acid sequence was obtained and synthetic oligonucleotides were used to screen a mouse kidney cDNA library. Two cDNA were isolated that encode the entire amino acid sequence of mouse somatic ACE.[2] This sequence contains 4838 nucleotides and encodes a protein of 1312 amino acids. Within the protein, there are two large areas of homologous sequence, each containing a potential zinc binding region and catalytic site (Fig. 1). The homologous regions are approximately half the size of the whole ACE protein and this suggests that the ACE gene arose by a tandom duplication of a smaller primordial gene. Northern analysis of mouse kidney and lung RNA demonstrates that somatic ACE is encoded by two message sizes, 5000 and 4300 nucleotides. These two forms of ACE mRNA differ in the lengths of the 3' untranslated regions.

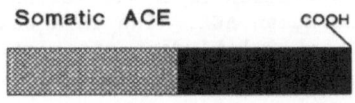

Fig. 1. Schematic of somatic ACE. The protein is composed of two homologous amino acid domains, each containing a catalytic site.

To understand the regulated expression of somatic ACE, genomic DNA 5' to the mouse and human ACE genes has been isolated and analyzed.[3] Sequence comparison identified two discrete regions of genomic DNA that are highly conserved between these two species. One region is found immediately 5' to the transcription initiation site and is shown in Figure 2 with mouse genomic sequence represented by CAPITOL letters and human sequence by lowercase. Gaps (indicated by a dash) have been inserted to maximize alignment and colons mark conserved nucleotides. The translation start site of somatic ACE is indicated by the position of the first two amino acids, methionine (Met) and glycine (Gly). The start of translation is at +1 while upstream DNA is indicated with negative numbers. In both species this immediate upstream region of DNA is a guanine-cytosine rich

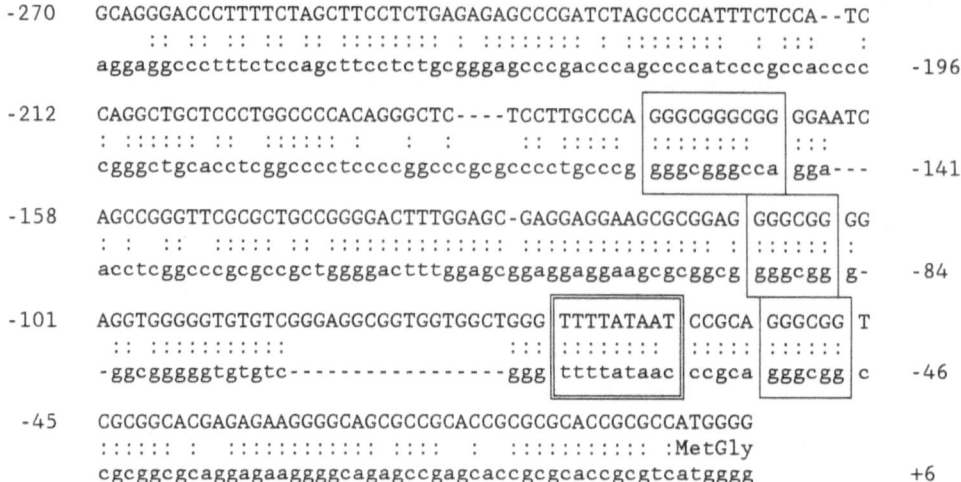

-270 GCAGGGACCCTTTTCTAGCTTCCTCTGAGAGAGCCCGATCTAGCCCCATTTCTCCA--TC
      :: :: :: :: :: ::::::::: : ::::::::: : ::::::::: : :::   :
      aggaggccctttctccagcttcctctgcggggagcccgacccagccccatcccgccacccc   -196

-212 CAGGCTGCTCCCTGGCCCCACAGGGCTC----TCCTTGCCCA GGGCGGGCGG GGAATC
      : :::::: :: ::::::: : :   :: ::::: :::::::: :::
      cgggctgcacctcggcccctccccggcccgcgcccctgcccg gggcgggcca gga---   -141

-158 AGCCGGGTTCGCGCTGCCGGGGACTTTGGAGC-GAGGAGGAAGCGCGGAG GGGCGG GG
      : : :: ::::: :: ::::::::::::: ::::::::::::: :: : ::::::: :
      acctcggcccgcgccgctggggactttggagcggaggaggaagcgcggcg gggcgg g-   -84

-101 AGGTGGGGGTGTGTCGGGAGGCGGTGGTGGCTGGG TTTTATAAT CCGCA GGGCGG T
      :: ::::::::::: ::: ::::::::: ::::: :::::::
      -ggcgggggtgtgtc----------------ggg ttttataac ccgca gggcgg c   -46

-45   CGCGGCACGAGAGAAGGGGCAGCGCCGCCACCGCGCGCACCGCGCCATGGGG
      :::::: : ::::::::::::: :::: : :::::::::: :MetGly
      cgcggcgcaggagaagggggcagagccgagcaccgcgcaccgcgtcatgggg   +6

Fig. 2. Comparison of genomic DNA 5' to the mouse (Capitol letters) and human (lowercase) ACE genes. Gaps have been added to maximize alignment. Sequence identity is indicated with a colon. The start of translation is at +1; Met and Gly indicate the first two amino acids of mouse and human ACE. The TATA box sequences are enclosed with a double line. Potential Sp1 binding sites are enclosed with a single line.

segment that contains a classical TATA box sequence (enclosed with a double line) and several potential Sp1 binding sites (enclosed with a single line). The second conserved region is found 600 base pairs 5' to that shown in Fig. 2. This upstream region contains several potential regulatory cis elements including a possible glucocorticoid responsive element. We have now undertaken studies to map in detail the promoter region of somatic ACE and to investigate the mechanisms controlling ACE expression by cultured bovine aortic endothelial cells. Analysis of these cells demonstrates that somatic ACE is only produced when the cultured endothelial cells reach a confluent state, suggesting that the ACE gene is only transcribed when the cells exit the cell cycle and enter a growth arrested state. Understanding the molecular mechanisms of ACE expression in non proliferating endothelial cells may lead to a better understanding of gene expression in growth arrested cells.

As mentioned above, a unique isozyme of ACE is produce by developing spermatozoa. Isolation and analysis of cDNA encoding this form of the enzyme demonstrates that mouse testis ACE is composed of 732 amino acids (Fig. 3).[4]

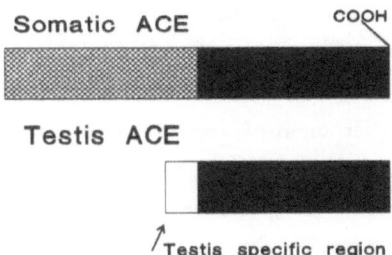

Fig. 3. Comparison of the two ACE isozymes. Testis ACE is composed of one catalytic domain identical to the carboxyl domain of somatic ACE. The first 60 amino acids of testis ACE are specific to this isozyme.

The amino terminal 66 amino acids are only expressed by the testis isozyme while the remainder of the molecule, 666 amino acids, is identical to the carboxyl half of mouse somatic ACE. Thus while somatic ACE contains two potential catalytic sights, testis ACE is composed of a single catalytic domain identical to that in the carboxyl half of somatic ACE. Primer extension and RNase protection experiments show that RNA transcription of the testis ACE isozyme begins 16 or 17 bases upstream from the translation start site. We have analyzed mouse genomic DNA and determined that both isozymes are encoded by a single gene. The amino terminal 53% of somatic ACE is encoded by 13 exons spanning approximately 10 kilobases of mouse genomic sequence (Fig. 4). Comparison of this genomic sequence to cDNA encoding the testis isozyme of ACE demonstrated that the testis specific amino terminal 66 amino acids of mouse

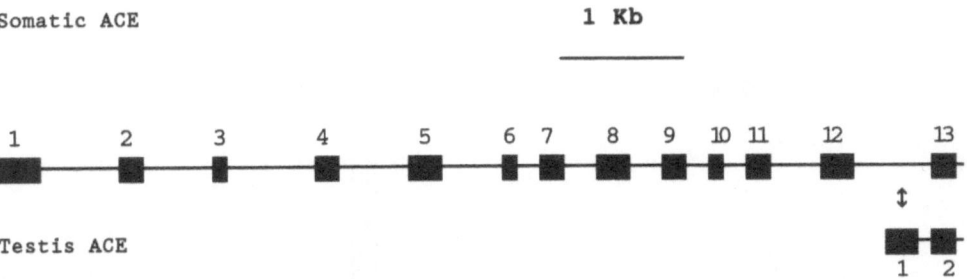

Fig. 4. Genomic organization of the ACE gene. Exons are indicated by boxes and introns by lines. This figure shows the relative sizes and positions of the first 13 exons of somatic ACE comprising the amino terminal 53% of the enzyme. The first two exons of the testis isozyme of ACE are also indicated. The first exon encodes amino acid sequence uniquely found in the testis ACE isozyme, Thereafter, the testis ACE isozyme is constructed from the identical exons used to construct the carboxyl terminal half of somatic ACE. The key point in this figure is that the DNA encoding the first exon of testis ACE is treated as the 12th intron of somatic ACE by somatic tissues.

testis ACE is encoded by a single exon within the mouse genome. This exon is
within sequence flanked by the 12th and 13th exons of somatic ACE (Fig. 4).   In
other words, the 12th intron of somatic ACE encodes the first exon of testis ACE.
The second exon of testis ACE is identical to the 13th exon of somatic ACE. Thus
testis ACE, after beginning RNA transcription within the 12th intron of somatic
ACE, starts to duplicate with its second exon the DNA sequences used to construct
the carboxyl domain of somatic ACE. These results raise the question of how a
single ACE gene can give rise to two transcription start sites. Because transcription of testis ACE begins approximately 7200 base pairs 3' of the transcription start site of somatic ACE, we hypothesized that developing spermatozoa must
recognize a different promoter region than that used by somatic tissues.[5] This
hypothesis was tested by cloning a portion of mouse genomic DNA extending from
position -683 of testis ACE (+1 is the start of testis ACE transcription) to +17
(the start of testis ACE translation) 5' to the coding region of the E. coli LacZ
gene. We call this construct tACE-pLacI. Mice were made transgenic for this
construct and analyzed for expression of β-galactosidase. As compared to
littermate control animals, only the testis expressed elevated levels of β-
galactosidase (9 times control levels) (Fig. 5). Confirmation of these findings

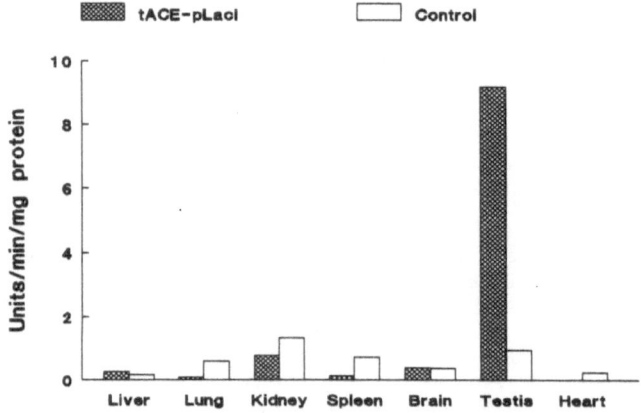

Fig. 5. Tissue expression of β-galactosidase in a mouse transgenic for tACE-pLacI
(dark bars) and a control animal (open bars). Only the testis of the transgenic
animal expresses elevated levels of enzyme.

was obtained through RNase protection analysis of mRNA expression which showed LacZ mRNA present only in the testes of transgenic animals. These experiments prove that the ACE gene is comprised of two transcription units controlled by two widely separated promoters. One promoter, located just 5' of the first exon of somatic ACE, is used by somatic tissues expressing angiotensin converting enzyme. The second promoter is located greater than 7200 base pairs 3' of the somatic promoter and is within the 12th intron of somatic ACE. This second promoter is only recognized and used by developing spermatozoa.

To further analyze the biochemistry of the testis specific promoter, we are using the technique of in vitro transcription. Here testes of mature rats are homogenized in such a fashion that cells are broken while cell nuclei remain intact. The nuclei are then isolated by ultracentrifugation through a dense sucrose cushion. After nuclear lysis, ammonium sulfate is added to precipitate DNA. What remains are nuclear proteins capable of recognizing and transcribing the ACE testis promoter region. We are presently testing deletion constructs to identify regulatory elements important in testis specific transcriptional regulation.

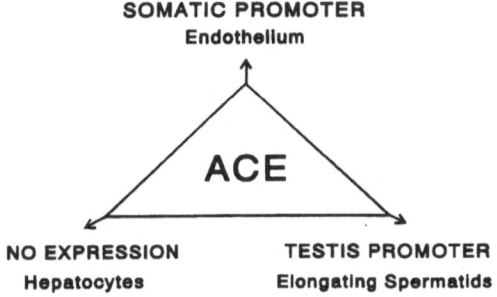

Fig. 6. A single gene encodes ACE. Tissues can be categorized into three patterns of ACE expression. Endothelium and several other somatic tissues use the somatic promoter. Developing sperm recognize the testis promoter. Many tissue types use neither promoter and do not express ACE.

DISCUSSION

It is within this century that the development of converting enzyme inhibitors allowed successful manipulation of the renin-angiotensin system.

Parallel to this important clinical advance has been an appreciation that the biochemistry and molecular biology of this system is also fascinating. In a reductionist sense, the renin-angiotensin system can be considered as a machine to maintain blood pressure, volume and electrolyte homeostasis. For this machine to function properly, and indeed for any machine to maintain homeostatic equilibrium, the machine itself must be quite dynamic. This is reflected in the regulated expression of renin, angiotensin converting enzyme and the receptor for angiotensin II. My laboratory is investigating tissue specific expression of ACE. It is now clear that this is the comparative analysis of three patterns of expression, tissues making no ACE, those tissues expressing the somatic form of the enzyme and developing spermatozoa that make testis ACE (Fig. 6). The discovery and the elucidation of the somatic and testis ACE promoters represents a first step. What remains is to understand promoter selection and utilization by individual tissue types. As these studies are extended further, ACE should serve not only as a locus for the pharmacologic reduction of blood pressure, but as a model of tissue specific gene expression, the phenomena that makes complex life on this planet possible.

ACKNOWLEDGEMENT

    This work was supported by Public Health Service grant DK39777. TEH is supported by the Harris Family Scholarship and the Helen Miller Scholarship Fund. KEB is an Established Investigator of the American Heart Association

REFERENCES

1. Bernstein KE, Martin BM, Striker L, and Striker G. Angiotensin-converting enzyme (ACE): Homology between mouse and bovine kidney ACE revealed by partial protein sequence. Kidney International 1988; 33:652-655.

2. Bernstein KE, Martin BM, Edwards AS, and Bernstein EA. Mouse angiotensin-converting enzyme is a protein composed of two homologous domains. J. Biol. Chem. 1989; 264:11945-11951.

3. Shai S-Y, Langford KG, Martin BM and Bernstein KE. Genomic DNA 5' to the Mouse and Human Angiotensin-Converting Enzyme Genes Contains Two Distinct Regions of Conserved Sequence. Biochem. Biophys. Res. Comm. 1990; 167:1128-1133.

4. Howard TE, Shai S-Y, Langford KG, Martin BM and Bernstein KE. Testis uses a unique promoter in the production of angiotensin-converting enzyme (ACE). Mol. Cell. Biol. 1990; 10:4294-4302.

5. Langford KG, Shai S-Y, Howard TE, Kovac MJ, Overbeek PA and Bernstein KE. Transgenic mice demonstrate a testis specific promoter for angiotensin converting enzyme (ACE). J. Biol. Chem 1991; 266:15559-15562.

AAS 38/I
Recent Progress on Kinins
© 1992 Birkhäuser Verlag Basel

DETECTION OF ANGIOTENSIN CONVERTING ENZYME MRNA IN THE RAT HEART BY USE OF THE POLYMERASE CHAIN REACTION (PCR)

M. Paul[1] and H. Schunkert[2]

[1]Pharmakologisches Institut, Universität Heidelberg, Im Neuenheimer Feld 366 and German Institute for High Blood Pressure Research, D-6900 Heidelberg and [2]Medizinische Klinik II, Universität Regensburg, Franz-Josef Strauß Allee, D-8400 Regensburg

SUMMARY: Previous work has shown that angiotensin converting enzyme (ACE) activity and mRNA are present in cardiac tissue. Since ACE appears to be a key enzyme in the regulation of the activity of the cardiac renin angiotensin system, the aim of the present study was to examine the expression and regulation of ACE mRNA in the heart. ACE is a membrane bound enzyme with low synthetic turnover. We therefore investigated whether the highly sensitive polymerase chain reaction (PCR) can serve as a tool for detection and quantification of ACE mRNA in small tissue samples of the heart. Enzymatic reverse transcription was performed using 1 mg total RNA of atrial as well as of right and left ventricular orgin. The resulting DNA was amplified in 25 cycles of PCR using Taq polymerase and specific primers. The amplification products were separated by agarose gel electrophoresis and detected by Southern blot analyses. Employing these methods, ACE mRNA was found in the atrium as well as right and left ventricles of rat hearts. Furthermore, PCR was useful to study the induction of ACE mRNA levels in left ventricles of hearts with experimental pressure overload hypertrophy as well right ventricles with compensatory hypertrophy after left ventricular infarction.

INTRODUCTION

Angiotensin converting enzyme (ACE) serves an important role in the regulation of cardiac function and metabolism by local generation of angiotensin II as well as local degradation of bradykinin. Angiotensin II has a wide variety of effects on target organs of the cardiovascular system including systemic and coronary vasoconstriction (1), stimulation of myocyte growth (2), as well as positive inotropy, chronotropy and negative lusitropy (3, 4, 5). Bradykinin, on the other hand, serves as a potent paracrine vasodilator (6). Components of the system such as ACE renin, angiotensinogen and angiotensin II-receptor mRNA's and proteins (7 - 12) have been detected in cardiac tissue and the intracardiac generation of angiotensin II and bradykinin has been demonstrated (5, 11, 13).The aim of the present study (5, 14) was to examine whether PCR is a useful tool to study the expression and regulation of cardiac ACE mRNA, which is present in low abundance in the heart and difficult to quantitate using conventional methods of mRNA measurements.

MATERIALS AND METHODS

Protocols. Eight-week-old male Wistar rats underwent ligation of the left coronary artery or open chest operation (sham) using standard methods (15) to induce left ventricular infarction and consecutive left ventricular failure and right ventricular hypertrophy. Left ventricular hypertrophy was induced by placing a stainless steel clip of 0.6 mm internal diameter on the ascending aorta in 3-4 week-old rats. Animals were studied 10-12 weeks after surgery.

ACE mRNA measurement. Total RNA was extracted using ultracentrifugation through a cesium chloride cushion after homogenization of tissues in guanidium thiocyanate and its concentration determined by photospectroscopy at 260 nm wavelenght. The RNA samples were kept in the -80 $^{\circ}$C freezer until further used for PCR amplification.The sense primer used for PCR was homologous to bases 492-512, the antisense primer complementary to bases 860-880 of the human ACE cDNA sequence. The amplification procedure consisted of two steps (Fig.1); first, total mRNA was subjected to cDNA first strand synthesis using reverse transcriptase, then the resulting double stranded fragments were amplified using the ACE specific primers as described above.For first strand synthesis 1 ug of rat heart total RNA was incubated in 20 ul of a reaction mixture containing 0.5 mM dATP, dCTP, dGTP, and dTTP, as well as 1 ul RNase inhibitor, 100 pmol of random hexamers and 200 units reverse transcriptase in PCR buffer (50 mM KCl, 100 mM Tris-Cl, 2.5 mM MgCl$_2$, 100 mg/ml bovine serum albumin, pH 8.4).

The samples were then incubated at room temperature for 10 minutes, followed by 45 minutes at 42 $^{\circ}$C. The reaction was stopped by heating the tubes to 95 $^{\circ}$C for five minutes.For PCR amplification, 50 pmol each of the upstream and downstream primers and 1 ml of Taq I polymerase in 80 ul PCR buffer were added to the reaction mixture. Twenty-five amplification cycles were run using a temperature cycler consiting of 30 seconds at 95 $^{\circ}$C, 30 seconds at 55 $^{\circ}$C, and 30 seconds at 72 $^{\circ}$C. At the end of the last cycle samples were again incubated for 7 minutes at 72 $^{\circ}$C, to allow complete extension of specific sequences. Amplified fragments of correct size (385 bp) were identified by agarose gel electrophoresis. To demonstrate the specificity of amplified sequences, gels were blotted on nylon membranes as described (15) and hybridized to P^{32} labeled fragments of human ACE cDNA. After hybridization, non-specific hybrids were removed and blots were exposed to X-ray films.

Statistical analysis. The intensity of the signals was measured by laser densitometry. Results are expressed as mean +/- standard errow. Differences observed between groups were analysed by Student's t-test for unpaired data. Statistical significance was accepted at the 95% confidence limit.

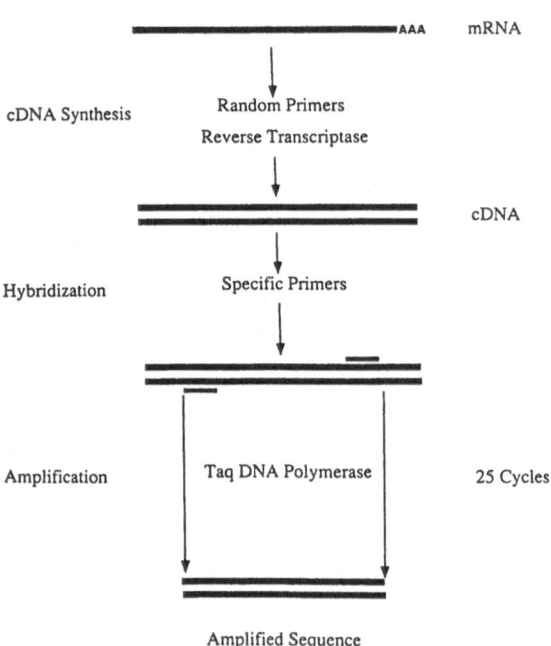

Figure 1: Schematic representation of PCR methodology. Total RNA is converted to a double stranded cDNA, which is then amplified by ACE specific primers.

RESULTS

The sequence of rat ACE cDNA is unpublished as of this writing. The positions of primers for PCR amplification were, therefore, searched among sequences which showed highest homology between the human and mouse cDNA sequences (assuming that these regions would be highly conserved in the rat ACE gene). PCR amplification of rat total RNA (subjected to cDNA first strand synthesis) indeed resulted in a product of correct lenght (385 basepairs) which gave a specific hybridization signal when hybridized to human ACE cDNA probe. Furthermore, the amplification product displayed a specific digestion pattern when incubated with selected restriction enzymes (data not shown). This gave conclusive evidence that primers which were designed upon the human ACE cDNA sequence can be successfully used for amplification of rat ACE.

ACE mRNA in right ventricle &   atrium

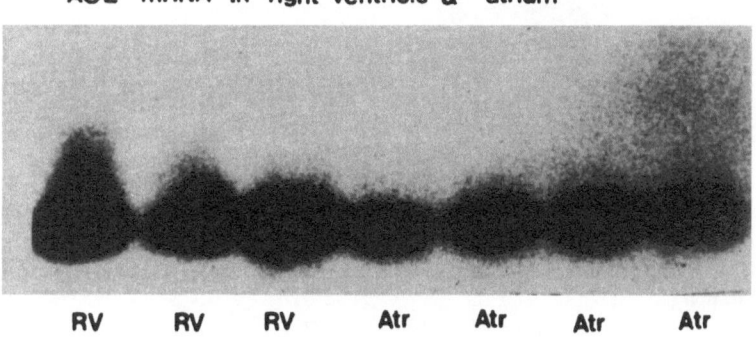

Figure 2: Distribution of ACE mRNA in rat heart atria (Atr) and right ventricles ventricles (RV) of Sprague-Dawley rats. 1 ug of total RNA was used for PCR amplification.

ACE mRNA signals were detected both in the rat heart atria and ventricles (Fig. 2) which suggests a widespread distribution of ACE in cardiac tissue. The cellular localization of cardiac ACE was not addressed by our study and remains to be defined but the levels of ACE mRNA appeared to be similar in all cardiac regions studied. In addition, these concentrations correlated well with levels found in human heart using PCR analysis (14). Preliminary studies carried out in our laboratory also showed high ACE mRNA levels in the rat vasculature and other organ involved in cardiovascular regulation (Paul, unpublished data), further illustrating the potential importance of ACE for local angiotensin II production in the cardiovascular system.

We furthermore studied the regulation of ACE mRNA in established left and right ventricular hypertrophy. Comparision of PCR amplified ACE mRNA levels in hearts with left ventricular hypertrophy (LVH) and sham operated controls revealed a four-fold induction of ACE mRNA when LVH was present (Fig. 3) (5). In parallel, ACE mRNA was amplified in hearts with right ventricular hypertrophy induced by left ventricular infarction and failure (15).

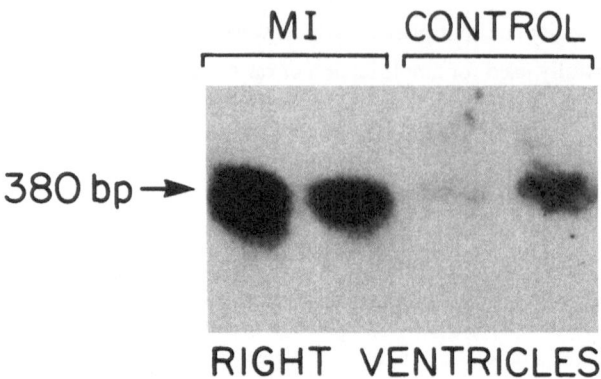

MI   CONTROL

380 bp →

RIGHT VENTRICLES

Figure 3: Regulation of cardiac ACE mRNA expression in heart failure. Note the difference in
infarcted (MI) and control hearts. 1 ug of total RNA from the right ventricles was used for
PCR amplification

CONCLUSION

A large body of data suggests the presence of local renin-angiotensin systems (RAS) in several
tissues, including the heart (11, 16, 17). Tissue ACE activity in the heart was first described in 1968
by Huggins and Thampi (18). In recent studies, the enzyme was localized by radiolabeled ACE-
inhibitors in the coronary arteries,the myocardium of atria and ventricles and valve leaflets (19).
Using 500 ug total RNA and subsequent poly $(A)^+$ purification cardiac ACE mRNA was detected by
Northern blot analysis (5). In the present study (5, 14), PCR permitted detection of cardiac ACE
mRNA in 1 ug total RNA, suggesting that this method is a sensitive technique better suited for
analysis of tissues with low abundance of ACE mRNA. PCR permitted detailed studies on
expression of ACE m RNA in atria, left and right ventricles (5). The functional importance of tissue
ACE was first demonstrated by intra-arterial infusion of angiotensin I to hindlimbs (20), kidneys,
mesenteric arteries and isolated hearts (21). More recently, the conversion rate of angiotensin I to
angiotensin II was measured biochemically in the rat hindleg (50%), kidney (5%) and heart (6.4%;
16). By local induction of the growth promoting peptide angiotensin II, cardiac ACE may play in
important role under pathophysiological conditions such as cardiac hypertrophy (5, 15). In the
present investigation (5, 14), we studied the regulation of the tissue ACE mRNA expression in left
ventricles with pressure overload left ventricular hypertrophy (LVH) (5). As compared with sham
operated controls, animals with LVH showed significantly higher ACE mRNA concentrations. In a

parallel study (15), tissue ACE mRNA was examined in rats with left heart failure after coronary ligation and subsequent hypertrophy of right ventricles (RVH). Similar to the situation in hearts with LVH, the noninfarcted but hypertrophied right ventricles of heart failure animals were found to express higher ACE mRNA levels than respective controls (15). The mechanism for the induction of ACE remains unclear.

The activation of tissue ACE under these pathophysiological conditions might result in locally increased levels of angiotensin II and decreased levels of bradykinin. In fact, the intracardiac generation of angiotensin II was found to be induced in hearts with pressure overload LVH (5) providing more evidence for an activation of the cardiac converting enzyme in pressure overload hypertrophy. Therefore, the system might participate in cardiac remodeling (22) by the growth promoting effects of angiotensin II (2, 23).

Recent studies demonstrated the efficacy of local or tissue ACE-inhibition for the prevention of local angiotensin I conversion (16,24). Another effect of tissue converting enzyme inhibition, demonstrated in the isolated hearts, is the deceleration of bradykinin metabolism, which improved the coronary hemodynamics (13). Both mechanisms may add to the benefial effects of ACE-inhibitors in the treatment of cardiac hypertrophy and failure (25, 26).

ACKNOWLEDGEMENTS

The ACE cDNA is a generous gift of Dr. P. Corvol and Dr. F. Soubrier, Paris.

REFERENCES

1. Xiang J, Linz W, Becker H, Ganten D, Lang RE, Schoelkens B, Unger T (1984) Effects of converting enzyme inhibitors ramipril and enalapril on peptide action and sympathetic neurotransmission in the isolated rat heart. Eur J Pharmacol 113:215-223.
2. Khairallah PA, Kanabus (1983) Angiotensin and myocardial protein synthesis. Perspect. Cardiovasc. Res 8: 337-347.
3. Koch-Weser J (1965) Nature of the inotropic action of angiotensin on ventricular myocardium. Circ Res 16:230-237 13.
4. Kobayashi M, Furukawa Y, Chiba S (1978). Positive chronotropic and inotropic effects of angiotensin II in the dog heart. Eur. J Pharmacol 50:17-25.
5. Schunkert H, Dzau VJ, Tang SS, Hirsch AT, Apstein C, Lorell B. Increased rat cardiac angiotensin converting enzyme activity and mRNA levels in pressure overload left ventricular hypertrophy: effects on coronary resistance, contractility and relaxation. J Clin Invest 1990; 86: 1913-1920.
6. van Gilst WH, deGraeff PA, Wessling H, deLangen CDJ (1987) Reduction of reperfusion arrhythmias in the ischemic isolated rat heart by angiotensin converting enzyme inhibitors: a comparison of captopril, enalapril and HOE 498. J Cardiovasc Pharm 9:254-255
7. Cushman DW, Cheung HS (1971). Concentrations of angiotensin converting enzyme in tissues of the rat. Biochem Biophys Acta 250: 261-265.
8. Dzau VJ, Ellison KE, Ouellette AJ (1985) Expression and regulation of renin in the mouse heart. Clin Res 33:181A (abst).
9. Paul M, Wagner D, Metzger R, Ganten D, Lang RE, Suzuki F, Murakami K, Burbach JHP, Ludwig G (1988) Quantification of renin mRNA in various mouse tissues by a novel hybridization assay. J. Hypertens. 6:247-252.
10. Baker KM, Cherin MI, Wixson SK, Aceto JF (1990) Renin angiotensin system involvement in pressure overload hypertrophy in rats. Am J Physiol 259: H324-332.
11. Lindpaintner K, Ganten D (1991). The cardiac renin-angiotensin system. Circ Res 68: 905-921
12. Murphy TJ, Alexander RW, Griendling KK, Bernstein KE. Isolation of a cDNA encoding the vascular type-1 angiotensin II receptor. Nature 1991; 351:233-236.
13. Linz W, Scholkens BA, Han YF (1986) Beneficial effects of the converting enzyme inhibitor, ramipril, in ischemic rat hearts. J Cardiovasc Pharm 8(suppl 10):S91-S99.
14. Paul M, Schunkert H, Allen PD, Dzau VJ (1990). Evidence for widespread expression of angiotensin converting enzyme mRNA in human tissues. J Hypertens 8 (Suppl 3): S36 (Abstr.).
15. Hirsch AT, Talsness CE, Schunkert H, Paul M, Dzau VJ (1991). Tissue-specific activation of cardiac angiotensin converting enzyme in experimental heart failure. Circ. Res. 69: 475-482
16. Lindpaintner K, Jin M, Wilhelm MJ, Susuki F, Linz W, Schoelkens BA, Ganten D (1988).Intracardiac generation of angiotensin and its physiologic role. Circulation (suppl I); I18-I24.
17. Dzau VJ, Burt DW, Pratt RE (1988). Molecular biology of the renin angiotensin system. Am J Physiol 255: F563-F573.
18. Huggins CG, Thampi NS (1968). A simple method for the determination of angiotensin I converting enzyme. Life Sciences 7: 633-639.
19. Yamada H, Fabris B, Allen AM, Jackson B, Johnston CI, Mendelsohn FAO (1991). Localisation of angiotensin converting enzyme in rat heart. Circ Res. 68: 141-149.
20. Ng KKF, Vane JR (1968). Fate of angiotensin I in the circulation. Nature 218:144-150.
21. Needleman P, Marshall GR, Sobel BE (1975). Hormone interactions in the isolated rabbit heart. Circ Res 37: 802-808.
22. Pfeffer MA, Lamas GA, Vaughn DE, Parisi AF, Braunwald E (1988) Effect of captopril on progressive ventricular dilatation after anterior myocardial infarction. N Engl J Med 319:80-86.
23. Geisterfer AAT, Peach M, Owens GK (1988) Hypertrophic response of cultured vascular smooth muscle cells to angiotensin II. Circ Res 62:749-756.

24. Schunkert H, Jackson B, Tang SS, Lorell BH. Localisation and functional significance of cardiac angiotensin converting enzyme (ACE) in hypertrophied rat hearts (abstract). Circulation (in press).
25. Hirsch AT, Pinto Y, Schunkert H, Dzau VJ (1990). Potential role of the tissue renin angiotensin system in the pathophysiology of congestive heart failure. Am J Cardiol 66 (Suppl): 22D-32D.
26. The CONSENSUS Trial Study Group (1987) Effects of enalapril on mortality in severe heart failure. N Engl J Med 316:1429-1431.

AAS 38/I
Recent Progress on Kinins
© 1992 Birkhäuser Verlag Basel

TONIN-LIKE ACTIVITY PRESENT IN THE HUMAN SUBMANDIBULAR GLAND

Maria P. Gualberto, Ronaldo L. Nunes, Wilson T. Beraldo and
Jorge L. Pesquero

Department of Physiology and Biophysics, Universidade Federal de Minas Gerais, Belo
Horizonte, 31270, Minas Gerais, Brazil.

SUMMARY: An enzyme which is able to liberate angiotensin II from angiotensin I,
angiotensinogen(1-14) fragment and angiotensinogen was purified from human submandibular
gland. Its molecular weight is 110,000; is inhibited by PMSF but not by EDTA or enalaprilat.
The pH optima for angiotensin II liberation were 4.0 for angiotensin I, 7.0 for
angiotensinogen(1-14) fragment and 8.0 for angiotensinogen. The total amount of angiotensin II
generating activity in the human submandibular gland is 5,000-times smaller than that in the rat
gland.

INTRODUCTION

Tonins are serine proteinases which present ability of generating the potent vasoactive
peptide angiotensin II (Ang II) from angiotensin I (Ang I), angiotensinogen (AG) or AG(1-14)
[1-2] by cleavage of Phe.His bond as illustrated in the following scheme:

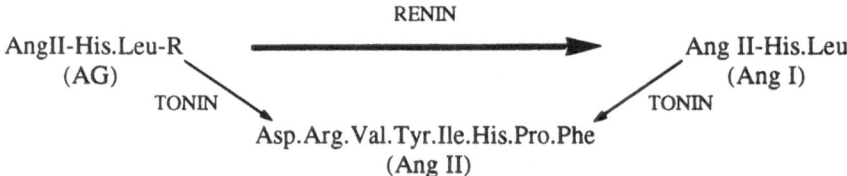

ABBREVIATIONS: AG, angiotensinogen; AG(1-14), angiotensinogen(1-14) fragment; BSA,
bovine serum albumin; HPLC, high performance liquid chromatography; SBTI, soybean trypsin
inhibitor; SDS, sodium dodecyl sulphate; RIA, radioimmunoassay; TFA, trifluoroacetic acid.

Despite its possible role in the regulation of blood pressure, its physiological function has not yet been established. Tonin is present in different rat tissues [2-4], however, it is found in large quantities in the submandibular gland, where it represents about 10% of protein content [5]. In the human tissue, only one serine proteinase possessing similar proteolytic properties has been described, being present in the prostate [6]. However, the human gene encoding proteins of the tonin and kallikrein family consists of four members, one of those present in the salivary gland [7]. Therefore, we decided to search for enzymes with tonin activity in the human submandibular gland.

MATERIALS and METHODS

All peptides used were synthesized by Paiva and Juliano, Escola Paulista de Medicina, Sao Paulo, Brasil. Antisera to angiotensin II were prepared in rabbits by immunization with (4-8)angiotensinamide coupled to BSA. Coupling and RIA according to Vieira et al. [8]. A standard curve was obtained by plotting the B/Bo against logarithm of angiotensin II concentration [9]. Electrophoretically homogeneous human renal renin was obtained by a single-step DEAE chromatography, after acid and ammonium sulphate treatment according to Shinagawa et al. [10]. Sephadex G-100, Sephacryl S-200, Mono Q HR 5/5 and MinoRPC S 5/20 columns were from Pharmacia (Uppsala, Sweden). DEAE-cellulose was from Whatman.

Enzyme purification

All solutions contained 1 mM EDTA. Submandibular glands, obtained from normotensive patients (Medical Legal Service), were extracted and perfused with 0.25 M sucrose, pH 7.0. After homogenization in the sucrose solution, the supernatant was collected by centrifugation and applied on a Sephadex G-100 column (2.7 x 73 cm), previously equilibrated with 75 mM phosphate buffer, pH 6.8. The fractions presenting angiotensin II liberating activity were pooled, dialysed for 12 h against 3 L of 20 mM Tris-HCl buffer, pH 7.5 and applied on a Mono Q column.

Angiotensinogen

Human AG was highly purified from plasma. Blood was collected into tubes containing EDTA to a final concentration of 5 mM. The plasma was fractionated by ammonium sulphate. The fraction containing AG, which precipitated between 1.5 and 2.4 M ammonium sulphate, was collected by centrifugation, ressuspended in water, and applied to a Sephacryl S-200 column (2.5 x 65 cm) previously equilibrated with 50 mM sodium phosphate buffer, pH 6.8 containing 1 mM EDTA and 300 mM sodium chloride. The fractions containing AG were pooled and dialysed for 12 h against 3 L of 20 mM Tris-HCl buffer, pH 8.4 containing 1 mM EDTA. After dialysis, the solution was applied to a DEAE-cellulose column (2.5 x 8.0 cm). The proteins eluted from the column by a sodium chloride gradient and the fractions containing AG appeared at 100 mM of the salt. When this material was incubated with 10 µg of human renal renin in 0.2 M sodium phosphate buffer, pH 6.0, containing 8.0 mM EDTA, 2.0 mM 8-hydroxyquinoline and 8.0 mM PMSF, yielded 21.2 µg of angiotensin I/mg of protein.

Tonin activity

Tonin activity was determined by incubating the sample (hSMT) either with 75 µM angiotensin I, 75 µM AG(1-14) or 420 µg of AG in a final volume of 250 µL of the following 0.1 M buffer solutions: sodium acetate, pH 4.0 for Ang I, sodium phosphate, pH 7.0 for AG(1-14) and Tris-HCl, pH 8.0 for AG. The mixture was incubated at 37° C for 60 min with angiotensin I or AG(1-14) and 18 h with AG. The reaction was terminated by adding 10 µL of 6 M HCl and the generated angiotensin II determined by RIA. Alternatively, the reaction was terminated by adding 100 µL of 20% TFA and the incubates applied on a reversed phase column in a HPLC system being the fractions analysed by RIA and biological assay.

To determine the effect of proteinase inhibitors, the enzyme was incubate with AG(1-14) as substrate in the absence and in the presence of the following inhibitors: EDTA (10 mM), enalaprilat (10 µM) or PMSF (1.6-20 mM).

The buffer solutions for optimun pH determinations were: 0.2 M sodium acetate pHs 5.0 and 5.5, 0.2 M sodium phosphate pHs 6.0, 6.5, 7.0 and 7.5 or 0.2 M Tris-HCl pHs 8.0, 8.5 and 9.0.

Biological assay

Bioassay was performed as described by Feitosa et al. [11], utilizing an isolated rat uterus. Isotonic contractions were recorded with a frontal writing lever and the oxytocic effect of samples were compared to those of synthetic standards of angiotensin II. The angiotensin II response was characterized by specific inhibition with 0.2 µM saralasin.

High performance liquid chromatography

The incubates, after addition of 20% TFA were filtered and applied on a MinoRPC column in a HPLC system. Peptides were eluted with a linear gradient of 3.7%/min of acetonitrile in 1% TFA.

Electrophoresis

Polyacrylamide gel electrophoresis was performed at pH 8.3 in 7.5% acrylamide gels with 0.1% SDS [12]. Samples (2-10 µg of protein) were prepared in buffer containing 2.9% 2-mercaptoethanol, 2.9% SDS and 5.8% glycerol. Gels were stained with silver nitrate. The molecular weight markers were BSA (Mr 67,000), ovalbumin (Mr 45,000), carbonic anhydrase (Mr 29,000) and SBTI (Mr 20,100).

RESULTS

One enzyme presenting angiotensin II generating activity was obtained after Mono Q chromatography. This enzyme presents tonin activity as evidenced by the ability of generating angiotensin II from angiotensin I, AG(1-14) and from AG and therefore was designated human submandibular tonin (hSMT). The enzyme was purified by a two chromatographic steps as showed in the figure 1. The enzyme appeared to be homogeneous by SDS-polyacrylamide gel electrophoresis (Fig. 2) and to have molecular weigh of 110,000. Under reduced conditions, tree protein bands with molecular weights of 60,000, 50,000 and 20,000 were detected. The results of the purification procedure are summarized in the table 1.

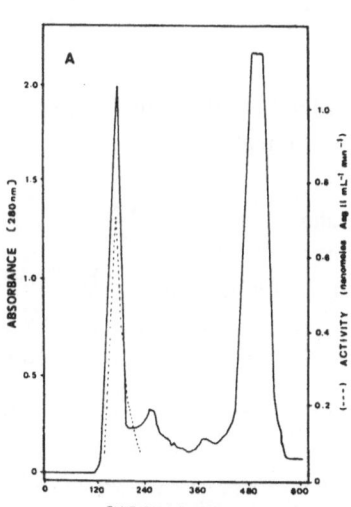
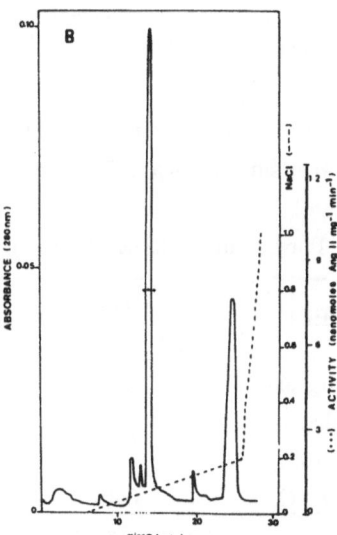

Figure 1. A) Gel filtration on Sephadex G-100. Samples were eluted at a flow rate of 12 mL/h, being collected fractions of 4.0 mL. B) Ionic exchange chromatography on a Mono Q column of the material from Sephadex G-100 chromatography. Activity determined by angiotensin II RIA utilizing AG(1-14) as substrate.

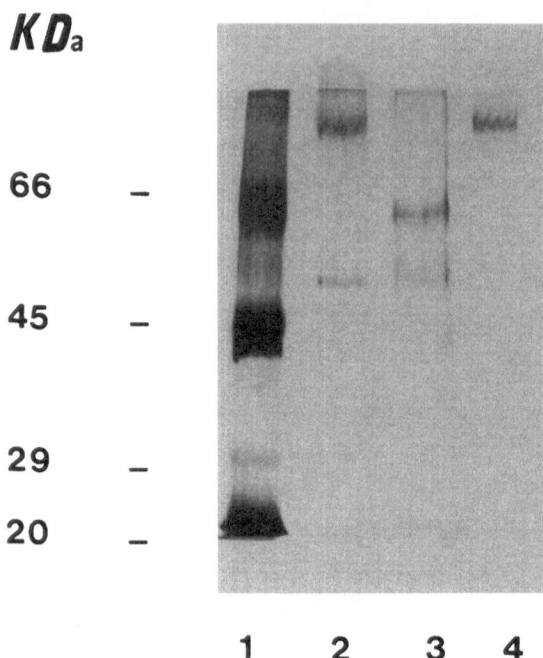

Figure 2. SDS-polyacrylamide gel electrophoresis of molecular weight markers (lane 1) and hSMT with (lane 3) or without (lane 4) 2-mercaptoethanol.

As can be seen in this table, the total tonin activity per gram of tissue, determined utilizing AG(1-14) as substrate was 2.72 nanomoles of angiotensin II per minute.

Table 1. Purification of hSMT from 1 g of submandibular gland

PROCEDURE	TOTAL ACTIVITY*	SPECIFIC ACTIVITY#	PURIFICATION	RECOVERY (%)
Homogenate	2.72	141	1	100
Sephadex G-100	1.29	295	2.1	47.3
Mono Q	0.46	8,050	57	16.8

* nanomoles of angiotensin II/min, # picomoles of angiotensin II/ min/mg of protein, determined by RIA using AG(1-14) as substrate.

The product released from the tree substrates tested was angiotensin II as evidenced by RIA associated to HPLC (Fig. 3).

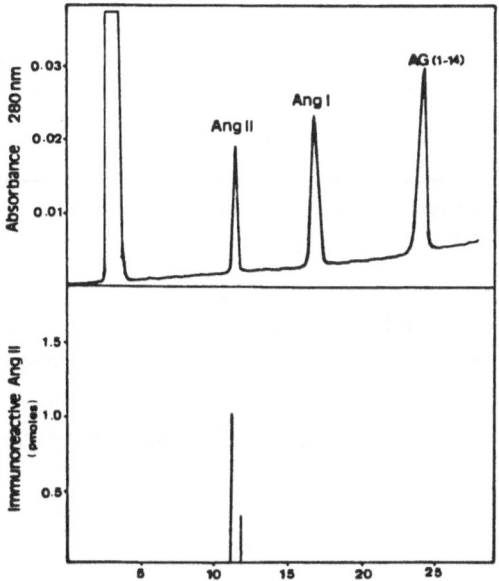

Figure 3. HPLC elution profiles of A) synthetic standards angiotensin I (Ang I), angiotensin II (Ang II) and AG(1-14), B) angiotensin II immunoreactivity of the fractions from hSMT-AG incubate, determined by RIA.

This product showed oxytocic activity which was inhibited by saralasin, an antagonist of angiotensin II (Fig. 4).

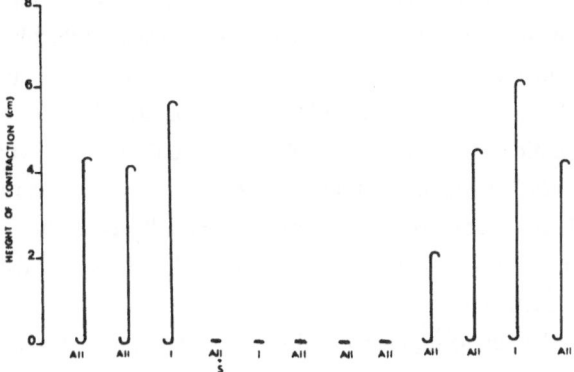

Figure 4. Effect of 0.2 µM saralasin (S) on the contraction induced by 0.73 nM angiotensin II (AII) or hSMT-AG incubate (I).

The specific activities and the pH optima for the action of hSMT upon the tree substrates are shown in the table 2.

Table 2. Physicochemical parameters for the action of hSMT upon different substrates

SUBSTRATE	SPECIFIC ACTIVITY*	pH OPTIMA
Angiotensin I	1.80	4.0
AG(1-14)	8.05	7.0
AG	34	8.0

* Amount of angiotensin II/min/mg of protein, expressed in nanomoles for angiotensin I and AG(1-14) or picomoles for AG.

The effect of proteinase inhibitors upon the activity of hSMT was tested using AG(1-14) as substrate. The enzyme was inhibited by PMSF a serine proteinase inhibitor but not by enalaprilat and EDTA, inhibitors of the angiotensin converting enzyme.
The activity of hSMT was inhibited 36, 76 and 85% by PMSF at concentrations 1.6, 12 and 20 mM, respectively.

DISCUSSION

An enzyme with angiotensin II generating activity was obtained from human submandibular gland. This enzyme, designated hSMT, is a tonin-like since it liberate angiotensin II from angiotensin I, AG(1-14) or from human AG. It is inhibited by PMSF but not by quelating inhibitors, so it is an enzyme of the serine proteinase family. hSMT presents different properties from rat submandibular gland tonins. Its estimated molecular weight is approximately 110,000 which under reducing conditions is separated into three polipeptide chains having molecular weights of 60, 50 and 20 kDa. This separation of the polipeptide chains by 2-mercaptoethanol indicated that they are linked by disulfide bonds. The pH aptima for AG and AG(1-14) hydrolysis 7.0 and 8.0 respectively, are close to that observed for rat tonin, however, for angiotensin I, optimum pH 4.0, is very different. It seens that the approximation of the negative charge of C-terminal end to the bond attacked by hSMT in the angiotensin I affects the interaction with the enzyme.

In the rat, the submandibular gland contains the highest levels of tonin. The total tonin activity observed in the human submandibular gland is approximatelly 5,000-times smaller than that of the rat gland [2]. The specific activities for hydrolysis of angiotensin I and AG(1-14), obtained with hSMT, at optima pH, are 1000- and 550-times smaller than that observed for rat tonin [2]. For the AG, we observed that hSMT is 2-times more active to liberate angiotensin II when compared to rat tonin acting upon rat AG [2]. This results show that the structural conformation of the AG is more important for human tonin.

Studies are undertaken in our laboratories in order to provide a better physicochemical and biological characterization of hSMT.

ACKNOWLEDGEMENTS

The competent technical assistance of Mercia P. Lima is gratefully acknowledged. This work was supported by grants from UFMG research Council (PRPq/UFMG), FINEP and FAPEMIG.

REFERENCES

1. Grisé C, Boucher R, Thibault G, Genest J. Formation of angiotensin II by tonin from partially purified human angiotensinogen. Can J Biochem 1981; 59:250-5.

2. Araujo GW, Pesquero JB, Lindsey CJ, Paiva ACM, Pesquero JL. Identification of serine proteinases with tonin-like activity in the rat submandibular and prostate glands. Biochim Biophys Acta 1991; 1074:167-71.

3. Woodley-Miller C, Chao J, Chao L. Identification of tonin in brain and exocrine tissues and in the cell-free translation products encoded by the mRNA of these tissues. Biochem J 1987; 248:477-81.

4. Johansen L, Berg T, Bergundhaugen H, Nustad K, Scicli AG, Carretero OA. Excess antibody immunoassay for measurement of tonin in rat tissues and plasma. J Immunonol Methods 1987; 98:257-65.

5. Thibault G, Genest J. Tonin, an esteroprotease from rat submaxillary glands. Biochim Biophys Acta 1981; 660:23-9.

6. Watt KWK, Lee PJ, M'Timkulu T, Chan WP, Loor R. Human prostate specific antigen: Structural and functional similarity with serine proteases. Proc Natl Acad Sci USA 1986; 83:3166-70.

7. Clements JA. The glandular kallikrein family of enzymes: Tissue-specific expression and hormonal regulation. Endocr Rev 1989; 10:393-419.

8. Vieira JGH, Noguti KO, Rosso EMK, Maciel RMB. Radioimmunoassay for the measurements of plasma renin activity: technical aspects. Rev Bras Pat Clin 1981; 17:195-200.

9. Rodbard D, Bridson W, Rayford PL. Rapid calculation of radioimmunoassay results. J Lab Clin Med 1969; 74:770-7.

10. Shinagawa T, Do Y-S, Tam H, Hsueh WA. Complete purification of human renal renin and sequence of the amino terminus. Biochem Biophys Res Commun 1986; 139:446-54.

11. Feitosa MH, Pesquero JL, Ferreira MAD, Oliveira GM, Rogana E, Beraldo WT. Tonin and kallikrein-kinin system. Adv Exp Med Biol 1989; 247A:573-80.

12. Laemmli UK. Cleavage of Structural proteins during the assembly of the head of bacteriophage T4. Nature (Lond) 1970; 227:680-5.

AAS 38/I
Recent Progress on Kinins
© 1992 Birkhäuser Verlag Basel

LOCALIZATION AND CHARACTERIZATION OF HUMAN SALIVARY KININASES

G. Porcelli[1], R. Raffaelli[2], A. Sacchi[2], A.R. Volpe[1] and C. Miani[2]

Center of Receptors Chemistry of the National Research Council (C.N.R.) and Institute of Chemistry[1],Medical Faculty of Catholic University, and School of Dentistry[2],Catholic University, Largo Francesco Vito 1, 00168 Rome,Italy

SUMMARY: The human saliva of normal subjects containing large amounts of basic carboxypeptidase produces decarboxylated non inflammatory peptides, for instance, kinins and anaphilotoxins C3a, C4a and C5a. A reduction of epithelial cell-bonded enzyme (carboxypeptidase M-type or kininase I), produces inflammations by the active intact kinins and the initiation of the alternative activating pathway of complement by active anaphilotoxins, which generate complement cleavage products,containing potential destructive mechanism.

INTRODUCTION

Kinins produce four cardinal signs of inflammation and it has been suggested that they may act as chemical mediators in inflammatory reactions[1]. The amount of kinins in an area at one time depends on the available amount of kinin-forming (kallikrein) and of the kinin-inactivating (kininases) present enzymes .

Using biological assay,a correlation was observed between the rate of bradykinin inactivation in human saliva and periodontal status of examined subjects . The inactivation proceeded at a more rapid rate in a group with definite signis of periodontal disease than in an apparently "normal"group[2].

When the human complement system (a defense mechanism of the host against foreign substances) is activated by immune complexes or by endotoxins, it produces enzymes with potent biological activity[3]. It is known that complement cascade induces chemotactic effect on polymorphonuclear leucocytes, which can release proteolytic enzymes and subsequently cause in turn cell lysis, and tissue destruction. In addition, oral complement activation causes degranulation of mast cells, increases vascular permeability andtimulatessteoclasticboneesorption[4]. Since tissue damage and bone destruction are the primary characteristics of periodontal diseases, complement activation may be considered the initial factor in periodontitis.

Carboxypeptidase M[5,6] and dipeptidyldipeptidases are the most important inactivators of kinins. Carboxypeptidase M is the arginine-carboxypeptidase (E.C.3.4.17.7) that cleaves the basic C-terminal amino acids, including the arginine (Arg) C-terminal sequence of bradykinin (BK), and the lisine (Lys) and Arg C-terminal sequences of anaphilotoxins C3a, C4a and C5a peptides, that activate the complement system. Kininases are also the dipeptidyldipeptidases (E.C.3.4.15.1) that inactivates bradykinin (BK) by cleaving the C-terminal dipeptide phenylalanylarginine (Phe-Arg), identical to the angiotensin I converting-enzyme (ACE) and neutral dipeptidase enzyme which inactives enkephalines[7].

Using incubation with shaking[2] can induce in human saliva an increase of kininase activity.

The purpose of the present study is to demonstrate that a quantitative analysis of carboxypeptidase M-type and dipeptidyldipeptidase, in diluted salivary samples, dialyzed and incubated under determinate conditions, may permit the differentiation of normal from pathological saliva.

MATERIALS AND METHODS

Fourteen subjects with relatively normal dentition and twelve patients with periodondal disease were studied. In order to determine the validity of data and to check variations among subjects, individual saliva samples from each volunteer were collected and assayed (three tests for each sample). The morning salivary samples of donors were taken before breakfast, smoking and brushing of teeth. The samples (0.5-1.0 ml) were collected in sterile polystyrene test tubes fitted with plastic caps and immediately frozen at - 20°C.

When salivary sample were thawed for determination of basic carboxipeptidase and dipeptidildipeptidase, a 0.5 ml aliquot of each homogeneous samples was diluted to 2.5 ml with 0.01 M TRIS-HCl, pH 7.0, and underwent overnight dialysis with magnetic stirring at 5°C against the same buffer (2 lt per 5 ml of saliva).

A 0.2 ml-aliquot of a diluted and dialyzed sample, preincubated for ten min with shaking in a water bath at 37°C, was added to 0.070 ml of a solution containing 5 mg of hippurylphenylalanylarginine (Hip-Phe-Arg) in 5 ml of 0.1 M TRIS-HCl pH 7.0 and incubated with shaking for 15 min at the same temperature. The reaction was stopped adding a mixture of 0.500 ml of acetonitrile:H_2SO_4 pH 3.0 (1:1) and 0.230 ml of 0.05 M TRIS-HCl pH 7.0.

Successively, the samples were purified of sediment, macromolecules, peptides, amino acids and substrate excess in a small pasteur column (0.3x1 cm) of AG-50W-X8, H^+ form, equilibrated with acetonitrile/H_2SO_4 (1:1). A 0.2 ml aliquot of the purified liquid,corresponding to 0.004 ml of the original salivary samples,was used for the HPLC analysis.

Quantification of separated hippurylphenylalanyl (Hip-Phe) and hippuric acid (Bz-Gly), formed respectively by caarboxypeptidase M and dipeptidyldipeptidases from the Hip-Phe-Arg substrate, was accomplished by using a peak height of 230 nm, according to 8.

The HPLC assay procedure, at the flow rate of 1.3 ml/min., was performed with ODS column equilibrated in water phase solution of H_2SO_4 at pH=3.0, eluted acenitrile/H_2SO_4 = (1:1) and washed with acetonitrile/H_2SO_4 = (8:2).

For the evaluation of oral health status 26 subjects were classified by dental investigators into three groups on the basis of a clinical dental examination and evaluation of x-rays.They were classified using the following scores: (' =normal or apparently normal oral conditions; 1 = gingivitis in localized areas or generalized marginal gingivitis with no evidence of bone loss or pocket formations; 2 = periodontitis with slight evidence of bone loss (horizzontal bone resorption <1,3 cm of root length).

RESULTS

The control of incubation and enzymatic reaction products (Hip-Phe and Bz-Gly) with and without incubated salivary samples were examined according to the method described in (8). The other results are summarized in three Tables.

Table 1 shows that the dialysis of salivary samples produces a significant increase of carboxypeptidase M and a not significant decrease of dipeptidyldipeptidase activity.

Table 1. Dialisis effects on carboxipeptidase M (Hip-Phe) and dipeptidase (Bz-Gly). The values represent the mean derived from the three samples preparations for each subjects examined.

Subjects	BEFORE DIALISIS		AFTER DIALISIS	
	Hip-Phe	Bz-Gly	Hip-Phe	Bz-Gly
No. 11	0.022±0.011	0.013±0.006	0.043±0.021	0.008±0.005

Significant decrease of carboxypeptidase M values after dialysis (p<0.05)

Table 2 demonstrates that centrifugation does not produce variations of dipeptidildases, while carboxypeptidase M activity is significant decreased.

Table 2. The effect of centrifugation on salivary samples. The enzymatic values represent the mean of three determinations.

Subjects	SAMPLE SUPERNATANTS		INTEGRAL SAMPLES	
	Hip-Phe	Bz-Gly	Hip-Phe	Bz-Gly
No. 11	0.004	0.009	0.432	0.009

Significant decrease of carboxipeptidase M activity (p<0.0001 after salivary sample.

The examination of kininases of each subjects,reported in Table 3, were performed after several determination. The study revealed large differences in carboxypeptidase M and dipeptidyldipeptidase activity among the subjects. In the 26 examined, kininase activities in saliva were correlated with the periodontal status of each partecipant.

Table 3. Enzymatic activity of subiects with dentition. Formation of Hip-Phe and Bz-Gly from Hip-Phe-Arg substrate. The values are reproduced in mmoli of hydrolized substrate per ml of saliva and per min of incubation.

Subject No.	Hip-Phe	Bz-Gly
1 (6)	0.031±0.026	0.013±0.100
2 (6)	0.017±0.049	0.009±0.003
0 (14)	0.060±0.024	0.013±0.007

The decrease of carboxipeptidase M activity in groups (1) and (2) in comparison to group (0) is significant (p<0.0001).

Carboxypeptidase M (sometimes also dipeptidyldipeptidase) values were significantly increased in normal subjects and in a single donor with gingivitis, whereas the other patients with gingivitis had lower carboxypeptidase and dipeptidyldipeptidase levels of activity, similar to the donors having levis periodontitis.

Carboxypeptidase M and dipeptidyldipeptidase activities increase proportionally with saliva concentration. With the incubation time,the kinetics of both enzymes after 15 min.appears prograssively inhibited. Using the Lineweaver-Burk method, the km values related to carboxypeptidase and dipeptidyldipeptidases of human saliva were respectively found to be 5.8×10^{-8} M and 6.05×10^{-7} M.

DISCUSSION

With biological assay all salivary kininase activity was found to be associated with sediment containing cellular elements[9]. In that study was demonstrated that the rate of bradykinin inactivation was accelerated by disintegration of desquamated epithelial cells from the oral mucous membranes. Previously[11] was observed that saliva of subjects with clinically active periodontitis contained a greater number of epithelial cells than the saliva of subjects without periodontal disease.

A correlation between the rate of bradykinin inactivation by saliva and periodontal status was observed[8]. In addition the rapid rate of bradykinin inactivation in patients with increasing severity of periodontal diseases was thought to be due to increased kininase activity with an increased number of damaged epithelial cells, serous exudates, blood, leucocytes and bacteria.

From preliminary studies[3,10] were found reduced levels of native complement C3 and increased amounts of the corresponding C3c product in gingivial fluid obtained from patients with severe periodontitis.

The conclusions of these studies suggested that complement activation may be an important mechanism in the local inflammatory process occurring in periodontal diseases. Utilizing special paper filter strips for sampling and multilayer crossed immunoelectrophoresis for assays,was demonstrated an incresed amout of complement cleavage products in single sites with minimal inflammation[11].

From Table 3 it is evident that the carboxypeptidase M and the dipeptidyldipeptidases are present in high amounts in the saliva of "normal" subjects and are significantly decreased in subjects having mild periodontal disease and by gingivitis. In addition, it has been observed that uniform the sampling of saliva and successive dialysis of diluted samples are essential to obtain very significant differences between "normal" and pathological salivary carboxypeptidase M values. The kinetics of both carboxypeptidase and dipeptidyldipeptidases, using the incubation with shaking appearedto be progressively inhibited after 15 minutes.

Carboxypeptidase M has been proposed to serve as a regulator of the action of various physiologically active peptides such C3a, C4a, C5a anaphilotoxins, kinins, fibrinopeptides and the plasmin-degradation products of fibrin by the removal of the C-terminal basic amino acid.

From our results,using the incubation with shaking, it appears that bonded carboxypeptidase M to solid phase of saliva in apparently "normal"subjects reaches its maximum enzymatic values, and the lower enzymatic values, corresponding to pathological oral liquids.

If the assay of C3c, C4c and C5c products of complement is most important to localize minimal inflammation area, the salivary carboxypeptidase activity should have diagnostic value of transient or irreversible oral inflammation.

ACKNOWLEDGMENTS

This work was supported by grant of CNR (Progetto Finalizzato Chimica Fine II).

REFERENCES

1. D.F. Elliot, E .W. Horton and G.P. Lewis. Actions of pure bradykinin. J. Physiol. 1960; 153: 473
2. J. Tonzetich, E. Eigen, A.R. Volpe and S. Weiss. Relationship of salivary kininase activity to periodontal status in humans. J. Periodontal. Res. 1969; 4: 118
3. H.A. Schenkein and R.J. Genco. Gingival fluid and serum in periodontal diseases. J . Periodontal.1977; 48: 772
4. H. A. Schenkein. In: Host-Parasite Interactions in Periodontal Disease. R. T. Genco and S.E Mergenhaben editors. Washington: American Society for Microbiology Press1982:299
5. R.A. Skidgel. Basic carboxypeptidase: regulators of peptide hormone activity. Trends Pharmacol. Sci. 1988; 9:299.
6. R. A. Skidgel, R. M. Davis, F. Tan. Carboxipeptidase M: purification and characterization of membrane-bound carboxypeptidase that cleaves peptide hormone. J. Biol. Chem. 1989; 264: 2236.
7. E.G. Erdos. In: Hand. Exp. Pharmacol.. E.G. Erdos editor.Springer-Verlag Berlin, Heidelberg, New York 1979: 427.
8. G. Porcelli, M. Di Iorio, A.R. Volpe. Determination of kininase I and kininase II activities in human urine. J. Chromatogr. 1989; 414: 423
9. E. Amundsen and K. Nustad. Kininase activity in human saliva. Nature 1964; 201: 1226.
10. R. Attstrom, A.B. Laurel, U. Lahsson and P.A. Ward. Complement factors in gingival crevice material from heath and inflammed gingiva in human . J. Periodontal. Res.1975;10:19.
11. C.E. Niekrash and M.R. Patters. Assessment of complement cleavage in gingival fluid in human with and without periodontal disease.J. Periodontal. Res. 1986; 21: 233.

AAS 38/I
Recent Progress on Kinins
© 1992 Birkhäuser Verlag Basel

HUMAN SERUM CARBOXYPEPTIDASE U: A NEW KININASE ?

Dirk Hendriks, Wei Wang, Marc van Sande and Simon Scharpé

Laboratory of Medical Biochemistry, Department of Pharmaceutical Sciences, University of Antwerp, Universiteitsplein 1 , B-2610 Wilrijk, Belgium

SUMMARY

A carboxypeptidase capable of cleaving basic amino acids from synthetic peptide substrates is present in fresh human serum, and not in human heparinized plasma. Its activity is generated during the process of coagulation. Because of its instability at room temperature and at 37°C, we named it "unstable carboxypeptidase" (carboxypeptidase U, CPU). The enzymatically active subunit of carboxypeptidase U was purified and exhibits a single band at 53 kDa on SDS-PAGE.

INTRODUCTION

Carboxypeptidase N (arginine carboxypeptidase, kininase I, anaphylatoxin-inactivator, serum carboxypeptidase B, EC 3.4.17.3) is a 280,000 M_r tetrameric enzyme present in human serum. It cleaves carboxyterminal arginine and lysine from various peptides. Some of the most interesting substrates for this enzyme are the kinins bradykinin and kallidin (1), the anaphylatoxins C_{3a}, C_{4a} C_{5a} (2,3), the fibrinopeptides 6A and 6D (4), the creatine-kinase MM-isoenzyme (5,6), the hexapeptide enkephalins (7) and the atrial natriuretic peptide atriopeptin II (8). Important differences in arginine carboxypeptidase activities between fresh serum, on the one hand, and older serum or heparinized plasma on the other, depending on the substrate used have been observed (9). We suggested the presence of an arginine carboxy-peptidase in fresh human serum, which differed from carboxypeptidase N in terms of substrate specificity with peptide substrates, esterase activity, pH optimum, and influence of various inhibitors and activators and named this activity CPU-activity, which stands for unstable carboxypeptidase activity (10).

Partially purified carboxypeptidase U has an apparent molecular weight of 435 kDa and proved to be very difficult to purify due to its instability characteristics (11). In this report we describe the purification of the enzymatically active subunit of carboxypeptidase U.

MATERIALS AND METHODS

Chemicals

Hippuryl-L-arginine and hippuryl-L-lysine were from Bachem Feinchemicalien (Bubendorf, Switzerland). HEPES was purchased from Calbiochem (La Jolla, CA). Diisopropylfluorophosphate (DFP) and human serum albumin were obtained from Sigma Chemical Company (St. Louis, MO). Arginine-Sepharose 4B, DEAE-Sepharose, Sephacryl S-300 and S-100, Mono-Q Sepharose, and molecular weight standard proteins were obtained from Pharmacia (Uppsala, Sweden). Hippuryl-L-argininic acid was kindly provided by Dr. Yehuda Levin of the Weizmann Institute of Science, Rehovot, Israël. *o*-Methylhippuric acid was synthesized from glycine and *o*-methylbenzoylchloride (UCB, Drogenbos, Belgium) by a procedure analogous to that used for the synthesis of hippuric acid (12). All other reagents used were of high purity grade and were from Merck (Darmstadt, FRG).

Instruments

The pipetting of serum samples and reagents was performed with a Dilutrend dispenser (Boehringer, Mannheim, FRG). The high pressure liquid chromatography system consisted of a 303 solvent delivery system, an 802 C manometric module, a model 231-401 autosampling injector (all from Gilson, Paris, France), an LKB 2140 diode-array UV detector (LKB, Bromma, Sweden), and a 100 x 8 mm (i.d.) C18 reversed-phase µ-Bondapak column fitted in a radial compression module (Millipore, Brussels, Belgium). The FPLC™-system (Fast Protein Liquid Chromatography), the SMART™-system, the columns for ion-exchange chromatography, gel permeation chromatography and affinity chromatography, and the ExcelGel™ for SDS-PAGE electrophoresis were obtained from Pharmacia (Uppsala, Sweden). Proteins were concentrated with Centricon-10 (Amicon, Danvers, MA) and Microsep-10 (Filtron, Northborough, MA) concentrators. Dialysis sacks (30 x 2.1 cm) were from Sigma Chemical Company (St. Louis, MO).

Enzyme assays

The enzyme activities with the substrates hippuryl-L-arginine and hippuryl-L-lysine were determined by a high pressure liquid chromatography assisted assay as described elsewhere (13), with the following modifications: the buffered substrate solutions were both prepared at pH 8.0 (pH measurements were made at room temperature, 18-21°C) and the incubation time was 30 min. The esterase activity, determined with the substrate hippuryl-argininic acid, was measured as follows: to 40 μl of substrate solution (10 mmol/l hippuryl-argininic acid, 50 mmol/l HEPES, pH 8.0) was added 10 μl of the sample; this mixture was incubated for 10 min at 37°C and the reaction was stopped with 50 μl 1 mol/l HCL. After addition of 10 μl of the internal standard *o*-methylhippuric acid, the hippuric acid was extracted and determined by liquid chromatography (13). Triplicate determinations were performed for all enzyme assays.

Protein determinations

Protein was measured with the Pierce BCA Protein Assay (Pierce Chemical Company, Rockford, IL). Human serum albumin was used as the standard.

Enzyme purifications

Carboxypeptidase N was purified from outdated human serum and carboxypeptidase U from fresh human serum as described before (11). The enzymatically active subunit of carboxypeptidase N was purified according to the procedure originally described by Levin et al. (14).

To obtain the enzymatically active subunit of human carboxypeptidase U, the following procedure was followed. Carboxypeptidase U in fresh human serum - containing 1 mmol/l diisopropylfluorophosphate - was separated from carboxypeptidase N by means of ion - exchange chromatography on DEAE-sepharose as described before (11). Fractions containing the CPU activity were concentrated on a Centriprep-10 concentrator and then loaded onto a Sephacryl S-300 column (1.6 x 65 cm) at a flow rate of 0.5 ml/min and eluted with Tris 20 mmol/l , NaCl 100 mmol/l , pH 7.4. Enzymatically active fractions are concentrated with Centriprep-10 concentrators to a volume of 2 ml. Guanidinium hydrochloride was added to a concentration of 3 mol/l and this solution was left at 4°C during 1 hour before applying it on a Sephacryl S-100 column (1.6 x 60 cm). The enzyme was eluted at a flow rate of 0.5 ml/min with Tris 20 mM, NaCl 100 mM, pH 7.4. Fractions containing CPU activity were pooled and applied onto a Mono-Q Sepharose column (0.16 x 5 cm) at a flow rate of 0.1 ml/min using the SMART™ protein purification system. Proteins were eluted in a linear gradient from 0 to 300 mmol/l NaCl in Tris 20 mmol/l pH 7.8. Fractions of 0.1 ml were collected. The fractions containing CPU activity were evaluated with SDS-PAGE using standard procedures from the manufacturer. All purification steps are performed at 4°C.

RESULTS AND DISCUSSION

It proved to be very difficult to purify intact carboxypeptidase U from fresh human serum due to the marked instability of the enzyme (11). The partially purified CPU has an apparent molecular weight of 435 kDa and therefore seems to be composed of subunits. In an effort to separate the subunits by using high concentrations of guanidinium hydrochloride, we noticed that the active subunits of carboxypeptidase U eluted after about one column volume using gelfiltration on Sephacryl media. This suggests a hydrofobic interaction between CPU subunits and the gelfiltration medium, as is the case for the active subunits of CPN (14). By using the above conditions, we were able to increase their purification of CPU subunits dramatically. The specific activity of the active subunits after this purification step is about 1500 times higher than the specific activity in fresh human serum. Still a number of contaminant proteins are present in the purified sample as was observed by SDS-PAGE. By applying this purified sample on Mono-Q Sepharose (Fig. 1), determining carboxypeptidase U activity in the fractions and performing SDS-PAGE electrophoresis with subsequent silver staining on each fraction, we were able to attribute the CPU activity to a single band at 53 kDa (Fig. 2).

The purified carboxypeptidase U subunit still exhibits the same differences in substrate specificity in comparison with the active subunit of carboxypeptidase N (Table 1) similar to the differences observed using the intact enzymes (11).

Table 1. Substrate specificity of carboxypeptidase N and carboxypeptidase U active subunit

	CPN-subunit	CPU-subunit
Hip-Arg (U/l)	19.1	32.4
Hip-Lys (U/l)	74.6	41.0
Lys/Arg ratio	3.9	1.3
Hip-Argininic acid (U/l)	160	< 5

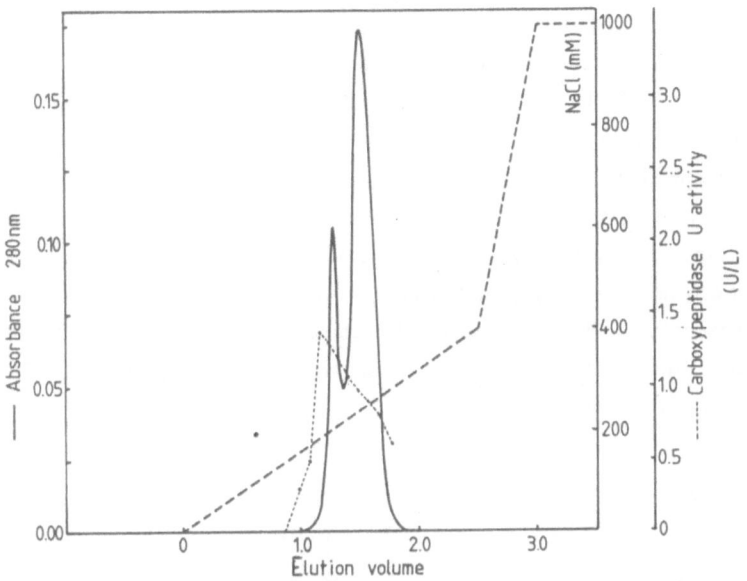

Fig. 1. Mono-Q-Sepharose chromatography of carboxypeptidase U subunits.

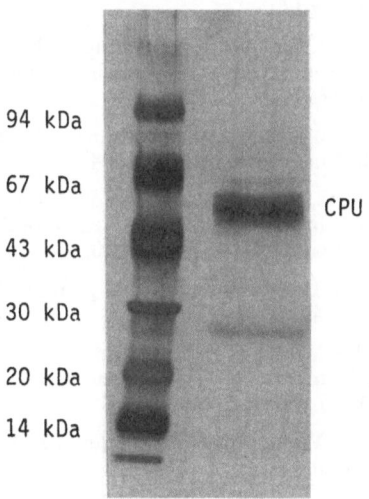

Fig. 2. SDS-polyacrylamide gel electrophoresis of the purified carboxypeptidase U subunit.
Left lane : molecular weight marker proteins; right lane : purified carboxypeptidase U subunit.

Purified carboxypeptidase U is also able to transform bradykinin to des-Arg^9-bradykinin (unpublished results). The presence of carboxypeptidase U is in agreement with the observations of Sheikh & Kaplan (15) who found that the degradation of bradykinin to des-Arg^9-bradykinin was slower in plasma compared to serum. Also in agreement with our findings are the results of Campbell et al. (16) who found an arginine specific carboxypeptidase in blood which is derived from plasma components and unrelated to carboxypeptidase N. Recently a plasminogen-binding 60 kDa protein was isolated from human plasma which proved to be an inactive precursor of a new carboxypeptidase which was named plasma carboxypeptidase B, a name which is very confusing because this name is also used to designate carboxypeptidase N (17). It will be interesting to find out if this carboxypeptidase is homologous or identical with carboxypeptidase U active subunit.

REFERENCES

1. Erdös, E.G. (1979) In: Bradykinin, Kallidin and Kallikrein, Handbook of Experimental Pharmacology (Erdös,E.G., ed) Vol.25 (Suppl), 427-487.

2. Bokish, V.A.& Müller-Eberhard, H.J. Anaphylatoxin inactivator of human plasma : its isolation and characterization as a carboxypeptidase. J Clin Invest 1970; 49 : 2427-2436.

3. Hugli, T., Gerard, C., Kawahara, M., Scheetz, M., Barton, R., Bruggs, S., Koppel, G. & Russell, S. Isolation of three separate anaphylatoxins from complement-activated human serum. Mol Cell Biochem 1981; 41 : 59-66.

4. Belew, M., Gerdin, B., Lindeberg, G., Porath, J, & Wallin, R. Structural-activity relationships of vasoactive peptides derived from fibrin or fibriongen degraded by plasmin. Biochim Biophys Acta 1980; 621: 169-178.

5. Perryman, M., Knell, D.& Roberts, R. Molecular mechanism for the production of multiple forms of MM creatine kinase. Clin Chem 1984; 30: 662-664.

6. Hendriks, D., Soons, J., Scharpé, S., Wevers, R., van Sande, M. & Holmquist, B. Identification of the carboxypeptidase responsible for the post-synthetic modification of creatine kinase in human serum. Clin Chim Acta 1988; 172: 253-260.

7. Skidgel, R.A., Johnson, A.R. & Erdös, E.G. Hydrolysis of opioid peptides by carboxypeptidase N. Biochem Pharmacol 1984; 33: 3471-3478.

8. Hendriks, D., Verkerk, R., Vanhoof, G., De Meester , I., van Sande, M., & Scharpé, S. Release of the carboxyterminal arginine from atriopeptin II by human plasma carboxypeptidase N. Biochem Soc Trans 1987; 16: 359-360.

9. Hendriks, D., Scharpé, S., Lommaert, M.P., Wang, W. & van Sande, M. A labile enzyme in fresh human serum interferes with the assay of carboxypeptidase N. Clin Chem 1989; 35:177.

10. Hendriks, D., Scharpé, S., van Sande, M. & Lommaert,M.P. Characterisation of a carboxypeptidase in human serum distinct from carboxypeptidase N. J Clin Chem Clin Biochem 1989; 27 : 277-285.

11. Hendriks, D., Wang, W., Scharpé, S., Lommaert, M. & van Sande M. Purification and characterization of a new arginine carboxypeptidase in human serum. Biochim Biophys Acta 1990; 1034 : 86-92.

12. Vogel, A.J. (1970) In: Practical Organic Chemistry, Longman, London, 584.

13. Hendriks, D., Scharpé, S. & van Sande, M. Assay of carboxypeptidase N activity in serum by liquid-chromatographic determination of hippuric acid. Clin Chem 1985; 31: 1936-1939.

14. Levin, Y., Skidgel, R.A. & Erdös, E.G. Isolation and characterization of the subunits of human plasma carboxypeptidase N. Proc Natl Acad Sci USA 1982; 79 : 4618-22.

15. Sheikh, J.A. & Kaplan, A.P.The mechanism of degradation of bradykinin in human serum. Biochem Pharmacol 1986; 35 : 1957-1963.

16. Campbell, W. & Okada, H. An arginine specific carboxypeptidase generated in blood during coagulation or inflammation which is unrelated to carboxypeptidase N or its subunits. Biochem Biophys Res Comm 1989; 162 : 933-939.

17. Eaton, D., Malloy, B., Tsai, S., Henzel, W. & Drayna, D. Isolation, molecular cloning, and partial characterization of a novel carboxypeptidase B from human plasma. J Biol Chem 1991; 32 : 21833-21838.

AAS 38/I
Recent Progress on Kinins
© 1992 Birkhäuser Verlag Basel

AMINOPEPTIDASE P: PURIFICATION OF A MEMBRANE-BOUND BRADYKININASE FROM RAT LUNG

Arthur T. Orawski and William H. Simmons

Department of Molecular and Cellular Biochemistry, Loyola University of Chicago Stritch School of Medicine, Maywood, IL 60153 USA

SUMMARY: Aminopeptidase P that hydrolyzes the Arg^1-Pro^2-bond of bradykinin was solubilized from rat lung microsomes using phosphatidylinositol-specific phospholipase C. The enzyme was purified 420-fold by chromatography on decyl-agarose (two steps), ω-aminodecyl-agarose and DEAE-Sephacel. A single stained band was observed following native gradient (4-15%) polyacrylamide gel electrophoresis. Dipeptidylaminopeptidase IV-like activity was also present in the final preparation and co-migrated with aminopeptidase P in the above gel system.

INTRODUCTION

Rat lung microsomes contain aminopeptidase P (aminoacylprolyl-peptide hydrolase) that can hydrolyze bradykinin at the Arg^1-Pro^2 bond (1-4). In the isolated rat lung, aminopeptidase P competes favorably with angiotensin converting enzyme in the degradation of perfused radiolabelled bradykinin (2,4-5). Aminopeptidase P may therefore be a physiologically important kininase with a high specificity for bradykinin (3). We have recently purified aminopeptidase P to homogeneity from bovine lung microsomes and extensively characterized this enzyme (3). This report describes the isolation of aminopeptidase P from rat lung microsomes.

MATERIALS AND METHODS

Enzyme assay: Aminopeptidase P activity was routinely measured using Arg-Pro-Pro as the substrate in a fluorescent assay described previously (3). Bradykinin degradation was determined by an HPLC method (1).

Hydrophobic interaction chromatography: Washed rat lung microsomes were prepared and treated with phosphatidylinositol-specific phospholipase C (Bacillus thurigiensis) (ICN Biomedicals) as previously described (3). Solubilized aminopeptidase P activity was applied at $4^{\circ}C$ to each of several different 2.5 ml prepacked chromatography columns of the series $CH_3-(CH_2)_n-NH$-agarose and $H_2N-(CH_2)_n-NH$-agarose (hydrophobic chromatography media Kits MAA-8 and DAA-8 from Sigma). Columns were equilibrated with 0.1 M potassium phosphate, pH 6.8. The percentage of applied activity which failed to bind to each column (% applied activity in breakthrough fractions) was determined as was the percentage of applied activity which both bound to the column and was elutable with 1 M NaCl in 0.1 M potassium phosphate, pH 6.8.

Enzyme purification: Aminopeptidase P was purified from 83g of rat lung tissue (Sprague-Dawley, 120-lobes) (Pel-Freez) by a modification of the method utilized previously to purify the same enzyme from bovine lung (3). Column chromatography on decyl-agarose (low ionic strength step) and on ω -aminodecyl-agarose were carried out as separate steps rather than sequentially in a single step as previously described. Enzyme collected from each column was concentrated to 200-500µl in the appropriate buffer with Centricon-30 ultrafiltration units prior to application to the next column. The final Centricon-100 ultrafiltration purification step was eliminated. Polyacrylamide gel electrophoresis (PAGE) was performed with a Pharmacia PhastSystem apparatus using Gradient 4-15 PhastGel precast gels under non-denaturing conditions. Gels were developed with silver stain according to the PhastSystem instructions.

RESULTS

Aminopeptidase P activity was associated with extensively washed rat lung
microsomes. When the washed microsomes were incubated with
phosphatidylinositol-specific phospholipase C (PI-PLC) (from Bacillus
thurigiensis) and then centrifuged at 40,000xg for 2 hours, about 70% of the
aminopeptidase P activity was recovered in the supernatant. The observation
that PI-PLC could solubilize aminopeptidase P suggested that the enzyme was
attached to membranes via a glycosyl-phosphatidylinositol anchor.

The ability of PI-PLC-solubilized aminopeptidase P to bind to
hydrophobic interaction chromatography columns at low ionic strength was
evaluated (Table 1).

Table 1.   Behavior of solubilized rat lung aminopeptidase P on hydrophobic
interaction chromatography columns

Column	% Applied Activity in Breakthrough Fractions	% Applied Activity Eluted with 1M NaCl
ethyl-agarose	88	1
propyl-agarose	83	1
butyl-agarose	65	0
pentyl-agarose	45	0
hexyl-agarose	56	0
octyl-agarose	68	0
decyl-agarose	61[a]	0
dodecyl-agarose	0	0
ω-aminoethyl-agarose	79	0
ω-aminopropyl-agarose	84	2
ω-aminobutyl-agarose	65	0
ω-aminopentyl-agarose	77	0
ω-aminohexyl-agarose	53	0
ω-aminooctyl-agarose	82	0
ω-aminodecyl-agarose	2	84[a]
ω-aminododecyl-agarose	22	61

[a] Fraction with the highest specific activity in the hydrophobic
interaction column series.

Two series of hydrophobic interaction column materials were tested. In the $CH_3(CH_2)_n$-NH-agarose series, 45-88% of the applied activity eluted in the breakthrough fractions (except for dodecyl-agarose which bound activity completely). Decyl-agarose (n=9) absorbed a significant amount of contaminating protein so that the specific activity of the breakthrough fractions was higher than for similar fractions from the other columns in the series. In the H_2N-$(CH_2)_n$-NH-agarose series, ω-aminodecyl-agarose absorbed most of the enzyme activity, and much of this bound activity could be subsequently eluted with 1 M NaCl. Both the percent recovery and specific activity of the salt-eluted enzyme were greater for ω-aminodecyl-agarose than for ω-aminododecyl-agarose. These results suggested that decyl-agarose and ω-aminodecyl-agarose might be effective in purifiying rat lung aminopeptidase P as had been the case for bovine lung aminopeptidase P (3).

Table 2. Scheme for purification of aminopeptidase P from rat lung microsomes

Step	Total activity (μmoles/min)	Protein (mg)	Specific activity (μmoles/min/mg)	Recovery (%)	Purification (-fold)
Crude microsomes	19	400	0.048	100	1.0
Washed microsomes	16	220	0.073	84	1.5
PI-PLC[a] treatment of microsomes	11	23	0.48	58	10.
Decyl-agarose	7.5	14	0.54	39	11.
ω-Aminodecyl-agarose	5.3	1.0	5.3	26	110.
Decyl-agarose (0.8 M NaCl)	6.4	0.69	9.3	34	190.
DEAE-Sephacel	6.1	0.31	20	32	420.

[a] phosphatidylinositol-specific phospholipase C from B. thuringiensis.

Table 2 shows the purification scheme developed for rat lung aminopeptidase P. The enzyme was purified 10-fold over crude microsomes by extensive washing of the membranes followed by solubilization with PI-PLC. An additional 10-fold purification was achieved by a combination of decyl-agarose and ω-aminodecyl-agarose hydrophobic interaction chromatography steps. The enzyme was further purified by decyl-agarose in the presence of 0.8 M NaCl and by ion exchange chromatography on DEAE-Sephacel. Aminopeptidase P was purified 420-fold over crude rat lung microsomes with 32% recovery of activity.

Figure 1. Polyacrylamide gel electrophoresis of purified rat lung aminopeptidase P on a native Gradient 4-15 PhastGel. The gel was developed with silver stain.

Polyacrylamide gel electrophoresis (PAGE) of the final enzyme product on native Gradient 4-15 PhastGels revealed a single stained band (Fig. 1). However, when the preparation was incubated with bradykinin, not only was N-terminal arginine removed as expected for aminopeptidase P, but the Pro^2-Pro^3 dipeptide was subsequently released from the bradykinin-2-9 product. Pro-Pro-release was inhibited by diisopropylphosphofluoridate and diprotin A (Ile-Pro-Ile) suggesting that this activity was due to dipeptidylpeptidase IV (1-2).

Gradient PAGE gels were cut into segments and assayed for aminopeptidase P activity (Arg-Pro-Pro as the substrate) and dipeptidylpeptidase IV activity (bradykinin-2-9 as the substrate). Both activities migrated in the gel to the same position which corresponded to the position of the single stained band. Other lung membrane-bound peptidases which can hydrolyze bradykinin or its fragments such as angiotensin converting enzyme, metalloendopeptidase 24.11, aminopeptidase M, and carboxypeptidase M (2) were absent from the final aminopeptidase P preparation.

Aminopeptidase P activity was optimal at pH 7. The release of arginine from both Arg-Pro-Pro and bradykinin was essentially completely inhibited by 1 mM 1,10-phenanthroline, 1 mM p-chloromercuriphenylsulfonic acid, and 4 mM 2-mercaptoethanol.

DISCUSSION

Aminopeptidase P from rat lung microsomes was shown to be attached to membranes via a glycosyl-phosphatidylinositol (GPI) anchor since phosphatidylinositol-specific phospholipase C could solubilize the enzyme from the lung microsomes. Aminopeptidase P from both bovine lung microsomes (3) and from pig kidney cortex membranes (6) have also been shown to be GPI-anchored. In contrast, non-anchored cytosolic and circulating forms of aminopeptidase P have been purified from rat brain (7) and guinea pig serum (8), respectively.

The structures and physical properties of microsomal rat lung and bovine lung aminopeptidase P must be very similar since they behaved similarly on a series of $CH_3(CH_2)_n$-NH-agarose and H_2N-$(CH_2)_n$-NH-agarose hydrophobic interaction columns. Essentially the same protocol was successful in purifying aminopeptidase P from both species (the bovine form to homogeneity (3) and the rat form to high purity but containing some dipeptidylaminopeptidase IV-like activity). Both enzymes failed to bind to decyl-agarose in the presence of either 0 or 0.8 M NaCl while both enzymes bound to ω-aminodecyl-agarose and DEAE-Sephacel and could be eluted from either column with a shallow NaCl gradient (0-0.2 M). Inhibition by 1,10-phenanthroline, p-chloromercuriphenylsulfonic acid, and 2-mercaptoethanol was also common to both enzymes (3).

Current efforts are being directed toward determining whether the dipeptidylpeptidase IV-like activity can be separated from aminopeptidase P or whether the two enzymes might exist as a multimeric complex in the rat.

ACKNOWLEDGEMENTS

This work was funded by USPHS grant RO1 HL45159 and a Loyola University Bane grant (2058). The authors thank Bridget M. Borja for typing the manuscript.

REFERENCES

1.   Orawski AT, Susz JP, Simmons WH. Aminopeptidase P from bovine lung: solubilization, properties, and potential role in bradykinin degradation. Mol Cell Biochem 1987; 75:123-132.

2.   Orawski AT, Susz JP, Simmons WH. Metabolism of bradykinin by multiple coexisting membrane-bound peptidases in lung: techniques for investigating the role of each peptidase using specific inhibitors. Adv Exp Med Biol 1989; 247B:355-364.

3.   Simmons WH, Orawski AT. Membrane-bound aminopeptidase P from bovine lung: its purification, properties, and degradation of bradykinin. J Biol Chem 1992; 267 (in press).

4.   Ryan JW. Peptidase enzymes of the pulmonary vascular surface. Am J Physiol 1989; 257:L53-L60.

5.   Baker CRF Jr., Little AD, Little GH, Canizaro PC, Behal FJ. Kinin metabolism in the perfused ventilated rat lung. I: bradykinin metabolism in a system modeling the normal, uninjured lung. Circ Shock 1991; 33:37-47.

6.   Hooper NM, Hryszko J, Turner AJ. Purification and characterization of pig kidney aminopeptidase P: a glycosyl-phosphatidylinositol-anchored ectoenzyme. Biochem J 1990; 267:509-515.

7.   Harbeck TH, Mentlein R. Aminopeptidase P from rat brain: purification
      and action on bioactive peptides. Eur J Biochem 1991; 198:451-458.

8.   Ryan JW, Valido F, Berryer P, Chung AYK, Ripka JE. Purification and
      characterization of guinea pig serum aminoacylproline hydrolase
      (aminopeptidase P) Biochem Biophys Acta 1991; (in press).

AAS 38/I
Recent Progress on Kinins
© 1992 Birkhäuser Verlag Basel

FURTHER CHARACTERIZATION OF ENDOPEPTIDASE H_2 A SERINE PROTEINASE FROM HUMAN URINE

Casarini, D.E.*; Fellows, C.E.**; Stella, R.C.R.***, Sampaio, C.A.M.***

* Disciplina de Nefrologia, Escola Paulista de Medicina, São Paulo, Brazil
** Laboratoire Aimé - Cotton, CNRS, Orsay, France
*** Disciplina de Bioquímica, Escola Paulista de Medicina, São Paulo, Brazil

SUMMARY: A human urine serine proteinase chymotrypsin like hydrolyzes the peptide bonds: Phe-Ser (kinin); Gly-Gly, Leu-Arg, Phe-Lys (neuropeptides) and Gln-Gln (substance P). Endopeptidase H_2 hydrolyzes better oligopeptides with 4 to 18 aminoacid résidues than larger peptides, it does not hydrolyzes kininogen or proenkephalin. The enzyme behaves as an oligoendopeptidase.

INTRODUCTION

Vasoactive peptides such as bradykinin, angiotensin, vasopressin and atrial natriuretic factor act as local hormones in renal tissue. Neuropeptides have in brain their likely target tissue, but have also been postulated as a possible mediate factor in some renal functions (1). Peptidases, exo or endoenzymes, are key enzymes concerned with the processing and inactivation of the peptide-hormones. These enzymes have no restrict specificity towards a hormone class, inactivating sometimes kinins and enkephalins (2) or kinins, angiotensin and atrial natriuretic peptides (3) or even inactivating a hormone and realeasing another, as endooligopeptide A (4) does towards bradykinin and enkephalin, or angiotensin converting enzyme (ACE) (2), does towards bradykinin and angiotensin.

In human urine the presence of exopeptidases as angiotensin converting enzyme (ACE) or carboxypeptidase N have been related sometime ago (5,6) and these enzymes are already well purified and studied (7,8,9,10). The references about urinary endopeptidases are more recent and only few have been purified (2,11).

In a previous study we purified a endopeptidase H_2 that is a 60 KDa serine proteinase with optimum pH 8.5 and 6.59 isoeletric point. This enzyme hydrolyzes the Phe^5-Ser^6 bond of bradykinin and also shows ability to hydrolyze enkephalins and enkephalin containing peptides (12). Following this observation, we report here on the ability of the endopeptidase H_2 to hydrolyze a range of bradykinin derivatives peptides, enkephalins and enkephalin containing peptides, substance P, LHRH, and also report some kinetic parameters of the interaction of the enzyme with bradykinin and substance P.

MATERIAL AND METHODS

ENZYME PREPARATION: Endopeptidase H_2 was purified by chromatography on DEAE cellulose, Sephadex G75, DEAE Protein pak (HPLC) and Iminodiacetic acid-epoxy activated sepharose 6 B fast flow columns (12).

This procedure resulted in a 202 - fold purification of the enzyme with 1,81% yield. The specific activity of purified enzyme upon BK as substrate is 1090U/mg. The enzyme was purified until homogeneity which was verified by 10% SDS-Page.

HYDROLYSIS OF PEPTIDES: Each peptide (10 nmol) used as substrate was incubated at $37^{o}C$ for two hours with the purified enzyme sample in 0,05M Tris-HCl buffer, pH 8,0, in a final volume of 250 ul. The reaction was stopped by addition of 10 ul of 10% H_3PO_4. HPLC analysis of the incubated was performed on a reverse phase C18 uBondopack column (4,6 x 250 mm; Millipore Corp) equilibrated with 0,1%. H_3PO_4 containing 5% acetonitrile on a Waters HPLC system. Peptides were eluted with a linear gradient of 0-30% (vol/vol) acetonitrile in 0,1% H_3PO_4 developed for 20 min at a flow rate of 2,0 ml/min. The effluent was monitored by absorbance at 214 nm. The following peptides studied were: BK, LBK, MLBK, BK-NH_2, Gly-Gly-Gly-Arg-BK, Gly-Arg-Met-Lys-BK, Succ-Bis-BK, AI, AII, Tyr-Gly-Gly-Phe, ME (Met-enkephalin), LE (Leu-enkephalin), LE-Arg, LE-Arg-Arg, ME-Lys-Lys, ME-Arg-Gly-Leu, LE-Arg-Arg-Ile, Dyn B (Dynorphin B), BAM 18 (Bovine Adrenal Medulla), BAM 22, Peptide E, B-endorphin, SP (Substance P), LHRH (Luteinizing hormone releasing hormone), NT (Neurotensin).

AMINOACID ANALYSIS OF HYDROLYSIS PRODUCTS OF ME, LE, LHRH, DYN B AND SP: The hydrolysis products of LE, ME, LHRH, Dyn B and SP, separated by HPLC, were eluted, and submitted to aminoacid analysis in automatic analyser, using ionic exchange PC-1A column as described by Alonzo et Hirs, 1968 (13).

KINETIC STUDIES: Bradykinin and substance P were incubated at 37°C in a final volume of 1 ml 0,05 M Tris/HCl, pH 8,5 with 0,15U of endooligopeptidase H2. The following concentrations of peptide were employed: 5, 10, 15, 20, 30, 40 and 50 uM. Each reaction was stopped by heating after incubation and the products analysed by HPLC.

ASSAY OF PROTEOLITIC ACTIVITY ON DOG KININOGEN: The dog kininogen solution was initially incubated with the H_2 enzyme and trypsin added in a second step to verify whether or not the first incubation had affected the kinin-moiety in the kininogen molecule. A mixture of 2.88 ml of dog kininogen (AE=4,8 ug BK/ml) in 0.35 M, sodium phosphate buffer, pH 7.5 and 0,3 ml of enzyme, was kept at 37°C for two hours and then boiled for 10 minutes. After, an aliquot of 0.5 ml of trypsin (2 mg/ml) was added to the tube and incubated during 20 minutes at 37°C, being stopped by heating during 15 minutes. A blank without H_2 enzyme was also run. The kinin liberated was assayed in guinea-pig-ileum using bradykinin as standard.

MET ENKEPHALIN RADIOIMUNOASSAY: The action of endopeptidase H_2 upon proenkephalin was verified by specific radioimunoassay for Met-enkephalin described by Stell et al, 1990 (14).

RESULTS

HYDROLYSIS OF BRADYKININ-RELATED PEPTIDES: Under the conditions employed, BK and LBK were better substrates than Met-Lys-BK. After two hours of incubation, under the same enzyme/substrate relation (1:200), synthetic substrates larger than bradykinin were poor substrates and so was bradykinin amide (Table I).

TABLE I: KININ HYDROLYSIS BY ENDOOLIGOPEPTIDASE H_2

PEPTIDES	AMINO ACID RESIDUES	PEPTIDE HYDROLIZED
BK	09	94%
BKNH2	09	71%
LBK	10	100%
MLBK	11	70%
Gly-Gly-Gly-Arg-BK	13	66%
Gly-Arg-Met-Lys-BK	13	72%
Suc-Bis-BK	18	0%

HYDROLYSIS OF PEPTIDE HORMONES OTHER THAN KININS: Among the substrates studied (Table II) the enzyme was able to hydrolyze Leu-enkephalin and Met-enkephalin. The LE or ME derivatives containing 4 to 18 amino acid residues were also enzyme substrates. Enkephalin precursors larger than BAM 18 were not hydrolyzed. Among the other peptide hormones studied, substance P and LHRH showed enzyme susceptibility, but angiotensins and neurotensin were not substrates.

IDENTIFICATION OF HYDROLYSIS PRODUCTS OTHER THAN BK: The peptide fragments produced by the enzyme degradation of BK, various neuropeptides and LHRH were separated by HPLC and eluted to determine the sequence of these fragments.

The sequence of each peptide fragment studied could be deduced

TABLE II: PEPTIDE SUBSTRATES HYDROLYSIS BY ENDOOLIGOPEPTIDASE H_2

PEPTIDES	AMINO ACID RESIDUES	PEPTIDE HYDROLYZED
Tyr-Gly-Gly-Phe	04	50%
LE	05	59%
ME	05	48%
LE-Arg	06	63%
LE-Arg-Arg	07	75%
ME-Lys-Lys	07	50%
ME-Arg-Gly-Leu	08	80%
LE-Arg-Arg-Ile	08	80%
Dyn B	13	75%
BAM 18	18	75%
SP	11	50%
LHRH	10	80%
NT	13	0%
AI	10	0%
AII	08	0%
BAM 22	22	0%
Peptide E	25	0%
B Endorfin	31	0%

from its amino acid composition and that in most cases the fragments were obtained in stoichiometric ratios. BK (Arg-Pro- -Pro-Gly-Phe-Ser-Pro-Phe-Arg) was cleaved at the Phe^5-Ser^6 bond, ME and LE (Tyr-Gly-Gly-Phe-Met and Tyr-Gly-Gly-Phe-Leu) were cleaved specifically at the Gly^2-Gly^3 bond, where as dynorphin B (Tyr-Gly-Gly-Phe-Leu-Arg-Arg-Gln-Phe-Lys-Val-Val-Thr) was cleaved at three sites Gly^2-Gly^3, Leu^5-Arg^6 and Phe^9-Lys^{10}, substance P and LHRH (Arg-Pro-Lys-Pro-Gln-Gln-Phe-Phe-Gly-Leu-Met) and p-Glu-His-Trp-Ser-Tyr-Gly-Leu-Arg-Pro-Gly-NH_2 were cleaved at the Leu^7-Arg^8 and Gln^5-Gln^6 respectivelly.

HYDROLYSIS OF KININOGEN AND PRO-ENKEPHALIN: Kininogen, which contains the bradykinin moiety in its structure, is not hydrolyzed and also the precursor of Met-enkephalin, pro-enkephalin.

KINETIC PARAMETERS: The Km obtained for bradykinin and substance P were 50 uM for both, the Vmax were 12500 and 2000 umol.min^{-1}.mg^{-1} respectevily and Vmax/km, 250 umol.min^{-1}.mg^{-1}.uM^{-1} for BK and 40 umol.min^{-1}.mg^{-1}.uM^{-1} for SP.

DISCUSSION

To further characterize the substrate specificity of enzyme H_2, three sets of experiments were made: hydrolysis of bradykinin related peptide, hydrolysis of other peptide hormones differently sized and hydrolysis of large molecules.

The peptide-bonds splited by enzyme H_2 in kinins, neuropeptides and LHRH; Phe-Ser, Gly-Gly, Leu-Arg, Phe-Lys, Gln-Gln were all refered as susceptible to the action of chymotrypsins (15).

The enzymatic efficiency was slightly better for bradykinin than substance P.

Among the 25 peptides tested only 7 peptides were not hydrolyzed by the enzyme. The hydrolyzed ones had 4 to 18 aminoacid residues. Larger peptides and the two proteins, kininogen and pro-enkephalin, were not substrates. It is possible to observe from the data that there is a size restriction to the enzyme action. The selectivity of a renal endopeptidase in the hydrolysis of small peptides was described in rabbit kidney by Kerr and Kenny (1974) (16). Later, the same selectivity was described in rabbit brain by Camargo et al (1979) (17) who proposed the designation of endooligopeptidase for these enzymes.

The synthetic peptide Succ-Bis-BK was not hydrolyzed by the enzyme. This fact could be an indication of another restriction, beside the size; the peptide conformation. It has already been shown that there is a Beta turn involving the Pro-Pro-Gly-Phe amino acid sequence in BK and its derivatives; in the N-terminus extremity of several neuropeptides (LE,ME, Dyn B and BAM 18) and also in the regions between Pro-Gln-Gln in SP (18, 19). Suc-Bis-BK does not have the Beta turn since the succinic-acid linkage between the two BK molecules permits their juxtaposition and inter molecular hydrophobic interactions.

The angiotensins which were not hydrolyzed, since in pH 8,5 the histidines are deprotonated thus, there is no protonated aminoacid in the Beta turn of the molecule (20).

Endopeptidase H_2 that acts upon different hormone peptides, is a possible modulator of the half life of these hormones in renal tissue. Further kinetic studies involving the other hormone substrates besides bradykinin and substance P, well contribute to the understanding of this possible role.

ACKNOWLEDGEMENTS

We are very grateful for Dr. Jean Roussier that permited the development of part of other work at his laboratory .

REFERENCES

1. SLIZGI, R.G. and LUDENS, J.H.   Displacement of 3H-Enc binding by opioids in rat kidney: a correlate to diuretic activity. Life Sciences 1985; 36: 2189-2193.

2. SKIDGEL, R.A., SCHULZ, W.W., TAM LEI-TING and ERDOS, E.G. Human renal angiotensin I converting enzyme and neutral endopeptidase. Kidney International, 1987; 31 (Suppl 20):545-548.

3. SEYMOUR, A.A., SWERDEL, J.N., FENNELL, S.A. and DELANEY, N.G. Atrial natriuretic peptides cleaved by endopeptidase are inactive in conscious spontaneously hypertensive rats. Life Sciences, 1988; 43: 2265-2274.

4. CAMARGO, A.C.M., OLIVEIRA, E.B., TOFFOLETTO, O, METTERS, K and ROSSIER, J. Brain endooligopeptidase A, a putative enkephalin converting enzyme. J. Neurochem, 1987; 48 (4): 1258-1263.

5. ERDOS., E.G., SLOANE., E.M., WOHLER., I.M. Carboxypeptidase in blood and other fluids - I - Properties, Distribution, and partial purification of the enzyme. Biochem. Pharmac. 1964; 13:893-905.

6. RYAN, J.W., OZA, M.B., MARTIN, L.C. and PENA, G. A. Components of the kallikrein kinin system in urine. In: Fuji S, Moryria H. e Suzuki T. (Editors), Kinin II. Biochemistry, Pathophysiology and Clinical Aspects. New York, Plenum Press. 1978; 10: 313-323.

7. KOKUBO, T., KATO, I., NISHIMURA, K., YOSHIDA, N., HIWADA, K.and UEDA, E. Angiotensin I converting enzyme in human urine. Clin. Chim. Acta, 1978; 89:375-379.

8. MARINKORVIC, D.V., WARD, P.E., ERDOS, E.G. and MELLO, I.H. Carboxypeptidase - type kininase of human kidney and urine. Proc. of the Soc. Exp. Biol. Med. 1980; 165 (1): 6-12.

9. SKIDGEL, R.A., DAVIS, R.M. and ERDOS, E.G. Purification of a human urinary carboxypeptidase (kininase) distinct from carboxipeptidase A, E, or N. Anatitical Biochemistry 1984; 140: 520-531.

10. CASARINI, D.E., and Stella, R.C.R. Estudos de distintas cininases de urina humana. Arq. Biol.Tecnol. 1982; 25 (1): 69.

11. CASARINI, D.E., ALVES, K.B., ARAUJO-VIEl, M.S., BRANDI, C.M.W. and STELLA, R.C.R. Human urine endopeptidase with kininase activity. Braz. J. Med. Biol. Res. 1986; 19 (4-5):585 A.

12. CASARINI, D.E., STELLA, R.C.R., ARAUJO, M.S. and SAMPAIO, C.A.M. Purification and characterization of an endooligopeptidase H2, a kinin inactivating serine proteinase (kininase) from human urine. Submmited, 1992.

13. ALONZO, N. and HIRS, V. Automation of sample application in amino acid analyzes. Anal. Biochem. 1968; 23: 272-288.

14. STELL, W.K.,CHAMINADE, M., METTERS, K.M., ROUGEOT, C., DRAY, F. and ROSSIER, J. Detection of synenkephalin, the amino-terminal portion of proenkephalin, by antisera directed against its carboxyl terminus Neurochemistry, 1990; 54 (2): 434-443.

15. NEIL, G.L. and NIEMANN, C. Structural specificity of alpha chymotrypsin: polypeptide substrates Nature. 1966; 5093, 903-907.

16. KERR, M.A. and KENNY, A.J. The purification and specificity of a neutral endopeptidase from rabbit kidney brush border. Biochem. J. 1974; 137: 477-488.

17. CAMARGO, A.C.M., CALDO, H. and REIS, M.L. Susceptibility of a peptide derived from bradykinin to hydrolysis by brain endo-oligopeptidases and pancreatic proteinases. J. Biol. Chem. 1979; 254 (12): 5304-5307.

18. CHOU, P.Y. and FASMAN, G.D. Prediction of protein conformation. Biochemistry, 1974; 13 (2): 222-245.

19. CHASSOUNG, G., CONVERT, O. and LAVIELLE, S. Preferencial conformation of substance P in solution. Eur. J. Biochem. 1986; 154: 77-85.

20. OLIVEIRA, M.C.F., JULIANO, L. and PAIVA, A.C.M. Conformation of synthetic tetradecapeptide renin substrate and of angiotensin in aqueous solution. Biochemistry 1977; 16 (12): 2606-2609.

AAS 38/I
Recent Progress on Kinins
© 1992 Birkhäuser Verlag Basel

THE KALLIKREIN, KININASE AND RELATED PEPTIDES ACTIVITIES IN CENTRAL ASIAN SNAKE VENOMS

L. Ya. Yukelson, V. M. L'vov, A. V. Shkinev, N. Sultanalieva

Institute of Biochemistry, Uzbek Academy of Sciences, Gorky street, 56, Tashkent, 700143, Republic Uzbekistan

SUMMARY: The quantitative content estimation of kininogenases, kininases and related peptides have been made for Central Asian snake venoms: V. lebetina turanica and E. multisquamatus (gen. Vipera and Echis, fam. Viperidae), Ag. halys halys (gen. Agkistrodon, fam. Crotalidae) and N. oxiana (gen. Naja, fam Elapidae). It has been demonstrated, that all venoms investigated cause the contractile effect, when acting on isolated smooth muscle preparations. Kinin-like contractile activity was found in the low molecular weight fraction of the cobra venom. This action has the prolonged character as compared with bradykinin, but apart from it, results in the inactivation of the rat uterus because of cytotoxic components presence. The specific bradykinin-potentiating effect of the low molecular weight fraction of the E. multisquamatus venom has been discovered. It has been found, that the effect is connected with inhibition of the kininase II (angiotensin I converting enzyme, ACE). Two peptide inhibitors was isolated and characterized from this fraction.

INTRODUCTION

Kallikrein-kinin system (KKS) is complex regulatory formation including biologically active peptides-kinins, as well as kinin-forming and kinin-inactivating enzymes, which determine the content of kinins in the medium. It is clear, that the factors stimulating or inhibiting the activity of these enzymes also affect the level of kinins.

Snake venoms contain the peptides and proteins, the structure and functions of which are similar to those of the components of

KKS. Upon this snake venoms belonging to various taxonomical groups have the compositional peculiarities of these components, affecting the character of their interaction both with each other and with other venom-forming protein-peptide substances.

The paper describes the presence of factors, possesing the properties characteristic of the KKS components in the venoms of Central Asian snakes belonging to various taxons of three main families: Viperidae, Crotalidae and Elapidae.

MATERIALS AND METHODS

The dried whole venoms of Agkisrodon halys halys Schn., Echis multisquamatus Ch., Naja oxiana Eichw., Vipera lebetina turanica C. were supplied by the Institute of Biochemistry, Uzbek Academy of Sciences, Tashkent, Republic Uzbekistan. Synthetic bradykinin and hippuryl-L-arginine were products of Reanal, Hungary. Sephadex G-75 & G-15 were products of Pharmacia, Sweden. Chromogenic substrates were received from Boehringer Mannheim, GMBH, Germany and Kabi Diagnostica, Sweden. Acrylamide and N,N'-methylene bisacrylamide twice-crystallized were products of Serva, Germany.

The determination of kallikrein content in venoms was performed by measuring of BAEE-esterase activity (1) and biological assay technique (2), by measuring of rat uterus contraction after incubation of kininogen with venom. Assay of amidolytic activity was used for the kallikrein determination too. Amidolytic activities towards the chromogenic substrates S2302, Chromozym PK were measured at 37 oC in a buffer containing 50 mM Tris, pH 7.9, 175 mM NaCl, 2 mM CaCl-2 and 200 μM substrate. Generation of p-nitroaniline was determined on a dual-wavelength spectrophotometer by measuring A 405-500 nm and using a molar extinction coefficient of 10,400 mol-1.cm-1 for p-nitroaniline.

The kininase activities were investigated using the biological method (4), by measuring of bradykinin contraction on rat uterus, after incubation with venom. The venom concentrations

3 orders (i.e. 1000-fold) lower than minimal venom amount causing the contractile effect were used for determination. The hippuryl-L-arginine was used for the determination of kininase I (carboxypeptidase N) in whole venoms (3).

The contactile activity of whole venoms was determined in a 12-ml organ bath by measuring contraction of guinea pig ileum in aerated Tyrode solution and estrus rat uterus in oxigenated de Jalon solution at 30 oC, as well as of rat aorta rings in Krebs-Hanselait solution oxigenated with carbogen. Bradykinin as standart was used.

Bradykinin-potentiating activity of venoms and fractions was investigated by the increasing of rat uterus bradykinin contraction (5). Peptides were added just before addition of a 0.05-0.5 ml of the standart bradykinin solution and the increase in size of contractions of the smooth muscles was estimated by comparison with that induced by a standard dose of synthetic bradykinin. As standard, a concentration of 0.1 μg/ml synthetic bradykinin was used for assay with rat uterus. The amounts (or concentrations) of peptides required to double the effect of bradykinin on smooth muscles, which were independent of the amount of standard bradykinin added, were measured (factor F).

The inhibitory activity of venom fractions was estimated by the capacity of them to block kininase II action (ACE from bovine kidney; dipeptidyl-carboxypeptidase from Latrodectus tredecimguttatus spider venom) (4,6). The amount (μg/ml) needed to inhibit 50% of the enzymatic activity is defined as the IC-50.

Gel filtrations of whole N. oxiana Eichw. and E. multisquamatus were performed at about 4 oC on Sephadex G-75 columns equilibrated with 0.05 M ammonium acetate buffers, pH 4.5 and pH 7.9 respectively, and eluted with the same buffers.

Paper chromatography was carried out on Whatman No 3MM paper. The solvent systems employed were 1-butanol-water-puridine-acetic acid (15:12:10:3, v/v) and 1-butanol-acetic acid-water (63:10:27, v/v). Thin-layer chromatograms on silica gel were developed in the same solvent systems. To locate the peptides, ninhydrin reagent, peptide reagent (tert-butyl hypochlorite-o-tolidine-KI) were used.

Elecrophoresis of venom fractions was carried out on the 10 to 24,5% linear gradient slab gels, containing 7 M urea with an acrylamide:bisacrylamide ratio of 20:1. Staining solution: 25% ethanol (w/v), 3.5% formaldehyde (v/v), 0.11% coomassie R-250 (w/v). Cyanogen bromide cleavage products of myoglobin were used as markers.

RESULTS AND DISCUSSION

The data demonstrating the kallikrein and kininase activities in Central Asian snake venoms are given in Table 1.

Table 1. Kininogenase and kininase activities of Central Asian snake venoms

Venoms	Enzyme activity (U/mg) of					
	Kallikreins by hydrolysis				Kininases by hydrolysis	
	BAEE	Chromozym PK	S-2302	Kinino-gen	Hippuryl-L-arginine	Bradykinin
Vipera le-betina tura-nica C.	17.75	n.d.	20.7	0.0076	0.29	13.488x10-3
Echis multi-squamatus Ch.	3.40	8.90	9.15	0.0066	0.27	-*
Agkistrodon halys halys Schn.	5.46	n.d.	7.96	0.0066	0.56	8.920x10-3
Naja oxiana Eichw.	abs.	n.d.	<0.02	abs.	0.55	-*

-* - Lack of kininase II activity. Bradykinin-potentiating effect is observed.

Activity of kallikrein (kininogenase) was found only in enzyme-rich high molecular weight venoms (according to the classification of H. W. Raudonat, 1963); these are the venoms from Viperidae and Crotalidae families. The presence of great number of various proteinases is characteristic feature of these venoms.

Enzyme-poor low molecular weight cobra venom (Elapidae family) differs from the other venoms by lacking the hydrolytic action on proteins and peptides, as well as on ether and p-nitroanilide amino acid and peptide derivatives used in the work.

The low kininase activity was detected only in V. lebetina turanica Ch. and A. halys halys Schn. venoms, also belonging to enzyme-rich high molecular weight venoms. In contrast to these venoms those of E. multisquamatus Ch. and N. oxiana Eichw. increased the contractile activity of bradykinin, i.e. posessed bradykinin-potentiating effect.

It must be noted, that the data presented in Table 1 like all other measurements performed using the crude venoms, can not be reliable enough to deny the presence of individual non-enzymatic factors or enzymes (for example, kininase) in these venoms, because of the interferention of venom-forming substances.

When acting on isolated smooth muscle preparations all venoms investigated cause the contractile effect. The venom of V. lebetina turanica C., like bradykinin, attacts rat uterus preparation, but it does not effect rat aorta rings. The contractile effect of all the rest venoms is accompanied by inactivation of nerve-muscle preparation and, apparently, provided by the same components, that induce the contraction of rat aorta rings (Table 2).

The crude venoms composition and the ratio of the venom-forming substances determine the specific mechanisms for realization of their contractile effect shown in Figure 1.

The great number of alternative mechanisms for realization of direct or mediated contractile effects corresponds to complex multicomponent composition of the venoms with the only one being capable of triggering several mechanisms at the same time.

The direct effect of the venoms on smooth muscles is caused by the action of kinins, the contractile agents of non-protein (non-peptide) nature, as well as by the action of specific peptides - cytotoxins, that interact with cell membrane lipid bilayers and induce their depolarization. Biomolecules (kininogens) or cells (mast cells) act as mediators of venom

Table 2.   Phospholipase A-2 activity, contractile and direct
           lytict effects of Central Asian snake venoms

Venoms investigated	Phospholipase A-2 activity (U/mg)	Contractile action on preparations			Bradykinin-potentiating activity (rat uterus)	Direct lytic effect
		rat uterus 100 mkg	200 mkg	rat aorta 100 mkg		
Vipera lebetina turanica C.	5165	+	+	-	-	abs.
Echis multisquamatus Ch.	1222	+	+	+	+	abs.
Agkistrodon halys halys Schn.	7250	-	+	+	-	abs.
Naja oxiana Eichw.	9198	-	+	+++	+	total lysis

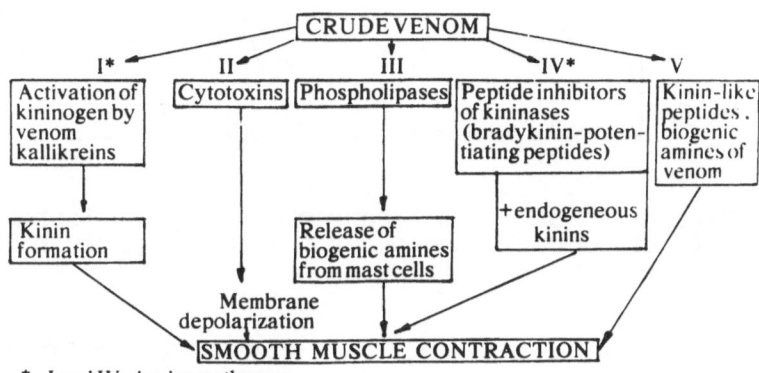

Figure 1. Possible mechanisms of contractile venoms effect on
smooth muscle.

contractile effects. The release of muscle-attacking substances
from   the   cell   is   connected   with   their   lysis,   caused   by

sinergistic action of cytotoxin and phospholipase A-2.

All venoms contractile effect associated with the action of kinins are blocked by kininase I (carboxipeptidase B) or kininase II (dipeptidyl-dipeptidase). The suppression of these enzymes by peptide inhibitors of kininase potentiates the effect of kinins.

The revealing, characterizing and using contractile-acting venom factors including the substances possessing the activity of KKS components is only possible after their separation and purification. Taking into consideration the substantial differences in venom composition, these problems are solved independently and in conformity with each venom.

The crude venom of Echis multisquamatus, with this aim in view, was fractionated on Sephadex G-75 column.

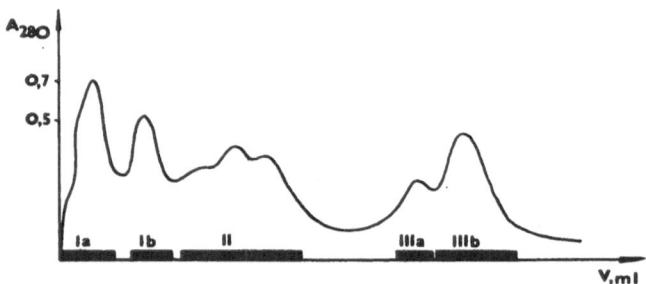

Figure 2. Separation of E. multisquamatus venom on Sephadex G-75. I - III - fraction collected according to the protein "peaks".

Distribution of biological activity among the fractions was as following: Ia - casein-hydrolysing enzyme, prothrombin-activating proteinase and BAEE-esterase; kallikrein by hydrolysis of chromogenic substrate. Ib - casein-hydrolysing enzyme, haemorrhagin, kallikrein by hydrolysis of chromogenic substrate. II - phospholipase A-2. IIIa-IIIb - bradykinin-potentiating activity, inhibitors of angiontensin-converting enzyme (ACE) from bovine kidney and dipeptidyl-carboxypeptidase from Latrodectus tredecimguttatus spider venom. Contractile activity of E. multisquamatus venom is separated from bradykinin-potentiating activity and is localized in fraction II. Fractions Ia and Ib hydrolyze kallikrein chromogenic substrate, but they do not manifest their contractile effect in the presence of kininogen. The lack of contractile activity in fractions Ia and Ib in the presence of kininogen might be associated with inactivation of mewly-formed bradykinin by kininase II freed from peptide inhibitors IIIa and IIIb during gelfiltration.

It was shown according to thin-layer chromatography data, using identification by ninhydrin and peptide reagent, that total low molecular weight fraction III contained at least 8 components.

Electrophoresis in PAAG in the presence of SDS-Na and urea demonstrated, that fractions IIIa and IIIb contained the peptides with Mr 1.0 - 8.0 kDa.

Potentiating effect of peptide fractions is specific for bradykinin, but it is not observed in the presence of other contractile agents (acetylcholine, histamin, serotonin) and it is probably connected with inhibition of ACE (Fig. 3).

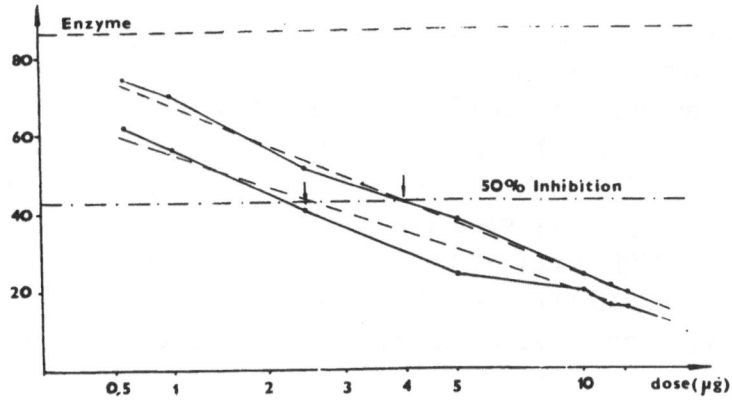

Figure 3. Characterization of inhibitory effect of fractions IIIa and IIIb on bovine kidney ACE.

Preliminary measurements established IC-50 for fractions IIIa and IIIb within the limits of 2.5x10-8 M - 2.5x10-9 M and 4.0x10-8 M - 4.0x10-9 M, respectively.

Analogously, the following results were received by fractionation of whole cobra venom on Sephadex G-75 column (Fig. 4).

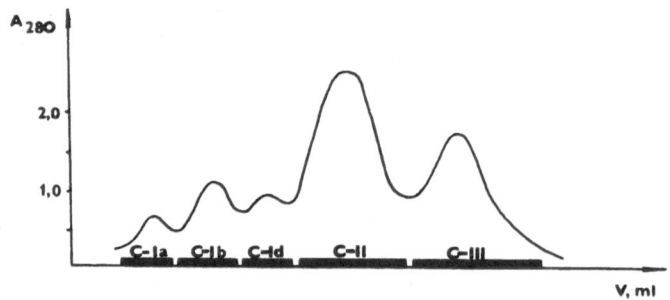

Figure 4.   Separation of N. oxiana Eichw. venom on Sephadex G-75. C-I - C-III - fractions, collected according to the protein "peaks".

Fraction C-II and to the less degree fraction C-III, exert the contractile action on rat uterus and rat aorta rings. This effect is more prolonged comparable to that of bradykinin, but unlike the latter, it leads to inactivation of rat uterus, apparently due to the presence of cytotoxic components. Two phospholipases A-2 (Mr 12.0 and 15.0 kDa respectively) and cytotoxins with primary structures: Vc-1 LKCNKLVPIAYKTCEGKNLCYKMF-MMSDLTIPVKRGCIDVCPKNSLLVKYVCCNTDRCN, Vc-5 LKCKKLVPLFSKTCPAGKNLC-YKMFMVAAPHVPVKRGCIDVCPKSSLLVKYVCCNTDRCN and Mr 6.5 and 7.0 respectively, were isolated from the fraction C-II in the pure form (7).

It is shown, that contractile activity is associated with cytotoxins potentiated by phospholipases A-2.

Fraction C-III is separated by gel-filtration on Sephadex G-15 into 5 fractions. Only C-III-1 retained its contractile effect on both smooth muscle preparations, that might be explained by their containing the same cytotoxins as contaminants.

Besides phospholipase A-2 and cytotoxins the neurotoxic polypeptides were purified and characterized as long (73, 5-S-S) and short (62, 4-S-S) ones. The specific interaction was established between both neurotoxins and choline receptor (8). These neurotoxins didn't affect on smooth and heart muscle preparations.

CONCLUSIONS

The snake venom contains the factors similar to those of KKS by their activity and mode of action. The snake venoms differ substantially each other by the content and ratio of these factors. KKS enzymes are found only in high molecular weight venoms of Viperidae and Crotalidae snakes, whereas bradykinin-potentiating activity is observed both in high and low molecular weight snake venoms. All venoms have contractile effect on smooth muscle preparations.

The alternative pathways for contractile effect of snake venoms, among which there are the mechanisms associated with activation-inactivation of kinins, were considered on the basis of the data on composition of snake venoms.

The interference of venom-forming substances prevents their identification, characterization and subsequent definition according to mechanism of their action. Therefore, it is necessary to separate the activities in conformity with each venom in order to provide its complete characterization.

Bradykinin-potentiating activity of E. multusquamatus venom was separated in accordance with Mr of components, and its role in kininase inactivation was shown. Both kininase and kallikrein were localized among high molecular weight componens.

N. oxiana Eichw. venom does not contain KKS enzymes, and its contractile activity is induced by cytotoxic components and phospholipases A-2 interacting with them. The participation of these components and particularly, phospholipase A-2, in contractile action of Viperidae and Crotalidae snake venoms is not excluded too.

REFERENCES

1.) Paskhina TS, Krinskaya AV Quantitative determination of kallikrein and kininogen in human blood serum (plasma). In: Update methods in Biochemistry. Orekhovich VN, editor. Moscow: Medicine, 1977: 157-163.
2.) Krinskaya AV, Paskhina TS. Obtaining of partial purified kallikrein preparation from human blood serum. In: Update methods in Biochemistry. Orekhovich VN, editor. Moscow: Medicine, 1977: 163-170.
3.) Trapeznikova CC, Rossinskaya EB, Krainova BL, Chaman ES, Paskhina TS. Determination of carboxipeptidase N (kininase I) esterase activity in human blood. In: Update methods in Biochemistry. Orekhovich VN, editor. Moscow: Medicine, 1977: 180-188.
4.) Paskhina TS, Egorova TL Chemical and biological methods of main blood kallikrein-kinin system components determination. In: Update methods in Biochemistry. Orekhovich VN, editor. Moscow: Medicine, 1968: 232-241.
5.) Kato H, Suzuki T. Bradykinin-potentiating peptides from the venom of Agkistrodon halys blomhoffii. Isolation of five bradykinin potentiators and the amino acid sequence of two of them, potentiators B and C. Biochemistry 1971; 10: 972-980.
6.) Akhunov A, Golubenko Z, Sadykov AS. Isolation of kininase from the Latrodectus tredecimguttatus spider venom. Dokl Acad Sci USSR 1981; 257: 1478-1481.
7.) Yukelson LYa. Membrane-active components from Naja oxiana Eichw. venom: cytotoxins and phospholipases A-2. DS diss Tashkent, 1977. - 331 P.
8.) Sorokin VM. Mechanisms of action of Central Asian cobra venom toxins. Uzb biol zurnal 1982; 1: 68-69

AAS 38/I
Recent Progress on Kinins
© 1992 Birkhäuser Verlag Basel

A USEFUL AND SENSITIVE METHOD FOR DEMONSTRATION OF THE INVOLVEMENT OF EITHER KALLIKREIN-KININ SYSTEM IN PATHOLOGICAL STATES

M. Majima, *N. Sunahara, Y. Uchida and M. Katori

Department of Pharmacology, Kitasato University School of Medicine, Sagamihara, Kanagawa 228, Japan and *Dainippon Pharmaceutical Co., Enoki, Osaka 661, Japan

Summary: In rat carrageenin-induced pleurisy, bradykinin (BK) was hardly able to be detected (<160 pg per rat) in the exudates. In contrast, des-Phe^8-Arg^9-BK (des-8,9-BK) level, determined by an enzyme immunoassay (EIA) newly developed, was larger in the exudate and the levels were kept throughout the entire course of this inflammation. Arg-Pro-Pro-Gly-Phe ([1-5] BK) level, measured by an EIA newly developed, was much higher than that of des-8,9-BK in the exudate. Intrapleural administration of soy bean trypsin inhibitor (0.3 mg per rat) reduced the levels of both des-8,9-BK and [1-5] BK in the exudates. Reduction in the residual levels of plasma prekallikrein (P-Kall) and high-molecular-weight-kininogen (HMW-K), not low-molecular-weight-kininogen (LMW-K), were accompanied with increase in these BK degradation products, indicating that plasma prekallikrein was activated in the pleural cavity. On the other hand, intravenous injection of acetaldehyde to rats pretreated with disulfiram resulted in the significant increase in the levels of [1-5] BK in the blood, which was accompanied with reduction in the residual levels of LMW-K, not of HMW-K and P-Kall in plasma. These results indicated that the detection of BK degradation products was a good marker for the kinin release *in vivo* and that the concomitant reduction of the precursor proteins allowed us to identify the type of kallikrein-kinin systems relevant to the kinin release.

INTRODUCTION

Detection of free kinin in body fluid is a strong evidence of the involvement of kallikrein-kinin systems in some pathological states. Development of an enzyme immunoassay for bradykinin (BK), made in our laboratory (1), however, did not guarantee the detection of free kinin, because of rapid destruction of the peptides in plasma and other biological fluids (2, 3). The studies on the degradation pathway of bradykinin in plasmas from several species (3) enabled us to find stable metabolites of this biologically active peptide and to develop sensitive enzyme immunoassays (EIAs) specific for des-Phe^8-Arg^9-BK (des-8,9-BK) and N-terminal pentapeptide of BK ([1-5] BK). The detection of these metabolites did not indicate which type of the kallikrein-kinin systems, plasma kallikrein-kinin system or tissue kallikrein-kinin system, may be a source of kinin released. We reported that plasma kallikrein preferentially consumes high-molecular-wight (HMW) kininogen and the activation of the plasma prekallikrein is accompanied with reduction of the residual levels of plasma prekallikrein and HMW kininogen in plasma and body fluid (4, 5), whereas release of tissue (glandular) kallikrein is accompanied with the reduced residual level of low-molecular-wight (LMW) kininogen, because of preferential consumption of LMW kininogen by glandular kallikrein. The measurement of the residual levels of kininogens in plasma or body fluids is useful, since the turn over rates of plasma prekallikrein or HMW kininogen were low and it takes over 72 hours in rats before the restoration to the previous levels after the depletion of these precursor proteins (6).

   In the present paper, we describe simply the development of EIAs for the degradation products of BK and report that the determination of the degradation products of BK is a useful maneuver to verify the kinin release *in vivo* and the concomitant reduction of the precursor proteins of the kallikrein-kinin system may identify the type of kallikrein-kinin system responsible for release of kinin.

MATERIALS AND METHODS

Development of enzyme immunoassays for degradation products of bradykinin
   Enzyme immunoassays (EIAs) for either des-Phe^8-Arg^9-BK (des-8,9-BK) or N-terminal pentapeptide of BK ([1-5] BK) were developed using antibodies to the peptides whose amino terminus were conjugated to bovine serum albumin (BSA, Fraction V) using glutalaldehyde (1). The solution of immunogens were emulsified with complete Freund's adjuvant, and then injected subcutaneously into male Japanese White rabbits (Shizuoka Laboratory Animal Center, Hamamatsu, Japan). Blood was collected from a central artery of the ear and allowed to clot completely, and serum was separated. The cross reactivity of the each antibody against BK, Lys-BK, Met-Lys-BK and T-kinin are very low

(under 1%). β-Galactosidase-labeled peptides were prepared according to the method reported previously (1). The antigen-antibody reactions were performed for 1 hour at 37°C. To separate the bind fraction from the free, insolubilized second antibodies from anti-rabbit IgG goat immunoglobulin, which was coupled chemically with cell walls of *Lactobacillus plantarum* as reported previously (7), were used. After centrifugation, the enzyme activities in the precipitate were measured with synthetic substrate (2-nitrophenyl-β-D-galactopyranoside). The values of the authentic peptides (10-100 nmol/ml) in physiological saline, determined by the corresponding EIA, were well correlated with those obtained by HPLC. The EIA specific for BK, developed previously, was also used.

Determination of the residual levels of plasma prekallikrein, HMW-kininogen and LMW-kininogen

The residual levels of plasma prekallikrein, HMW-kininogen and LMW-kiniinogen in citrated plasma or inflammatory exudate were determined by the method reported previously (4, 5).

Experimental models

Male Sprague-Dawley rats (8 weeks old, specific pathogen free) were anesthetized lightly with ether and 0.1 ml of λ-carrageenin solution (2% (W/V) in sterile physiological saline, Picnin-A) was injected into the right pleural cavity as previously reported (8). After exsanguination at a fixed time until 24 hour, 5 ml of absolute ethanol was injected into the pleural cavity for prevention of further degradation to smaller peptides. The fluid in the pleural cavity was collected to a siliconized glass tube and after heating at 70 °C for 10 min centrifuged for 15 min at 1500 x g at 4 °C. The ethanol extracts (supernatants) were evaporated to dryness under reduced pressure and the residues were dissolved with 2 ml of distilled water, acidified with 0.1 ml of 0.01N HCl, and washed twice with 10 ml of diethylether to remove the lipid (3). The aqueous phase was evaporated to dryness under reduced pressure and the dried sample was dissolved with 4 ml of distilled water acidified with 0.2 ml of 0.01N HCl and applied Sep-Pak C_{18} cartridge column. After washing the column with 12 ml of distilled water and 4 ml of 0.1 M acetic acid, BK and BK degradation products were eluted with 6 ml of 80% (V/V) acetonitrile containing 0.1 M acetic acid (9). Kinin fraction was evaporated under reduced pressure and the residue was resolved with the assay buffer for EIA to determine the levels of BK and BK degradation products. From another group of animals, the pleural exudate and blood from the carotid artery were collected into the plastic tubes containing

1/10 volume of 3.8% sodium citrate and centrifuge at 1500g at 20°C for 15 min. The supernatants were used as samples for the determinations of the precursor proteins described above. To inhibit the generation of BK from HMW-kininogen by plasma kallikrein, 0.3 ml of soy bean trypsin inhibitor (SBTI) solution (1 mg/ml in physiological saline) was injected into the pleural cavity 30 min before the collection of pleural exudates. The plasma exudation rates were determined to measure the dye amount exuded into the pleural cavity for 20 min after intravenous injection of the pontamine sky blue. For a control rat, only saline (0.3 ml) was injected into the pleural cavity.

Disulfiram (150 mg/kg, Nakarai Chemical Corp.,Osaka), an inhibitor of aldehyde dehydrogenase, was given orally to male Sprague-Dawley rats (8 weeks old, specific pathogen free) and 24 hours later rats were administered by acetaldehyde (10 mg/kg, i.v.) under light ether anesthesia. Fifteen min later, blood was collected directly into the ice-cold absolute ethanol and the levels of [1-5] BK in blood was determined by the method reported previously (10). Thirty min after the acetaldehyde administration, citrated plasma was prepared and the levels of the precursor proteins were determined.

RESULTS AND DISCUSSION

Changes in the levels of BK, BK degradation products and precursor proteins in the exudates of carrageenin-induced pleurisy

The administration of carrageenin into the pleural cavity resulted in increase in the plasma exudation rate and the volume of exudate over 24 hours. The volume of the exudate was increased up to 19 hours and then gradually decreased thereafter. The plasma exudation rates, determined by dye leakage for 20 min, increased rapidly up to 5 hours and then decreased gradually.

As shown in the left panel of Figure 1, the levels of BK, des-8,9-BK and [1-5] BK in the wash of the pleural cavity of normal rats were below the detection limit of EIA (below 160 pg per rat). The BK level in the pleural exudate collected 3 hours after carrageenin was not different from that in normal rats and was below the detection limit. In contrast, the des-8,9-BK level was larger in the exudate and the levels were kept throughout the entire course of this inflammation. As shown in Figure 1, the [1-5] BK level in the 3 hour exudate was much higher than that of des-8,9-BK and showed a peak at 5 hours after carrageenin injection. The level was gradually reduced, but the higher was maintained over 24 hours. SBTI (soy bean trypsin inhibitor) treatments resulted

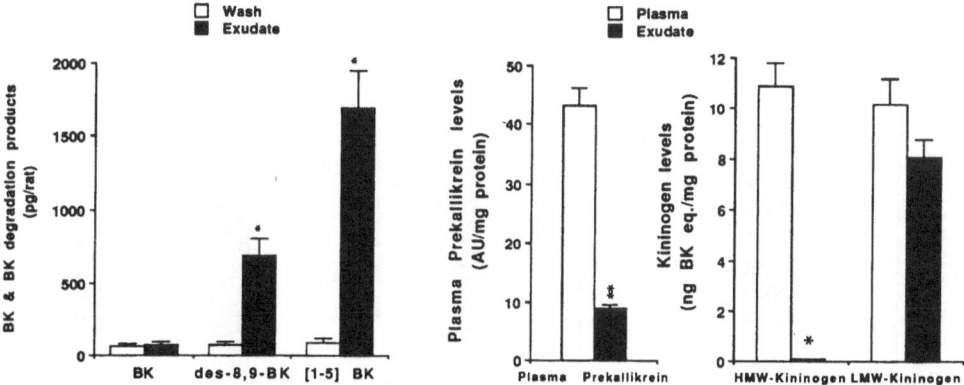

Figure 1. The levels of BK degradation products and the residual levels of the precursor proteins in the exudate of carrageenin-induced pleurisy in rats.

The levels of the BK and its degradation products in the exudates (Exudate) 3 hours after carrageenin were compared with those in the washings of the pleural cavity of normal rats (Wash). The residual levels of the precursor proteins, plasma prekallikrein, high molecular wight (HMW) and low molecular wight (LMW) kininogens in the exudates (Exudate) 3 hours after carrageenin were compared with those in their own plasma (Plasma) in the carrageenin-injected rats. The residual levels of the precursor proteins were expressed in terms of protein concentrations. Each value shows the mean ± s.e. mean from four to six experiments. *, p<0.05; **, p<0.01.

in the significant reduction in the levels of [1-5] BK and des-8,9-BK 3, 7 and 19 hours after carrageenin, suggesting these metabolites were generated from BK released.

The right two panels of Figure 1 depict the residual levels of plasma prekallikrein, HMW-kininogen and LMW-kininogen in the exudates and plasma, expressed in terms of protein concentrations. The HMW-kininogen level in the 3 hours exudate was not detectable and that of plasma prekallikrein was reduced significantly, compared with those in their own plasma. The residual level of LMW-kininogen in the 3 hours exudate was not significantly different from that in plasma. These results clearly indicated that the levels of the degradation products, des-8,9-BK and [1-5] BK, were detectable in the pleural exudate of pleurisy and the release of the degradation products was accompanied with reduction in the residual kininogen level and both changes showed a mirror-immage. Furthermore, the residual levels of plasma prekallikrein and HMW-kininogen, not of LMW-kininogen, clearly indicated that plasma prekallikrein was activated in the pleural cavity, indicatnig the source of the kinin released. In

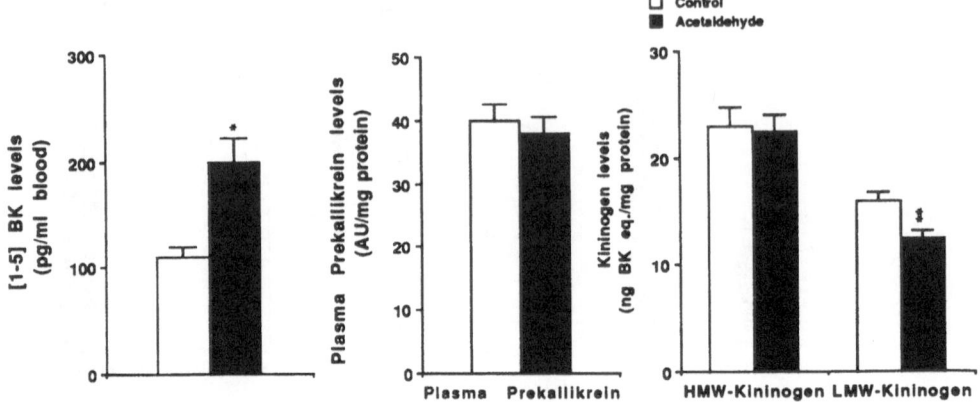

Figure 2. The levels of BK degradation products and the residual levels of the precursor proteins in the blood after intravenous injection of actaldehyde with disulfiram in rats.

The levels of BK degradation product ([1-5] BK) 15 min. after actaldehyde (Acetaldehyde) were compared with those of the control rats recieved only saline (Control). The residual levels of the precursor proteins, plasma prekallikrein, high molecular wight (HMW) and low molecular wight (LMW) kininogens in the plasma 30 min after acetaldehyde (Acetaldehyde) were compared with those in control rats recieved only saline (Control). The residual levels of the precursor proteins were expressed in terms of protein concentrations. Each value shows the mean ± s.e. mean from five to six experiments. *, p<0.05; **, p<0.01.

fact, we reported that λ-carrageenin activates Hageman factor in plasma (8). Thus, we conclude that λ-carrageenin contacts with Hageman factor in plasma exuded in the pleural cavity.

Changes in the levels of BK degradation product and precursor proteins in the blood after intravenous injection of actaldehyde to rats pretreated with disulfiram

Intravenous injection of acetaldehyde induced the gradual hypotensive responses in rats pretreated with disulfiram. As shown on the left panel of Figure 2, the levels of [1-5] BK 15 min after the acetaldehyde injection was increased significantly by this treatment, as compared with those determined under saline treatments. Concomitantly, the residual levels of LMW-kininogen, not plasma prekallikrein and HMW-kininogen, in the plasma 30 min after acetaldehyde were significantly reduced from the control levels, which recieved only saline (the right two panels of Figure 2).

The intravenous injection of acetaldehyde to the disulfiram-treated rats resulted in increase in the [1-5] BK level in blood, suggesting the kinin release, but it is not plausible to identify the plasma kallikrein-kinin system as a source of the kinin release, since the residual levels of plasma prekallikrein and HMW-kininogen were not changed.   Instead, the LMW-kininogen level was significantly reduced, as comfirmed with our previous report (11). This results indicated that the tissue or glandular kallikrein was released, which may be glandular-kallikrein from sweat gland (12).

In conclusion, the plasma kallikrein-kinin system act independently in the body and the detection of the degradation products, particularly [1-5] BK, enables us to verify the kinin release and the differential determination of HMW-kininogen and LMW-kininogen indicate the source of kinin released.

ACKNOWLEDGEMENTS

The authors thank Ms. Harue Mihara and Mr. Osamu Yoshida for taking care of rats, and Mr. Hiroshi Ishikawa, Ms. Chikako Shima, Ms. Michiko Takahara and Ms. Maki Saito for skillful technical assistance. The part of this work was supported by Uehara Memorial Foundation and a Grant-in-Aid from the Ministry of Education, Science and Culture (#02454497).

REFERENCES

1.   UENO, A., OH-ISHI, S., KITAGAWA, T., KATORI, M. Enzyme immunoassay of bradykinin using β-D-galactosidase as a labeling enzyme. Biochem. Pharmacol. 1981; 30, 1659-1664.
2.   FERREIRA, S.H. and VANE, J.R. The disappearance of bradykinin and eledoisin in the circulation and vascular beds of the cat. Br. J. Pharmacol., 1967; 30, 417-424.
3. MAJIMA, M., UENO, A., SUNAHARA, N. & KATORI, M. Measurement of des-Phe8-Arg9-bradykinin by enzyme immunoassay---A useful parameter of plasma kinin release. In "Kinin V" Part b, 1989; pp.331-335, Adv. Exp. Med. Biol., Plenum Press, New York.
4.   OH-ISHI, S., KATORI, M. Fluorometric assay method for plasma prekallikrein using peptidylmethyl-coumariylamide as a substrate. Thromb. Res. 1979; 14, 665-672.

5. UCHIDA, Y., MAJIMA, M., KATORI, M. A method of determination of human plasma HMW and LMW kininogen levels by bradykinin enzyme immunoassay. Pharmacol. Res. Commun. 1986; 18, 831-846.

6. OH-ISHI, S., UCHIDA, Y., UENO, A., KATORI, M. Bromelain, a thiolprotease from pineapple stem, depletes high molecular weight kininogen by activation of Hageman factor (factor XII). Throm. res. 1979; 14, 665-672.

7. SUNAHARA, N., KUROOKA, S., KAIBE, K., OHKARU, Y., NISHIMURA, S., NAKANO, K., SOHMURA, Y., IIDA, M. Simple enzyme immunoassay methods for recombinant human tumor necrosis factor α and its antibodies using a bacterial cell wall carrier. J. Immunol. Methods, 1988; 109, 203-214.

8. UCHIDA, Y., TANAKA, K., HARADA, Y., UENO, A., KATORI, M. Activation of plasma kallikrein-kinin system and its significant role in pleural fluid accumulation of rat carrageenin-induced pleurisy. Inflammation, 1983; 7, 121-131.

9. MAJIMA, M., KATORI, M., HANAZUKA, M., MIZOGAMI, S., NAKANO, T., NAKAO, Y., MIKAMI, R., URYU, H., OKAMURA, R., MOHSIN, S., OH-ISHI, S. Suppression of rat deoxycorticosterone-salt hypertension by kallikrein-kinin system. Hypertension, 1991; 17, 806-813.

10. KATORI, M., MAJIMA, M., ODI-ADOME, R., SUNSHARA, N. & UCHIDA, Y. Evidence for the involvement of a plasma kallikrein-kinin system in the immediate hypotension produced by endotoxin in anaesthetized rats. Br. J. Pharmacol. 1989; 78, 1383-1391.

11. UCHIDA, Y., KATORI, M. Independent consumption of high and low molecular weight kininogens in vivo. In "Kinin IV" Part a, 1986; pp.113-117, Adv. Exp. Med. Biol., Plenum Press, New York.

12. FRAKI, J., JANSEN, C., HOPSU-HAVU, V. Human aweat kallikrein. Acta Derm.-Vereol. (Stockh.) 1970; 50, 321-326.

AAS 38/I
Recent Progress on Kinins
© 1992 Birkhäuser Verlag Basel

QUANTIFICATION OF ILE-SER-BRADYKININ DEGRADATION IN HUMAN SERUM AND ASCITES

J. Rehbock, C. Steinhauser and A. Hermann

1. Frauenklinik der Universität München
(Direktor Prof. Dr. G. Kindermann)
Maistr. 11, D-8000 München 2, Deutschland

SUMMARY: A leucine aminopeptidase (LAP) and a carboxypeptidase (CP) activity in human serum and malignant ascites degrade Ile-Ser-Bradykinin (ISB = T-Kinin) in two catalytic steps to desArg9Bradykinin. The catalytic activity in serum is always higher than in ascites. In serum the carboxypeptidase activity is higher than the LAP activity whereas in ascites the two activities are not different.

INTRODUCTION

Large amounts of Ile-Ser-Bradykinin (ISB = T-Kinin) have been reported to occur in a few cases of human malignant ascites (1). As kinins are very effective in enhancing vascular permeability they are supposed to play a role in the pathophysiology of ascites generation (1,2). To find ISB is surprising as kinins are normally degraded rapidly in vivo (3). Experiments concerning the degradation of Ile-Ser-BK elucidated the role of a leucine aminopeptidase (LAP) and a carboxypeptidase activity (CP) (4). Further experiments were now performed to quantify these two enzymatic activities in several paired samples of serum and ascites from tumor patients.

MATERIALS AND METHODS

We collected paired samples of serum and ascites of eight patients suffering from different carcinoma (six with ovarian

and two with cervix carcinoma). The samples were taken freshly
for the incubation studies. 5 nmol ISB in 100 ul PBS were
incubated at 37°C with 100 ul serum or ascites, respectivly.
Incubation was stopped by adding hot methanol after 10, 20, and
30 min.

The reaction products were measured by reversed phase HPLC
method using an isocratic system. Column: Ultrasphere C8, 5 u,
0.46 x 15 cm. Eluent: 0.05% TFA and 0.025% TEA in acetonitrile
20% (v/v) and water. Flow 1 ml/min.

Specific inhibitors (Amastatin 25 uM, MGTA 1 mM, captopril 25
uM) were studied in order to further characterize the enzymes.

RESULTS

A LAP and a CP activity could be constantly found in each
malignant ascites or serum. Added ISB (T-Kinin) was degraded by
these enzymatic activities as shown in Figure 1 and 2.

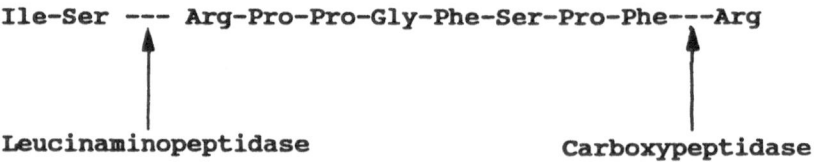

Figure 1. Amino acid sequence of Ile-Ser-BK with the cleaving
sites for LAP and CP.

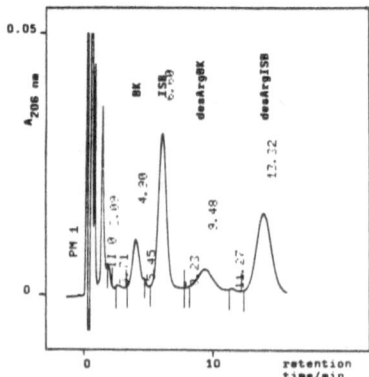

Figure 2. HPLC chromatogramm after having incubated ISB with
serum for 20 min. ISB is partly degraded to BK and desArgISB and
finally to desArgBK.

LAP was blocked by 50-90% by amastatin 25 uM. CP was almost completely blocked by MGTA 330 uM. An influence of captopril could not be demonstrated. In every patient the catalytic activity in serum was higher than in ascites. In serum CP activity was always higher than LAP activity. In ascites the two activities were not different. The interindividual activities differed considerably (Table 1).

Table 1. CP and LAP activities (nmol/min) in serum and ascites of eight tumor patients

| | SERUM | | | ASCITES | | |
	CP	AP	total	CP	AP	total
Cervix Ca.	1.4	1.2	2.6	0.2	0.7	0.9
Ovarian-Ca.	1.4	0.3	1.7	0.3	0.7	1.0
Ovarian-Ca.	1.1	0.4	1.5	0.3	0.3	0.6
Ovarian-Ca.	1.1	0.6	1.7	0.3	0.2	0.5
Cervix-Ca.	1.8	0.2	2.0	0.2	0.1	0.3
Ovarian-Ca.	1.0	0.5	1.5	0.4	0.3	0.7
Ovarian-Ca.	1.0	0.1	1.1	0.3	0.2	0.5
Ovarian-Ca.	1.1	0.3	1.4	0.5	0.3	0.8
mean	1.2	0.5	1.7	0.3	0.4	0.7
±SEM	0.1	0.12	0.16	0.04	0.08	0.08

statistics: unpaired t-test
CP-activity Serum vs Ascites $p < 0.001$
AP-activity Serum vs Ascites N.S.
total enzyme activity Serum vs Ascites $p < 0.001$
Serum CP-activity vs Serum AP-activity $p < 0.001$
Ascites CP-activity vs Ascites AP-activity N.S.

DISCUSSION

The kininase activities of the studied tumor patients are higher in serum than in ascites. Many factors may be involved: different sites of synthesis, different distribution, dilution and a different half time in the different compartments. Extended further studies are necessary to investigate these factors.

Kininases are synthesised in many tissues in mammals (3). The also may diffuse or be secreted into the peritoneal cavity and into the circulation by solid tumors which are one site of production as shown by Deddish et al. This group detected the enhanced production of neutral endopeptidase (NEP) in solid tumors. Carboxypeptidase M occured also in the tumor, but was not enhanced in the same way as NEP. (5)

Matsumura et al. performed digestion studies with BK and (Hyp3)BK or fragments of these peptides as subtrates and with much longer incubation times. They observed also a carboxypeptidase activitiy and besides that an angiotensin converting enzyme (ACE) activity and other unidentified metalloproteases responsible for kinin degradation. A LAP activity in malignant ascites was not described.(6). In another study by Sheik and Kaplan carboxypeptidase N and B and ACE were shown to degrade kinins in serum, whereas ACE activity was detected with prolonged incubation time(7).

Taking ISB as substrate no influence of other enzymes was observed during thirty minutes of incubation as the sum of the remaining ISB and the formed degradation products was nearly constant .Therefore it seems to be unlikely that other enzymes contribute significantly to the degrading of ISB under the conditions of this study in the first 30 min of incubation.

CONCLUSION

Ile-Ser-Bradykinin (T-Kinin) is more rapidly degraded in human serum than in ascites. For the few cases where ISB was detected in ascites it must be assumed that synthesis of ISB in vivo exceeded degradation. The higher enzymatic activity in human serum may be the cause that ISB was not found in serum.

ACKNOWLEDGEMENTS

This work was supported by the Wilhelm Sander-Stiftung.

REFERENCES

1. Wunderer G, Walter I, Eschenbacher B, Lang M, Kellerman J, Kindermann G. Ile-Ser-Bradykinin is an aberrant permeability factor in various human malignant effusions. Biol Chem Hoppe-Seyler 1990; 371: 977-981.

2. Matsumura Y, Kimura M, Yamamoto T, Maeda H. Involvement of the Kinin-generating Cascade in Enhanced Vascular Permeability in Tumor Tissue. Jpn J Cancer Res (Gann) 1988; 79: 1327-1334.

3. Erdös EG. Kininases. In: Bradykinin, Kallidin and Kallikrein. Erdös EG, editor. Berlin: Springer, 1979; 25: 428-487.

4. Rehbock J, Wunderer G. Degradation of Ile-Ser-Bradykinin by enzymes in human serum and ascites. Biochem Pharmacol 1991; 41: 1081-1083.

5. Deddish PA, Dragovic T, Erdös EG, Weber G. High Concentration of Neutral Endopeptidase (Enkephalinase E.C. 3.4.24.11) in a malignant Tumor: Rat Hepatoma 3924A. BBRC 1990; 169: 81-86.

6. Matsumura Y, Maeda H, Kato H. Degradation pathway of kinins in tumor ascites and inhibition by kininase inhibitors: Analysis by HPLC. Agents Actions 1990; 29: 172-180.

7. Sheik IA, Kaplan AP.Mechanism of Digestion of Bradykinin and Lysylbradykinin (Kallidin) in Human Serum. Biochem Pharmacol, 1989; 38: 993-1000.

AAS 38/I
Recent Progress on Kinins
© 1992 Birkhäuser Verlag Basel

INHIBITORS OF SOME RECENTLY CHARACTERIZED KININ-METABOLIZING ENZYMES: A BRIEF OVERVIEW

Ervin G. Erdös

Depts. of Pharmacol. and Anesthesiol. U. of Illinois, Coll. Med. Chicago, IL 60612

SUMMARY: The brief review surveys some of the recent advances in studies on kininases and their inhibitors.

INTRODUCTION

The rapid inactivation of kallidin in plasma was noted simultaneously with its discovery (1-3). The history of the release and inactivation of bradykinin, that followed its release, was quite similar. Bradykinin and kallidin having 8 or 9 peptide bonds, are susceptible to a variety of peptidases that can convert kallidin to bradykinin, inactivate kinins, or modify their receptor selectivity. These kininases - as they are called collectively and possibly erroneously - were extensively reviewed in 1970 and 1979 (1,2). The reviews also list many inhibitors of these enzymes. This contribution is certainly not a detailed examination of the topic. My aim in writing it was not to present an extensive survey but to point only to some recent developments.

The current interest in the subject, in the inactivation of kinins, may be due to newly revealed information stemming from the purification and subsequent cloning of some of these kininases and somewhat paradoxically, that none of them is specific to a single substrate. It follows that their inhibitors can have multiple effects. For example, inhibitors of angiotensin I converting enzyme (ACE), obviously block the action of the identical kininase

II on bradykinin (1-5). Besides inhibiting the release of angiotensin II, ACE inhibitors may owe some of their beneficial effects to prolonging the half-life of bradykinin. This action has been the subject of extensive investigations, with special emphasis on the heart (6,7). Inhibitors of another kininase II type enzyme, neutral endopeptidase 24.11 or enkephalinase (NEP), prolong the renal action of the atrial natriuretic peptide, which is cleaved by this enzyme (8,9). Inhibitors of NEP can also protect endogenous kinins, released in the kidney, against inactivation by NEP (10).

Ideally, an inhibitor could be considered important in kinin metabolism, if the enzyme it reacts with is widely distributed, if it acts in vivo, and if it can prolong the half-life of kinins in several species. Besides the inhibitors of ACE and NEP, few others would fit into that category.

Among the caveats worth considering is the simple fact that the specificity of inhibitors is relative to their concentration. If raised beyond a certain level they can inhibit other enzymes. In studies in vivo, the dilution of the samples to be assayed in vitro and the possible dissociation of the enzyme and a reversible inhibitor, hence the lowering of available inhibitor concentration in vitro, should be considered. Furthermore, when the potency of tight-binding inhibitors is compared, the molar enzyme concentrations should be paid attention to, and possibly adjusted to the same level.

It was reported three decades ago (1) that in blood plasma, kallidin was rapidly converted to bradykinin by the hydrolysis of Lys^1-Arg^2 bond by an aminopeptidase. Bradykinin was inactivated by the removal of N-terminal Arg^1 by an erythrocyte enzyme which was called at that time, prolidase or imidopeptidase. Later, the same reaction was described to occur in kidney and lung (1). Both of these enzymes, aminopeptidase M and P, have been further characterized and purified (11-13). The former enzyme is inhibited, for example, by amastatin and the latter by Pro-Pro-Ala. Obviously, all metallopeptidases are inhibited by sequestering agents that bind metal cofactors, such as o-phenanthroline.

Kinins are substrates, at least in vitro, of other

endopeptidases. One of them is the so called prolylendopeptidase, a serine protease. It is inhibited by dipeptides related to its substrate (e.g. Z-Pro-Pro) and noncompetitively by prolinal (Z-Pro-Prolinal; 14-17). Another endopeptidase that cleaves bradykinin at Phe[5]-Ser[6] bond is endopeptidase 24.15, which is identical with the brain oligoendopeptidase or Pz-peptidase (18-20). This is a thiol dependent metalloendopeptidase, thus it is inhibited by metal chelators and thiol blocking agents. The specific inhibitor N-[1-R,S]carboxy-3-phenylpropyl-Ala-Ala-Phe-p-aminobenzoic acid potentiates the hypotensive effect of bradykinin in rat (21).

Meprin, an enzyme discovered in mouse proximal tubules, also cleaves bradykinin at Phe[5]-Ser[6]. Based on that finding, Phe[5]-4-nitrobradykinin (22,23) was synthesized as a substrate.

The enzymes we studied most are kininase I or II-type, thus they either split off Arg[9] or Phe[8]-Arg[9] of bradykinin or equivalent bonds in kallidin. Although originally these terms referred to human plasma carboxypeptidase N and ACE (1,2), by now several other enzymes are known to catalyze the reaction (Table 1). Besides ACE, NEP is a major enzyme that releases the C-terminal dipeptide (4), for example, it is the kininase on the plasma membrane of neutrophils (24). NEP is inhibited by phosphoramidon, a thermolysin inhibitor, by thiorphan and by other agents synthesized with possible clinical application in mind (9).

The C-terminal arginine of kinins is released by carboxypeptidase B of the pancreas, N of blood plasma, and by M that is present on the plasma membrane of many cells (25). An entirely different enzyme, the so called deamidase (26) or lysosomal protective protein (27) also cleaves this arginine. The properties of this protein distinguish it from the metallopeptidases mentioned above, and it has many similarities to cathepsin A. Depending on the pH, it has three activities; it liberates free and protected C-terminal amino acids, cleaves esters, and deamidates peptides such as tachykinins, converting them to free acid. It is not inhibited by carboxypeptidase inhibitors, but by DFP, p-chloromercuriphenylsulfonate and chymostatin; thus, it is a serine protease-type enzyme. Although it is inhibited by compounds which react with SH groups, it is not a cathepsin since the specific cathepsin inhibitor E64 does not inhibit it. It has an acid pH optimum for peptidase activity, but in contrast to short dipeptide substrates which are not significantly hydrolyzed at pH 7, it cleaves bradykinin at neutral pH only about 30% slower than at pH 5.5. Although we purified the enzyme from human platelets, it is present in many other cell types, for example, in smooth muscles (28).

The inhibitors of these kininase I and II-type enzymes vary in their specificity a great deal. Caboxypeptidases, NEP and ACE have zinc cofactors, consequently, they are inhibited by sequestering agents. The basic carboxypeptidases (25) are also inhibited by 2-mercaptomethyl-3-guanidinoethyl thiopropanoic acid (MGTA) and by guanidinoethylmercaptosuccinic acid (GEMSA) or by E-amino-n-caproic acid (1-5). The latter compound is structurally closely related to a split product of the reaction.

The inhibition of carboxypeptidase B, N and M is also pH and structure dependent. GEMSA is a more potent inhibitor of the membrane-bound form of carboxypeptidase M than of the purified soluble enzyme. It also inhibits carboxypeptidases more at an acid pH (e.g. 5.5) than above neutrality, which is optimal for the enzymes (29). Carboxypeptidase N and M activity, however, cannot be distinguished by these inhibitors, but by immunopreciptation with specific antibodies raised to the purified enzymes (Abe, et al., submitted).

The successful clinical application of ACE inhibitors to millions of patients in various countries is well accepted. The exact contributions of the increased half-life of bradykinin to the beneficial effects of ACE inhibitors have yet to be established. There are many ACE inhibitors in clinical use by now enalapril, lysinopril, captopril, quinilapril and ramipril are among them. Some NEP inhibitors are undergoing clinical trials.

Recently, the synthesis of two new, potentially very useful inihibitors was reported. These compounds have a dual action. One, besides inhibiting NEP, also blocks aminopeptidase N (30), thus it should prolong the half-life of enkephalins and maybe other peptides which are cleaved by the two enzymes. The other compound is targeted to inhibit both NEP and ACE (31), consequently, it may potentiate bradykinin in organs where both NEP and ACE act as kininases, such as the kidney (10). Hypothetically, this mixed inhibitor may facilitate the diuretic and natriuretic actions of intrarenal kinins (31).

Very likely, the continued use of inhibitors will help to reveal new information on the enzymatic metabolism of kinins and on their functions in various tissues.

Table 1.   INHIBITORS OF KININASE I AND II-TYPE ENZYMES

Enzyme Group	Name	Inhibitor
	Carboxypeptidase N	Sequestering Agents GEMSA, MGTA
Kininase I	Carboxypeptidase M	Sequestering Agents GEMSA, MGTA
	Deamidase (Cathepsin A ?; Protective Protein)	Chymostatin, DFP Z-G-L-F-CH$_2$Cl[1], PCMS[2]
	ACE	Sequestering Agents ACE Inhibitors
Kininase II	Neutral Endopeptidase 24.11 (Enkephalinase, Calla[3])	Sequestering Agents Phosphoramidon, Thiorphan

1.   Cbz-Glycyl-Leucyl-Phenylalanine-CH$_2$Cl.
2.   p-Chloromercuriphenylsulfonate.
3.   Common acute lymphoblastic leukemia antigen.

1. Erdös EG, Yang HYT. Kininases. In Bradykinin, Kallidin and Kallikrein. Handbook of Experim Pharmacology. Erdös EG, editor. Springer-Verlag, Heidelberg. 1970; Vol XXV:289-323.

2. Erdös EG. Kininases. In Bradykinin, Kallidin and Kallikrein. Handbook of Experim Pharmacol. Erdös EG, editor. Springer-Verlag, Heidelberg. 1979; Supplement to Vol. XXV, 427-487.

3. Erdös EG. From measuring the blood pressure to mapping the gene: the development of ideas of Frey and Werle. In The Kallikrein and Kinin System in Health and Disease. EK Frey and E Werle Memorial Volume. Fritz H, Schmidt I and Dietze G editors. Limbach-Verlag, Braunschweig. 1989; 261-276.

4. Erdös EG. Some old and some new ideas on kinin metabolism. J Cardiovascular Pharmacol. 1990; 15(Suppl 6):S20-S24.

5. Erdös EG. Angiotensin I converting enzyme and the changes in our concepts through the years. LK Dahl Memorial Lecture. Hypertension. 1990; 16:363-370.

6. Schölkens BA, Linz W, Lindpaintner K, and Ganten D. Angiotensin deteriorates but bradykinin improves cardiac function following ischaemia in isolated rat hearts. J Hypertension. 1987; 5(suppl 5):S7-S9.

7. Linz W, Martorana PA, Grötsch H, Bei-Yin Q, and Schölkens BA. Antagonizing bradykinin (BK) obliterates the cardioprotective effects of bradykinin and angiotensin-converting enzyme (ACE) inhibitors in ischemic hearts. Drug Develop Res. 1990; 19:393-408.

8. Richards AM, Wittert G, Espiner EA, Yandle TG, Frampton C, and Ikram H. EC 24.11 Inhibition in man alters clearance of atrial natriuretic peptide. J Clinical Endocrinol and Metabol. 1991; 72:1317-1322.

9. Schwartz J-C, Gros C, Lecomte J-M, and Bralet J. Enkephalinase (EC 3.4.24.11) inhibitors: Protection of endogenous ANF against inactivation and potential therapeutic applications. Life Sci. 1990; 47:1279-1297.

10. Ura N, Carretero OA, Erdös EG. The role of renal endopeptidase 24.11 in kinin metabolism. Kidney Internat. 1987; 32:507-513.

11. Himmelhoch SR, and Peterson EA. Preparation of leucine aminopeptidase free of endopeptidase activity. Biochem. 1968; 7:2085-2093.

12. Ward PE, Chow A, Drapeau G. Metabolism of bradykinin agonists and antagonists by plasma aminopeptidase P. Biochem Pharmacol. 1991; 42:721-727.

13. Simmons WH, and Orawski AT. Membrane-bound aminopeptidase P from bovine lung. Its purification, properties, and degradation of bradykinin. J Biol Chem. 1992; 257: in press.

14. Koida M, and Walter R. Post-proline cleaving enzyme. Purification of this endopeptidase by affinity chromatography. J Biol Chem. 1978; 261:7593-7599.

15. Wilk S. Prolyl endopeptidase. Life Sci. 1983; 33:2149-2157.

16. Orlowski M, Wilk E, Pearce S, and Wilk S. Purification and properties of a prolyl endopeptidase from rabbit brain. J Neurochem. 1979; 33:461-469.

17. Wilk S, and Orlowski M. Inhibition of rabbit brain prolyl endopeptidase by N-benzyloxycarbonyl-prolyl-prolinal, a transition state aldehyde inhibitor. J Neurochem. 1983; 69-75.

18. Orlowski M, Reznik S, Ayala J, and Pierotti AR. Endopeptidase 24.15 from rat testes. Isolation of the enzyme and its specificity toward synthetic and natural peptides, including enkephalin-containing peptides. Biochem J. 1989; 261:951-958.

19. Camargo ACM, Caldo H, and Reis ML. Susceptibility of a peptide derived from bradykinin to hydrolysis by brain endo-oligopeptidases and pancreatic proteinases. J Biol Chem. 1979; 254:5304-5307.

20. Barrett AJ, and Brown MA. Chicken liver Pz-peptidase, a thiol-dependent metallo-endopeptidase. Biochem J. 1990; 271:701-706.

21. Genden EM, and Molineaux CJ. Inhibition of endopeptidase-24.15 decreases blood pressure in normotensive rats. Hypertension. 1991; 18:360-365.

22. Kounnas MZ, Wolz RL, Gorbea CM, and Bond JS. Meprin-A and -B. Cell surface endopeptidases of the mouse kidney. J Biol Chem. 1991; 266:17350-17357.

23. Wolz RL, and Bond JS. Phe[5](4-nitro)-bradykinin: A chromogenic substrate for assay and kinetics of the metalloendopeptidase meprin. Anal Biochem. 1990; 191:314-320.

24. Skidgel RA, Jackman HL, Erdös EG. Metabolism of substance P and bradykinin by human neutrophils. Biochem Pharmacol. 1991; 41:1335-1344.

25. Skidgel RA. Basic carboxypeptidases: regulators of peptide hormone activity. Trends Pharmacol Sci. 1988; 9:299-304.

26. Jackman HL, Tan F, Tamei H, Erdös, EG, Beurling-Harbury C, Li X-Y, Skidgel RA.   A peptidase in human platelets that deamidates tachykinins: probable identity with the lysosomal "protective protein." J Biol Chem. 1990; 265:272.

27. Galjart NJ, Gillemans N, Harris A. van der Horst GTJ, Verheijen FW, Galjaard H, and d'Azzo A. Expression of cDNA encoding the human "protective protein" associated with lysosomal β-galactosidase and neuraminidase: homology to yeast proteases. Cell. 1988; 54:755-764.

28. Jackman HL, Morris PW, Deddish PA, Skidgel RA, and Erdös EG. Inactivation of endothelin I by deamidase (lysosomal protective protein). J Biol Chem. 1992; in press.

29. Deddish PA, Skidgel RA, Erdös EG. Enhanced cobalt activation and inhibitor binding of carboxypeptidase M at low pH: similarity to carboxypeptidase H (enkephalin convertase). Biochem J. 1989; 261:289-291.

30. Roques BP, and Beaumont A.   Neutral endopeptidase-24.11 inhibitors: from analgesics to antihypertensives?   Trends Pharmacol Sci. 1990; 11:245-249.

31. Gros C, Noël N, Souque A, Schwartz J-C, Danvy D, Plaquevent J-C, Duhamel L, Duhamel P, Lecomte J-M, and Bralet J. Mixed inhibitors of angiotensin-converting enzyme (EC 3.4.15.1) and enkephalinase (EC 3.4.24.11): Rational design, properties, and potential cardiovascular applications of glycopril and alatriopril. Proc Natl Acad Sci. 1991; 88:4210-4214.

AAS 38/I
Recent Progress on Kinins
© 1992 Birkhäuser Verlag Basel

ISOLATION OF A BRADYKININ-POTENTIATING FACTOR FROM SCORPION TITYUS SERRULATUS VENOM

L.A.F. Ferreira and O.B. Henriques

Department of Biochemistry, Butantan Institute, Sao Paulo, Brasil

SUMMARY: A bradykinin-potentiating factor was isolated and characterized from the scorpion TITYUS SERRULATUS venom by chromatographic techniques and reverse phase followed by biological assays. This factor showed to be able to potentiate the contractile activity of the isolated guinea-pig ileum, inhibited the angiotensin-converting enzyme and potentiated the bradykinin-induced lowering of the arterial blood pressure in the rat.

INTRODUCTION

At least four kinins have been isolated from mammalian blood plasma: Bradykinin (BK), Lys-bradykinin (LBK) or kallidin, Met-Lys-bradykinin (MLB) and T-kinin. These kinins act on several smooth muscles with dose-dependent contractions or relaxation (7).

Snake venoms usually contain a considerable number of inhibitor peptides of angiotensin-converting enzyme (ACE) and kininases. As they potentiate the smooth-muscle contracting activity of bradykinin, they are called bradykinin-potentiating peptides (BPF). They were first reported in *Bothrops jararaca* venom by Ferreira & Rocha e Silva 1963 (2), who observed that the venom itself had a strong potentiating activity upon the contractions elicited by bradykinin (1).

Nassar et al 1989 (6) isolated bradykinin-potentiating peptides showing an activity similar to that of the synthetic B and C from *Buthus occitanus*, and *Leiurus quiquestriatus* scorpion venoms. This paper reports the isolation and biological activity of a bradykinin-potentiating factor from *Tityus serrulatus* venom.

MATERIALS AND METHODS

Tityus serrulatus dried venom was obtained from the Butantan Institute, Sao Paulo, Brasil. *Bothrops jararaca* plasma was a gift from the Laboratory of Pharmacology from Butantan Institute. Adult male rats (300-320 g) and female guinea-pigs (160-180 g) were used. Sephadex G-25 M and Sephadex G-10 were obtained from Pharmacia Fine Chemicals, Uppsala. Bradykinin, Captopril and BPF_{5a} (pGlu-Lys-Trp-Ala-Pro) were purchased from Sigma Chemical Co, St. Louis, Mo. Angiotensin-converting enzyme was partially purified from *B. jararaca* plasma (5). Other reagents were from Merck, Darmstadt, F.R.G.

Factor purification. The crude venom (500 mg) was dissolved in 2.5 ml of ammonium acetate buffer 50 mM, pH4.7, and chromatographed on a G-25 M Sephadex column (2 x 190 cm) previously equilibrated with the same buffer at a flow rate of 40 ml/hr. The fractions (3 ml) were tested on the isolated guinea-pig ileum for bradykinin-potentiation, pooled and then lyophilized. The lyophilized residue (85 mg) was dissolved in 3 ml of the ammonium acetate buffer chromatographed on a Sephadex G-10 column (1 x 120 cm), previously equilibrated with the same buffer, at the rate of 20 ml/hr, in fractions of 2 ml. The active fractions were pooled (peak 1, Fig. 1) and analysed by HPLC. These analyses were performed with a Waters instrument using a reverse phase column (Ultropac TSK ODS 120 P, 5 μm) of 30 x 0.38 cm. Two gradient systems were used: 20% acetonitrile/80% and 15% ortho-phosphoric acid, followed by 10% acetonitrile/90 % and 0.1 % trifluoracetic acid.

Potentiating activity. The potentiating activity of the fractions was measured on the isolated guinea-pig ileum. One potentiating "unit" was defined as the amount of peptide per ml of incubation solution, able to double the activity of a single dose of bradykinin (3). In order to determine potentiation, a log-dose response curve of the effect of bradykinin on the isolated guinea-pig ileum was made. The isolated peptide was then tested by measuring the effect of an established amount of bradykinin plus increasing amounts of peptide, in order to determine the dose of potentiator beyond which no further increase of the ileum response to bradykinin occured. The maximal potentiation of bradykinin by increasing amounts of peptide is measured on a log-dose response curve obtained using an established dose (5 ng) of bradykinin (Fig. 3).

Angiotensin-converting enzyme (ACE) inhibition. To measure inhibition of ACE from *B. jararaca* plasma (50 μg), factor (1.4 μg) and bradykinin (100 μg) in 500 μl of Tyrode solution, were incubated at 37°C, pH7 for 15 and 30 min. The residual activity was calculated using a log-dose response curve for spontaneous bradykinin hydrolysis in the absence of ACE under the same conditions of assay on the isolated guinea-pig ileum. The factor was omitted from control samples.

Arterial blood pressure. The carotide artery blood pressure of an adult male rat (300 g), anesthetized with nembutal (90 mg/kg) i.p. was recorded by a mercury manometer on a smoked drum. Injection of the drugs into the iliac was made through a polyethylene catheter.

RESULTS AND DISCUSSION

A bradykinin-potentiating factor was isolated from *Tityus serrulatus* venom by gel filtration and HPLC chromatography, Fig. 1 and 2.

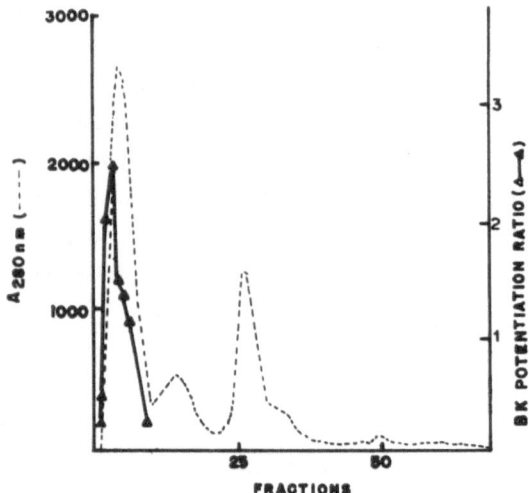

Fig.1. Gel filtration on Sephadex G-10 of the lyophilized active pool obtained from the Sephadex G-25 M.
Gel filtration Sephadex G-10 column (0.9 x 118 cm) of 85 mg active pool (Sephadex G-25): Buffer was 50 mM ammonium acetate (pH4.7) and fractions were 1.5 ml. Absorbance at 280 μm (----). Bradykinin (BK) potentiation ratio ($\triangle$——$\triangle$). Similar results to those were obtained in three separate experiments.

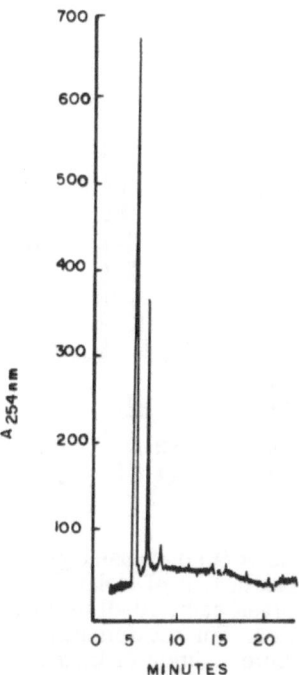

Fig.2. HPLC separation of the active peptide eluted on the peak I of the Sephadex G-10 column.
Separation of 100 μg of the peak I (Fig. 1), on reverse-phase HPLC column (Ultropac TSK ODS) of 30 x 0.38 cm. Eluent was 10% acetonitrile/90% and 0.1% trifluoracetic acid. Flow rate was 1 ml/min. This experiment is representive of four similar results.

Our results show that this isolated factor from scorpion venom (400 μg) potentiated two times the bradykinin potentiating unit, when it was submitted on the guinea-pig ileum, Fig. 3. The factor was also assayed to inhibit the angiotensin-converting enzyme (ACE) from *B. jararaca* plasma; an incubation of the factor and ACE was made, see Methods. The inhibition of the ACE showed to be total after 30 min. of incubation, Fig. 4.

Fisher & Ryan (4) have observed that the C-terminal carboxyl group seems to be an absolute requirement for binding of an inhibitor to the enzyme and appears to be most advantageous when the C-terminal residue is proline or isoleucine.

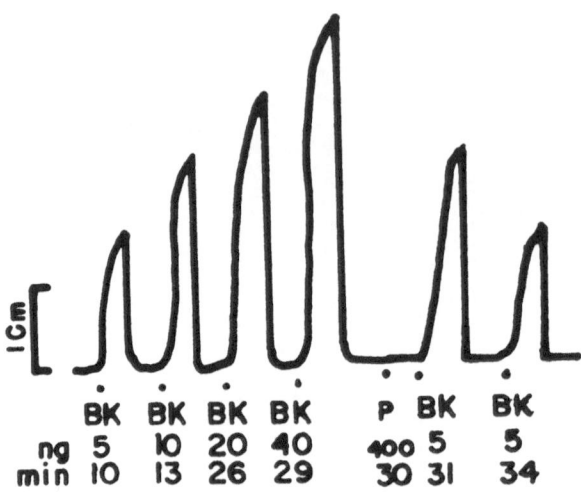

Fig.3. Potentiation of bradykinin by factor (P) on isolated guinea-pig ileum.
Bradykinin activity was assayed by contraction of isolated guinea-pig ileum in aerated tyrode solution at 35°C. To a 5 ml organ bath, 10-40 ng of synthetic bradykinin were added at 3 min. intervals, as indicated. For measurement of bradykinin potentiating activity, the factor was added just before addition of bradykinin (BK), P (400 ng) and BK (5 ng). Similar results to those shown were obtained in four separate experiments.

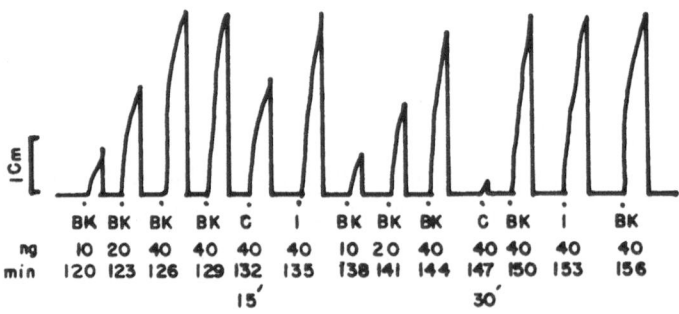

Fig.4 Inhibition of the angiotensin-converting enzyme by purified factor.
Inhibition was obtained by assay on isolated guinea-pig ileum. Factor (1.2 µg) was incubated with 100 µg of angiotensin-converting enzyme (ACE) at pH 7 at 37°C for 15 and 30 min. using 100 µg of bradykinin as substrate (I). Controls were performed in the same conditions, except that the factor was substituted by Tyrode solution (c). Similar results to those shown were obtained in three separate experiments, means ± SE.

On the other hand, this factor was tested to potentiate the effect hypotensive of the bradykinin upon the rat arterial blood pressure. When the factor (1.5 μg/kg) was injected intravenously into the iliac vein rat followed by bradkinin (20 μg/kg), a decrease of 30 mm Hg from the usual basal pressure of 110 mm Hg was observed showing to be two times greater than produced by bradykinin, Fig. 5. The results here presented may help to explain the mechanism of the potentiating effect of the inhibitory actions on bradykinin-destroying enzymes.

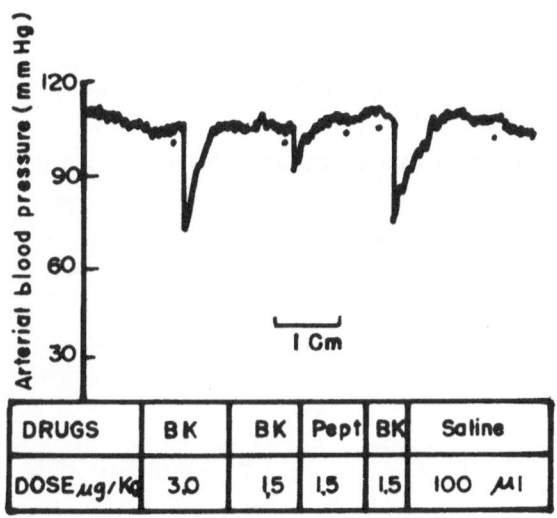

Fig.5. Action of factor on hypotensive action of bradykinin.
Bradykinin (BK) hypotensive potentiating activity of the factor (Pep) was found to be 1.5 μg/kg upon rat arterial blood pressure. Similar results to those shown were obtained in four separate experiments.

ACKNOLEDGEMENT

This work was supported by FAPESP and CNPq.

REFERENCES

1.   Cintra ACO, Vieira CV, Giglio JR. Primary structure and biologiacal activity of
     bradykinin-potentiating peptides from *Bothrops insularis* snake venom. J Protein
     Chemistry 1990; 9: 221.

2.   Ferreira SH, Rocha e Silva M. Potenciacao de polipeptidios (bradicinina, angiotensina, ocitocina, etc.) por um fator presente no veneno de *B. jararaca*. Ciencia e Cultura 1963; 15:276.

3.   Ferreira SH, Bartelt DC, Greene LJ. Isolation of bradykinin-potentiating peptides from *Bothrops jararaca* venom. Biochemistry 1970; 9:2583.

4.   Fisher GH, Ryan JW. Distant binding sites of kininase II. Adv Exp Med Biol 1981; 156B:813.

5.   Nishimura K, Yoshida N, Hiwada K, Ueda E, Kokubu T. Purification of angiotensin converting-enzyme from human lung. Biochim Biophys Acta 1977; 483:398.

6.   Nassar AY, Abu-Sinna G, Abu-Amra S. Isolated fractions from toxins of egyptian scorpions and cobra, activated smooth muscle contraction and glomerular filtration (Abstract). Toxicon 1989; 27:65.

7.   Piek T. Neurotoxic kinins from wasp and antivenoms. Toxicon 1991; 29:139.

AAS 38/I
Recent Progress on Kinins
© 1992 Birkhäuser Verlag Basel

ISOLATION AND CHARACTERIZATION OF BIOLOGICAL PROPERTIES
OF INHIBITORS ANGIOTENSIN-1-CONVERTING ENZYME FROM THE
SPIDER VENOM LATRODECTUS TREDECIMGUTTATUS

A.A. Akchunov, Z. Golubenko, N. Sosnina

Institute of Bioorganic Chemistry
named after A.S. Sadykov AS RUz, Tashkent, Uzbekistan

SUMMARY: For the first time by method of gel-filtration and ionexchange chromatography two bradykinin-potentiating peptides have been isolated in homogeneous state from Latrodectus tredecimguttatus spider venom. The homogeneity was proved by disk-electrophoresis, isoelectrical focusing, analysis of aminoacid content and rechromatography. Peptides are acid proteins with molecular mass 10,000 and 2500 D. Peptides prolong depressor effects of bradykinin, stimulate histamine releasing from cells, decrease blood pressure in rats.

INTRODUCTION

Kinins have the wide spectrum of biological action and take part in some processes, occurring in the body. Peptides, which were promoting and prolonging bradykinin's action in the experiments in vivo and in vitro, have been isolated from the venoms of some species of spiders.

Nine different bradykinin-potentiating peptides, containing from 5 to 13 aminoacid residues have been isolated from the venom of the Southamerican snake (1). In the Japanese snake Agistrodon halys venom five bradykinin-potentiating peptides have been observed. For the first time we've established that not only snakes venoms, but Lotrodectus tredecimguttatus spider venom contain peptides, prossessing bradykinin-potentiating activity (2).

MATERIALS AND METHODS

Latrodectus tredecimguttatus venom has been used in our work. Sephadexes G-10, G-50 (Pharmacia, Sweden), DEAE-cellulose DE-52 (Whatman, Great Britain), TSR-HW-55F (Toyo Soda, Japan), plates with ampholine gradient (LKB, Sweden) carboxypeptidase Y (Sigma, USA) have been utilised.

Carboxycatepsine activity has been determined by fluorometric method with the use as substrate of C-end tripeptide angiotensin I, Phe-His-Leu (3). The homogeneity of the received peptides was proved by the method of gradient electrophoresis in denaturating conditions (4), electrofocusing on standard PAAG-plates with gradient of ampholines in pH grade from 3.5 to 9.5 (LKB, Sweden) according to Karason's method (5) on "Multifor" apparatus and TCH which was carried on the plates with silica-gel Merck (FRG) in the system of solvents butanol-acetic acid-water (63:10:27), developing by 0.2 % ninhydrin in acetone.

For synthesizing bradykinin-potentiating peptides from the venom the method of gelfiltration on the column with TSK-HW-55F ionexchange chromatography with DEAE-Toyopearl and further refining of the active fraction on the column with "Ultrasphere C-18" have been used.

Peptides influence on the hydrolysis of bradykinin kininase of the venom spider has been studied according to the bradykinin inactivation speed (6).

RESULTS

Preparative separation of Latrodectus tredecimguttatus spider venom has been performed on the column with hydrophilic gel TSK-HW-55F. Venom elution was carried in 0.05 M Tris-buffer, pH 8.0. We've succeeded to separate spider venom in 6 fractions. As a result of testing bradykinin-potentiating activity was observed in fractions 3 and 4. Further refining has been carried on the column with DEAE-Toyopearl 650 M in Tris-HCl-buffer at pH 8.0 in 0.05 - 0.2 M NaCl gradient. Three peaks each have been received on the chromatograms, fractions 3-2, 4-1 having potentiating activity. The refining of the fraction 3-2 has been carried on the column "Ultrapak G-2000 SW" at moderate pressure using as eluent 0.5 % acetonytrylphthorant buffer (Fig. 1). The fraction 4-1 has been chromatographed on the column "Ultrasphere C-18" eluing by 0.1 % ammony-phthoracetate buffer (Fig. 2). Both fractions were eluated from the columns as one symmetric peak, at repeated chromatography in the same conditions. At the chromatography in the thin layer of silikagel each fraction gave one spot after staining by ninhydrin, BPP.

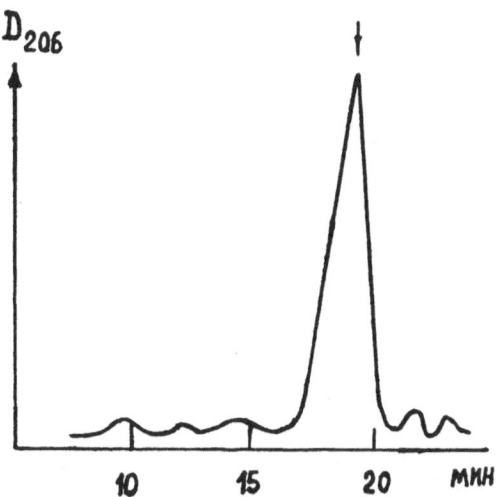

Figure 1. Higheffective liquid chromatography of fractions 3-2. Elution speed 3 ml/h. Arrow marks the fraction containing biological activity

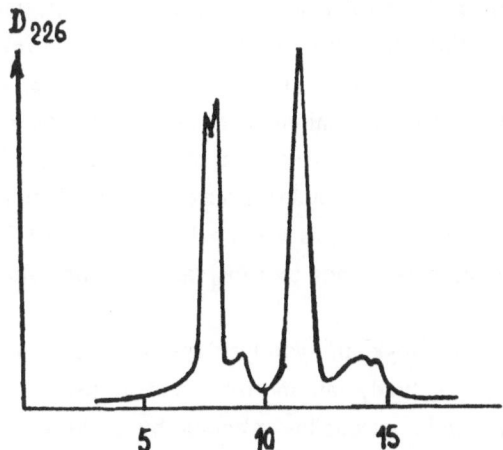

Figure 2. Reverse phase chromatography at high pressure of fractions 4-1. Elution speed 0.7 ml/min. Arrow marks the active fraction

Isolated peptides were marked as BPP_1 (Rf = 0.25) and BPP_2 (Rf = 0.43). According to BPP_1 and BPP_2 electrophoresis and isoelectrofocusing data, acid proteins with isoelectric point 4.7 ± 0.3; 3.5 ± 0.5 and molecular mass 10,000 ± 200 are equal to 2500 ± 300 DA, accordingly. Aminoacid content of the peptides is shown on Table 1.

Table 1. Aminoacid content of BPP_1 and BPP_2 from the spider venom.

Aminoacids	Residues number, mol on mol protein	
	BPP_1	BPP_2
Aspartic acid or asparagine	-	1
Threonine	1	1
Serine	1	1
Glutamic acid	40	1
Proline	1	-
Glycine	23	1
Alanine	1	1
Valine	2	1
Methionine	1	1
Isoleucine	1	1
Leucine	-	1
Tyrosine	-	2
Phenylalanine	1	1
Histidine	20	3
Arginine	-	3
Lysine	2	-
Total	94	19
N-end aminoacid	Glutaminic acid	Glycin

It is established that BPP_1 has N-end glutamic acid and BPP_2 - glycine. According to aminoacid analysis data, polypeptide chain BPP_1 contains 94 aminoacid residues. Glutamic acid, glycine, histidine predominate among them and tyrosine, arginine, leucine, aspartic acid residues are absent. BPP_2 contains 19 aminoacid residues. We should pay attention to the availability of methionine in its content, high content of histidine, aspartic acid, that distinguish them from bradykinin-potentiating peptides, isolated from other animals venoms.

On the basis of the kinetic curves analysis we should consider that C-end aminoacid consequence Tre-Val-Ala-Gly-OH corresponds to BPP_1 and Tre-Met-Glu-Leu-Ala-OH to BPP_2.

BPP_1 and BPP_2 influence on bradykinin hydrolysis and also kininase of spider venom effect have been studied according to bradykinin inactivation speed (3).

Kinetic constants of bradykinin uncoupling reaction by kininase of spider venom Latrodectus tredecimguttatus in the peptides presence were determined by Lineweaver-Burk (7) method and is equal 1.08 mkM.

Data on carboxycatepsin activity inhibition from bull's kidneys by two peptides are shown on Fig. 3. The first peptide is stronger inhibitor, that follows from the values IC_{50}, accordingly equal for BPP_1 and BPP_2 as $1 \cdot 10^{-7}$ and $1 \cdot 10^{-4}$M.

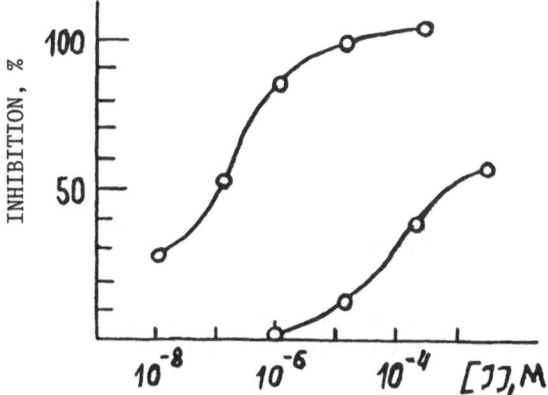

Fig. 3. Influence of BPP_1 and BPP_2 from Latrodectus tredecimguttatus spider venom on carboxycatepsine activity from the bull's kidneys

The studies showed that intravenous injection of bradykinin-potentiating peptides (0.1 mg/kg) doesn't change arterial pressure. At intravenous injection of bradykinin after injected to the animal BPP_1 and BPP_2 in doses 15 mkg/kg, his hypotensive effect increased to 45 - 50 % and to 20 - 25 %, accordingly and prolongation of the bradykinin depressor effect was observed depending on the used dose. Hypotension depth, caused by bradykinin injection before and after the injection of potentiating peptides, shows that BPP_1, which hinders carboxycatepsine activity more powerfully than BPP_2 prolongs and potentiates hypotensive bradykinin effect in greater extent.

Bradykinin-potentiating property of the peptides has specific character because they don't influence the spasmogenic effect of acetylcholine, histamine and serotine.

DISCUSSION

The received data show that potentiating of bradykinin hypotensive action takes place probably owing to the hindrance of carboxycatepsine activity. We should notice that inhibition of kininases isn't the only mechanism, lying in the basis of bradykinin contractile effect increase by the peptides from the venom. That's why the second peptide having expressed bradykinin-potentiating properties appeared less active inhibitor of kininases.

Thus, two peptides isolated for the first time are able to effectively inhibit activity both from the bull's kidneys carboxycatepsine, and kininase from the spider venom that decreases the rates of kinins metabolism in the body and this leads to pharmacological effects increase.

REFERENCES

1.   Kato H, Suzuki T. Bradykinin potentiating peptides from the venom of Agistradon halys blomhoffii. Isolation of five bradykinin potentiators B and C. Biochemistry 1971; 10:972-980.

2.   Akchunov A, Golubenko Z, Sadykov AS. Isolation of kininase from Latrodectus tredecimguttatus spider venom. USSR Acad Sci Rep 1981; 257:1478-1481.

3.   Eliseeva YuE, Orekchovich VN, Pavlichina LV. Property and specificity of action of bull's kidneys carboxycatepsine. Problems of Medical Chemistry 1976; 22:81-82.

4.   Weber R, Osborn M. The reliability of molecular weight determination by dodecyl sulfate polyacrylamide gel electrophoresis. J Biol Chem 1969; 244.

5.   Karlsson C. LKB Application Note 1973; N 75.

6.   Eliseeva YuE, Orekchovich VN, Pavlikina LV. Carboxycatepsine (peptidyl-dipeptidase) isolation. USSR Acad Sci Rep 1974; 217:953-956.

7.   Yakovlev VA. Kinetics of the fermentative catalysis. M Sci 1965; 248.

Kinin Receptors and Kinin Antagonists

KININ RECEPTOR CLASSIFICATION

D. Regoli, D. Jukic, C. Tousignant and N.-E. Rhaleb

Department of Pharmacology, Medical School, University of Sherbrooke, Sherbrooke, Québec, J1H 5N4, Canada

ABSTRACT

Apparent affinities of kinin agonists and antagonists were determined in terms of pD_2 and pA_2 respectively, on three isolated smooth muscles: rabbit jugular vein (Rb.J.V.), rabbit aorta (Rb.A.) and guinea pig ileum (G.P.I.). Both kinin agonists and antagonists were evaluated for their ability to induce the release of histamine from rat mastocytes. Our results indicate that the kininase I metabolites (desArg^9-BK and desArg^{10}-KD) were inactive on Rb.J.V. and G.P.I. (B_2 preparations) and were full agonists on Rb.A. (B_1) while [Tyr(Me)^8]-BK and [Hyp^3,Tyr(Me)^8]-BK were inactive on Rb.A. and maintain a high affinity on Rb.J.V. and G.P.I. In addition, [Hyp^3]-BK was a potent agonist on Rb.J.V. (pD_2 = 8.88) and was of a moderate affinity on G.P.I. (pD_2 = 7.27). On the other hand, the affinity of [Aib^7]-BK was identical to that of BK on G.P.I. (pD_2 = 7.90) but drastically reduced in Rb.J.V. (pD_2 = 6.28). Contractile effects of kinins in the Rb.J.V. and G.P.I. were reduced or eliminated by B_2 receptor antagonists but at different concentration levels (e.g. DArg[Hyp^3,DPhe^7,Leu^8]-BK showed pA_2 values of 8.86 on Rb.J.V., but only 6.77 on G.P.I. DArg[Hyp^3,Gly^6,Leu^8]BK showed high affinity on Rb.J.V. (pA_2 = 7.60) but was a full agonist on G.P.I. Conversely, DArg[Tyr^3,DPhe^7,Leu^8,BK] showed high agonistic activity on Rb.J.V. (pD_2 = 8.30, α^E = 1.0) and showed a pA_2 value of 6.80 on G.P.I. All compounds (agonists and antagonists) were quite potent on histamine release induced in rat mastocytes. [Arg^1(Tos),Hyp^3,Thi^5,DTic^7,Oic^8]-BK and DArg[Hyp^3,Thi^5,DTic^7,Oic^8]-BK showed almost similar pA_2 values on both Rb.J.V. and G.P.I., but were inactive on Rb.A. (B_1). These results suggest that kinins act on at least four functional sites: B_1 (Rb.A.), B_{2A} (Rb.J.V.), B_{2B} (G.P.I.) and B_H. However, there is no clear evidence of a kinin receptor on rat mast cells and the release of histamine may simply be a non-receptor phenomenon. Our data also show that B_{2A} and B_{2B} receptor subtypes might simply be variations of the B_2 receptor in different species.

INTRODUCTION

Bradykinin and related kinins are released in body fluids to act as autacoids in peripheral blood vessels and in a variety of target cells such as smooth muscles, epithelia, exocrine and endocrine glands [1,2,3]. The biological activities of these peptides are mediated by two different receptor types, named B_1 and B_2, of which the former is present only in some species (e.g. the renal vessels of the dog [4] and is generally generated in pathological conditions [5], while the B_2 appears to be a stable component of the plasma membrane of a variety of cells and subserves the majority of the kinin biological effects [3]. Recently, potent antagonists have been identified that block the effects of kinins *in vivo*, on the rat blood pressure [6], the bronchoconstriction in the guinea pig [7], plasma extravasation and pain in man [8]. Some of these compounds have been found to act as agonists instead of antagonists in the isolated guinea pig trachea [9] and the existence of a third kinin receptor (B_3) in this tissue has been proposed [10]. The existence of this new site has been questioned after the discovery of potent B_2 receptor antagonists (e.g. Hoe 140, D-Arg[Hyp^3,Thi^5,D-Tic^7,Oic^8]BK) which blocks the effect of BK on the isolated guinea pig trachea and does not show any agonistic activity [11]. In the present paper, an analysis of the kinin functional sites will be presented by comparing the activities of several agonists and antagonists in an attempt to provide an up-to-date classification of the kinin receptors.

MATERIALS AND METHODS

Pharmacological assays were performed in six isolated organs, taken from rabbits and guinea pigs killed by stunning and exsanguination. The tissues were prepared according to methods previously described: the rabbit jugular vein (Rb.J.V.) and the vena cava (Rb.V.C.) according to Gaudreau *et al.* [12], the rabbit aorta (Rb.A.) according to Furchgott and Bhadrakom [13], the guinea pig ileum (G.P.I.) according to Rang *et al.* [14], the rabbit and guinea pig urinary bladders (Rb.U.B., G.P.U.B) by using the method described by Nakahata [15] and the guinea pig pulmonary artery (G.P.P.A.) according to Hock et al. [11].

The tissues were suspended in 10 ml organ baths containing warm Krebs solution (37°C) oxygenated with a mixture of 95% O_2 and 5% CO_2 for Rb.J.V., Rb.V.C., Rb.A., G.P.I. and G.P.P.A., Tyrode's solution at 32°C for the G.P.U.B. and Rb.U.B. The urinary bladders were stretched with an initial tension of 1 g for all tissues except the isolated veins and ileum which were given 0.5 g. Changes of tension produced by the various agents were measured with Grass isometric transducers (FT 03C, Grass Instrument Co., Quincy, Mass.), calibrated to 1 g = 30 mm. Contractions were displayed on an a Grass polygraph (Model 7D). Before testing the drugs, the preparations were allowed to equilibrate for 45-90 min.

Experimental protocols for kinin agonist activities have been recently described by Rhaleb et al. [16] and those of kinin antagonists by Rhaleb et al. [17]. Assays of histamine release were performed on rat mastocytes according to the method and the experimental protocols previously described by Devillier et al. [18].

All peptides, except Hoe 140 and S1368, were prepared by solid-phase synthesis procedure described by Drapeau and Regoli [19]. Hoe 140 (D-Arg[Hyp³,Thi⁵,D-Tic⁷,Oic⁸]-BK) and S1368 ([Arg¹(Tos),Hyp³,Thi⁵,D-Tic⁷,Oic⁸]-BK were made available from Hoechst AC (Frankfürt, Germany). Concentrated solutions (1-5 mg/ml) of peptides and other agents were made in water and kept at -20°C.

The peptides used in the present experiments, namely bradykinin (BK: 1060.2 M.W.), Lys-BK (kallidin: 1188.4 M.W.), D-Arg-BK (1216.4 M.W.), Sar-BK (1131.3 M.W.), Ile-Ser-BK (T-Kinin: 1260.6 M.W.), [Aib⁷]-BK (1048.3 M.W.), [Tyr(Me)⁸]-BK (1106.3 M.W.), [Hyp³,Tyr(Me)⁸]-BK (1118.4 M.W.), [Hyp³]-BK (1076.4 M.W.), |Arg⁴]BK(4-9) (809.9 M.W.), desPhe⁸,DesArg⁹-BK (757.00 M.W.), Lys,DesPhe⁸,DesArg⁹-BK (885.2 M.W.), DesArg⁹-BK (904.2), [DPhe⁷]-BK (1110.4), D-Arg[D-Phe⁷]-BK (1266.6), [Hyp³,D-Phe⁷]-BK (1125.4), D-Arg[Hyp³,DPhe⁷]-BK (1282.6), D-Arg[Hyp³,Leu⁸]-BK (1198.6), D-Arg[Hyp³,Gly⁶,Leu⁸]-BK (1168.6), D-Arg[Hyp³,D-Phe⁷,Leu⁸]-BK (1248.7), D-Arg[Tyr³,D-Phe⁷,Leu⁸]-BK (1298.7), [Hyp³,D-Phe⁷,Leu⁸]-BK (1102.5) were all synthesized in our laboratory by the solid-phase method and purified by high pressure chromatography [19] and the molecular weight (M.W.) of each peptide was determined by fast atomic bombardment (FAB) mass spectrometry.

Concentration-response curves were measured for bradykinin and its analogues on the four preparations to determine the apparent affinity of the peptides in terms of pD_2 (the negative logarithm of the concentration of agonist that produces 50% of the maximal effect) for isolated smooth muscle and in terms of EC_{50} for histamine release by rat mast cells. Affinites of B_2 antagonists were estimated in terms of pA_2 (-log of the concentration of antagonist that reduces the effect of a double dose of agonist to that of a single dose) [20]. The antagonists were applied 5-10 min before the myotropic effect of bradykinin was measured in their presence. All kinin antagonists were initially applied to tissues at concentrations of 10-100 µg/ml to measure their potential agonistic activites in comparison with BK or desArg⁹-BK. Residual effects of antagonists will be expressed quantitatively in terms of α^E. To compare the competition of two antagonists, Hoe 140 and D-Arg[Hyp³,D-Phe⁷,Leu⁸]-BK, non cumulative concentration-response curves were recorded for BK in the absence and the presence of increasing concentrations of each compound, in order to build a Schild plot [17].

D. Regoli et al.

RESULTS AND DISCUSSION

1. Analysis of four functional sites with agonists

Data summarized in Table 1 indicate that kinins act on at least four functional sites that can be differentiated (even B_{2A} and B_{2B} to some extent) with agonists.

Table 1. Apparent affinities (pD_2) and relative activities of kinin agonists in four functional sites.

COMPOUND	B_1 Rb.A.			B_{2A} Rb.J.V.			B_{2B} G.P.I.			B_H R.M.*
	pD2	Rb.A.	α^E	pD2	Rb.A.	α^E	pD2	Rb.A.	α^E	R.P.
1. BK	6.22	9	1.0	8.48	100	1.0	7.90	100	1.0	100
2. Lys-BK	7.27	96	1.0	8.63	141	1.0	7.88	95	1.0	165
3. DesArg⁹-BK	7.29	100	1.0		Inac.			Inac.		42
4. DesArg⁹-BK	8.60	2042	1.0		Inac.			Inac.		58
5. DesPhe⁸,desArg⁹-BK		Inac.			Inac.			Inac.		--
6. DesPhe⁸,desArg⁹-BK	--	--	--		Inac.			Inac.		--
7. DArg-BK	6.56	19	1.0	8.70	166	1.1	7.41	33	0.9	170
8. Sar-BK	6.39	13	1.2	8.41	85	1.0	7.60	51	1.0	--
9. Ile-Ser-BK (T-kinin)	5.97	5	0.7	8.18	50	0.7	7.58	47	1.0	78
10. [Hyp³]-BK	6.17	8	1.0	8.88	254	1.0	7.27	23	1.1	115
11. [Tyr(Me)⁸]-BK		Inac.		8.59	129	1.1	7.93	107	1.0	58
12. [Hyp³,Tyr(Me)⁸]-BK		Inac.		8.56	123	1.1	7.82	84	1.1	44
13. [Aib⁷]-BK	<4.5	<0.1	0.3	6.28	0.6	0.6	7.90	100	1.3	--
14. [Arg⁴]BK(4-9)		Inac.			Inac.			Inac.	175	

-pD_2 -Log of molar concentration of agonist that produces 50% of the maximal effect of BK.
Rb.A.   Relative activity.
α^E Intrinsic activity (BK = 1.0).
R.P.   Relative potency.
Rb.A.   Rabbit aorta; Rb.J.V.: Rabbit jugular vein; G.P.I.: Guinea pig ileum; R.M.: Rat mastocyte.
Inac.   Inactive
*   Data taken from Devillier et al. [18] or communicated by Landry et al. [24].

A series of compounds that include naturally-occuring kinins and their metabolites form kininase I and kininase II, as well as kinins extended at the N-terminal or substituted (with Hyp) in position 3 or in position 7, are presented in Table 1. A C-terminal BK fragment (4-9) in which Gly^4 was replaced by Arg is also included. The naturally-occurring peptides (compounds 1-6 of Table 1) differentiate between B_1, B_2 (B_{2A} and B_{2B}) and B_H since kinins are active on B_1, B_2 and B_H, the kininase I metabolites on B_1 and B_H and the kininase II metabolites only on B_H. These compounds do not discriminate between B_{2A} and B_{2B}. The same is true for the three analogues extended at the N-terminal, while $[Hyp^3]BK$ is more potent than BK on the B_{2A} but much less on the B_{2B}. Conversely, $[Aib^7]BK$ is more potent than BK on the B_{2B} but much less on the B_{2A}, suggesting that Pro^3 and Pro^7 may play a role in discriminating between the B_2 receptor subtypes. Work is underway with analogues of BK to consolidate this hypothesis. Results obtained with antagonist point in the same direction (see results below). The molecular requirements for receptor activation can be schematically summarized as follows:

$$\text{H-Lys-Arg-Pro-Pro-Gly-Phe-Ser-Pro-Phe-Arg-OH}$$

$$\underline{\quad\quad B_H \quad\quad} \qquad\qquad\qquad B_1 \quad \overline{B_{2A}, B_{2B}}$$

whereby the N-terminal positive changes are needed for B_H (histamine release). The C-terminal Arg is essential for B_2 (B_{2A} and B_{2B}) and is not required for B_1 activation, for which Phe^8 is essential. Differentiation between B_{2A} and B_{2B} appears to be faisible with agonists in which the key proline residues in position 3 and 7 have been adequately replaced.

2. Differentiation of kinin functional sites with antagonists

B_1 antagonists

Fairly potent and selective antagonists for the B_1 receptor were identified at the end of the seventies [21,3] and used by many investigators to differentiate B_1 and B_2 receptor functions [21,22,7]. Results obtained with the most active compounds (Table 2), $[Leu^8]desArg^9BK$ and Lys-

[Leu^8]desArg^{9}BK, are summarized in Table 2.

Table 2. B$_1$ antagonist features

	B$_1$ Rb.A.	B$_{2A}$ Rb.J.V.	B$_{2B}$ G.P.I.	B$_H$ * R.M.
Selectivity				
15. [Leu^8]-desArg^{9}BK	ANTAGONIST	INACTIVE	INACTIVE	++
16. [Leu^8]-desArg^{9}BK	ANTAGONIST	INACTIVE	INACTIVE	+++
Competitivity	pA2-pA10 1.0 on the Rb.A.			
Specificity	INACTIVE agonist Angiotensin II			
	INACTIVE agonist Substance P			

Rb.A.   Rabbit aorta
Rb.J.V. Rabbit jugular vein
R.M.   Rat mastocyte
G.P.I. Guinea pig ileum
*   Data taken from Devillier et al. [18]

The compounds are potent antagonists of the B$_1$ receptors of the rabbit aorta [21], inactive on the B$_2$ receptor of the rabbit jugular vein [12] and therefore selective for the B$_1$ receptor. They exert a competitive type of antagonism since the difference pA$_2$-pA$_{10}$ is near unity. Because they contain N-terminal groups (Arg or Lys-Arg), the compounds are able to induce histamine release. The B$_1$ antagonists are specific since they do not affect the responses of the Rb.A. to angiotensin II and substance P. The data presented in Table 2 support the hypothesis of the functional sites, namely B$_1$, in which the compounds act as antagonists, B$_{2A}$ and B$_{2B}$, in which the compounds are inactive and B$_H$, in which they act as agonists. B$_1$ receptor antagonists do not differentiate between B$_{2A}$ and B$_{2B}$.

B$_2$ antagonists

A structure-activity study of B$_2$ antagonists is summarized in Table 3. [D-Phe^7]BK was reported as a first B$_2$ receptor antagonist [23]; it is however a weak antagonist, active on the G.P.I. and on the Rb.A.: it is non selective for B$_2$. It is an agonist on the Rb.J.V. and on other B$_2$ preparations [9]. Antagonistic activities on the G.P.I. (and on the Rb.A., the B$_1$ receptor system)

Table 3. Structure-activity relationships of bradykinin receptor antagonists on isolated smooth muscles and rat mast cells.

COMPOUND	B_1	B_{2A}		B_{2B}		B_H
	Rb.A.	Rb.J.V.		G.P.I.		R.M.
	pA2	pA_2	α^E	pA_2	α^E	R.P.
17. [DPhe^7]-BK	5.94	N.M.	0.4	5.85	0.2	1248
18. DArg[DPhe^7]-BK	6.16	N.M.	0.5	6.46	0.1	294
19. [Hyp^3,DPhe^7]-BK	N.D.	N.M.	0.7	Inac.	0.2	678
20. DArg[Hyp^3,DPhe^7]-BK	6.41	8.01	0.7	5.41	0.1	85
21. [Hyp^3,DPhe^7,Leu^8]-BK	5.10	8.40	0.3	6.56	0.2	185
22. DArg[Hyp^3,DPhe^7,Leu^8]-BK	5.76	8.86	0.1	6.77	0.1	197
23. DArg[Hyp^3,Leu^8]-BK	<5.0	7.45	0.7	<5.0	0.2	---
24. DArg[Hyp^3,Gly^6,Leu^8]-BK	<5.0	7.60	0.3	N.M.	>0.5	---
25. DArg[Tyr^3,DPhe^7,Leu^8]-BK	<5.0	F.Ag.	1.0	6.80	0.3	---
26. [Arg^1(Tos),Hyp^3,Thi^5, DTic^7,Oic^8]-BK	Inac.	9.19	0	8.17	0	224
27. DArg[Hyp^3,Thi^5,DTic^7, Oic^8]-BK	Inac.	9.17	0	8.94	0	385

Rb.A., Rb.J.V., G.P.I., R.M. as in Table 1.
pA_2: -log of the concentration of antagonist that reduces the effect of a double dose of agonist to that of a single dose (Schild, 1947).
α^E: Residual agonistic activity as a fraction of that of BK.
pD_2: As in Table 1; Inac.: Inactive; R.P.: Relative activity in percent of that of BK; N.D.: Not determined; N.M.: Antagonism is not measurable because of high residual agonistic effect; F.Ag.: Full agonist.

are improved by the extension of the C-terminal by a D-Arg residue, while the replacement of Pro^3 with Hyp is not sufficient to increase antagonist affinity (compound n° 19 is an agonist). The combination of the three substitutions as in D-Arg[Hyp^3,D-Phe^7]BK leads to a potent antagonist on the Rb.J.V. (B_{2A}), which is however much weaker (by more than 2 log units) on the G.P.I. (B_{2B}). Such a difference of antagonist affinity suggests that the two tissues contain different receptors. Antagonist affinity is further increased by the replacement of Phe^8 by Leu: D-Arg[Hyp^3,D-Phe^7,Leu^8]BK shows pA_2 values of almost 8.9, is very selective for the B_{2A} site with respect to B_1 site (pA_2 values differ by more than 3 log units) and also with respect to the B_{2B}

site (pA$_2$ values differ by more than 2 log units). The presence of Leu in position 8 favours the occupation of B$_{2A}$ and this is demonstrated by the fairly high antagonistic affinity of D-Arg[Hyp^3,Leu^8] (compound n° 23) for the B$_{2A}$. This compound is almost inactive on B$_1$ and B$_{2B}$ sites and is of particular interest since it is selective for B$_{2A}$ and it does not contain any D residue, in position 7. It maintains, however, a fairly strong agonistic residual effect when applied at high concentrations on the B$_{2A}$ system, suggesting that a conformational change (contributed by D-Phe^7) might be important for pure antagonism. This interpretation is supported by the finding that D-Arg [Hyp^3,Gly^6,Leu^8]BK (compound n° 24) has much less agonistic activity than compound n° 23. The absence of D-Phe^7 eliminates all antagonism on the G.P.I., suggesting that a drastic change of conformation is required by B$_{2B}$ more than by B$_{2A}$ for antagonism. The two sites are further differentiated by the residue in the third position, whereby the presence of Hyp favours occupation of B$_{2A}$ and that of an aromatic residue (Tyr) (compound n° 25) leads to elimination of all antagonistic

D-Arg-Arg-Pro-**Hyp**-Gly-Phe-Ser-**D-Phe-Leu**-Arg-OH

activity on this site. D-Arg [Tyr^3,D-Phe^7,Leu^8]BK is a full agonist (pD$_2$: 8.30) on the B$_{2A}$ and a pure antagonist on the B$_{2B}$ receptor subtype. The compound is inactive on the B$_1$ site and is therefore a selective antagonist for the B$_{2B}$ receptor. The new compounds described by Hock et al. [11] at Hoechst are very active, pure B$_2$ antagonists, inactive on the B$_1$ site, equally active on B$_{2A}$ and B$_{2B}$ and therefore non discriminative of the two sites. One of these compounds, D-Arg[Hyp^3,Thi^5,D-Tic^7,Oic^8]BK, shows very similar pA$_2$ values on the Rb.J.V. and the G.P.I. and by this fact, it proves that B$_{2A}$ and B$_{2B}$ sites are subtypes of the same receptors, rather than distinct receptors.

As to the histamine release (B$_{II}$), all compounds presented in Table 3 are agonists [24]. Those containing an extended N-terminal (by the D-Arg) are more active than the others and compounds 26 and 27 are more active than the others, probably because they are more resistant to enzymatic degradation. Because of strong agonistic activities, none of the compounds could be tested for antagonism of histamine release [24].

Difference between B$_{2A}$ and B$_{2B}$ receptor subtypes is further supported by the data summarized in Table 4, in which five compounds were tested in three tissues (the ileum, pulmonary artery

Table 4. B_2 Receptor subtypes - pA_2 values of antagonists

COMPOUND	GUINEA PIG			HAMSTER	RABBIT		
	Ileum	Pulmon. Artery	Urin. Blad.	Urin. Blad.	Jug. Vein	Vena Cava	Urin. Blad.
DArg[Hyp³,Gly⁶,Leu⁸]BK	P.Ag.	Inac.	P.Ag.	P.Ag.	7.60	7.44	7.44
DArg[Tyr³,DPhe⁷,Leu⁸]BK	6.80	<5.0	--	6.18	P.Ag.	P.Ag.	P.Ag.
DArg[Hyp³,DPhe⁷,Leu⁸]BK	6.77	5.76	6.76	7.16	8.86	8.92	8.68
DArg[Hyp³,Thi⁵,DTic⁷, Oic⁸]BK (Hoe 140)	8.92	8.27*	8.81	8.81	9.17	9.24	9.24

P.Ag. Partial agonist
* Log of the IC_{50}
Inac. Inactive

and urinary bladder) from the guinea pig and three tissues (jugular vein, vena cava, urinary bladder) from the rabbit. This data indicates that the compound D-Arg[Hyp³,Gly⁶,Leu⁸]BK without D-Phe⁷ is either inactive or is a partial agonist with a fairly strong residual activity in the preparations from the guinea pig, and is an antagonist in the preparations from the rabbit. Conversely, D-Arg[Tyr³,D-Phe⁷,Leu⁸]BK is a partial agonist on the preparations from the rabbits and an antagonist in those of the guinea pig. When D-Phe is included as in D-Arg[Hyp³,D-Phe⁷,Leu⁸]BK, the compound is an antagonist (fairly pure) much more active (by 2-3 log units) in the rabbit than in the guinea pig tissues. The pA_2 difference is highly significant. The potent compounds (n°s 26 and 27) from Hoechst show high affinity in all preparations and does not discriminate between B_{2A} and B_{2B} receptor subtypes.

The type of antagonism exerted by D-Arg[Hyp³,D-Phe⁷,Leu⁸]BK and by Hoe 140 was assessed by measuring concentration-response curves of BK in the presence of increasing doses of the antagonists. It was found [17] that the first compound exerts a competitive antagonism since the curves of BK are displaced to the right, remain parallel to the control and reach the maximum, while Hoe 140 is non competitive because the maximum of the BK curve is progressively depressed (in parallel with the increase of antagonist concentration) and the curves loose parallelism with the control. Hoe 140 exerts an apparent non-competitive type of antagonism because it occupies the receptors for a prolonged period of time and hinders the access of BK to the receptor sites. Hoe 140 appears therefore to act as a "non-equilibrium" antagonist.

CONCLUSION

Four functional sites for kinins have been described and differentiated by measuring the biological activities of kinin agonists in four pharmacological preparations. The sites are B_1 in the rabbit aorta, B_{2A} in the rabbit jugular vein, B_{2B} in the guinea pig ileum and B_H (H is for histamine) in the rat mast cell. Elimination of the C-terminal Arg favors B_1 occupation and activation, while the presence of this residue is essential for B_{2A} and B_{2B} receptor function and the N-terminal positively-charged residues (Lys^0 and Arg^1) are instrumental for histamine release. B_1 receptor antagonists block the B_1 receptor, are inactive on B_{2A} and B_{2B} and act as agonists on the B_H. B_2 receptor antagonists of different affinities have been found to act as antagonists on B_1 and on B_{2A} and B_{2B} receptor sites, while maintaining some residual agonistic activities on both B_2 subtypes and a strong activity as histamine releasers. B_2 antagonists have been progressively improved with respect to affinity, selectivity for B_2 sites compared to B_1, and reduction of the residual agonistic activities on smooth muscle by 1) extending the N-terminal with a D-Arg, b) replacing Pro^3 with Hyp and Phe^8 with Leu. The presence of D-Phe in position 7 leads to increase of antagonist affinity but is not essential for antagonism on B_{2A}, while being important for antagonism on B_{2B}. Crucial for B_{2A} antagonism is the presence of Pro or Hyp in position 3, while a pure B_{2B} antagonist has been obtained with an aromatic residue (Tyr) in this position. Thus a distinciton between B_{2A} and B_{2B} that was emerging with agonists (see $[Aib^7]BK$) has been validated by the use of antagonists such as $D-Arg[Tyr^3,D-Phe^7,Leu^8]BK$ which is a potent agonist on the B_{2A} and a potent antagonist on the B_{2B}. The two receptor subytpes are blocked by compounds (e.g. Hoe 140) containing strong hydrophobic residues that improve receptor occupation and appear to be present in different species.

ACKNOWLEDGEMENTS

We thank H. Morin for her excellent secretarial work and R. Laprise for technical assistance. We are very grateful to Prof. Y. Landry and J.L. Bueb for allowing the reproduction of some unpublished results on histamine release in Tables 1 and 3. The work was performed with the financial support of the Medical Research Council of Canada (MRCC). N.-E.R. and C.T. are fellows of the Fonds de la recherche en santé du Québec (FRSQ) and the MRCC, respectively. D.R. is a career investigator for the MRCC.

REFERENCES

[1]   Frey, E.K., Kraut, H., Werle, E., Vogel, R., Zickgraf-Rudel, G. and Trautschold, I. (Eds.) *Das kallikrein-kinin system und seine inhibitoren*. F. Enke-Verlag, Stuttgart, 1968.

[2]   Pisano, J.J. *Chemistry and biology of the kallikrein-kinin system*. In: Proteases and biological control, E. Reich, D.B. Rifkin and E. Shaw (Eds). Cold Spring Harbour Lab. 2: 199-222, 1975.

[3]   Regoli, D. and Barabé, J. *Pharmacology of bradykinin and related kinins*. Pharmacol. Rev. 32 (1): 1-46, 1980.

[4]   Rhaleb, N.-E., Dion, S., Barabé, J., Rouissi, N., Jukic, D., Drapeau, G. and Regoli,D. *Receptors for kinins in dog isolated arterial vessels*. Eur. J. Pharmacol 162: 419-427, 1989.

[5]   Marceau, F., Lussier, A., Regoli, D. and Giroud, J.P. *Pharmacology of kinins: their relevance to tissue injury and inflammation*. Gen. Pharmacol 14: 209-229, 1983.

[6]   Carbonell, L.F., Carretero, O.., Madeddu, P. and Seicli, A.G. *Effects of a kinin antagonist on mean blood pressure*. Hypertension II (suppl. I) I: 84-88.

[7]   Jin, L.S., Seeds, E., Page, C.P. and Schachter, M. *Inhibition of bradykinin-induced bronchoconstriction in the guinea pig by a synthetic B_2 receptor blocker*. Br. J. Pharmacol. 97: 598-602, 1989.

[8]   Steranka, L.R. and Burch, R.M. *Bradykinin antagonists in pain and inflammatory*. In: Bradykinin antagonists, Burch, R.M. (Ed.), Marcel Dekker Inc., 191-212, 1991.

[9]   Regoli, D., Rhaleb, N.-E., Dion, S. and Drapeau, G. *New selective bradykinin receptor antagonists and bradykinin B_2 receptors characterization*. Trends Pharmacol. Sci. 11: 156-161, 1990.

[10]   Farmer, S.G., Burch, R.M., Meeker, S.N. and Wilkins, D.. *Evidence for a pulmonary bradykinin B_3 receptor*. Mol. Pharmacol. 36: 1-8, 1989.

[11]   Hock, F.J., Wirth, K., Albus, U., Linz, W., Gerhards, H.J., Wiemer, G., Henke, S., Breipohl, G., König, W., Knolle, J. and Schölkens, B.A. *Hoe 140, a new potent and long-acting bradykinin antagonist: in vitro studies*. Br. J. Pharmacol. 102: 769-773, 1991.

[12]   Gaudreau, P., St-Pierre, S. & Regoli, D. *Pharmacological studies of kinins on venous smooth muscles*. Can. J. Physiol. Pharmacol. 59, 371-379.

[13]   Furchgott, R.F. and Bhadrakom, S. *Reaction of strips of rabbit aorta to epinephrin isopropyl-arterenol, sodium nitrate and other drugs*. J. Pharmacol. Exp. Ther 108: 124-143, 1953.

[14]   Rang, H.P. *Stimulant actions of volatile anesthesics on smooth muscle*. Br. J. Pharmacol. 22: 356-365, 1965.

[15]   Nakahata, H. Ono, T. and Nakanishi, H. *Contribution of prostaglandin E₂ to bradykinin-induced contraction in rabbit urinary detrusor.* Jap. J. Pharmacol. **43**: 351-359.

[16]   Rhaleb, N.-E., Drapeau, G., Jukic, D., Rouissi, N., and Regoli, D. *Structure-activity studies on bradykinin and and related peptides.* Agonists. Br. J. Pharmacol. **99**: 445-448, 1990.

[17]   Rhaleb, N.-E., Rouissi, N., Jukic, D., Regoli, D., Henke, S., Breiphol, G. and Knolle, J. *Pharmacological characterization of a new higly potent B₂ receptor antagonist (Hoe 140): D-Arg[Hyp³,Thi⁵,D-Tic⁷,Oic⁸]-BK.* Eur. J. Pharmacol., 1991 (in press).

[18]   Devillier, P., Renoux, M., Drapeau, G. and Regoli, D. *Histamine release from rat peritoneal mast cells by kinin antagonists.* Eur. J. Pharmacol. **149**: 137-140, 1988.

[19]   Drapeau, G. and Regoli, D. *Synthesis of bradykinin analogs.* In: Immunochemical techniques: Part M. Chemotaxis and Inflammation Methods Enzymol. **163**: 263-272, 1988.

[20]   Schild, H.O. *pA₂, a new scale for the measurement of drug antagonism.* Br. J. Pharmacol. **2**: 189-206, 1947.

[21]   Regoli, D., Barabé, J. and Park, W.K. *Receptors for bradykinin in rabbit aortae.* Can. J. Physiol. Pharmacol. **55**: 855-867, 1977.

[22]   Stewart, J.M. and Vavrek, R.J. *Chemistry of peptide B₂ bradykinin antagonists.* In: Bradykinin antagonists, Burch, R.M. (Ed.), Marcel Dekker Inc., 51-96, 1991.

[23]   Vavrek, R.J. and Stewart, J.M. *Competitive antagonists of bradykinin.* Peptides **6**: 161-164, 1985.

[24]   Landry et al., personal communication.

CLONING OF A B$_2$ BRADYKININ RECEPTOR: EXAMINATION OF THE
BRADYKININ BINDING SITE BY SITE DIRECTED MUTAGENESIS

Richard Freedman and Kurt Jarnagin

Syntex Research, 3401 Hillview Ave., Palo Alto, CA, U.S.A. 94304

Summary: A cDNA encoding a bradykinin receptor has been isolated. In oocytes expressing the receptor, bradykinin-induced chloride current is blocked by [Thi^{5,8} dPhe^7]BK and is unaffected by des-Arg^9-BK suggesting that the cDNA encodes a classical B$_2$ type receptor. The predicted protein sequence is homologous to other G protein-coupled receptors. Preliminary models of the receptor and BK have been built. Data from mutagenesis experiments designed to test the models is reported.

INTRODUCTION

We set out to clone bradykinin receptors (BK-R). We felt that knowledge of the nucleotide and protein sequence of a BK receptor would lead to identification of subtypes, and expression and purification of large amounts of receptor protein. The cDNA sequence could also lead to identification of the BK binding site via the use of protein chemistry and mutagenesis.

After several false starts, in which we made unsuccessful attempts to isolate BK receptor protein or to clone the BK receptor using fluorescence activated cell sorting of transfected mammalian cells loaded with INDO-1 and activated by BK; we succeeded in cloning a B$_2$ BK receptor using sib selection procedures and the *Xenopus* oocyte expression-chloride current detection method.

METHODS

Cloning Procedure: Size selected mRNA from rat uterus was assayed by injecting each fraction into oocytes and then measuring BK induced chloride currents (1) (Fig 1.1). A fraction of ≈4 kb was found to be enriched for BK induced currents; from this fraction a λzapII cDNA library was made. The 100,000 member library was divided into 5 pools each pool was amplified and cRNA was made using T7 RNA polymerase and the λzapII T7 polymerase promoter. The cRNA's from each pool were injected into several oocytes and BK induced Cl⁻ currents of measured. These procedures identified a pool which conferred BK inducible Cl⁻ currents (Fig 1.2). This pool was further divided into 10 pools, each pool was amplified and analyzed as in the first round. After seven rounds of selection a single clone had been purified (clone #60).

Figure 1. Bradykinin induced Cl⁻ currents in oocytes injected with RNA.

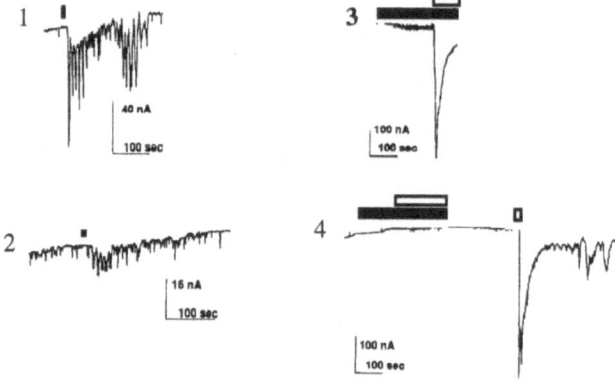

Figure 1; Subpanels 1 and 2: cells were continuously perfused and 1 μM bradykinin was applied at the time indicated by the solid bar to oocytes injected with the following RNAs: (.1). total poly–A⁺RNA from rat uterus; (.2), cRNA from the first library division. Subpanel 3: the response of an oocyte to treatment with 10 μM des-Arg⁹-BK (for the duration of the solid bar, no perfusion) followed by application of 10 nM bradykinin (open bar) and 10 μM des-Arg⁹-Bk. Subpanel 4: the response of an oocyte to treatment with 1 μM [Thi⁵,⁸, dPhe⁷]BK (for the duration of the solid bar, no perfusion) followed by application of 10 nM bradykinin (open bar) and 1 μM [Thi⁵,⁸, dPhe⁷]BK; finally the cell was washed and 10nM BK was added (small open bar). The oocytes in subpanels 3 and 4 were injected with cRNA from clone #60.

Binding Site Models: Models of the BK molecule were built based on the NMR results of Lee et al. (2), in which the most stable conformations of BK in SDS micelles were proposed. NMR data collected at Syntex (Joe Pease, personal communication), which suggest that HOE-140 may favor some of the same conformations as reported by Lee et al., contributed to our BK models. Models of the BK-R were based on the electron-cryo microscopic picture of bacteriorhodopsin developed by Henderson et al (3). Our first model was a simple residue by residue replacement of the bacteriorhodopsin sequence with the BK-R sequence within transmembrane regions; extra residues found in the BK-R were placed in extramembrane loops.

Mutagenesis: BK-R mutants were made by a modification of the PCR mutagenesis method (4). The mutagenesis was performed on a cassette encompassing the unique Bgl II and Pvu II sites of the protein coding region. All mutagenesis cassettes were completely sequenced; only results from mutants in which the sequence was confirmed are reported.

Mammalian cell expression: Expression was achieved by subcloning each mutant into an expression vector driven by the SR-alpha promoter (5) and transiently transfecting COS-7 cells using the Lipofectin reagent (BRL-Gibco, Bethesda, MD). Membranes were prepared from the transfected cells after 72 hours and assayed immediately for [^{3}H]-Bradykinin binding (1).

RESULTS AND DISCUSSION

Cloning and sequence: A single clone has been purified from a rat uterus cDNA library by sib selection; in order to further clarify the nature of this clone (#60) the effect of BK analogs and antagonists on binding and Cl$^-$ current in Cos-7 cells and oocytes expressing clone #60 was measured. The rank order of potency was similar in all three assays suggesting that the cDNA encodes the same BK receptor which is measured in rat uterus.

The clone does not encode a B$_1$ BK receptor since des-Arg^9 BK does not stimulate a Cl$^-$ current nor does des-Arg^9 BK inhibit BK induced chloride currents (Fig.1.3) (6, 7). Clone #60 does not encode a neuronal subtype of the BK receptor since [Thi^{5,8} dPhe^7]BK is an antagonist and not an agonist. (Fig1.4) (8, 9).

The rank order of potencies, the lack of affect of des-Arg^9 BK, and the antagonism without any agonism of [Thi^{5,8} dPhe^7]BK suggests that clone 60 encodes a classical B$_2$ BK receptor.

We examined the tissue distribution of RNAs encoding the BK-R. The following rat tissues contain significant amounts of receptor: uterus, lung, kidney, heart, brain, testis

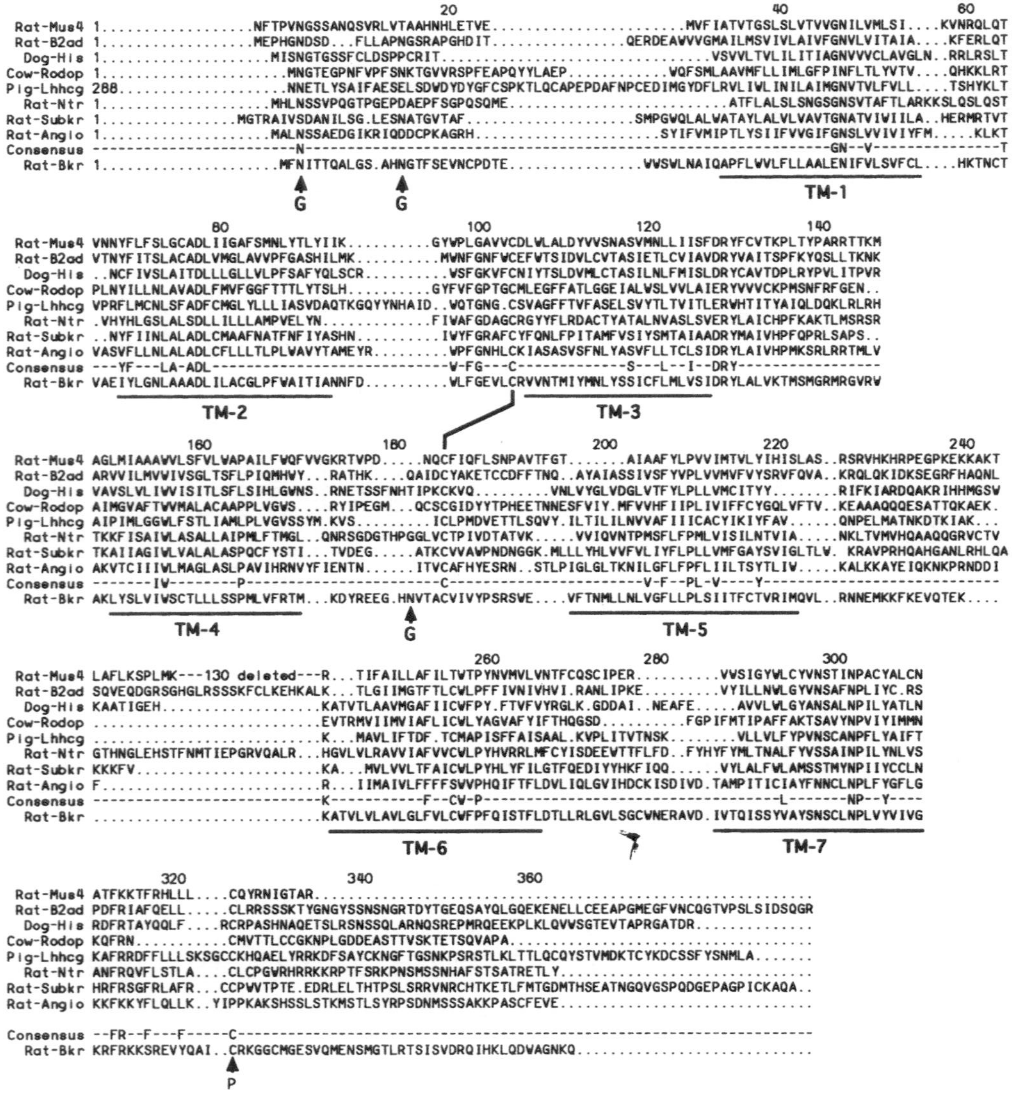

Figure 2. The predicted amino acid sequences of bradykinin and other (rat m4 muscarinic, rat β2-adrenergic, cow rhodopsin, pig luteinizing hormone/human chorionic gonadotropin, rat neurotensin, rat substance k, rat angiotensin II) receptors were aligned using the algorithm of Needleman and Wunsch, and a consensus sequence was generated, all as described previously (1). The symbols are as follows: G, putative asparagine linked glycosylation site; P, putative palmitoylation site; the line connecting Cysteine 105 and 186 represents a putative disulfide bond. The solid bars represent approximate positions of transmembrane regions. The numbering is correct for bradykinin receptor.

(weak), vas deferens, and ileum. Our results suggests that uterus may have as much as 5 times more BK-R mRNA than any other tissue and that the testis has very little; the small amount of mRNA in testis may be easily explained by contamination by vascular tissue. The tissue distribution of mRNAs encoding the BK-R is consistent with that reported for B$_2$ BK-R.

Sequencing of the BK-R clone revealed an open reading frame of 1266 bp. which encodes a protein which is homologous to the G-protein coupled (GPC) superfamily of receptors. An alignment of the predicted BK-R protein sequence is shown in Figure 2. There are 7 stretches of hydrophobic residues which contain several of the "signature" sequences found in G-protein coupled receptors (Fig. 2). Interestingly, the receptors for BK and angiotensin II (AII-R) have significant identities, 31.2%, and similarities, 54.1% (Fig 2.). The GPCR superfamily averages less than 20% identity for 37 pairs. Transmembrane 5, 6, and 7 share especially strong identities, 30-52%; identities in these regions are weak among other members of the superfamily. This homology is especially notable because of the opposite nature of BK's and angiotensin's action on blood pressure, their shared metabolic enzyme, ACE, and their parallelism of synthetic mechanism -- by proteolytic cleavage from large molecular weight protease inhibitors.

Models and Mutagenesis: Work in the last 15 years examining the structure and function of bacteriorhodopsin, visual opsins , and receptors for biogenic amines has suggested a model in which the 7 hydrophobic stretches are arranged in alpha helices which each transverse the membrane (transmembrane regions, TM1-7). These protein have there amino terminus outside the cell and the protein carboxy terminus in the cytosol. The helices are arranged in a kidney shape when viewed from the top, with TM-1 and TM-4/5 at opposite ends of the kidney, TM-2,3,4 on the concave side and TM-5, 6, 7 on the convex side. The retinal or amine binds in a central region about 1/3 of the way through the membrane.

The above conclusions are based on the three dimensional structure of bacteriorhodopsin as determined by electron cryo-microscopy (3). Other work which suggest that the bacteriorhodopsin structure is similar to the opsin and adrenergic case includes studies examining chemical labeling patterns, sequence specific antibody binding, and sites of proteolytic cleavage (summarized in (10, 11)).

Results derived from adrenergic receptor mutation experiments have lead to the hypothesis that the amine portion of the catecholamine interacts with an aspartic acid on TM-3 which is conserved in all amine binding receptors (12). Work by Dixion and Strader have suggested that two serine residues on TM-5 interact with the vicinal catechol hydroxyl groups (13). In addition TM-6 is thought to contribute a phenylalanine to an aromatic-aromatic interaction with the catechol ring in the adrenergic receptors (11). Muscarinic receptors have been postulated to bind acetylcholine in a manner similar to that which epinephrine binds to adrenergic receptors (14, 15). An aspartic acid on TM-3 interacts with the amine of acetylcholine while hydroxyls contributed by threonines on TM-5 and tyrosines on TM-6 and -7 contact agonists at their ester linkage. In the visual opsins retinal is bound via a Schiff's base to a lysine on TM-7 and the polyene side chain radiates toward TM-5 crossing the face of TM-6. Covalent attachment of the retinal to the opsin is not necessary for signal transmission to transducin, the visual system G-protein (16). Mutations made in visual opsins implicate a glutamic acid from TM-3 as the Schiff's base charge neutralizing residue and possibly another glutamic acid, E122 from TM-3, has a point charge near the polyene chain of retinal (17, 18).

No peptide binding G-protein coupled receptor has been examined by mutagenesis, thus, in order to begin our examination of the BK binding site we built a model of the BK-R using the electron cryo-microscopy model of bacteriorhodopsin and incorporated the data about opsin, adrenergic receptors and muscarinic receptors. We also examined the structure activity data for BK and its analogs (19), the NMR studies of BK in SDS micelles (2), and used multidimensional NMR to examine the solution conformation of HOE-140 in micelles (Joe Pease personal communication).

From these results we made first version models and derived the following hypotheses (Fig. 3): **1.** Active conformations of BK and HOE-140 have a β –turn at the carboxy terminus encompassing residues 6-9. **2.** Because amino terminal extensions of BK are fairly well tolerated the amino terminus of BK is not deep in the receptor binding pocket. Our initial crude model of the receptor bound BK is a "fish hook" with the point and barb being Arg^9, the hook the β –turn of residues 6-9, and the shank being residues 1-5. **3.** The beta turn of BK is deep in the binding pocket and is in a loose sense an analog of epinephrine, retinal or acetylcholine. **4.** We have initially assumed that the guanido function of Arg^9 is the charge anchor for binding as is the amine of epinephrine, acetylcholine or the Shifts base of retinal. **5.** TM-3 of the BK-R has no negatively charged amino acids thus we positioned the "fish hook" with the point and barb, Arg9, near the top of TM-6 interacting with an aspartic acid, D268. **6.** The BK hook was located near TM-5 with two asparagines, N200 and N204, being the analog of the serines and threonines of the adrenergic and muscarinic receptors respectively. We postulated that N200 and/or N204 may hydrogen bond with the carbonyl or amide nitrogen of the BK Pro-Phe peptide bond. **7.** The carbonyl of the Phe-Arg peptide bond was positioned to interact with hydrogen bond capable residues from TM-4, either S164, S165 or S158. **8.**

The serine hydroxyl, Ser^6, was postulated to be interacting with hydrogen bond capable residues on TM-3, either N109, T110, or Y113.

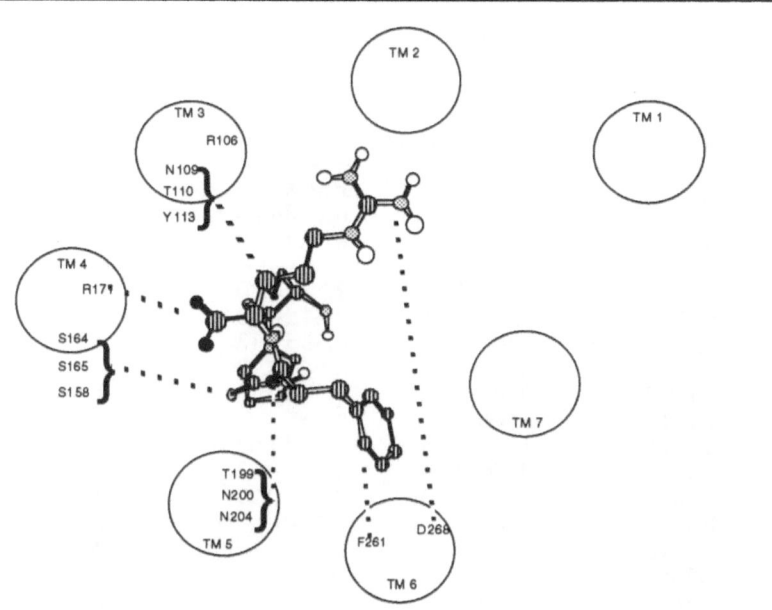

Figure 3. Initial Model of BkR Binding Site. The four C-terminal residues of BK are shown. The 7 transmembrane domains of BkR are shown, top view and distrorted for presentation clarity. Putative interactions are indicated by dashed lines.

Based on the this model 12 initial mutations were made and tested for their ability to bind [^{3}H]-BK (Table 1). Most of the mutations had little or no effect on [^{3}H]–BK binding. Three mutations yielded receptors which do not bind BK. The lack of binding by these mutants suggests that there is ≥ 100 fold decrease in affinity compared to the wild type receptor, or that the mutated receptor is not correctly transcribed, translated, folded, and/or sub-cellularly localized. Future studies using [^{125}I]HOE-140 to increase the determinable range of Kds, or antibodies to asses the ability of the mutant to be translated, folded or transported will be done. These "negative" mutants yield no interpretable data.

We postulated that N200 or N204 was contributing a hydrogen bond to a backbone peptide bond. Change of N204 to alanine had no effect of BK affinity. However, change of N200 to alanine may have altered the affinity of BK by ≈4 fold.

None of our mutants have been tested more than three times; thus, confirmation of the significance of a 4 fold affinity shift awaits more careful experiments. The loss of a single hydrogen bond in adrenergic receptors caused an 8.3-50 fold decrease in Kd and reduced by ≈50% the ability of the receptor to stimulate downstream events (13), thus our observed effect is smaller than we would have anticipated and may suggest that our model needs modification.

Table 1. Binding Affinity of BK-R Mutants.

MUTANT	Kd (nM) Mean ±SD	Bmax (pmol/mg) Mean ±SD	N
WT	1.35 ±1.09	2.72 ±0.30	6
R106A	1.81 ±0.57	2.84 ±0.18	2
R106Q	2.02 ±0.57	0.45 ±0.13	2
T110A	0.88 ±0.89	2.64 ±3.30	2
Y113F	0.60 ±0.11	3.30 ±0.13	1
R171Q	NONE	NONE	2
T199A	1.40 ±0.66	2.20 ±1.63	2
N200A	4.89 ±4.99	1.65 ±0.73	2
N204A	1.13 ±1.20	1.01 ±0.29	2
F261A	NONE	NONE	3
Q262A	NONE	NONE	2
D268A	1.80 ±1.33	0.59 ±0.09	3
D268R	NONE	NONE	2

One of the sites which yielded a "negative" mutant, D268, when mutated to R, arginine, produced a mutant with normal binding of [^{3}H]-BK when that position was changed to alanine. This result could imply that large steric bulk is not tolerated in position 268. Since D268 was our initial candidate for the guanido, Arg[9], binding site and Alanine at this position yielded a receptor with normal binding constants we can conclude that D268 is not the guanido binding acid, thus our initial model needs modification.

We hope that a new understanding of bradykinin's mechanism of action will develop as a result of the cloning of a B$_2$ BkR and our attemps to identify the binding site. Soon a molecular and possibly atomic level view of bradykinin-bradykinin receptor interaction may be available.

ACKNOWLEDGEMENTS
    We would like to thank Joe Pease, Aaron Miller for their many helpful discussions, preliminary data, and aid in building our first models. We would also like to

thank Hardy Chan and John Nestor for their support and encouragement. Earl Shelton, Adrienne McEachern, and Rick Aldrich are the giants upon whose shoulders we stand.

REFERENCES

1. McEachern AE, et al. Expression cloning of a rat B$_2$-bradykinin receptor. Proc Natl Acad Sci USA 1991; 88:7724-7728.

2. Lee SC, Russell AF, Laidig WD. Three-dimensional structure of bradykinin in SDS micelles. Int. J. Peptide Protein Res. 1990; 35:367-377.

3. Henderson R, Baldwin JM, Ceska TA, Zemlin F, Beckmann E, Downing KH. Model for the structure of bacteriorhodopsin based on high-resolution electron cryo-microscopy. J. Mol. Biol. 1990; 213:899-929.

4. Higuchi R. In: PCR Technonology. Erlich HA, editor. New York: Stockton Press,1989: 61-70.

5. Takebe Y, Seiki M, Fujisawa J-I, Hoy P, Yokota K, Arai K-I, Yoshida M, Arai N. SRα promoter: an efficient and versatile mammalian cDNA expression system composed of the simian virus 40 early Promoter and the R–U5 segment of human T–cell leukemia virus type 1 long terminal repeat. Mol. Cell. Biol. 1988; 8:466-472.

6. Churchill L, Ward PE. Relaxation of isolated mesenteric arteries by des–Arg^9-bradykinin stimulatin of B$_1$ receptors. Eur. J. Pharmacol. 1986; 130:11-18.

7. Regoli D, Barabé J. Pharmacology of bradykinin and related kinins. Pharmacol Rev. 1980; 32:1-46.

8. Braas KM, Manning DC, Perry DC, Snyder SH. Bradykinin analogues: differential agonist and antagonist activities suggesting multiple receptors. Br. J. Pharmacol. 1988; 94:3-5.

9. Llona I, Vavrek R, Stewart J, Huidobro-Toro JP. Identification of pre- and postsynaptic bradykinin receptor sites in the vas deferens: evidence for different structural prerequisites. J. Pharmacol. Exp.Therap. 1987; 241:608-614.

10. Findlay JBC, Pappin DJC. The opsin family of proteins. Biochem. J. 1986; 238:625-642.

11. Strader CD, Sigal IS, Dixon RAF. Structural basis of β-adrenergic receptor function. FASEB J. 1989; 3:1825-1832.

12. Strader CD, Sigal IS, Candelore MR, Rands E, Hill WS, Dixon RAF. Conserved aspartic acid residues 79 and 113 of the β-adrenergic receptor have different roles in receptor function. . Biol. Chem. 1988; 263:10267-10271.

13. Strader CD, Candelore MR, Hill WS, Sigal IS, Dixon RAF. Identification of two serine residues involved in agonist activation of β-adrenergic receptor. J. Biol. Chem. 1989; 264:13572-13578.

14.   Fraser CM, Wang C-D, Robinson DA, Gocayne JD, Venter JC. Site-directed
       mutagenesis of m1 muscarinic receptors: conserved aspartic acids play important
       roles in receptor function. Mol. Pharmacol. 1989; 36:840-847.

15.   Wess J, Gdula D, Brann MR. Site-directed mutagenesis of the m3 muscarinic
       receptor - identification of a series of threonine and tyrosine residues involved in
       agonist but not antagonist binding. EMBO J 1991; 10:3729-3734.

16.   Zhukovsky EA, Robinson PR, Oprian DD. Transducin activation by rhodopsin
       without a covalent bond to the 11-cis-retinal chromophore. Science 1991;
       251:558-560.

17.   Nathans J. Determinants of visual pigment absorbance: role of charged amino
       acids in the putative transmembrane segments. Biochem. 1990; 29:937-942.

18.   Zhukovsky EA, Oprian DD. Effect of carboxylic acid side chains on the
       absoption maximum of visual pigments. Science 1989; 246:928-930.

19.   Manning DC, Vavrek R, Stewart JM, Snyder SH. Two bradykinin binding sites
       with picomolar affinities. J. Pharmacol.Exp.Therap. 1986; 237:504-512.

AAS 38/I
Recent Progress on Kinins
© 1992 Birkhäuser Verlag Basel

ANTI-IDIOTYPIC ANTIBODIES AGAINST THE KININ RECEPTOR[1]

M. Haasemann[1], J. Buschko[1], A. Faussner[2], A.A. Roscher[2], J. Hoebeke[3,] R. Burch[4] and W. Müller-Esterl[1]

[1]Institute for Physiological Chemistry and Pathobiochemistry, University of Mainz, Duesbergweg 6, W-6500 Mainz, Germany; [2] Department of Clinical Biochemistry, Children's Hospital, University of Munich, Lindwurmstrasse 4, W-8000 Munich 2, Germany; [3]Laboratory for Enzymology and Protein Chemistry, University Francois-Rabelais, 2 bis Boulevard Tonelle, F-37032 Tours, France; [4]Nova Pharmaceuticals Corporation, 6200 Freeport Centre, Baltimore, MD 21224-2788, U.S.A.

SUMMARY: Three sets of monoclonal antibodies against bradykinin (MBK1, MBK2, MBK3) were generated by somatic cell fusion, characterized by their peptide specificity and compared to the known ligand specificity of the kinin receptor subtypes. By these criteria the paratope of MBK3 resembled the B2 receptor binding site whereas MBK1 shared principal binding characteristics with the B1 receptor. Anti-idiotypic antibodies against MBK1, MBK2 and MBK3 were raised in rabbit and sheep. Specificity of the network components was verified by inhibition experiments on the level of peptide, idiotype and anti-idiotype. Anti-idiotypic antibodies against MBK3 recognized a conformation-dependent epitope which was binding site-related. Binding studies on human foreskin fibroblasts and guinea pig ileum showed mutual displacement of the anti-idiotypic antibody and bradykinin at the binding site pointing to a specific interaction of the antibody with the receptor from various species. An agonist activity of the antibodies, demonstrated in human (inositolphosphate pathway) and mouse (prostaglandin pathway) fibroblasts indicated that the anti-idiotypes bear an internal image of the ligand epitope. This molecular mimicry, which was further substantiated by the detection of bradykinin specific anti-anti-idiotypic antibodies, provides the structural basis for the observed cross-reactivity over species borders.

INTRODUCTION

Anti-idiotypic antibodies have been contributing essentially to the analyses of structure and function of a wide spectrum of recipient sites, especially of differ-

---

[1] reprinted from J Cardiovasc Pharmacol (1992) with permission of Raven Press

ent kinds of receptors (1) and plasma proteins (2). The underlying priciple, the molecular mimicry of the receptor by an antibody against the ligand allows the production of these powerful immunological tools prior to receptor isolation. The anti-idiotypic route was applied successfully for the characterization of many receptors for biologically active peptides including angiotensin II (3), substance P (4), and insulin (5). It proved especially useful when size and conformation of the active peptide do not allow modifications such as the introduction of a reporter group without a drastic decrease of the receptor affinity; a situation encountered in the course of the isolation of the kinin receptor (Haasemann and Faussner, unpublished results). The generation of cross-reactive anti-idiotypic antibodies usually requires a two -step procedure initiated by the generation of a precise image of a receptor binding site by an anti-ligand antibody, which serves as an antigen in the second immunization step to obtain anti-idiotypic antibodies. Anti-idiotypic antibodies are classified in three major categories (6): the first type (α) is directed against the framework of the V region; the second type (γ) reacts with regions associated with the antigen combining site; and the third type (β), where the idiotope is congruent with the paratope and the anti-idiotype apparently mimics the antigen.

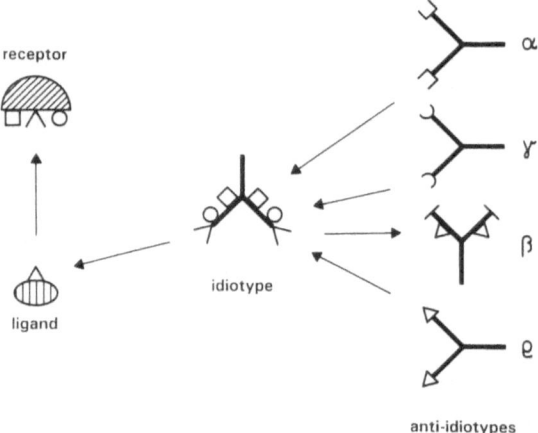

Figure 1. Anti-receptor antibodies via the anti-idiotypic approach. Schematic presentation of different classes of anti-idiotypic antibodies.

Observed receptor cross-reactivity, interspecies cross-reactivity and functional activity of anti-idiotypic antibodies may indicate that their idiotypes/paratopes bear internal images of the original ligand (antigen). Moreover, the cross-reactivity of anti-idiotypic antibodies with receptors may reflect common structural features of those two macromolecules, which have common binding characteristics with respect to ligand binding. Limitations of the anti-idiotypic approach are foreseen where cross-reactivities with unrelated proteins may occur (7). Therefore an in-depth characterization of the various components of the anti-idiotypic system is mandatory to exclude nonspecific interactions on the level of the immunological probes.

Here we report on the application of the anti-idiotypic approach for the creation of antibodies against the bradykinin receptors. A comparison of the affinity of distinct peptides from the kinin family towards three anti-bradykinin antibodies (MBK1, MBK2, MBK3) and the kinin receptor was performed defining MBK3 as a model for the B2 receptor. The specificity of anti-idiotypic antibodies, which were raised against MBK1, MBK2 and MBK3 was demonstrated by an extensive immunological characterization. The observed interaction of the corresponding anti-idiotypic antibodies with the kinin receptor on a structural and functional level provided definite evidence for the molecular mimicry of kinin by anti-idiotypic antibodies.

MATERIALS AND METHODS[1]

Antigen preparation and immunizations. To prepare immunogenic peptide conjugates, synthetic bradykinin was coupled to bovine serum albumin using 1-ethyl-3-(3-dimethylaminopropyl)carbodiimide HCL (8). Female BALB/c mice were immunized s.c. in 4 week intervals with 100 µg of conjugate in Freund's adjuvant. Four days before the fusion experiment 100 µg of conjugate and 50 µg of unmodified peptide dissolved in 250 µl of 0.15M NaCl were injected i.p. Polyclonal antibodies were elicited in female New Zealand White rabbits or sheep following standard immunization protocols (9). Affinity purified monoclonal antibodies (from mouse) were used as antigen for the production of anti-idiotypic antibodies in rabbits and sheep, and affinity-purified anti-idiotypes from rabbit were administered in mice to elicit anti-anti-idiotypic antibodies.

Production, purification and modification of antibodies. The fusion of $2 \cdot 10^8$ immune spleen cells with $5 \cdot 10^7$ X63/Ag8.653 myeloma cells was performed using 50% (w/v) polyethylene glycol 4000 as fusogenic agent (10). Screening for anti-bradykinin Ig was done by the indirect ELISA. Colonies secreting antibodies were subcloned three times by the limiting dilution method. Multiple mye-

---

[1] for a complete description of the applied methods see also: Haasemann et al. J Immunol 1991; 147:3882-92

loma were induced by i.p. injections of 10^7 hybrid cells in BALB/c mice primed with 2,6,4,10-tetramethylpentadecane (pristane). Monoclonal antibodies were purified from ascites by 45% (w/v) ammonium sulfate precipitation, anion exchange chromatography (DE52 cellulose) and affinity chromatography on immobilized bradykinin-BSA conjugates (Affigel 10). Anti-idiotypic antibodies were purified by preabsorption of sera with polyclonal and monoclonal (unrelated IgG1,κ) mouse Ig immobilized on CNBr-activated Sepharose followed by affinity chromatography on Sepharose-bound idiotypic Ig. Antibodies were labeled with biotin and ^{125}I as described elsewhere (11). Fab fragments were generated by limited proteolyses of the antibodies with papain.

Indirect ELISA. The indirect Elisa in 96-well microtiter plates using peptide conjugates was done according to established procedures (9). For membrane binding studies crude membrane fractions from the human foreskin fibroblast cell-line HF15, harvested as decribed previously (12), were immobilized (100 µg/ml protein) on polylysine-coated microtiter plates by fixation with 0.025% (w/v) glutardialdehyd (13).

Competitive ELISA. The ELISA in competitive version was performed under the same conditions as the indirect version except for a preincubation (90 min in the assay determining the peptide specificty of MBK1) or simultanous (membrane binding of anti-idiotypes) incubation of the antibody with the competing peptide.

Radioimmunoassay. Peptide specificity of antibodies MBK2 and MBK3 was assesed by a RIA developed for quantification of kinins (14). Briefly, antibodies (20 µg/ml), serial dilutions (2^n) of kinin peptides and a constant concentration of tracer peptide $[^{125}I]Tyr^0$ -bradykinin ($4 \cdot 10^5$ cpm/ml) were incubated overnight at 4^0 C in equivolumes (50 µl). The separation of free and bound peptide was achieved by precipitation of the antibodies with antiserum against mouse IgG in presence of 3% (w/v) polyethyleneglycol 6000.

SDS electrophoresis and Western blotting. Analytical electrophoreses was performed on 5 to 15% (w/v) linear polyacrylamide gradient gels in presence of 5% (w/v) dithiothreitol and 0.1% (w/v) SDS at 30 mA for 150 min. Proteins were electrotransferred to nitrocellulose (0.45 µm) by the semidry blotting technique for 90 min at 100 mA. Immunoprinting of the transferred proteins was done as detailed previously (11).

Receptor binding of anti-idiotypic antibodies. Binding of antibodies to human fibroblasts was tested by direct binding studies on intact cells. Cells were preincubated with modified Hank' buffer for 15 min, washed and incubated for 4h at 4^0 C with a 50 µg/ml solution of the antibodies in the same buffer. After extensive washing, 500 µl of ^{125}I-labeled anti-rabbit Ig (from sheep; $3 \cdot 10^5$

cpm/ml) were added and incubated for 2h at 4°C. After washing the cells were detached by trypsination and bound radioactivity was quantified. Binding of anti-idiotypic antibodies to guinea pig ileum was tested in a miniaturized version of a previously published assay (15).

Induction of the second messenger pathways. Stimulation of inositol phosphate pathway of intact fibroblasts via the B2 receptor was done as recently described (16). For metabolic labeling of the cells, 0.5 µCi/ml myo-[2-^{3}H]inositol (sp.act.15 Ci/mmol) was used. Two days later labeled cells were pretreated with 10 mM LiCl and stimulated for 1 to 5 min with 1 µM bradykinin or anti-idiotypic antibody. The stimulation was terminated by addition of TCA and freezing. Inositol phosphates present in cell lysates were separated by anion exchange chromatography and quantified in a liquid scintillation counter. Stimulation of PG synthesis in SV-T2 mouse fibroblasts by anti-idiotypic antibodies was measured as described previously (17).

RESULTS

Characterization of monoclonal anti-bradykinin antibodies. The fusion of myeloma cells with splenocytes of Balb/c mice immunized with bradykinin-BSA conjugate resulted in three individual clones secreting kinin specific monoclonal antibodies (MBK1,MBK2, MBK3). The antibodies were subtyped as Ig1, κ. The purity of large scale preparations of the immunoglobulins was assessed by SDS electrophoresis and isoelectric focussing, revealing distinct pIs: 6.4-6.6 (MBK1), 6.5-6.7 (MBK2) and 5.6-5.8 (MBK3). The characterization of their epitopes was achieved by determination of their affinity towards a panel of kinins and derivatives (Table 1). The resultant binding characteristics (determined by RIA for MBK2/MBK3 and ELISA for MBK1) was compared to the known potencies of the peptides that bind to (18) or activate the kinin receptor (19).

Antibody MBK1 showed specificity for the carboxyterminally truncated kinins desArg^9-bradykinin (4.0 ± 0.1 nM) and desArg^{10}-Lys-bradykinin (15 ± 0.7 nM) whereas the affinity towards bradykinin, kallidin, desArg^1-bradykinin, Hyp^3-bradykinin, shorter kinin fragments (desPhe^8-desArg^9-bradykinin) as well as bradykinin antagonists was low (>50 µM). A significant decrease of affinity following an extension of the target peptides suggests an exposure of distinct conformational epitopes in bradykinin and truncated versions thereof.

Our findings are reminiscent of pharmacological studies demonstrating an extreme selectivity of the two kinin receptors for kinins and their carboxyterminally truncated ligands. MBK1 shares the principal binding characteristics of the B1 receptor for which desArg^9-bradykinin and desArg^{10}-Lys-Bradykinin are the most potent agonists. Major differences are seen in the superagonistic activity of desArg^{10}-Lys-bradykinin which is less obvious in the binding to MBK1, and in the significant biological activity of Lys-bradykinin which is not reflected by its immunological affinity.

By contrast, antibody MBK3 showed high affinity towards bradykinin (180 ± 10 nM), Lys-bradykinin (220 ± 20 nM), desArg^1-bradykinin (320 ± 30 nM), and Hyp^3-bradykinin (310 ± 30 nM), but not to desArg^9-bradykinin and desPhe^8-desArg^9-bradykinin (>200 μm) or kinin antagonists. The carboxyterminal arginine residue obviously forms part of an essential contact site within the combining region or allows the generation of a conformational epitope recognized by the antibody. A striking correlation between MBK3 and the B2 receptor system was obvious for all the ligands tested with the exception of desArg^1-bradykinin, that is readily recognized by MBK3 but weakly bound by the B2 receptor.

peptide	imm. act. MBK1	biol.act. B1 receptor	imm.act. MBK2	imm. act. MBK3	pharm. act. B2 receptor	biol. act. B2 receptor
bradykinin	<0.1	8	100	100	100	100
Lys-bradykinin	<0.1	95	13	82	60	64
Hyp^3-bradykinin	<0.1	n.d.	71	58	100	n.d.
desArg^1-bk	<0.1	n.d.	14	56	n.d.	<0.01
desArg^9-bk	100	100	91	< 0.1	<0.03	<0.01
desArg^9-desPhe^8-bk	<0.1	<0.1	0.1	< 0.1	n.d.	<0.01
desArg^{10}-Lys-bk	25	2100	n.d.	n.d.	n.d.	n.d.
angiotensin II	<0.1	n.d.	< 0.1	< 0.1	<0.03	n.d.

Table 1. Comparison of immunological , pharmacological, and biological activities of bradykinin and its derivatives. Immunological activity was determined by measurement of the relative affinities (IC$_{50}$) by competitve ELISA (MBK1) and RIA (MBK2/MBK3 using (^{125}I)Tyr^0-bradykinin as the tracer peptide. Values indicate the relative activities normalized for bradykinin (B2 receptor system) and desArg^9-bradykinin (B1 receptor system). Pharmacological activity represents binding of the peptides to intact human fibroblasts (data taken from 18); data for biological activity were taken from standard assay systems i.e. rabbit jugular vein (B2 receptor system) and rabbit aorta (B1 receptor system), (19).

Antibody MBK2 bound strongly to bradykinin (27.0 ± 2.0 nM), desArg^9-bradykinin (39.0 ± 4.4 nM) and Hyp^3-bradykinin (30.6 ± 2.7 nM). Aminoterminal modifications resulted in slightly reduced affinities (desArg^1-bradykinin 191 ± 26 nM; Lys-bradykinin 213 ± 27 nM). This points to an epitope located in the center portion of the peptide, which required neither of the terminal arginines. Cross-reactivity with H-kininogen and L-kininogen across species shows that this epitope is also present when the peptide is integrated in the large peptide precursor. The binding profile of MBK2 does not resemble the characteristics of any known kinin binding molecule whereas the comparison between MBK1 and the B1 receptor, and MBK3 and the B2 receptor suggests a structural similarity in the binding regions of the recipient proteins, thereby defining these antibodies as receptor model structures.

Production and characterization of polyclonal anti-idiotypic antibodies. Purified monoclonal antibodies (MBK1, MBK2, MBK3) were used as antigens for the production of polyclonal anti-idiotypic antibodies (AIA1, AIA2, AIA3, respectively). A differentiated analysis of the immune reponse with respect to the appearance and regulation of anti-idiotypic antibodies was done by the anti-idiotype-detection assay (AIDA). The assay is based on the competition of anti-diotypic antibody and ligand for binding to the idiotypic region of the antibody used as the antigen. Application of antisera against MBK3 showed high titers in individual rabbits and sheep which varied during the course of immunization. To isolate anti-idiotypic antibodies, immune sera were extensively preabsorbed on mouse polyclonal Ig/monoclonal Ig1-Sepharose to remove anti-isotypic and anti-allotypic antibodies. The remaining anti-idiotypic antibodies were positively selected by affinity chromatography on MBK3-Sepharose. The specificity of anti-idiotypic antibodies was assessed by immunoprint analysis (Fig. 2). Anti-idiotypic antibodies specifically recognized MBK3 and the Fab fragment thereof, whereas neither unrelated Ig nor MBK1 or MBK2 were recognized by the anti-idiotypic probe, proving that both anti-isotypes and anti-allotypes were efficiently removed by the purification procedure. Our data further point to the existence of a private epitope on MBK3, which is not shared by the other antibradykinin antibodies. The requirement for defined conformation of the idiotypic region was demonstrated by the complete lack of binding of the anti-idiotypic antibodies to reduced MBK3. To characterize the conformation-dependent idiotope the interference of the authentic antigen with the idiotype-antiidiotype binding was analysed by competitive ELISA (Fig. 3). Application of increasing concentrations of bradykinin, but not desArg^9-bradykinin or angiotensin II, inhibited the formation of the idiotype anti-idiotype complex in a dose-dependent manner. The large molar excess (1500 fold) of the peptide that is required for displacement of the anti-idiotypes suggests that the anti-idiotypic antibodies have a remarkably high affinity for the antigen combining site of the idiotype.

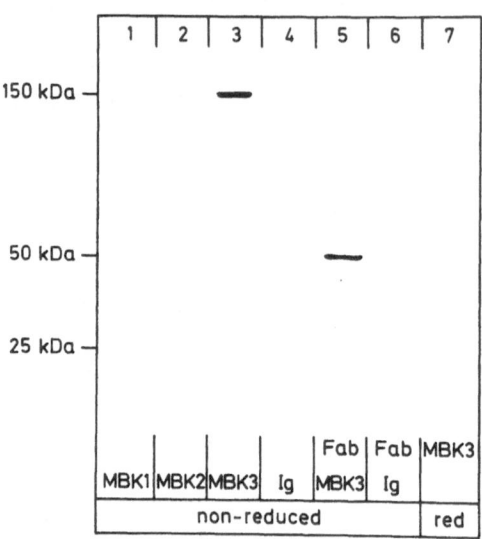

Figure 2. Verification of the specificity of anti-idiotypic antibodies AIA3 against MBK3 by immunoprint analyses. Murine antibodies MBK1 (lane 1), MBK2 (lane 2), MBK3 (lane 3), unrelated mouse Ig (lane 4), the Fab fragment of MBK3 (lane 5), unrelated Fab (lane 6), and the reduced heavy and light chains of MBK3 (lane 7) were run on 5-15% polyacrylamide gels including 1 % (w/v) of SDS. The resolved proteins were electrotransferred to nitrocellulose and probed with 1 µg/ml AIA3 (from rabbit). Bound anti-idiotypes were detected by biotinylated anti-rabbit Ig, the preformed biotin-avidin peroxidase complex, and 4-chloro-naphthol/H_2O_2. Marker proteins were run simultanously: their relative molecular masses are indicated on the left.

Together these data implicate, that the dominant idiotope of MBK3 is juxtaposed to if not congruent with the paratope and further point to a molecular mimicry of the ligand by (a fraction of) the anti-idiotypic antibodies. Characterization of anti-idiotypic antibodies against MBK1 and MBK2 revealed a different situation: anti-idiotypes AIA1 and AIA2 bound to single chains of their corresponding idiotypic antibodies to varying degrees whereas the interaction with their corresponding idiotope was only partially inhibited by kinins. These results classify the majority of the anti-idiotypic antibodies AIA1/AIA2 as α subclass being directed against framework regions of their corresponding idiotypes.

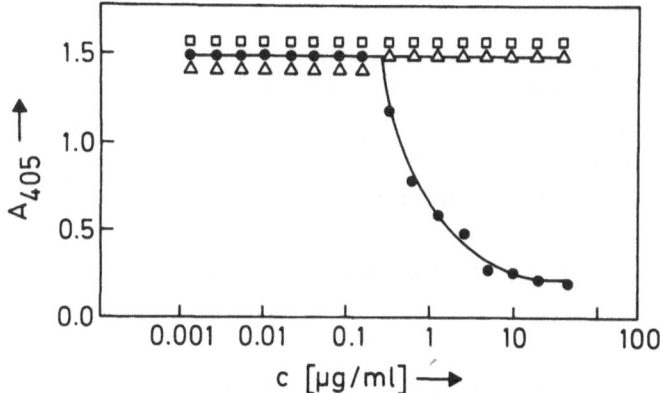

Figure 3. Competitive ELISA to probe for the relation of idiotope and paratope. Idiotypic antibody MBK3 was immobilized on ELISA plates (0.5 mg/ml). Serial dilutions (2^n) of peptide (starting concentration 100 mg/ml) were prepared and aliquots (100 ml) were applied with an equivolume of anti-idiotypic antibody AIA3 (optimized concentration of 0.02 mg/ml). Bound AIA was detected by a peroxidase labeled sheep anti-rabbit Ig (0.5 mg/ml). Competing peptides were: (•) bradykinin, (o) desArg[9]-bradykinin, (▲) angiotensin II.

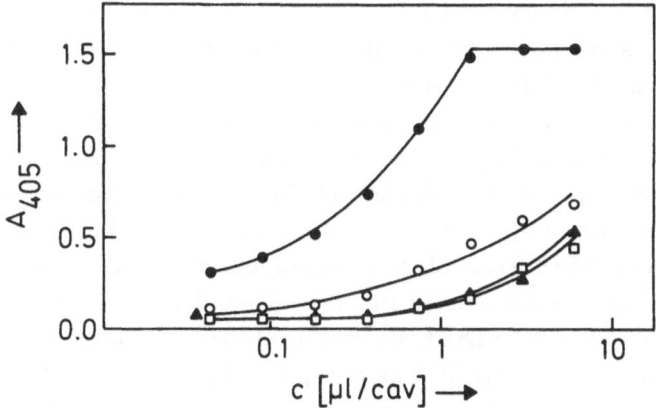

Figure 4. Indirect ELISA to define the specificity of antibodies of the third generation. Microtiter plates were coated with (0.5 µg/ml) of peptide conjugated to bovine serum albumin (BSA): (•) bradykinin-BSA, (o) desArg[9]-bradykinin-BSA, (o) angiotensin II-BSA. Serial dilutions of mouse immune serum were applied and bound anti- anti-idiotypes cross-reactive with bradykinin were detected with peroxidase labeled rabbit anti mouse Ig. For control, bradykinin-BSA was probed by a preimmune serum (▲).

Antibodies of the third generation. To confirm the display of an internal image of a bradykinin epitope, affinity purified AIA3 was used as antigen to elicit anti-anti-idiotypic antibodies in mice. Resultant probing of the sera for anti-kinin activity revealed a low, but significant titer of antibodies cross-reactive with bradykinin, but not desArg^9-bradykinin or angiotensin II (Fig. 4). Transmission of the fine specificity from the first to the third generation of antibodies reinforces our conclusion that the anti-idiotypes of the second generation harbor the internal image of an epitope associated with the authentic antigen, bradykinin.

Cross-reactivity of the anti-idiotypes with the kinin receptor. Given the immunological characterization of the anti-idiotypes suggesting a precise molecular mimicry of the ligand we tested the structural and functional interference of the anti-idiotypic antibodies with kinin receptors of different cells, which were pharmacologically well characterized with respect to the expression of B2 receptors (Table 2). Direct binding studies were performed with intact human fibroblasts under conditions avoiding receptor internalisation, with membrane fractions thereof and with homogenized intestinal cells from guinea pig ileum. Anti-idiotypic antibodies AIA2 and AIA3, but not AIA1 or non immune rabbit IgG, bound in a concentration dependent manner to intact fibroblasts as probed by ^{125}I-labeled secondary antibodies. The complex formation was also demonstrated for the same antibodies using immobilized cell membranes as the targets. The specificity of the interaction was further assessed by a competitive version of the assay in presence of bradykinin. Binding of AIA2 and AIA3 was significantly reduced in the presence of the natural ligand. A "reversed" competition assay testing for the potency of the anti-idiotypes to displace ^{3}H-bradykinin from the receptor was done at the homogenized intestinal cells from guinea pig ileum. AIA3 from rabbit or sheep, but not AIA2 from rabbit inhibited binding of the natural agonist in a dose-dependent manner. At an antibody concentration of 10 µg/ml AIA3 from rabbit inhibited ^{3}H-bradykinin binding to the receptor by 62%, and AIA3 from sheep by 39%, whereas AIA2 from rabbit and non immune Ig failed to displace the ligand. These results demonstrate that AIA3 binds to receptors from different species thereby favouring the view that the anti-idiotypes bear an internal image of the ligand rather than recognizing a common epitope shared by the idiotypic antibody and the kinin receptors.

As anti-idiotypic antibodies of the β subtype can act as agonists or antagonists in the corresponding receptor systems we tested the anti-idiotypic antibodies for stimulation of the second messenger pathways triggered by the kinin receptor.

In human foreskin fibroblasts bearing the B2 receptor, anti-idiotypic antibodies AIA2 and AIA3 proved to induce an intracellular accumulation of inositolphosphates in presence of LiCl. At an antibody concentration of 1 μM, the inositolphosphate turnover was stimulated by 20% over normal (buffer and non-immun IgG). The effect of the antibodies was clearly time-dependent , which can be explained by the slow diffusion rate of the antibody molecule. AIA2 reached a maximal inositolphosphate accumulation (37% of the maximum bradykinin effect after 5 minutes) whereas the bradykinin activity peaked after 1 minute.

	conc.	AIA2 (R)	AIA3 (R)	AIA3 (S)	Ig (R)	Ig (S)
A. Binding to intact fibroblasts [dpm]	300 nM	12124	11413		5862	
B. Binding to membranes						
without bradykinin [A_{405}]	66 nM	1.209	1.106		0.231	
with bradykinin [A_{405}]	"	0.497	0. 765		0.223	
C. Binding to guinea pig ileum (comp ^{3}H-bk)	μg/ml					
	0	3218	3218	3218	3218	3218
	1	3242	2754	3184	3168	3190
	2	3148	2570	3178	3224	3086
	5	3167	1743	2257	3196	3125
	10	3114	1221	1949	3255	3058

Table 2. Structural cross-reactivity of anti-idiotypic antibodies with B2 receptors. A. Human fibroblast were grown to confluency and probed by affinity-purified anti-idiotypes or control antibody (incubation 4h for at 4^0 C). After application of ^{125}I labeled secondary antibody against rabbit Ig, the washed cells were trypsinized and bound radioactivity (given in dpm) was counted in the suspension. B. Membrane fractions (100 μg/ml) were immobilized on poly-lysine coated titer plates by glutaraldehyd fixation and binding of the anti-idiotypes was tested in an indirect ELISA (absence of bradykinin) or competitive ELISA (presence of 300 fold molar excess of bradykinin). Binding of the antiidiotype was detected by a peroxidase labeled secondary antibody; values given represent absorbance read at 405 nm. C. Competition of anti-idiotypes for ^{3}H-bradykinin binding to B2 receptors of isolated guinea pig ileum cells. Binding of ^{3}H-bradykinin is given in dpm. Total radioactivity in each tube was 15 438 dpm. Increasing concentrations of anti-idiotypes or non immune Ig were added. Non- specific binding in the presence of 1 μM NPC567 was 186 dpm/tube.

Murine SV-T2 cells were used to test the induction of the eicosanoid pathway. A dose dependent increase in PGE2 secretion was recorded for AIA3 from rabbit and sheep, i.e. the same antibodies which showed a structural cross-reactivity across species borders, but not for AIA2 (not shown) and preimmune Ig (Fig.5). By application of a specific kinin receptor antagonist NPC567 the agonist effect of AIA3 from both species could be reduced almost to control level. These findings reinforce our previous conclusion that induction of antibodies bearing the internal image of a bradykinin epitope is a species-independent event. Together these data suggest that the antibody is likely to exploit the same molecular mechanism of agonism and antagonism as the authentic antigen bradykinin.

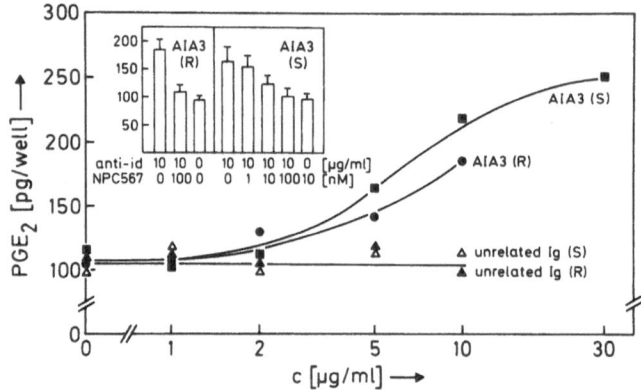

Figure 5. Stimulation of PG synthesis in murine SV-T2 fibroblasts. Secretion of PGE2 into the medium as a result of stimulation of cells with and AIA3 ($\bullet$) from rabbit , AIA3 from sheep ($\blacksquare$) and non immune Ig from rabbit ($\blacktriangle$) and sheep ($\triangle$) was measured by RIA. Media blanks were less than 5 pg/tube. The data are means of three determinations. SD were < 15% throughout. Inset: Inhibition of the antibody-induced PGE2 synthesis by increasing amounts of the kinin receptor antagonist NPC567 (0 to 100 nM). The experiments were carried out as above except that the antibody concentration was constant at 10 µg/ml. For control PGE2 concentrations were measured in the presence and absence of 10 µM NPC567 in absence of anti-idiotypes. Data are mean + SEM for three determinations.

DISCUSSION

Dichotomy within the agonist pathway of the kallikrein-kinin system has been observed on the level of different peptide conformations of bradykinin and des-Arg[9]-bradykinin (20, 21) and the correponding receptors, B1 and B2 which discriminate between the two kinins (22). Our results provide an extension of this dualism at the immunological level. The generation of antibodies specific for bradykinin (MBK3) and desArg^9-bradykinin (MBK1), which parallel the specificities of the two kinin receptors implicate that the molecular binding properties with respect to the differential ligand conformation are similar for both types of kinin binding molecules. The fact that antibody MBK1 is specific for desArg^9-bradykinin although the immunization was done with a bradykinin conjugate might be due to impurities of the peptide preparation and/or in vivo degradation of the antigen by kininases prior to induction of the immune response. We anticipate that the defined specificity of MBK1 and MBK3 could be exploited for the localization of the various kinin receptors using the corresponding ligand and anti-ligand antibody as immunological probes. Furthermore, quantitative analyses of intact versus kinin-free forms of the precursor molecules should be feasible with the antibody MBK2.

Intensive immunological characterization of the idiotypic network on the level of the ligand, idiotypic antibody, and anti-idiotypic antibody established the congruence of idiotope and paratope, and furthermore the display of a bradykinin epitope by the anti-idiotypic antibody. This notion was verified in several independent ways: 1) structural cross-reactivity of the anti-idiotypes with the B2 receptor; 2) agonism of the anti-idiotypes and antagonism by substance NPC 567; 3) structural and functional cross-reactivity of the anti-idiotypes across species borders; 4) maintenance of the peptide specificity over three generations of antibodies, and 5) failure of anti-idiotypes against MBK1 to cross-react with the B2 receptor. The question whether this molecular mimicry is reflected at the level of the sequence and/or on a conformational level remains to be solved. Recent analyses of an idiotype-antiidiotype complex by x-ray diffraction (23) displays an idiotope which is formed by contributions of both heavy and light chains; an analogous situation is seen in the immunological characterization of MBK3. The molecular configuration of the binding site of an anti-idiotypic antibody was characterized in a reovirus system, where the idiotope binding domain was also found to be colocalized on the light and heavy chains of the antiidiotype (24); Investigation into the paratope structure of anti-idiotypic antibodies cross-reactive with the kinin receptor awaits the development of monoclonal antibodies bearing the internal image of a bradykinin epitope.

Using an assay system devised to specifically screen for anti-idiotypes of the β-type we observed a cyclic appearance of this subspecies of antibodies in rabbits immunized with MBK antibodies. The detection of anti-antiidiotypic antibodies (third generation) in hyperimmunsera of the rabbit, which resemble the anti-ligand antibodies (first generation) in their peptide specificity, gives evidence that the anti-idiotypic response is highly regulated by the immune system generating a network of precise images. Appearance of internal image antibodies upon immunization may also induce an autoimmune response against the receptor as observed in the case of experimentally induced myasthenia gravis (25). Hence the regulatory events may be interpreted as a protective mechanism against the physiological activity of induced network antibodies (26). Interestingly, a potential autoimmune effect against the kinin receptor were observed, when mice were immunized with MBK3-BSA conjugates in an attempt to produce syngenic anti-idiotypic antibodies. Some of those mice developing an anti-idiotypic titer showed an intensive, prolonged inflammatory reaction following retroorbital bleedings, which were never observed in mice immunized with unrelated antibodies.

CONCLUSION

Anti-idiotypic antibodies AIA3 raised against anti-bradykinin antibody MBK3 display an internal image of a bradykinin epitope and cross-react with the B2 kinin receptor on a structural and functional level. Cross-reactive anti-idiotypic antibodies will serve as suitable probes for the immunolocalization of the receptor, for the purification of the receptor by immunoprecipitation and affinity chromatography, and for the identification of the ligand binding site formed by the receptor.

REFERENCES

1. Köhler H, Kaveri S, Kieber-Emmons T, Morrow WJW, Müller S, Raychaudhuri S. Idiotypic networks and nature of molecular mimicry: an overview. Methods Enzymol 1989; 178:3-35.

2. Vogel R, Kaufmann J, Chung DW, Kellermann J, Müller-Esterl W. Mapping of the prekallikrein binding site of human H-kininogen by ligand screening of lambda gt11 expression libraries. Mimicking of the predicted binding site by anti-idiotypic antibodies. J Biol Chem 1990; 265:12494-502.

3. Couraud PO. Anti-angiotensin II anti-idiotypic antibodies bind to angiotensin II receptor. J Immunol 1987; 138:1164-68.

4. Couraud JY, Escher E, Regoli D, Imhoff V, Rossignol B, Pradelles P. Anti-substance P anti-idiotypic antibodies characterization and biological activities. J Biol Chem 1985; 260: 9461-69.

5. Sege K, Petersen PA. Use of anti-idiotypic antibodies as cell surface receptor probes. Proc Natl Acad Sci USA 1978; 75:2443-7.

6. Bona CA, Kang CY, Köhler H, Monestier M. Epibody: the image of the network created by a single antibody. Immunol Rev 1986; 90:115-27.

7. Meyer DI. Receptor antiidiotypes. Mimics - or gimmicks. Nature 1990; 347:424-5.

8. Goodfriend TL, Levine L, Fasman GD. Antibodies to bradykinin and angiotensin: a use of carbodiimides in immunology. Science (Washington DC) 1964; 144:1344-6.

9. Müller-Esterl W, Johnson DA, Salvesen G, Barret AJ. Human Kininogens Methods Enzymol 1988; 163:240-56.

10. Galfre G, Milstein C. Preparation of monoclonal antibodies: strategies and procedures. Methods Enzymol 1981; 73:3-46.

11. Hock J, Vogel R, Linke RP, Müller-Esterl W. High molecular weight kininogen-binding site of prekallikrein probed by monoclonal antibodies. J Biol Chem 1990; 265:12005-11.

12. Faussner A, Heinz-Erian P, Klier C, Roscher A. Solubilization and characterization of B2 bradykinin receptors from cultured human fibroblasts. J Biol Chem 1991; 266:9442-6.

13. Andre C, Guillet JG, De Backer JP, Vanderhyden P, Hoebeke J, Strosberg AD. Monoclonal antibodies against the native or denatured forms of muscarinic acetylcholine receptors. EMBO J 1984; 3:17-22.

14. Fink E, Schill WB, Fiedler F, Krassnigg F, Geiger R, Shimamoto K. Tissue kallikrein of human seminal plasma is secreted by the prostate gland. Biol Chem Hoppe-Seyler 1985; 366:917-924.

15. Farmer SG, Burch RM, DeHaas DJ, Togo J, Steranka LR. [Arg^{1}DPhe^7]-substituted analogs of bradykinin inhibit vasopressin- and bradykinin-induced contractions of uterine smooth muscle. J Pharmacol Exp Ther 1989; 248:667-74

16. Griffin HD, Hawthorne JN. Calcium activated hydrolysis of phosphatidyl-myo-inositol 4-phosphate and phosphatidyl-myo-inositol 4,5-biphosphate in guinea-pig synaptosomes. Biochem J 1978; 176:541-52.

17. Burch RM, Axelrod J. Dissociation of bradykinin induced prostacyclin formation from phosphatidylinositol turnover in Swiss 3T3 fibroblasts. Evidence for a G protein regulation of phospholipase A2. Proc Natl Acad Sci USA 1987; 84:6374-6378.

18. Roscher AA, Manganiello VC, Jelsema CL, Moss J. Receptors for bradykinin in intact human fibroblasts.. Identification and characterization by direct binding studies. J Clin Invest 1983; 72:626-35.

19. Regoli D, Barabe J. Kinin receptors. Methods Enzymol 1988; 163:210-30.

20. Kyle DJ, Hicks RP, Blake PR, Klimkowski VJ. Conformational properties of bradykinin and bradykinin antagonists. In: Bradykinin Antagonists. Basic and Clinical research. Burch RM, editor. Marcel Dekker, New York. 1991; 131-46.

21. Dive VK, Lintner S, Fermandjian S, Pierre SS, Regoli D. Preferred solution

conformation of desArg^9-bradykinin and analysis of structure-confirmation-activity relationships in the series [Ala^n]des-Arg^9-bradykinin. Eur J Pharmacol 1982; 123:179-90.

22. Regoli D, Barabe J. Pharmacology of bradykinin and related kinins. J. Pharmacol Rev 1980; 32:1-45.

23. Bentley GA, Boulot G, Riottot MM, Poljak RJ. Three-dimensional structure of an idiotope-anti-idiotope complex. Nature (Lond) 1990; 348:254-7.

24. Williams WV, Weiner DB, Cohen JC, Greene MI. Development and use of receptor binding peptides derived from anti-receptor antibodies. Biotechnology 1989; 7:471-5.

25. Wassermann NH, Penn AS, Freimuth PI, Treptow N, Wentzel S, Cleveland WL, Erlanger BF. Anti-idiotypic route to anti-acetylcholine receptor antibodies and experimental myasthenia gravis. Proc Natl Acad Sci USA 1982; 79:4810-4.

26. Strosberg AD. Anti-idiotype and anti-hormone receptor antibodies. Springer Semin Immunpathol 1983; 6:67-78

AAS 38/I
Recent Progress on Kinins
© 1992 Birkhäuser Verlag Basel

PROBING THE BRADYKININ RECEPTOR:
MAPPING THE GEOMETRIC TOPOGRAPHY USING
ETHERS OF HYDROXYPROLINE IN NOVEL PEPTIDES

Donald J. Kyle,[*] Jennifer A. Martin, Ronald M. Burch, John P. Carter, Songfeng Lu, Sonya Meeker, Judith C. Prosser, James P. Sullivan, James Togo, Lalita Noronha-Blob, Jacqueline A. Sinsko, Robert F. Walters, Louis W. Whaley, Roger N. Hiner

Nova Pharmaceutical Corporation. 6200 Freeport Centre. Baltimore, Maryland 21224

SUMMARY: Five decapeptides were prepared, each having the generic primary sequence D-Arg^0-Arg^1-Pro^2-Hyp^3-Gly^4-Thi^5-Ser^6-X^7-Y^8-Arg^9. A C-terminal β-turn was anticipated when X was an alkyl ether of D-4-hydroxyproline in either the cis or trans geometric state and Y was either a Tic or Oic residue. Whereas cis ethers have only very weak receptor affinities, the trans ethers are significantly more potent in binding to guinea pig smooth muscle having K_i values as low as 0.16 nM. Notably, these peptides do not contain a D-aromatic amino acid at position 7 of the primary sequence.

INTRODUCTION

The approach of preparing conformationally constrained peptide analogues of a natural peptide ligand in order to obtain insight about its bioactive conformation has become widely accepted in pharmaceutical research. The rationale is particularly appropriate in those cases where neither X-ray crystallographic nor NMR data pertaining to the receptor or ligand-receptor complex are available as is the case for the nonapeptide hormone, bradykinin (Arg^1-Pro^2-Pro^3-Gly^4-Phe^5-Ser^6-Pro^7-Phe^8-Arg^9). Since bradykinin has been implicated in such a variety of pathophysiological processes (1,2) including pain (3) and symptoms of the common cold (4), a bradykinin receptor antagonist could have significant therapeutic value. Despite the recent developments toward improved peptide antagonists, there are no potent and selective nonpeptide antagonists of the bradykinin receptor (5). The challenge of deriving one *ad hoc* may ultimately rely on precise knowledge about the receptor binding environment. A portion of this knowledge could be obtained from conformationally constrained peptides.

Several bradykinin analogues containing conformational constraints such as N-methyl (6), C^α-methyl (7), and α,β-unsaturated (8) amino acids have been reported over the past several years, but until recently, none were credited with any improvement in binding affinity with respect to the bradykinin antagonist NPC 567 [D-Arg[0]-Arg[1]-Pro[2]-Hyp[3]-Gly[4]-Phe[5]-Ser[6]-D-Phe[7]-Phe[8]-Arg[9]] (9). Hence, information about the receptor structure deduced from a preferred conformation of a peptide ligand could not be extracted. The most recent examples of conformationally constrained bradykinin antagonist peptides with a dramatic increase in binding affinity have been described by Hock *et al.* (10) On the basis of conformational analyses using empirical calculations incorporating the CHARMm (11) force field, Kyle *et al.* (12) has suggested that several of these molecules are likely to adopt a β-turn (13) in the backbone of the four C-terminal residues. This hypothesis is consistent with observations made previously using two-dimensional NMR experiments at 500 MHz in which a β-turn was reported in bradykinin and the bradykinin receptor antagonist, NPC 567 (14). These turns were reported to span the residues Ser[6]-Pro[7]-Phe[8]-Arg[9] and Ser[6]-D-Phe[7]-Phe[8]-Arg[9] respectively. The studies were performed in solvents including dioxane/water (90:10), and SDS micelles (15) as mimics of the amphiphilic membrane-embedded receptor environment.

METHODS

In order to pursue the hypothesis that a β-turn in the four C-terminal amino acid residues of bradykinin analogues might be a prerequisite for high receptor affinity, a simple chemical surrogate was sought which would not only induce the turn in a decapeptide, but could also be functionalized with a variety of groups which would serve as "probes" of the allowed steric binding environment. Such a system would be valuable in mapping the geometric and electronic topography about the β-turn accepting portion of the bradykinin receptor.

Initially, five decapeptides were prepared[1], each having the generic primary sequence D-Arg[0]-Arg[1]-Pro[2]-Hyp[3]-Gly[4]-Thi[5]-Ser[6]-X[7]-Y[8]-Arg[9] as shown in Figure 1. The desired β-turn was anticipated when X was an alkyl ether of D-4-hydroxyproline in either the cis or trans geometric state and Y was either a Tic (1,2,3,4-tetrahydroisoquinoline-3-carboxylic acid) or Oic (octahydroindole-2-carboxylic acid) residue. The B[2] receptor affinities of these decapeptides and NPC 567 are presented in Table 1 as determined by K_i and pA_2 values. The latter were determined

---

[1]All peptides were synthesized by the solid phase method of Merrifield (19) using standard procedures on a MilliGen Biosearch 9600 peptide synthesizer. Protected (t-butyloxycarbonyl) amino acids were purchased from Bachem Bioscience (Philadelphia, PA.) with the exception of Boc-protected methyl and propyl ethers of hydroxyproline. The D-cis-4-hydroxyproline ethers were prepared by the method of Smith *et al* (20). The D-trans-4-hydroxyproline ethers were prepared in the same manner using D-trans-4-hydroxyproline prepared by the method of Braish and Fox (21). The amino acid Oic was also prepared by a modification of the literature method (22). Boc protected amino acid PAM (phenylacetamidomethyl) resins were purchased from Applied Biosystems (Foster City, CA). Single diisopropylcarbodiimide mediated coupling reactions were run on the automatic synthesizer with the first amino acid routinely recoupled to the resin . Peptides were cleaved from the resin by anhydrous liquid HF (10 mL/g of resin) containing 10% anisole at 0°C for 1 hr. All peptides were purified by RPHPLC on a Vydac C[18] column using an CH3CN/H2O (0.1% TFA) gradient. All peptides were characterized by analytical HPLC, amino acid analysis, and FABMS.

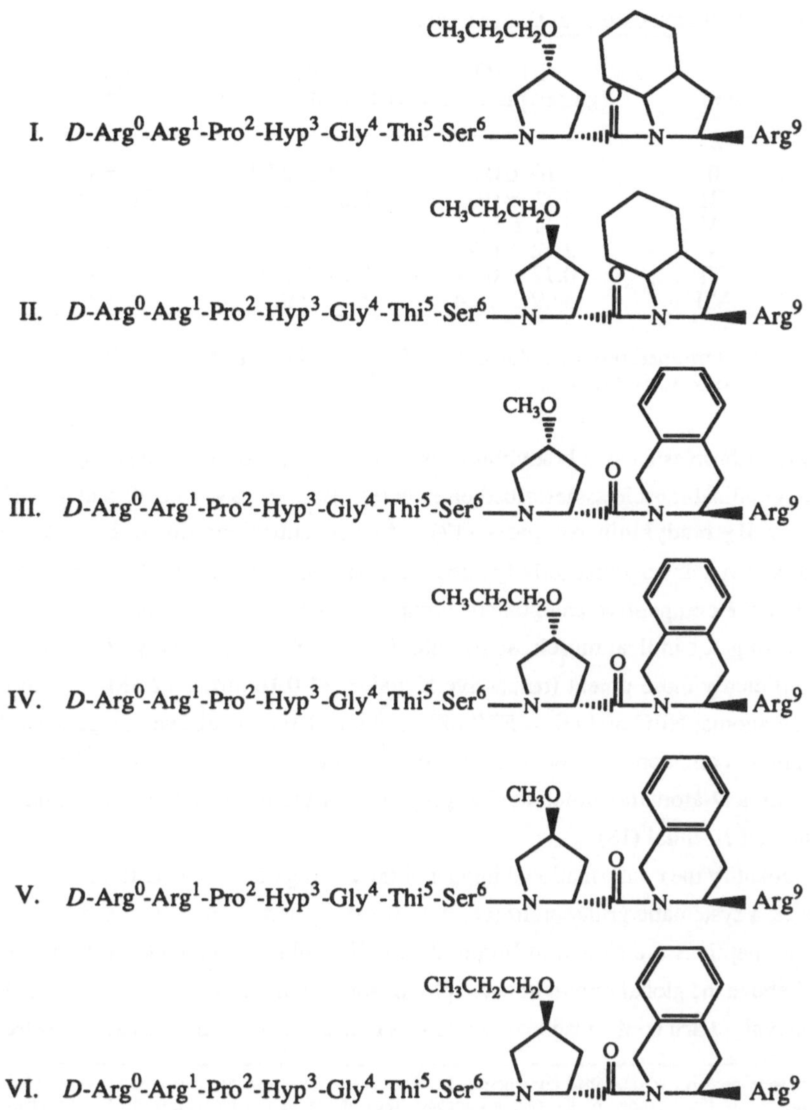

Figure 1.   Constrained decapeptides prepared as probes of the bradykinin receptor

Table 1. Pharmacological Data measured for Peptides II-VI and VII (NPC 567)

Peptide	K_i (nM) (guinea pig ileum)	pA_2 (guinea pig ileum)	pA_2 (SV-T_2 cells)
II	0.16 ± 0.03	8.54 ± 0.02	9.6 ± 0.3
III	102 ± 19.0	5.05 ± 0.03	6.6 ± 0.4
IV	144 ± 37.0	5.24 ± 0.01	6.8 ± 0.5
V	2.12 ± 0.23	6.73 ± 0.03	8.4 ± 0.2
VI	0.77 ± 0.27	7.61 ± 0.03	8.8 ± 0.2
VII	57.9 ± 12.4	5.82 ± 0.12	8.0 ± 0.1

Experimentally determined pharmacological profile of peptides. K_i units are 10^{-9} (nM). Peptide VII corresponds to NPC 567 (added for comparison).

in both SV-T_2 fibroblasts using bradykinin stimulated prostaglandin synthesis (16) and in guinea pig ileal longitudinal muscle as described elsewhere[2]. Both the SV-T_2 cells and guinea pig ileum express only B_2 bradykinin receptors (17). At concentrations up to 10 μM, none of the compounds showed any agonist activity either on tissues or in the cells. The results indicate that, although they are competitive antagonists, compounds III and IV have only very weak receptor affinities, having K_is in ileal muscle of 102 nM and 144 nM, respectively. However, II, V, and VI are significantly more potent (respective K_i values of 0.16 nM, 2.12 nM, 0.77 nM) than the reference antagonist NPC 567 (K_i = 57.9 nM) and are also competitive antagonists. It is worth noting that these compounds are the first examples of bradykinin antagonists to be reported which do not contain a *D*-aromatic amino acid at position 7 of the primary sequence as had previously been considered essential (18).

To quantify the conformational impact of these dipeptides at the C-terminus of their parent decapeptides, a systematic grid search[3] was performed on model dipeptides corresponding to each. These model peptides are shown in Figure 2. Contour plots corresponding to not more than 5 Kcal mol^{-1} above the global minimum were plotted for each model dipeptide with a 0.5 Kcal mol^{-1} contour interval. Each conformational search was repeated twice. In one case, the electrostatic

---

[2]Tissue strips were prepared as described elsewhere (23). Cumulative dose response curves were constructed to bradykinin in the absence and in the presence of increasing concentrations of bradykinin antagonists (0.1 - 0.3 micromolar). The EC_{50} of bradykinin was ca.20 nM.

[3]All energy calculations were performed using the program CHARMm (11), version 21 on a Silicon Graphics 4D120GTXB workstation. In each case all amide bonds were assumed to exist in the trans geometry in conformity with the observations made in previous NMR experiments (14). Since the dihedral angles corresponding to ϕ_1, ϕ_2 in each model peptide are incorporated into either a five- or six-membered ring thereby limiting their rotational degrees of freedom, the grid search was performed on those angles corresponding to ψ_1 and ψ_2 which dominate the overall backbone conformational states. At each grid point the ψ_1, ψ_2 dihedral angles were constrained to the specific grid value and 500 cycles of conjugate gradients energy minimization were performed. For each tetrahydroisoquinoline carboxylic acid (Tic) residue, both *endo*- and *exo*-boat forms of the saturated ring were considered explicitly.

contribution in the overall potential energy was neglected by assigning no partial charges to any of the atoms. In the other case, the default charges assigned by the program CHARMm were used such that the overall potential energy included an electrostatic contribution. In each case the two respective contour plots were identical suggesting that the conformational preferences were being driven by steric interactions, not by poorly represented partial charges assigned to each atom. For those dipeptides containing the Tic residue, the ψ_1, ψ_2 (where ψ_i corresponds to the backbone dihedral angle for residue i defined by the four adjacent amino acid backbone atoms N_i-C^α_i-C_i-N_{i+1}) coordinate values corresponding to the local minima were the same regardless of the Tic residue being in the *endo*- or *exo*-boat form. Hence, where appropriate, contour plots shown in this report were derived from the *endo* conformation of this residue, but for each local minimum it was assumed that either an *endo*- or *exo*-boat Tic conformation is possible. Shown in Figures 3 and 4 are the four respective contour plots corresponding to conformational searches done on Tic-containing model compounds. Figure 3 depicts the cis-hydroxyproline ether-containing peptides IIIA, IVA and Figure 4 depicts the trans-hydroxyproline ether-containing peptides VA, and VIA.

DISCUSSION

Most striking in Figures 3 and 4 is that all plots are identical, regardless of whether the alkyl ether is methyl or propyl, or more importantly, in the cis or trans geometry with respect to the carbonyl group. This suggests that for an ether of *D*-4-hydroxyproline adjacent to an *L*-Tic amino acid, the preferred backbone conformational state is the same, regardless of the ether being cis or trans. More significant is the allowed range for the dihedral angle ψ_1, which lies between -90° and -170° for each Tic-containing model. With the exception of another small local energy minimum centered about $\psi_1 = +36°$, $\psi_2 = \pm 48°$, there are no other allowed states for this dihedral angle. The inherent conformational constraints on the backbone dihedral angles ϕ_1 and ϕ_2 in conjunction with this relatively narrow, preferred range of values for the dihedral angle ψ_1, leads to the conclusion that a β-turn like structure is highly favored in the backbone of these dipeptide models. Analysis of the binding affinities for the decapeptides containing these amino acid pairs at position 7-8 reveals that the receptor has a zone of steric intolerance adjacent to the backbone at position 7 and cis to the carbonyl group. In contrast, there is a zone of steric tolerance on the opposite side of the backbone at position 7 (trans to the carbonyl group). This conclusion is based on the relative low affinity of cis ethers *versus* the very high affinity of the trans ethers. Furthermore, the size of the zone of steric tolerance is better approximated by the propyl group rather than the smaller methyl group based on their relative affinities. Currently in our laboratories, a variety of ether "probes" are being tested to more accurately map these two zones. Representative conformations ($\psi_1 = -140°$, $\psi_2 = -60°$) taken from within the region of broad local energy minimum for both the cis propyl ether of hydroxyproline-Tic, and the trans propyl ether of hydroxyproline-Tic dipeptide models are shown in Figure 5a.

IA
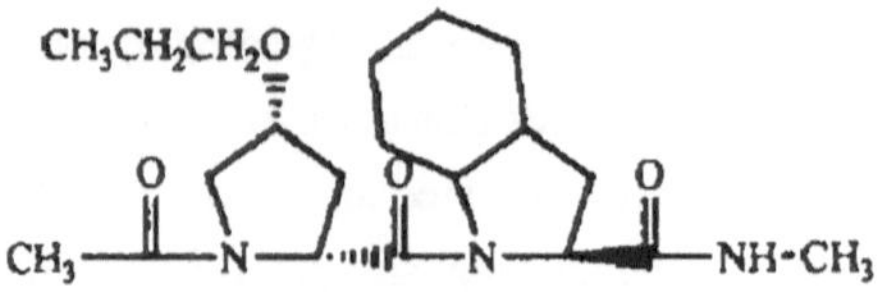

IIA
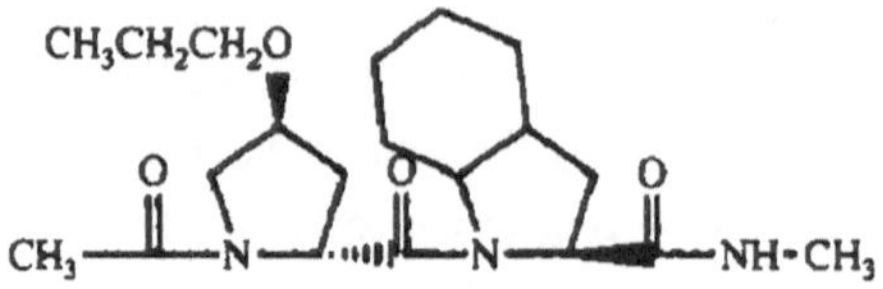

IIIA
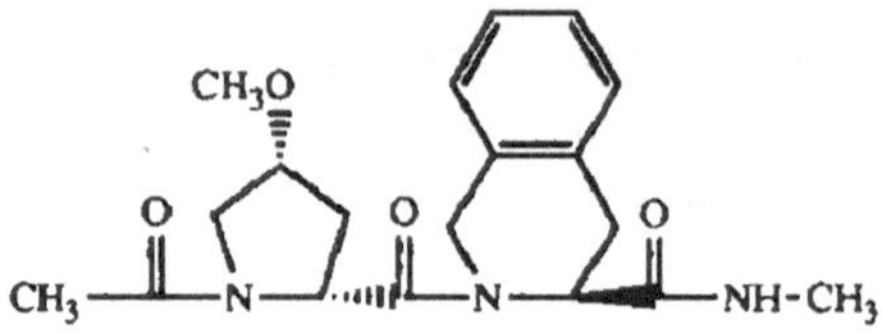

IVA
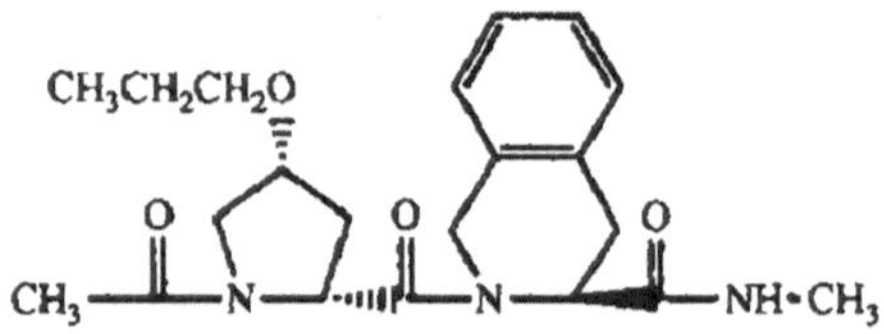

VA
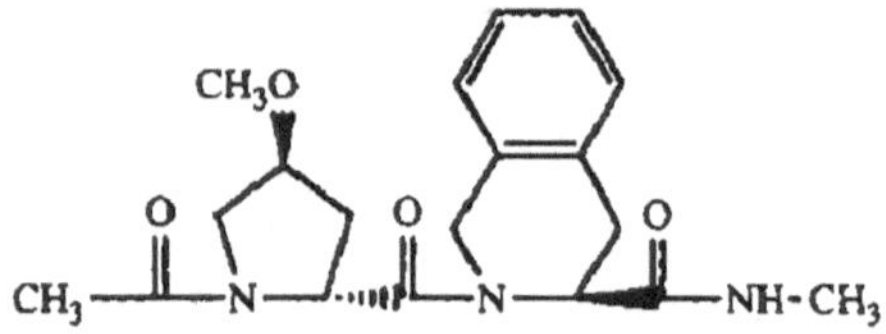

VIA
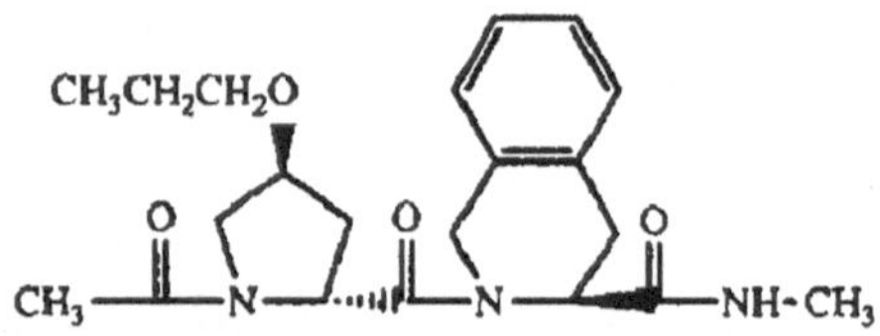

Figure 2. Model dipeptides expected to enforce β-turn conformations when incorporated as replacements for X-Y in the generic peptide *D*-Arg^0-Arg^1-Pro^2-Hyp^3-Gly^4-Thi^5-Ser^6-X^7-Y^8-Arg^9. IA is N-acetyl-(*D*-4-hydroxyproline *cis* propyl ether)-(Oic)-N'-methyl amide, IIA is N-acetyl-(*D*-4-hydroxyproline *trans* propyl ether)- (Oic)-N'-methyl amide, IIIA is N-acetyl-(*D*-4-hydroxyproline *cis* methyl ether)- (Tic)-N'-methyl amide, IVA is N-acetyl-(*D*-4-hydroxyproline *cis* propyl ether)- (Tic)-N'-methyl amide, VA is N-acetyl-(*D*-4-hydroxyproline *trans* methyl ether)-(Tic)-N'-methyl amide, VIA is N-acetyl-(*D*-4-hydroxyproline *trans* propyl ether)-(Tic)-N'-methyl amide.

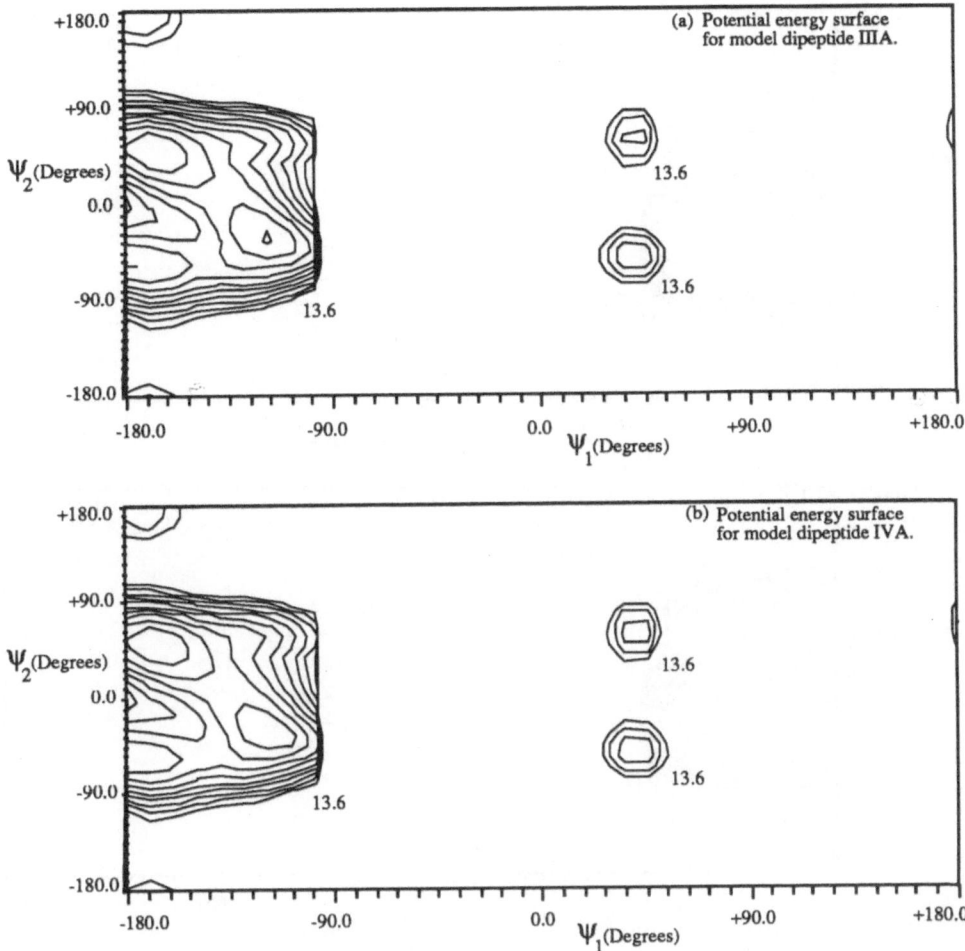

Figure 3.   Potential energy contour plots corresponding to the two respective conformational searches done on cis-hydroxyproline ether-containing model compounds (a) IIIA, (b) IVA. Energy units are Kcal mol⁻¹ and the highest value contour intervals are shown on the plots. The contour interval is 0.5 Kcal mol⁻¹.

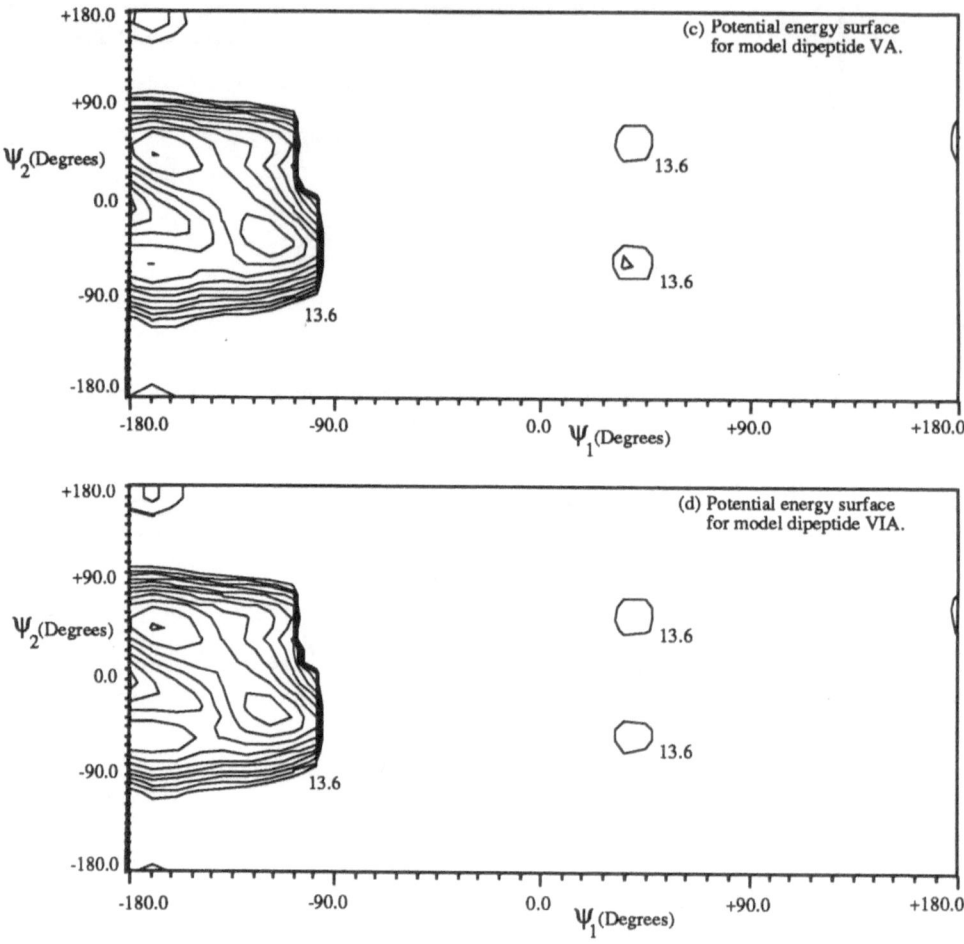

Figure 4. Potential energy contour plots corresponding to the two respective conformational searches done on trans-hydroxyproline ether-containing model compounds (c) VA, (d) VIA. Energy units are Kcal mol^{-1} and the highest value contour intervals are shown on the plots. The contour interval is 0.5 Kcal mol^{-1}.

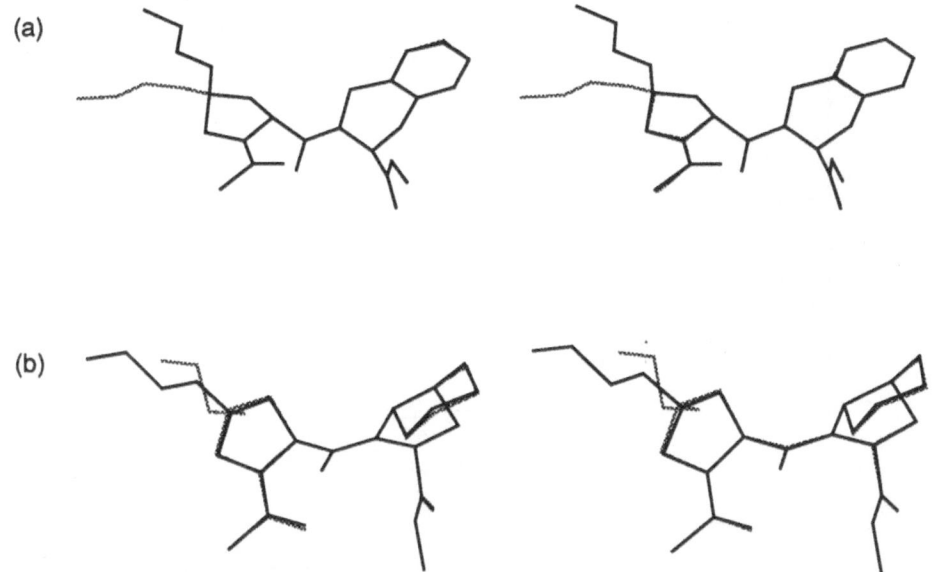

Figure 5. (a) Representative conformations extracted from the potential energy wells corresponding to the preferred β-turn in model peptides IVA (grey) and VIA (black). (b) Representative conformations extracted from the potential energy wells corresponding to the preferred β-turn in model peptides IA (grey) and IIA (black).

Shown in Figure 6 are the contour plots corresponding to conformational searches done on model compounds IA and IIA, wherein the second residue of the dipeptide corresponds to Oic. As was observed for the Tic-containing models, these are highly constrained with similar regions of local minima. However, in these examples, the allowed range for the dihedral angle ψ_1 is between -120° and -170°, slightly compressed from the allowed range in the Tic-containing analogues. Furthermore, in contrast to the broad minimum observed for the Tic-containing models, there are two well defined local minima, both having $\psi_1 = -140°$. These contour plots indicate that the propyl ether of the hydroxyproline-Oic dipeptide will adopt, with higher probability than did the Tic-containing analogues, the β-turn proposed to be required for optimal receptor binding to occur. This backbone state is independent of the geometry, cis or trans, of the ether itself since the overall contour plots are identical. Shown in Figure 5b are representative conformations extracted from the potential energy well centered about $\psi_1 = -140°$, $\psi_2 = -40°$.

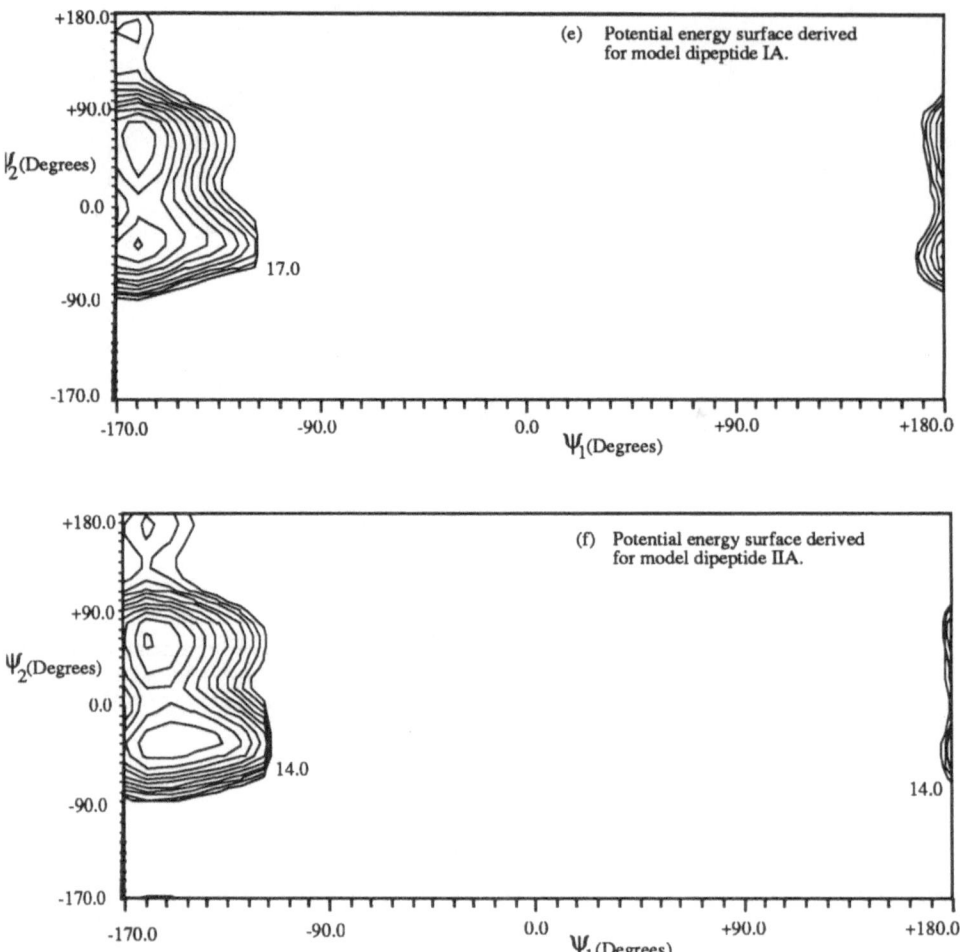

Figure 6.   Potential energy contour plots corresponding to the two respective conformational searches done on model compounds IA (e) and IIA (f). Energy units are Kcal mol^{-1} and the highest value contour intervals are shown on the plots. The contour interval is 0.5 Kcal mol^{-1}.

Based on the SAR developed from the Tic-containing decapeptides wherein alkyl ethers cis to the carbonyl had poor affinities while trans ethers had high affinities, only a trans propyl ether of hydroxyproline was coupled to an Oic residue in a complete decapeptide. As shown in Table 1, this combination of amino acids at the C-terminus, which greatly enhances the probability of forming a β-turn results in a peptide with a K_i measured in guinea pig ileum of 0.16 nM, making it amongst the most potent bradykinin antagonists yet reported. In addition, it has increased potency over the Tic-containing analog which is consistent with its increased probability of adopting the β-turn in its backbone.

In summary, several novel decapeptides were designed to energetically favor a β–turn about the four C-terminal amino acid residues, while providing an available functional group useful for attaching different sized alkyl groups as probes of the receptor topography. Two different steric zones at the receptor binding site, one on either side of the amino acid backbone at position 7 were discovered. The zone cis to the carbonyl at position 7 apparently has only slight steric tolerance since methyl and propyl ether probes of that zone exhibited very weak binding affinity. The zone trans to the carbonyl however, is proposed to be more readily able to accommodate the steric bulk, of at least a propyl group, since the peptide containing the trans propyl ether was so highly potent. Previously reported peptides containing a (D)Tic-Oic pair in positions "X" and "Y" respectively of the primary sequence also represent highly potent B_2 receptor antagonists. These compounds, also proposed to adopt a C-terminal β-turn, indicate that the zone trans to the carbonyl could be large enough to accomodate a phenyl ring.

Finally, while it is generally accepted that the conformation adopted by a small dipeptide will be different than when incorporated into a larger peptide due to changes in the local chemical environment. On the basis of the calculated conformational preferences dictated by steric factors and preliminary (unpublished) NMR results the aforementioned generality does not appear to be valid for these highly constrained dipeptides which adopt a limited number of discrete conformations despite the local environment. In this regard we have demonstrated the utility of this novel amino acid pair for forcing the backbone of a peptide into a β-turn, while providing an available hydroxyl group which lends itself to synthetic modification. Ultimate verification of the geometric states proposed in this report reside in either an X-ray crystallographic study or a high field NMR investigation of the peptides, the latter is underway in our laboratories. However, these preliminary results on such highly potent peptides are of significant value in our ongoing efforts to understand the, as yet unknown, topographical features of the bradykinin receptor.

REFERENCES

1. Regoli, D, Barabe, JC. Pharmacology of bradykinin and related kinins. J. Pharmacol. Rev. 1980; 32: 1-46.
2. Farmer, SG, Burch, R.M. The pharmacology of bradykinin receptors. In: Bradykinin Antagonists: Basic and Clinical Research. Burch, RM., Ed. New York: Marcel-Dekker, 1990: 1-31.
3. Proud, D, Reynolds, CJ, Lacapra, S, Kagey-Sobotka, A., Lichtenstein, LM, Naclerio, R. M. Nasal provocation with bradykinin induces symptoms of rhinovirus and a sore throat. Am. Rev. Respir. Dis. 1988; 137: 613-616.
4. Naclerio, RM, Proud, D, Lichtenstein, LM, Sobotka-Kagey, A., Hemdley, JO, Sorrentino, J, Gwaltney, JM. Kinins are generated during experimental rhinovius colds. J. Infect. Dis. 1988; 157: 133-142.
5. Calixto, J.B, Yunes, RA, Rae, GA. Nonpeptide bradykinin antagonists. In: Bradykinin Antagonists: Basic and Clinical Research. Burch, RM., Ed. New York: Marcel-Dekker, 1990: 97-129.
6. Turk, J, Needleman, P, Marshall, GR. Analogues of bradykinin with restricted conformational freedom. J. Med. Chem. 1975; 18: 1139-1144.
7. Mazur, RH, Jamer, PA, Tyner, DA, Halliman, EA, Sanner, JH, Schulze, R. Bradykinin analogues containing N^{α}-methyl amino acids. J. Med. Chem. 1980; 23: 758-764.
8. Fisher, GH, Berryer, P, Ryan, JW, Chauhan, V, Stammer, CH. Dehydrophenylalanyl analogues of bradykinin: Synthesis and biological activities. Arch. Biochem. Biophys. 1981; 211: 269-275.
9. Steranka, LR, Farmer, SG, Burch, RM. Antagonists of B_2 bradykinin receptors. FASEB J. 1989; 3: 2019-2025.
10. (a) Hock, FJ, Wirth, K, Albus, U, Linz, W, Gerhards, HJ, Wiemer, G, Henke, St., Breipohl, G, Knoig, W, Knolle, J, Scholkens, BA. HOE 140 a new potent and long acting bradykinin antagonist: *in vitro* studies. Brit. J. Pharmacol. 1991; 102: 769-773. (b) Wirth, K, Hock, FJ, Albus, U, Linz, W, Alpermann, HG, Anagnostopoulos, H, Henke, St., Breipohl, G, Knoig, Knolle, J, Scholkens, BA. HOE 140 a new potent and long acting bradykinin antagonist: *in vivo* studies. Brit. J. Pharmacol. 1991; 102: 774-777.
11. (a) Brooks, BR, Bruccoleri, RE, Olafson, BD, States, DJ, Swaminathon, S, Karplus, M. J. CHARMM: A program for macromolecular energy, minimization, and dynamics calculations. J. Comp. Chem. 1983; 4: 187-217. (b) Polygen Corporation, 200 Fifth Avenue, Waltham, MA 12254.
12. Kyle, DJ, Martin, J.A, Farmer, SG, Burch, RM. Design and conformational analysis of several highly potent bradykinin receptor antagonists. J. Med. Chem. 1991; 34: 1230-1233.
13. Rose, GD, Gierasch, LM, Smith, JA. Turns in peptides and proteins. Adv. Protein Chem. 1985; 37: 1-109.
14. Kyle, DJ, Hicks, RP, Blake, PR, Klimkowski, VJ. Conformational properties of bradykinin and bradykinin antagonists. In: Bradykinin Antagonists: Basic and Clinical Research. Burch, RM., Ed. New York: Marcel-Dekker, 1990: 131-146.
15. Lee, SC, Russell, AF, Laidig, WD. Three-dimensional structure of bradykinin in SDS micelles. Int. J. Peptide Protein Res. 1990; 35: 367-371.
16. Conklin, BR, Burch, RM, Steranka, LR, Axelrod, J. Distinct bradykinin receptors mediate stimulation of prostaglandin synthesis by endothelial cells and fibroblasts. J. Pharmacol. Exp. Ther. 1988; 244: 646-649.
17. Mahan, LC, Burch, RM. Functional expression of B_2 bradykinin receptors from Balb/c cell mRNA in Xenopus Oocytes. Mol. Pharmacol. 1990; 37: 785-792.

18. Stewart, JM, Vavrek, RJ. Chemistry of peptide B2 bradykinin antagonists. In: Bradykinin Antagonists: Basic and Clinical Research. Burch, RM., Ed. New York: Marcel-Dekker, 1990: 51-96.
19. Merrifield, RB. Solid phase peptide synthesis. I. The synthesis of a tetrapeptide. J. Am. Chem. Soc. 1963; 85: 2149-2154.
20. Smith, EM, Swiss, GF, Neustadt, BR, Gold, EH, Sommer, JA, Brown, AD, Chiu, PJ, Moran, R, Sybertz, EJ, Thomas, B. Synthesis and pharmacological activity of angiotensin-converting enzyme inhibitors: N-(mercaptoacyl)-4-substituted-(S)-prolines. J. Med. Chem. 1988; 31: 875-885.
21. Braish, TF, Fox, DE. Synthesis of (S,S)- and (R,R)-2-Alkyl-2,5-diazobicyclo[2.2.1]heptanes. J. Org. Chem. 1990; 55: 1684-1687.
22. Vincent, M, Remond, G, Portevin, B, Serkiz, B, Laubie, M. Stereoselective synthesis of a new perhydroindole derivative of chiral iminodiacid, a potent inhibitor of angiotensin converting enzyme. Tetrahedron Lett. 1982; 23: 1677-1680.
23. Noronha-Blob, L, Sturm, BL, Lowe, VC., Jackson, KN, Kachur, JF. In vitro and in vivo antimuscarinic effects of (-)cis-2,3-dihydro-3-(4-methylpiperazinylmethyl)-2-phenyl-1,5-benzothiazepin-4-(5H)one HCl (BTM-1086) in guinea pig peripheral tissues. Life Sci. 1990; 46: 1223-1231.

AAS 38/I
Recent Progress on Kinins
© 1992 Birkhäuser Verlag Basel

^{125}I-TYR,D-ARG[HYP^3,D-PHE^7,LEU^8]BK, A RADIOLABELLED B$_2$ ANTAGONIST SPECIFICALLY INTERACTS WITH TWO DISTINCT BINDING SITES ON EPITHELIAL MEMBRANES OF GUINEA PIG ILEUM

C. Tousignant, D. Regoli, N.E. Rhaleb, D. Jukic and G. Guillemette

Department of Pharmacology, Medical School, University of Sherbrooke, Sherbrooke, Québec, J1H 5N4, Canada

ABSTRACT

Kinins are endogenously formed peptides that have diverse biological actions, including effects on the gastrointestinal tract. In the search of selective ligands, we studied the binding properties of a selective B$_2$ radioiodinated antagonist (Tyr,D-Arg[Hyp^3,D-Phe^7,Leu^8]BK) on epithelial membranes of guinea pig ileum. Equilibrium binding experiments showed that ^{125}I-Tyr,D-Arg[Hyp^3,D-Phe^7,Leu^8]BK specifically labells two different sites. One of these sites is the conventional B$_2$ receptor. The new tracer recognized this site with a K$_d$ of 34.7 nM and revealed a B$_{max}$ of 156 fmol/mg protein. In equilibrium binding experiments ^{125}I-Tyr,D-Arg[Hyp^3,D-Phe^7,Leu^8]BK also recognized a second specific site. Scatchard analysis showed that this second site was of high affinity (K$_d$ of 16.8 nM) and very abundant (B$_{max}$ of 2.08 pmol/mg protein). Surprisingly, the natural B$_2$ agonists bradykinin and kallidin were unable to inhibit the specific binding of ^{125}I-Tyr,D-Arg[Hyp^3,D-Phe^7,Leu^8]BK to the second site. A series of B$_2$ antagonists failed to inhibit the specific binding of the new radiolabelled peptide. As expected, non related peptides such as angiotensin II, neurokinin A and B, substance P, vasopressin, calcitonin gene related peptide and bombesin were also inactive. These results show that the new tracer is interacting with two distinct binding sites in epithelial membranes of guinea pig ileum. One is the well known bradykinin B$_2$ receptor and the other is a new, non characterized binding site that interacts exclusively with bradykinin receptor antagonists.

INTRODUCTION

Bradykinin (Arg-Pro-Pro-Gly-Phe-Ser-Pro-Phe-Arg) is an endogenous peptide that is involved in the pathophysiology of inflammation and of other pathological states such as the carcinoid syndrome [1], the postgastrectomy dumping syndrome [2] and the Crohn's disease [3]. Various studies using different methodologies have been performed to characterize kinin B$_2$ receptors *in vitro* on isolated smooth muscles [4], intact cells, membrane preparations and solubilized receptors using ^{3}H-BK [5,6], [^{125}I-Tyr^1]Kallidin [7], [^{125}I-Tyr^0]BK [8] and [^{125}I-Tyr^8]BK [9]. Autoradiographic studies using ^{3}H-BK have shown that B$_2$ receptors may be present in the muscle and the epithelium of guinea pig ileum [10]. Interestingly, BK exerts at least two different effects on this tissue, since it contracts the longitudinal muscle layer [11] and stimulates active Cl$^-$ secretion [10] through activation of arachidonic acid metabolism [12].

Recently, we showed that the receptor for [^{125}I-Tyr^8]BK of guinea pig epithelial and smooth muscle membranes were identical [9]. We also reported that the B$_2$ receptor antagonist D-Arg[Hyp^3,D-Phe^7,Leu^8]BK shows a good affinity for epithelial (K$_i$ = 32.4 nM) and smooth muscle membranes (K$_i$ = 36.0 nM) [9].

To further characterize B$_2$ receptor in guinea pig ileum epithelial membranes we have radioiodinated the B$_2$ receptor antagonist, Tyr,D-Arg[Hyp^3,D-Phe^7,Leu^8]BK. We performed a full characterization of the binding properties of the new tracer on epithelial membranes and compared the results with those obtained with [^{125}I-Tyr^8]BK. Results show that ^{125}I-Tyr,D-Arg[X]BK labels two binding sites. One of these sites has been identified as the conventional bradykinin B$_2$ receptor. The second site recognized exclusively some bradykinin antagonists.

MATERIALS AND METHODS

Radioiodination of [Tyr^8]BK and Tyr,D-Arg[Hyp^3,D-Phe^7,Leu^8]BK (Tyr,D-Arg[X]BK)

[^{125}I-Tyr^8]BK was prepared as already described by Tousignant et al. [9]. For the preparation of ^{125}I-Tyr,D-Arg[X]BK, 10 µg of Tyr,D-Arg[X]BK and 1 mCi of Na^{125}I were incubated with 10 µg of iodogen, for 20 min at 25 °C, in 50 µl of borate buffer (0.05 M, pH 7.5). The reaction mixture was applied to a Waters C$_{18}$ µBondapak column and purified by reverse phase HPLC. Elution was started with a 1:1 mixture of ammonium acetate and methanol at pH 7.5 for 20 min, followed by a linear gradient for the next 20 min. Fractions of 1 ml were collected every minute. The final product was dissolved in water with 1 mg/ml of bovine serum albumin (BSA) and stored at -60°C. The specific radioactivity of the peptide varied between 50-250 Ci/mmol.

Preparation of epithelial membranes

Epithelium guinea pig membranes were prepared according to Tousignant et al. [9].

Binding experiments

For the kinetic studies, 0.8 nM of ^{125}I-Tyr,D-Arg[X]BK was incubated with epithelial membranes (0.5 mg of proteins / ml) in a medium containing 25 mM PIPES (pH 6.8, 4°C), 1 mM dithiotreitol, 1 mM 1,10-phenantroline, 140 μg/ml bacitracin, 1 mM captopril and 0.1% bovine serum albumin. The various constituents were incubated at 4°C in a final volume of 400 μl. All assays were run in duplicate and non specific binding was defined as the amount of labelled ligand bound in the presence of 10^{-5} M Tyr,D-Arg[X]BK. The incubation were terminated by filtration through GF/C filters (presoaked in 0.3% polyethyleneimine for three hours at 4°C) followed by three rapid washing with cold buffer (25 mM PIPES, pH 6.8 at 4°C).

Dissociation experiments were performed by allowing the membranes to preincubate with radioligand for 1 hr at 4°C (equilibrium conditions). Bound radioactivity was estimated with a LKB gamma counter at 70-75% efficiency.

Competitive binding studies were performed under the same conditions (0.5 mg of protein/ml, 1hr, 4°C) using concentrations of ^{125}I-Tyr,D-Arg[X]BK varying from 0.6 to 0.9 nM. Competitive inhibitions of [^{125}I-Tyr^8]BK binding to epithelial membranes with bradykinin and related peptides were performed as already described by Tousignant et al. [9].

For the saturation studies, epithelial membranes (0.25 mg of protein /ml) were incubated in the presence of 0.8 nM to 32 nM of ^{125}I-Tyr,D-Arg[X]BK under the same conditions as described for the kinetic studies. The second saturation studies using ^{125}I-Tyr,D-Arg[X]BK as a radioligand were performed in the absence or the presence of an excess unlabelled BK (10^{-5} M). A third saturation experiment was done with [^{125}I-Tyr^8]BK, a radiolabelled B_2 agonist. Epithelial membranes (0.25 mg of protein / ml) were incubated at 4°C for 90 min with increasing amounts of [^{125}I-Tyr^8]BK (1 - 41 nM) in the same buffer described for competitive binding studies.

Chemicals

Radiolabelled Na^{125}I was purchased from Amersham. PIPES (Piperazine-N, N'-bis[2-ethane-sulfonic acid]), sodium borate, bovine serum albumin (BSA), 1,10-phenantroline, dithiotreitol (DTT), bacitracin and polyethyleneimine were purchased from Sigma. Captopril was a generous gift of Squibb Canada.

Peptides

The following peptides were used: Bradykinin (BK), [Tyr^8]BK, D-Arg[Hyp^3]BK, Kallidin (KD), DesArg^{9}BK, D-Arg[Hyp^3,Leu^{5,8},D-Phe^7]BK, D-Arg[Hyp^3,D-Phe^7,Leu^8]BK, [Hyp^3,D-Phe^7,Leu^8]BK, Tyr,D-Arg[Hyp^3,D-Phe^7,Leu^8]BK, [Leu^8]BK, [Thi^{5,8},D-Phe^7]BK, D-Arg[Hyp^3,Thi^{5,8},D-Phe^7]BK, D-Arg[Hyp^2,Thi^{5,8},D-Phe^7]BK, [Leu^8]desArg^{9}BK, substance P, neurokinin A, bombesin and angiotensin II. All these peptides were prepared in our laboratory using the solid-phase method according to Drapeau and Regoli [13]. Calcitonin gene related peptide and vasopressin were purchased from Peninsula.

RESULTS

Binding characteristics of ^{125}I-Tyr,D-Arg[Hyp^3,D-Phe^7,Leu^8]BK to guinea pig ileum epithelial membranes

The specific binding of ^{125}I-Tyr,D-Arg[X]BK increased linearly with protein concentrations up to 0.5 mg/ml. Therefore a protein concentration of 0.5 mg/ml was used routinely, at which the non-specific binding was 50% of total binding and approximately 8% of the total radioactivity added. The specific binding was maximal from pH 6.4 to 6.8 and rapidly declined at pH > 6.8. A pH of 6.8 was chosen for all the experiments described in the present study. HPLC analyses reveals that ^{125}I-Tyr,D-Arg[X]BK was stable for up to 1 hour during incubations, at 4^0 C, with the membrane suspension in the presence of peptidase inhibitors.

Equilibrium binding studies with epithelial membranes of guinea pig ileum

In saturation studies, specific binding of ^{125}I-Tyr,D-Arg[X]BK increased as a function of the tracer concentration. The saturation curve of the radiolabelled B$_2$ antagonist is illustrated in figure 1 (upper panel, filled triangles). ^{125}I-Tyr,D-Arg[X]BK binding sites were near saturated in the presence of 33 nM of tracer. Scatchard analysis of these data was consistent with a single class of high-affinity sites with a K$_d$ of 18.5 nM and a maximal binding capacity of 2.29 pmol/mg protein (Fig. 1, lower panel, filled triangles).

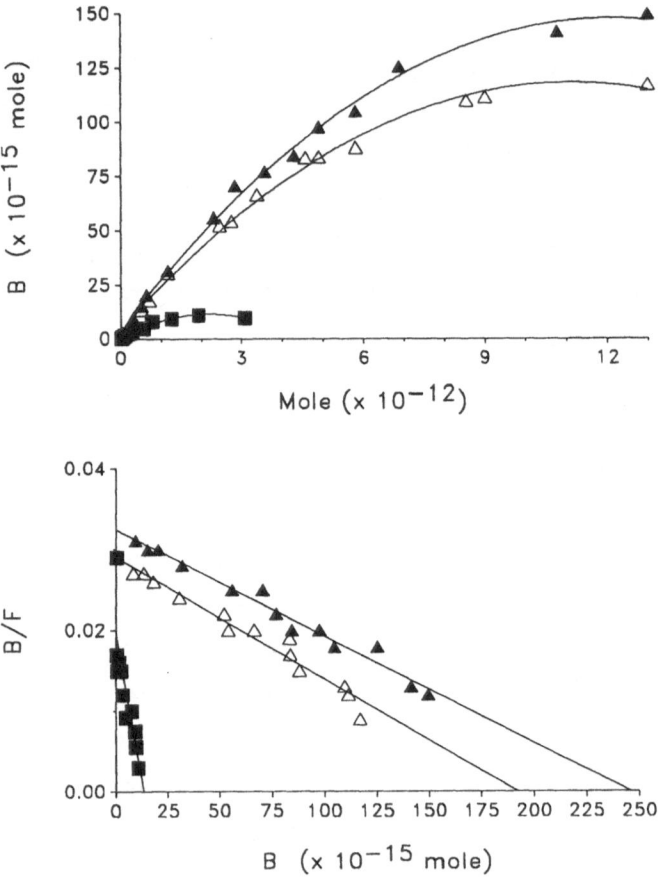

Figure 1. Saturation of ^{125}I-Tyr,D-Arg[X]BK and [^{125}I-Tyr^8]BK binding sites in epithelial membranes of guinea pig ileum. Upper panel, epithelial membranes (100 µg of protein) were incubated at 4°C in a medium containing: 1) increasing concentrations of ^{125}I-Tyr,D-Arg[X]BK (0.8 to 32 nM) (fill triangles) 2) increasing concentrations of ^{125}I-Tyr,D-Arg[X]BK (0.8 to 32 nM) in the presence of 10^{-5} M BK (empty triangles) or 3) increasing concentrations of [^{125}I-Tyr^8]BK (1 to 41 nM) (squares) . After 60 minutes (^{125}I-Tyr,D-Arg[X]BK) or 90 minutes ([^{125}I-Tyr^8]BK) the incubations were stopped as indicated under "Materials and Methods". This experiment performed in triplicate is representative of four such observations. The scatchard plots of the same binding data are shown in the lower panel.

In consideration of the unexpectedly high number of binding sites found with the radiolabelled B$_2$ antagonist, we performed a saturation study using the well characterized tracer [^{125}I-Tyr^8]BK in order to verify whether the high amount of binding sites for ^{125}I-Tyr,D-Arg[X]BK was due to a membrane preparation containing exceptionally high concentrations of B$_2$ receptors or to the presence of a novel site. B$_2$ receptors were near saturated in the presence of about 10 nM of [^{125}I-Tyr^8]BK (Fig. 1, upper panel, squares). Scatchard analysis (Fig. 1, lower panel, squares) of these data was consistent with a single class of high affinity binding sites with a K$_d$ of 1.6 nM and a B$_{max}$ of 156 fmol/mg protein. The K$_d$ value of [^{125}I-Tyr^8]BK (1.6 nM) was about ten times lower than that of ^{125}I-Tyr,D-Arg[X]BK (18.5 nM). Suprisingly, the number of ^{125}I-Tyr,D-Arg[X]BK binding sites on epithelial membranes of guinea pig ileum was about 15 times higher than that of [^{125}I-Tyr^8]BK (3 independent assays). These results suggest that the radiolabelled antagonist interacts with a site that is different from the B$_2$ receptor. To verify this hypothesis, we performed a saturation experiment using increasing concentrations of the new tracer in the presence of an excess (10^{-5} M) of unlabelled BK, a condition under which the B$_2$ receptor is saturated. This saturation curve presented in the upper panel (empty triangles) of fig. 1. shows that specific binding sites for ^{125}I-Tyr,D-Arg[X]BK were still available. Scatchard analysis (Fig. 1., lower panel, empty triangles) of this saturation curve indicated the presence of a single class of high affinity sites with a K$_d$ of 16.8 nM and a B$_{max}$ of 2.08 pmol/mg protein. The affinity of the new tracer was found to be identical when the saturation experiments were done in the presence (16.8 nM) or the absence (18.5 nM) of a high concentration of BK. These results suggest that the radiolabelled B$_2$ antagonist is interacting with two distinct binding sites, one of these being the B$_2$ receptor.

Structure-activity study of ^{125}I-Tyr,D-Arg[X]BK binding sites

Tyr,D-Arg[X]BK and [Thi^{5,8},D-Phe^7]BK (two B$_2$ antagonists) and BK (a B$_2$ agonist) were used as competitors of ^{125}I-Tyr,D-Arg[X]BK and [^{125}I-Tyr^8]BK binding to epithelial membranes (Fig. 2).

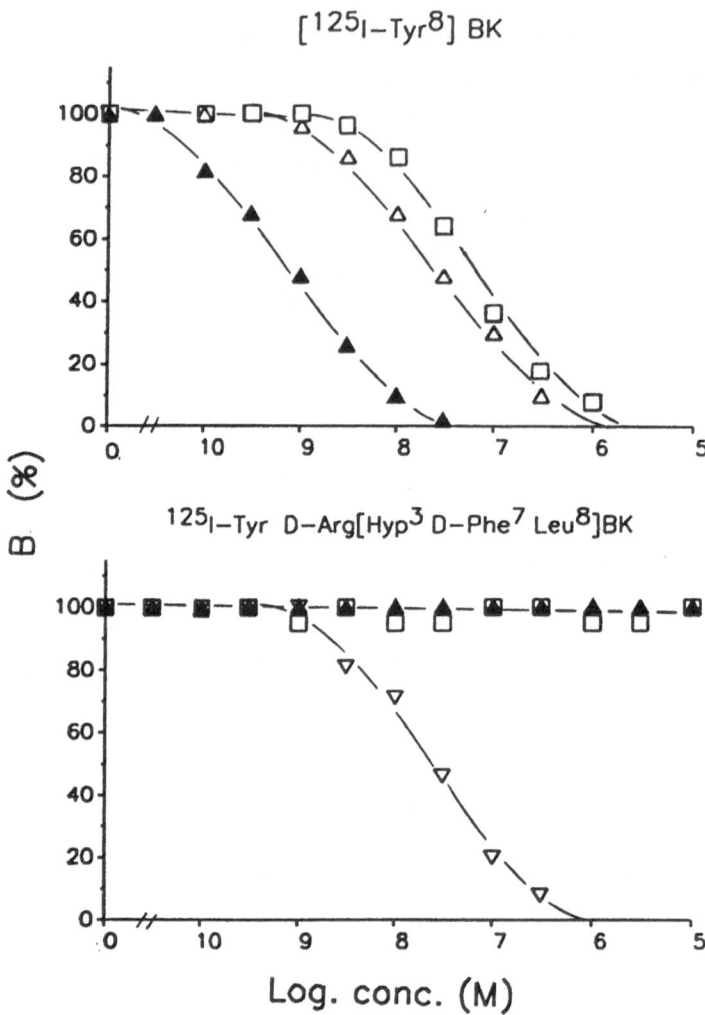

Figure 2. Competitive binding of ^{125}I-Tyr,D-Arg[X]BK and [^{125}I-Tyr^8]BK with related compounds in epithelium guinea pig ileum. Epithelial membranes (200 μg of protein) were incubated at 4°C in a medium containing [^{125}I-Tyr^8]BK (100 000 cpm) and ^{125}I-Tyr,D-Arg[X]BK (100 000 cpm) with increasing concentrations of Tyr,D-Arg[X]BK (empty triangle), [Thi^{5,8},D-Phe^7]BK (empty square) and BK (filled triangle). After 90 min ([^{125}I-Tyr^8]BK) and 60 min. (^{125}I-Tyr,D-Arg[X]BK) the incubations were stopped and analyzed as indicated under "Materials and Methods". This experiment performed in duplicate is representative of three such observations.

Tyr,D-Arg[X]BK inhibited the specific binding of ^{125}I-Tyr,D-Arg[X]BK with a K_i value of 25 nM (lower panel, open triangles) and that of [^{125}I-Tyr^8]BK with approximately the same potency (K_i of 35 nM) (upper panel, open triangles), suggesting that ^{125}I-Tyr,D-Arg[X]BK recognizes both sites with the same affinity. BK (K_i= 0.9 nM) and [Thi^{5,8},D-Phe^7]BK (K_i= 53.7 nM) inhibited [^{125}I-Tyr^8]-BK binding but not ^{125}I-Tyr,D-Arg[X]BK binding. These results further support the suggestion that ^{125}I-Tyr,D-Arg[ ]BK is interacting with two different binding sites on epithelial membranes of guinea pig ileum.

Other kinin agonists and antagonists were tested as potential inhibitors of ^{125}I-Tyr,D-Arg[X]BK binding. The affinities of these peptides are presented in Table 1. BK, [Tyr^8]BK, [Leu^8]BK, D-Arg[Hyp^3]BK and KD failed to inhibit ^{125}I-Tyr,D-Arg[X]BK binding but were effective inhibitors of [^{125}I-Tyr^8]BK binding. DesArg^{9}BK, a B$_1$ receptor agonists, wase inactive.

In order to further characterize ^{125}I-Tyr,D-Arg[X]BK binding sites, we evaluated the affinity of numerous BK analogues (Table 1). Tyr,D-Arg[Hyp^3,D-Phe^7,Leu^8]BK inhibited ^{125}I-Tyr,D-Arg[X]BK binding and [^{125}I-Tyr^8]BK binding with K_i values of 25.0 and 34.7 nM respectively. The presence of a Leu at position 8 favoured the binding and the concomitttent presence of a Leu at 5 and 8 further increased the affinity (see compound 10).

Antagonists containing Thi in positions 5 and 8 were either inactive or very weak inhibitors of ^{125}I-Tyr,D-Arg[X]BK (compounds 11 and 12), but fairly good inhibitors of [^{125}I-Tyr^8]BK binding (see below). It does appear that binding of ^{125}I-Tyr,D-Arg[X]BK is: a) optimal when positions 5 and 8 are occupied by Leu residues and b) very weak when they are occupied by Thi.

B$_1$ antagonist ([Leu^8]DesArg^{9}BK) is unable to inhibit the binding of ^{125}I-Tyr,D-Arg[X]-BK.

Table 1. Inhibition of ^{125}I-Tyr,D-Arg[Hyp^3,D-Phe^7,Leu^8]BK and [^{125}I-Tyr^8]BK by B$_2$ agonists and antagonists on guinea pig ileum epithelium membranes.

	^{125}I-Tyr,D-Arg[X]-BK		[^{125}I-Tyr^8]-BK*	
	K$_i$ nM	R.A. %	K$_i$ nM	R.A. %
Agonists^A				
1. BK	Inactive		0.9	100
2. [Tyr^8]-BK	Inactive		1.8	50
3. [Leu^8]-BK	Inactive		29	3
4. D-Arg[Hyp^3]-BK	15135	-	3.1	29
5. KD	Inactive		5.2	17
6. Des-Arg^9-BK	Inactive		Inactive	
Antagonists^B				
7. Tyr,D-Arg[Hyp^3,D-Phe^7,Leu^8]-BK	25	100	34.7	100
8. [Hyp^3,D-Phe^7,Leu^8]-BK	170	15	70	21
9. D-Arg[Hyp^3,D-Phe^7,Leu^8]-BK	20.9	120	32.4	108
10. D-Arg[Hyp^3,Leu^{5,8},D-Phe^7]-BK	15.8	158	15.8	222
11. [Thi^{5,8},D-Phe^7]-BK	Inactive		53.7	65
12. D-Arg[Hyp^3,Thi^{5,8},D-Phe^7]-BK	6606.9	0.4	912	4
13. D-Arg[Hyp^2,Thi^{5,8},D-Phe^7]-BK	1000	2.5	50	70
14. Leu^8,Des-Arg^9-BK	Inactive		Inactive	

*   Tousignant *et al.* [9].
K$_i$ The nanomolar concentration that inhibits 50% of the total specific binding.
A   Relative affinity expressed as a percentage of that of BK.
B   Relative affinity expressed as a percentage of Tyr,D-Arg[Hyp^3,D-Phe^7,Leu^8]-BK.

Likewise other kinin unrelated peptides such as substance P, neurokinin A, neurokinin B, bombesin, angiotensin II, calcitonin gene related peptide and vasopressin (applied at concentrations up 10^{-5} M) were unable to inhibit the binding of ^{125}I-Tyr,D-Arg[X]BK to epithelial membranes.

DISCUSSION

Relying on affinities of various B$_2$ antagonists, obtained from competition studies with [^{125}I-Tyr^8]BK on epithelial membranes of guinea pig ileum, we decided to prepared Tyr,D-Arg[Hyp^3,D-Phe^7,Leu^8]BK, a high affinity BK antagonist suitable for iodination. Addition of a Tyr at the N-terminal of D-Arg[Hyp^3,D-Phe^7,Leu^8]BK caused only a slight decrease of antagonist affinity for sites labelled by [^{125}I-Tyr^8]BK. In binding studies, we demonstrated that ^{125}I-Tyr,D-Arg[X]BK was interacting with B$_2$ receptor and with another site that appears to recognize exclusively some bradykinin antagonists. The existence of this new sites is based on saturation studies with ^{125}I-Tyr,D-Arg[X]BK performed in the presence of an excess BK (10^{-5} M). These assays have shown the presence of a saturable binding site with a K$_d$ value of 16.8 nM and a B$_{max}$ of 2.08 pmol/mg protein. In the absence of BK, the K$_d$ (18.5 nM) was similar and the maximal number of binding sites was 2.29 pmol/mg protein. Therefore BK displaces only a small fraction of binding. The difference between the two B$_{max}$ values corresponds approximately to the maximal number of [^{125}I-Tyr^8]BK binding sites in the preparation [9], suggesting that ^{125}I-Tyr,D-Arg[X]BK binds to two different sites. Several others B$_2$ agonists were used to inhibit tracer binding and were found to be inactive. It is therefore suggested that a small fraction of the ^{125}I-Tyr,D-Arg[X]BK binding is to B$_2$ receptors and a larger fraction (more than 90 %) is to another site still not identified.

In dose-displacement experiments, ^{125}I-Tyr,D-Arg[X]BK binding was not inhibited by BK. Although the tracer recognized the B$_2$ receptor with the same apparent affinity as it recognized the novel receptor, the large discrepancy between the densities of these two sites (210 fmol/mg protein as compared with 2.1 pmol/mg protein) could explain why, under the experimental conditions used (tracer and tissue concentrations), only the most abundant site was detected. It could also explain why, in dose-displacement experiments, binding to the B_2 receptor could not be visualized. Deblasi et al. [14] recently discussed the theoretical basis supporting this interpretation. Metabolism could not either be taken into account for this phenomenon, since degradation of the ligand, particularly by the kininase II which is present on gut epithelial cells [15], was prevented by 1mM captopril and by other enzyme inhibitors (1mM 1,10-phenantroline and 140 ug/ml bacitracin). Furthermore, in kinetic studies, binding was rapid and reached equilibrium after 60 minutes; then it remained stable for at least 60 more minutes.

The existence of multiple receptors or binding sites for BK is not a new concept. Two years ago, Farmer et al. [16] described a B_3 receptor in the tracheal tissue of the guinea pig. These authors based their suggestion on the fact that B_2 antagonists were virtually unable to inhibit BK-induced airway smooth muscle contraction and rather acted as agonists. Other workers have proposed the existence of B_2 receptor subtypes, based on agonists orders of potency [17], affinities of antagonists [4], residual agonistic effects of antagonists [18, 19] or differential affinities (K_d) of tracers on membranes preparations [5]. The novel ^{125}I-Tyr,D-Arg[X]BK binding site described in the present study cannot be classified as a B_3 receptor or a B_2 receptor subtype according to the criteria of these authors for the very striking reason that it does not recognize the natural agonists BK or kallidin.

Moreover, ^{125}I-Tyr,D-Arg[X]BK binding was found to be saturable, reversible and of high affinity (16.8 nM). If it was not for a lack of demonstrated physiological relevance these properties would suggest that ^{125}I-Tyr,D-Arg[X]BK binding site is a true receptor. Since no biological

response could be related to the activation of this receptor, it is rather difficult to predict whether

Tyr,D-Arg[X]BK is an agonist or an antagonist of this new site. All the attempts that we made

to assign a physiological role for Tyr,D-Arg[X]BK revealed that it was acting as a pure B_2

antagonist. This conclusion is based on results of biological assays in which it has been shown

that Tyr,D-Arg[X]BK acts as a potent antagonist of B_2 receptors in several organs [20]. In

isolated smooth muscle, the compound did not induce any agonistic effect, suggesting that the

binding site is not directly involved in smooth muscle contraction or relaxation. Some hints on

the new sites hypothetical function could be obtained by looking of second messengers generated

upon activation of this receptor. But then again the success of such an approach is contingent

upon the agonistic nature of the ligand.

Binding of kinins to enzymes rather than to functional membrane receptors has been proposed

by Odya et al. [21] some years ago and again demonstrated recently by Snell et al. [22] in the

rat uterus. To avoid such phenomenon, captopril (1 mM) and other enzyme inhibitors were used

in the present experiments. These inhibitors did not prevent ^{125}I-Tyr,D-Arg[X]BK binding to

epithelial membranes suggesting that the ligand does not interact with the same site as captopril.

Moreover, ^{125}I-Tyr,D-Arg[X]BK binding was not inhibited by substance P, neurokinin A,

neurokinin B, angiotensin II, bombesin, vasopressin and calcitonin gene related peptide. Thus,

Tyr,D-Arg[X]BK is a potent B_2 antagonist that blocks kinins biological effects in vitro and in

vivo and interacts with B_2 receptors in binding assays. This compound however binds to another

high capacity site, which is not common either to kinins or to various other peptides and is apparently without functional role. The new site could therefore be characterized only with

biochemical criteria to show that it is a high affinity site showing specificity, saturability,

reversibility similar to other sites demonstrated for atrial natriuretic factor (ANF-R$_2$) [22],

angiotensin (AT$_2$) [23] and other peptides.

ACKNOWLEDGEMENTS

This work was supported by grants from the Medical Research Council of Canada. C.T. is

recipient of a M.R.C.-Ciba Geigy Studentship. D.R. is a career investigator of the M.R.C. and

G.G. is Scholar of Le Fonds de la Recherche en Santé du Québec.

REFERENCES

[1]   J.A. Oates, A. Pettinger, and R.B. Doctor, *Evidence for the release of bradykinin in carcinoid syndrome.* J. Clin. Invest. 45:173-178 (1966).

[2]   P.Y. Wong, R.C. Talamo, B.M. Babior, G.G. Raymond and R.W. Colman, *Kallikrein-kinin system in postgastrectomy dumping syndrome.* Ann. Int. Med. 80:577-581 (1974).

[3]   E. Silverstein, S.M. Fierst, M.R. Simon, J.V. Weinstock, and J. Friedland, *Angiotensin-converting enzyme in Crohn's disease and ulcerative colitis.* J. Clin. Pathol. 75:175-178 (1981).

[4]   D. Regoli, N.-E. Rhaleb, S. Dion, and G. Drapeau, *New selective bradykinin antagonists and bradykinin B$_2$ receptor characterization.* Trends in Pharmacol. Sci. 11:156-161 (1990).

[5]   D.C. Manning, R. Vavrek, J.M. Stewart and S.H. Snyder, *Two bradykinin binding sites with picomolar affinities.* J. Pharmacol. Exp. Ther. 237:504-512 (1986).

[6]   C-P. Sung, A.J. Arleth, K. Shikano and B.A. Berkowitz, *Characterization and function of bradykinin receptors in vascular endothelial cells.* J. Pharmacol. Exp. Ther. 247:8-13 (1988).

[7]   M.J. Fredrick, and C.E. Odya, *Characterization of soluble bradykinin receptor-like binding sites.* Eur. J. Pharmacol. 134:45-52 (1987).

[8]   R. Lewis, S.R. Childers, and M. Ian Phillips, *[^{125}I]Tyr-Bradykinin binding in primary rat brain cultures.* Brain Research 346:263-272 (1985).

[9]   C. Tousignant, G. Guillemette, J. Barabé, N.-E. Rhaleb, and D. Regoli, *Characterization of kinins binding sites: identity of B₂ receptors in the epithelium and the smooth muscle of the guinea pig ileum.* Can. J. Physiol. Pharmacol. 69:818-825 (1991).

[10]   D.C. Manning, S.H. Snyder, J. Kachur, R.J. Miller and M. Field, *Bradykinin receptor-mediated chloride secretion in intestinal function.* Nature 299:256-259 (1982).

[11]   D. Regoli, and J. Barabé. *Pharmacology of bradykinin and related kinins.* Pharmacol. Rev. 32:1-45 (1980).

[12]   M.W. Musch, J.F. Kachur, R.J. Miller and M. Field, *Bradykinin-stimulated electrolyte secretion in rabbit and guinea pig intestine.* J. Clin. Invest. 71: 1073-1083 (1983).

[13]   G. Drapeau, and D. Regoli, *Synthesis of bradykinin analogues.* Methods in enzymology 163: 263-272 (1988).

[14]   A. DeBlasi, K. O'Reilly, H.J. Motulsky. *Calculating receptor number from binding experiments using same compound as radioligand and competitor.* Trends in Pharmacol. Sci. 10: 227-229 (1989).

[15]   E.G. Erdos, *Kininases.* In Handbook of experimental pharmacology. Vol. XXV, pp. 427-487 (Ed. E. G. Erdos). Springer-Verlag, Berlin 1979.

[16]   S.G. Farmer, R.M. Burch, S.A. Meeker and D.E. Wilkins, *Evidence for a pulmonary B₃ bradykinin receptor.* Mol. Pharmacol.36: 1-8 (1989).

[17]   D. Regoli, N.-E. Rhaleb, G. Drapeau and S. Dion, *Kinin receptor subtypes.* J. Cardiovasc. Pharmacol. 15: S30-S38 (1990).

[18]   R.J. Vavrek and J.M. Stewart, *Competitive antagonists of bradykinin.* Peptides 6: 161-164 (1985).

[19]   Y. Fujiwara, C.R. Mantione, R.J. Vavrek, J.M. Stewart and H.I. Yamamura. *Characterization of [³H]Bradykinin binding sites in guinea pig central nervous system: possible existence of B₂ subtypes.* Life Sci. 44: 1645-1653 (1989).

[20]   D. Regoli, N.-E. Rhaleb, S. Dion and G. Drapeau, *New selective bradykinin receptor antagonists and bradykinin B₂ receptor characterization.* Trends in Pharmacol. Sci. 11: 156-161 (1990).

[21]   C.E. Odya, F.P. Wilgis, R.J. Vavrek and J.M. Stewart, *Interactions of kinins with angiotensin I converting enzyme (Kininase II).* Biochem. Pharmacol. 32: 3839-3847 (1983).

[22]   C.R. Snell, M. Yaqoob and M. Webb, *The purification of the Bradykinin Receptor from Rat Uterus.* International Conference KININ 91, Munich, Germany, september 8-14, p. 91.

[23]   R. Quirion, M. Dalpé and A. DeLéan, *Characterization, distribution, and plasticity of atrial natriuretic factor binding sites in brain.* Can J. Phys. Pharmacol. 66: 280-287 (1988).

[24]   D.T. Dudley, R.L. Panek, T.C. Major, G.H. Lu, R.F., Bruns, B.A. Klinkefus, J.C. Hodges and R.E. Weishaar, *Subclasses of angiotensin II binding sites and their functional significance.* Mol. Pharmacol. 38: 370-377 (1990).

AAS 38/I
Recent Progress on Kinins
© 1992 Birkhäuser Verlag Basel

PUTATIVE NOVEL BRADYKININ B$_3$ RECEPTORS IN THE SMOOTH MUSCLE OF THE GUINEA-PIG TAENIA CAECI AND TRACHEA

Julie L Field, Judith M Hall and Ian K M Morton

Pharmacology Group, Biomedical Sciences Division, King's College London, Manresa Road, London SW3 6LX, UK

SUMMARY: The bradykinin receptors mediating contraction in smooth muscle of the guinea-pig taenia caeci were compared with the proposed novel B$_3$ receptors of the guinea-pig trachea. The activities of several antagonists in functional and binding studies were found to be very similar between these two guinea-pig preparations, but pK$_B$S were markedly lower than in a number of typical B$_2$ preparations from other species, suggesting that the characteristics of the proposed B$_3$ receptor may be in part species-related.

INTRODUCTION

Originally, the receptors for bradykinin (BK) were divided into B$_1$ and B$_2$ subtypes (1), on the basis of activity or inactivity, respectively, of BK analogues with deleted C-terminal arginine residues. Recently, Farmer and colleagues (2) reported that both the selective B$_1$ receptor antagonist [des-Arg^9,Leu^8]-BK (1), and also certain B$_2$ antagonists of the [D-Phe^7]-BK substituted series (3) lacked activity against BK-evoked contraction of the epithelium-denuded guinea-pig trachea and, further, did not displace [^{3}H]-BK binding in tracheal smooth muscle membrane preparations (2). These observations led to the proposal by this group, of a novel BK receptor subtype which they termed B$_3$ (2).

We showed in earlier studies (4,5,6) that a number of B$_2$ antagonists of the [D-Phe^7]-BK series (3), as well as the B$_1$ antagonist [des-Arg^9,Leu^8]-BK), similarly had low affinities in the guinea-pig taenia caeci longitudinal smooth muscle preparation, in marked contrast to a number of preparations from other species. Therefore, we have gone on to compare, in functional and binding studies, the recognition properties of the BK receptors in the guinea-pig taenia caeci with the proposed B$_3$ receptors of the guinea-pig trachea, making use of several BK receptor antagonists including the novel analogue D-Arg-[Hyp^3,Thi^5,D-Tic^7,Oic^8]-BK (HOE 140) (7,8).

METHODS

As described in detail elsewhere (9), for functional studies strips of taenia caeci or transverse strips of epithelium-denuded trachea from guinea-pigs were mounted isometrically at $37°C$ in Krebs' solution containing atropine, mepyramine, cimetidine, guanethidine, (all 1 μM) and hexamethonium (10 μM). BK was applied in serial doses in a randomised design, and paired preparations were used where one served as control whilst the other was exposed to antagonist (10 min preincubation). Responses were expressed in terms of % maximum response to carbachol. Estimates of pK_B (for 6-12 preparations) were calculated from individual dose-ratios using the Gaddum-Schild equation for competitive antagonism. Radio-ligand displacement studies of $[^3H]$-BK used membrane preparations from both these tissues, essentially according to the protocols already described for trachea (2).

RESULTS

In functional studies both preparations contracted to BK in a concentration-related manner. In contrast to the trachea, in high-tone taenia caeci preparations there was a biphasic response with an initial relaxation, which was found to be inhibited by antagonists in a similar manner to the contractile phase (data not shown). In terms of tension produced, maximum responses in taenia were greater than trachea (approximately 4 g or 500 mg respectively), and also the responses in the taenia proved more reproducible.

The selective BK B_1 receptor agonist [des-Arg^9]-BK (1-30 μM) was inactive (data not shown) and the B_1 receptor antagonist [des-Arg^9,Leu^8]-BK (1 - 10 μM; partial agonist activity at higher concentrations) did not antagonise responses to BK in either the guinea-pig trachea or taenia caeci preparations (**Figure 1** & **Table 1**).

The established BK B_2 receptor antagonist analogues D-Arg-[Hyp^3,D-Phe^7]-BK and D-Arg-[Hyp^3,$Thi^{5,8}$,D-Phe^7]-BK, both produced small rightward shifts of BK log concentration-response curves in both preparations (**Figure 1**), and the apparent pK_B values estimated from individual shifts are shown in **Table 1**. Estimates of pK_B for D-Arg-[Hyp^3,D-Phe^7]-BK did not differ significantly when estimated in the presence of peptidase inhibitors: mergetpa for carboxypeptidases, enalaprilat for kininase II, and phosphoramidon for neutral endopeptidase (each 1 μM; n = 4 ; $P > 0.05$; data not shown).

The potent novel BK B_2 antagonist D-Arg-[Hyp^3,Thi^5,D-Tic^7,Oic^8]-BK (HOE140) (30 - 300 nM) more markedly antagonised contractile responses to BK both in the guinea-pig taenia caeci and trachea (**Figure 1**), though at 300 nM, D-Arg-[Hyp^3,Thi^5,D-Tic^7,Oic^8]-BK showed insurmountable behaviour in depression of the maximal BK response. This antagonist appeared selective, since it was inactive (1 μM) against submaximal responses to substance P, neurokinin A, carbachol and angiotensin II (data not shown).

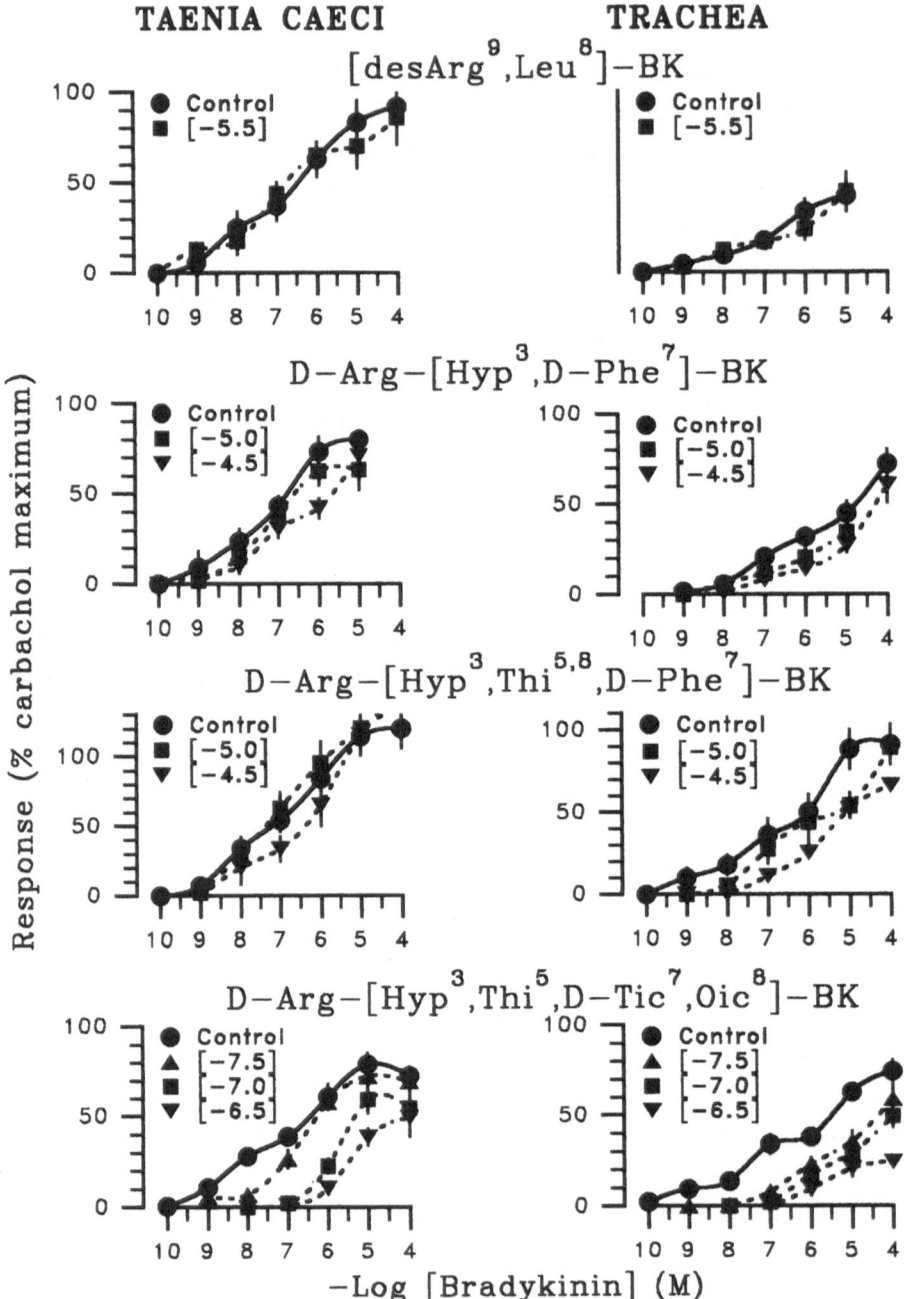

Figure 1. Comparison of the degrees of antagonism shown by four analogues [log M], on the contractile responses to bradykinin in two preparations, (see text). Each point is the mean taken from 9-12 preparations; s.e.mean shown by vertical lines.

Table 1. BK receptor antagonists affinity estimates in guinea-pig trachea and taenia caeci

Antagonist	Apparent pK_B		
	Taenia caeci	Trachea	Difference
	($\pm$ s.e.mean; n)	($\pm$ s.e.mean; n)	($\pm$ s.e.mean; P)
[des-Arg⁹,Leu⁸]-BK	<5.0	<5.0	
	(9)	(9)	
D-Arg-[Hyp³,D-Phe⁷]-BK	5.89	5.94	0.05
	(0.32; 11)	(0.31; 10)	(0.45; >0.05)
D-Arg-[Hyp³,Thi⁵,⁸,D-Phe⁷]-BK	5.81	5.87	0.06
	(0.35; 8)	(0.22; 7)	(0.36; >0.05)
D-Arg-[Hyp³,Thi⁵,D-Tic⁷,Oic⁸]-BK	8.42	8.94	0.52
	(0.15; 12)	(0.16; 14)	(0.21; <0.05)

The results of preliminary binding experiments are shown in **Figure 2**, and it can be seen that the relative pK_i values for the three B₂ antagonists in displacing [³H]-BK are similar to relative pK_Bs found in the functional studies, in that in both preparations the two [D-Phe⁷]-BK analogues show affinities about two orders of magnitude less that of D-Arg-[Hyp³,Thi⁵,D-Tic⁷,Oic⁸]-BK. Although the absolute pK_i values suggest higher affinities than might be expected from the functional experiment, for a given antagonist these values are very similar between the two preparations.

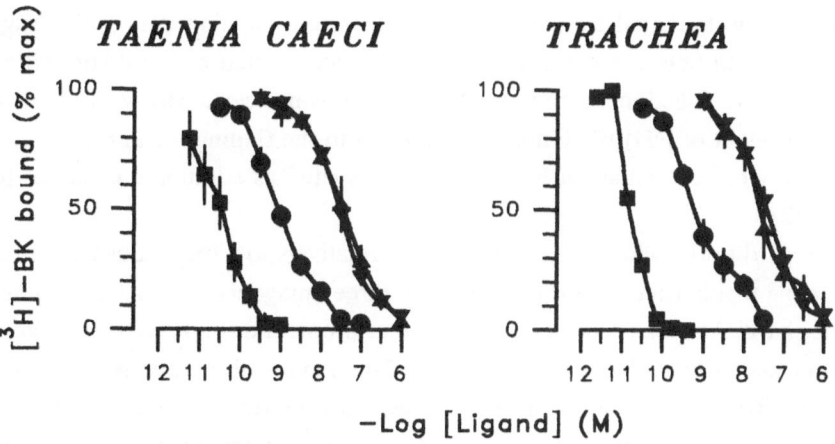

Figure 2. Binding-displacement curves for BK (●), D-Arg-[Hyp³,Thi⁵,D-Tic⁷,Oic⁸]-BK (■), D-Arg-[Hyp³,D-Phe⁷]-BK (▼), and D-Arg-[Hyp³,Thi⁵,⁸,D-Phe⁷]-BK (▲) determined in taenia and trachea membrane fragment preparations using [³H]-BK.

DISCUSSION and CONCLUSION

Bradykinin receptors in the guinea-pig taenia caeci were compared with those of the guinea-pig trachea, a preparation proposed to possess novel B_3 receptors. In neither preparation did B_1 receptors seem involved in responses to BK, since specific B_1 receptor ligands were relatively inactive. The B_2 receptor antagonists, D-Arg-[Hyp^3,D-Phe^7]-BK and D-Arg-[Hyp^3,Thi^{5,8},D-Phe^7]-BK were both shown to have affinities (pK$_B$ < 6) that are markedly low as compared to their affinities measured in a wide variety of preparations regarded as expressing B_2 receptors (pK$_B$ > 7) (3,4,5,6,10,13). These low pK$_B$ values are unlikely to be due to degradation by peptidases since peptidase inhibitors had no effect on antagonist affinity.

The novel antagonist D-Arg-[Hyp^3,Thi^5,D-Tic^7,Oic^8]-BK (HOE 140) antagonised responses to bradykinin in the taenia caeci and trachea preparations with a high affinity (pK$_B$ = 8.42 ± 0.15 and 8.94 ± 0.16, respectively) as compared to the [D-Phe^7]-BK analogues. This antagonist has a high affinity in all B_2 systems so far tested (e.g. rat uterus and rabbit iris; 7,8,11,12): nevertheless in the preparations studied here, the functional pK$_B$ values are about two order of magnitude lower than most other preparations.

Since the affinity profiles for the three B_2 antagonists that we have studied are very similar between the trachea and taenia preparations, but markedly low as compared to a number of other preparations, our data appear to support the proposal by Farmer et al (2) that BK receptors with properties differing from typical B_2 receptors do indeed exist. This conclusion seems substantiated by the pK$_i$ values from our binding data which suggest relative affinities, both between antagonists and preparations, that are in accord with the corresponding relative functional affinities. However, it is not clear why we were able to show full displacement of [^{3}H]-BK binding, in contrast to the findings of Farmer et al (2), where the inability of such antagonists to displace was cited as additional evidence for a distinct B_3 site (2).

With regard to the wider significance of the relatively low pK$_B$ values determined here in guinea-pig taenia caeci and trachea for the three antagonists, it is of great interest that low values have also been reported in some other preparations taken from the guinea-pig; the ileum and urinary bladder (11,13,14). Thus, these observations highlight the possibility that differences in antagonist affinities may in turn reflect species-related differences in bradykinin receptor subtypes (4,5,9), such that the proposed B_3 receptor might perhaps be regarded as a B_2 receptor from a guinea-pig; a species having receptors with characteristics at one end of the spectrum of affinities for a given antagonist.

In conclusion, when data are available for further antagonists and species, and also when other receptor characteristics including sequence analysis and second-messenger coupling-mechanisms have been elucidated, it will be easier to decide whether sufficient criteria can be met for the creation of a distinct B$_3$ receptor class.

ACKNOWLEDGEMENTS

We thank the Wellcome Trust, and the Sandoz Institute for Medical Research, for support.

REFERENCES

(1) Regoli D, Barabé J. Pharmacology of bradykinin and related peptides. Pharmacol Rev 1980; **32**:1-46.

(2) Farmer SG, Burch RM, Meeker SA, Wilkins, DE. Evidence for a pulmonary B$_3$ bradykinin receptor. Mol Pharmacol 1989; **36**:1-8.

(3) Vavrek R, Stewart JM. Competitive antagonists of bradykinin. Peptides 1985; **6**:161-164.

(4) Field JL, Fox AJ, Hall JM, Magbagbeola AO, Morton IKM. Multiple bradykinin B$_2$ receptors in smooth muscle preparations ? Br J Pharmacol 1988; **93**:284P.

(5) Hall JM, Field JL, Mitchell D, Morton, IKM. Putative bradykinin BK$_3$ receptors in the guinea-pig taenia caeci and trachea. Br J Pharmacol 1991; **104**:149P.

(6) Hall JM, Morton IKM. Bradykinin B$_2$ receptor evoked K$^+$ permeability increase mediates relaxation in the rat duodenum. Eur J Pharmacol 1991; **193**:231-238.

(7) Hock FJ, Wirth K, Albus U, Linz W, Gerhards HJ, Wiemer G, Henke G, Breipohl G, König W, Knolle J, Schölkens BA. HOE 140 a new potent and long acting bradykinin-antagonist: *in vitro* studies. Br J Pharmacol 1991; **102**:769-773.

(8) Lembeck F, Griesbacher T, Eckhardt M, Henke S, Briepohl G, Knolle J., New, long-acting, potent bradykinin antagonists. Br J Pharmacol 1991; **102**:297-304.

(9) Field JL, Hall JM, and Morton IKM. Bradykinin receptors in the guinea-pig taenia caeci are similar to proposed BK$_3$ receptors in the guinea-pig trachea, and are blocked by HOE140. Br J Pharmacol 1992; **105**:293-296.

(10) Griesbacher T, Lembeck F. Actions of bradykinin antagonists on bradykinin-induced plasma extravasation, prostaglandin E$_2$ release, nociceptor stimulation and contraction of the rabbit iris sphincter muscle of the rabbit. Br J Pharmacol 1987; **92**:333-340.

(11) Perkins MN, Burgess GM, Campbell EA, Hallett A, Murphy RJ, Naeem S, Patel IA, Patel S, Rueff A, Dray A. HOE 140: a novel bradykinin analogue that is a potent antagonist at both B$_2$ and B$_3$ receptors *in vitro*. Br J Pharmacol 1991; **102**:171P.

(12) Everett CM, Hall JM, Mitchell D, Morton IKM. Contrasting properties of bradykinin receptor subtypes mediating contractions of the rabbit and pig isolated iris sphincter pupillae preparations. Br J Pharmacol 1991; **104**:160P.

(13) Birch PJ, Fernandez L, Harrison SM, Wilkinson A. Pharmacological characterisation of the receptors mediating the contractile response to bradykinin in the guinea-pig ileum and rat uterus. Br J Pharmacol 1991; **102**:170P.

(14) Maggi CA, Patacchini R, Santicioli P, Geppetti P, Cecconi R, Giuliani S, Meli A. Multiple mechanisms in the motor responses of the guinea-pig isolated urinary bladder to bradykinin. Br J Pharmacol 1989; **98**:619-629.

AAS 38/I
Recent Progress on Kinins
© 1992 Birkhäuser Verlag Basel

BRADYKININ ANTAGONISTS: THE STATE OF THE ART

John M. Stewart

Department of Biochemistry, University of Colorado School of Medicine
4200 East 9th Avenue, Denver, Colorado 80262, USA

SUMMARY: The availability of practical bradykinin antagonists has revolutionized research in the kinin field. Development of the first antagonists and progress to the present time are reviewed.

INTRODUCTION

Progress of research in the kallikrein-kinin field, even after determination of the principal components of the system and of the structures of the kinins, was seriously hampered by instability of the kinins *in vivo*, rapid kinetics of the entire system, and multiple interactions with other mediator systems. Involvement of kinins in pathological processes could usually only be estimated by measurement of disappearance of kininogens, and participation of kinins in normal physiological regulatory processes could at best be only guessed. A major change in this state of affairs came in 1984, when analogs of bradykinin that could antagonize its actions on classical kinin assay systems were announced at the Kinin Congress in Savannah. Availability of competitive, selective and reversible braykinin antagonists made possible the rapid advances in understanding of the kinin system that have come since then. It is now apparent that kinins participate in regulation of every major physiological system, and that they are likely the initiators of most inflammatory responses in the body. The prospects for development of drugs based on kinin antagonists effective for treatment of many pathological processes are good.

FIRST GENERATION ANTAGONISTS

The first competitive antagonists of bradykinin effective on classical kinin systems - those that contain receptors previously categorized by Regoli as "B2" - were developed by replacement of the aliphatic proline residue at sequence position 7 by a D-aromatic amino acid, usually phenylalanine (1,2). An important additional modification was replacement of the two phenylalanine residues at positions five and eight by thienylalanine. This modification, made possible by a gift of thienylalanine from Floyd Dunn, had earlier been shown to increase the potency and receptor affinity of bradykinin agonist analogs (3,4). The addition of basic amino acids, especially Lys-Lys- or D-Arg-, to the amino end of bradykinin had been found to inhibit destruction of bradykinin in the pulmonary circulation, and application of this modification to the first weak antagonists greatly increased their potency and spectrum of activity. The other major modification of the early bradykinin antagonists was incorporation of 4-hydroxyproline at position 3 and/or 4. This modification, earlier found to confer some tissue selectivity on bradykinin (5), was later found to occur naturally in humans. These modifications have continued to be used in essentially all bradykinin antagonists reported to this time, and DArg-[Hyp^3,Thi^{5,8},DPhe^7]-bradykinin and DArg-[Hyp^3,DPhe^7]-bradykinin have been used in a wide variety of studies by many investigators. Much has been learned from application of these and other antagonists (6,7).

The discovery of [DPhe^7]-bradykinin as an antagonist came as a consequence of a study of bradykinin analogs in which proline residues were replaced by α-aminoisobutyric acid (Aib; α-methylalanine). Prompted by a report of Balaram that Aib is an acceptable substitute for proline in certain biologically active peptides, we replaced each and all proline residues of bradykinin by Aib and found that [Aib^7]-bradykinin was a potent agonist. Since Aib is achiral (it has no asymmetric center), this result suggested a further investigation of D-amino acids in position 7 of bradykinin analogs. One of the earliest systematic modifications of the bradykinin structure was replacement of each residue by its D-enantiomer, and "All-D-bradykinin" and "all-D-retro-bradykinin" had been synthesized in the search for antagonists (8). All those analogs were biologically inactive. The surprising finding of the potent agonist activity of [Aib^7]-bradykinin prompted synthesis of a series of bradykinin analogs having a wide variety of D-residue substitutions at position seven; one of these was the first antagonist, [DPhe^7]-bradykinin.

Resistance to enzymic degradation is an important consideration in development of useful pharmacological tools and especially for drugs based on peptides. Several studies have helped clarify roles of the various enzymes that degrade bradykinin (9,10), and development of analogs resistant to action of these enzymes has been a major feature of antagonist research. The primary structure modification that yields antagonists, incorporation of D-phenylalanine at position seven, confers resistance to angiotensin converting enzyme (11), and addition of the D-arginine residue to the N-terminus blocks aminopeptidase action. Prevention of cleavage by kininase I (plasma carboxypeptidase N) has been more difficult. Reduction of the Phe-Arg bond in bradykinin prevents this degradation (12), but exploration of this kind of modification in bradykinin antagonists has given disappointing results (13). Resistance to enzyme degradation seems not to be the only factor in achieving long-lasting activity *in vivo*. Hydrophobic character, particularly of the C-terminal part of the peptide, seems also very important. This goal remains a challenge for future development.

THE SECOND GENERATION

The "second generation" of bradykinin antagonists can be said to have begun with discovery of the potent Hoechst antagonist, HOE-140. We had found that the combination of a D-aromatic amino acid residue at position 7 with an L-proline residue replacing the normal phenylalanine residue at position 8 gave good antagonists (14,15). The Hoechst antagonist incorporated these features, but modified the D-phenylalanine and proline residues by additional cyclization:

DArg-Arg-Pro-Hyp-Gly-Thi-Ser-DTic-Oic-Arg   HOE-140

Tic   Oic

These further modifications gave HOE-140 its particular high potency and nearly irreversible activity (16). These modifications also clearly confer enzyme resistance on this analog. The implications of these amino acid residues for conformation of the antagonists have been examined in detail; this approach offers promise for facilitation of the search for improved antagonists (17).

The first bradykinin antagonists to break out of the traditional D-aromatic-7 pattern were developed simultaneously and independently in our laboratory in Denver and at Nova in Baltimore. Extending our work on bradykinin antagonists having proline at position eight, we found that very potent antagonists could be obtained among analogs having a D-aliphatic or D-alicyclic residue at position seven combined with an aliphatic L-residue at position eight (18). Particularly useful in these positions are residues having a branch at the β-position of the chain. Certain of these analogs are extremely potent and long-acting. Recently bradykinin analogs having 4-propoxy-D-proline at position 7, combined with a similar L-residue at position 8, have been reported to be potent antagonists of bradykinin (19).

Cyclopentyl glycine (Cpg)   Propoxy proline

Most recently, potent and long-acting dimeric bradykinin antagonists have been reported (20):

DArg-Arg-Pro-Hyp-Gly-Phe-Cys-DPhe-Leu-Arg
                                |
                         S—Succinimide
                                |
                            $(CH_2)_6$ CP-0127
                                |
                         S—Succinimide
                                |
DArg-Arg-Pro-Hyp-Gly-Phe-Cys-DPhe-Leu-Arg

This and related antagonists are reported to prevent mortality caused by lipopolysaccharide endotoxin, an action earlier found with "first generation" bradykinin anagonists. These antagonist structures are a logical development from the cystine and succinyl agonist dimers of bradykinin synthesized earlier in this laboratory (21).

The discoveries of these new classes of potent antagonists open the way for many new developments in the kinin antagonist field.

ACKNOWLEDGEMENTS

Kinin research in this laboratory has been supported by grant #HL-26284 from the US-NIH, and by Nova Pharmaceutical Corporation. Most synthesis of antagonists has been done by Raymond Vavrek, and synthesis of unusual amino acids and peptide derivatives by Lajos Gera. The technical excellence and dedication of an important group of people in the Stewart laboratory have made all the work possible. Gifts of thienylalanine and other unusual amino acids by Dr. Floyd Dunn have been extremely important for progress in this work.

REFERENCES

1. Vavrek RJ, Stewart JM. Bradykinin competitive antagonists for classical kinin systems. In: Kinins IV. Greenbaum LM, Margolius HS, editors. New York: Plenum. 1986: 537-42. (Adv. Exp. Med. Biol. 1986: 198A).

2. Vavrek RJ, Stewart JM. Competitive antagonists of bradykinin. Peptides 1985: 6:161-5.

3. Dunn FW, Stewart JM. Analogs of bradykinin containing β-2-thienyl-L-alanine. J. Med. Chem. 1971: 14: 779-81.

4. Fredrick MJ, Vavrek RJ, Stewart JM, Odya CE. Further studies of myometrial bradykinin receptor-like binding. Biochem. Pharmacol. 1984: 33: 2887-92.

5. Stewart JM, Ryan JW, Brady AH. Hydroxyproline analogs of bradykinin. J. Med. Chem. 1974: 17: 537-9.

6. Stewart JM, Vavrek RJ. Chemistry of peptide B2 bradykinin antagonists. In: Bradykinin Antagonists; Basic and Clinical Aspects. Burch RM, editor. New York: Marcel Dekker. 1991: 51-96.

7. Rhaleb N-E, Telemaque S, Rouissi N, Dion S, Jukic D, Drapeau G, Regoli D. Structure-activity studies of bradykinin and related peptides. Hypertension 1991: 17: 107-15.

8. Stewart JM, Woolley DW. All-D-bradykinin and the problem of peptide antimetabolites. Nature 1965: 206: 619.

9. Erdös EG. Some old and some new ideas on kinin metabolism. J. Cardiovasc. Pharmacol. Supp. 1990: 15: S20-4.

10. Ward PE. Metabolism of bradykinin and bradykinin analogs. In: Bradykinin Antagonists; Basic and Clinical Aspects. Burch RM, editor. New York: Marcel Dekker. 1991: 147-70.

11. Togo J, Burch RM, DeHaas CJ, Connor JR, Steranka LR. D-Phe-7 substituted peptide bradykinin antagonists are not substrates for kininase II. Peptides 1989: 10: 109-11.

12. Drapeau G, Rhaleb N-E, Dion S, Jukic D, Regoli D. [Phe^8(CH$_2$NH)Arg^9]bradykinin, a B2 receptor selective agonist which is not broken down by either kininase I or kininase II. Eur. J. Pharmacol. 1988: 155: 193-5.

13. Vavrek RJ, Gera L, Stewart JM. Pseudopeptide analogs of bradykinin and bradykinin antagonists. 1992 (This volume)

14. Stewart JM, Vavrek RJ. Applications for bradykinin antagonists. In: Peptides 1988. Jung G, Bayer E, editors. Berlin: Walter de Gruyter. 1989: 559-61.

15. Vavrek RJ, Stewart JM. Development of bradykinin antagonists: Structure-activity relationships for new categories of antagonist sequences. In: Kinins V. Abe K, Moriya H, Fujii S, editors. New York: Plenum. 1989: 395-400. (Adv. Exp. Med. Biol. 1989: 247B).

16. Lembeck F, Griesbacher T, Eckhardt M, Henke S, Breipohl G, Knolle J. New, long-acting, potent bradykinin antagonists. Brit. J. Pharmacol. 1991: 102: 297-304.

17. Kyle DJ, Martin JA, Farmer SG, Burch RM. Design and conformational analysis of several highly potent bradykinin antagonists. J. Med. Chem. 1991: 34: 1230-3.

18. Vavrek RJ, Gera L, Stewart JM. Bradykinin antagonists do not require a D-aromatic residue at position 7. 1992 (This volume).

19. Kyle DJ, Martin JA, Burch RM, Carter JP, Lu S, Meeker S, Prosser JC, Sullivan JP, Togo J, Noronha-Blob L, Sinsko JA, Walters RF, Whaley LW, Hiner RN. Probing the bradykinin receptor: Mapping the geometric topography using ethers of hydroxyproline in novel peptides. J. Med. Chem. 1991: 34: 2649-53.

20. Cheronis JC, Whalley ET. Kinin antagonists. Lancet 1991: 338: 1011. Also this volume.

21. Vavrek RJ, Stewart JM. Succinyl bis-bradykinins: potent agonists with exceptional resistance to enzymatic degradation. In: Peptides 1983. Hruby VJ, Rich DH, editors. 1983: Rockford, IL 1983: 381-4.

AAS 38/I
Recent Progress on Kinins
© 1992 Birkhäuser Verlag Basel

BRADYKININ ANTAGONISTS: SYNTHESIS AND *IN VITRO* ACTIVITY OF BISSUCCINIMIDOALKANE PEPTIDE DIMERS[*]

J.C. Cheronis, E.T. Whalley, and J.K. Blodgett

Cortech, Inc., 6840 North Broadway, Denver, Colorado 80221

SUMMARY: A systematic study on dimerization of the bradykinin (BK) antagonist D-Arg^0-Arg^1-Pro^2-Hyp^3-Gly^4-Phe^5-Ser^6- D-Phe^7-Leu^8-Arg^9 has been performed. Several of the dimeric BK antagonists displayed remarkable activities and long durations of action. Rank order of antagonist potency as a function of dimerization position is as follows: rat uterus 6>5>0>2>1>3>>4,7,8,9; guinea pig ileum 6>5>3>2>1>0>>4,7,8,9. These results suggest that the development of BK antagonists of significant therapeutic potential may be possible using a dimerization strategy that can overcome the heretofore limiting problems of potency and *in vivo* duration of action.

INTRODUCTION

The design and synthesis of potent, stable and specific bradykinin antagonists has long been considered a desirable goal in medicinal chemistry. Up until now, however, most antagonists have been plagued with the dual problem of relatively low potency and poor *in vivo* stability. Several studies have previously reported that dimerization can result in an increase in potency and/or resistance to inactivation for peptide agonists[1-8] and antagonists.[9] To our knowledge, however, this approach has not been employed in the design and synthesis of bradykinin antagonists. Described herein are two series of compounds that were produced using a standardized and systematic design strategy, involving the synthesis of peptide antagonist dimers based upon the introduction of cysteine residues in the parent peptide (D-Arg^0-[Hyp^3, D-Phe^7, Leu^8]-bradykinin)[10] at

---

[*] A more complete description of the synthesis and characterization of these and related compounds has been accepted for publication in the Journal of Medicinal Chemistry.

certain defined positions followed by dimerization utilizing various bismaleimidoalkane linkers. The resulting bissuccinimidoalkane dimers were found to have a number of surprising pharmacologic characteristics that appear to have resolved the heretofore limiting problems of potency and stability. Illustrated in Figure 1 is a representative compound from these series of dimers that has been shown to have remarkable potency and *in vivo* efficacy in a number of animal models of bradykinin activity (see Whalley, *et al.*, this volume).

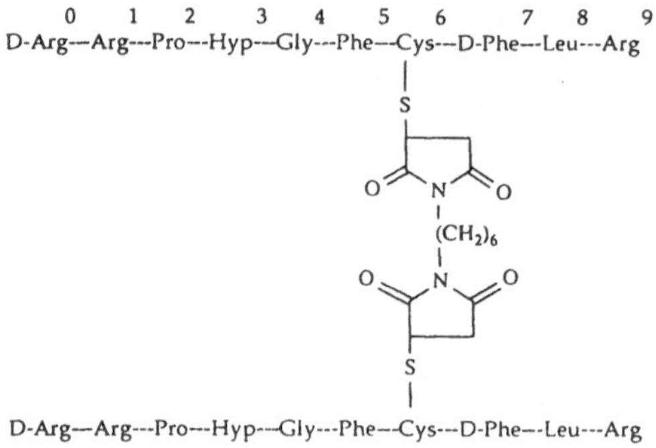

Figure 1. Chemical structure of CP-0127, the bissuccinimidohexane dimer of the peptide monomer D-Arg^0-[Hyp^3,Cys^6,D-Phe^7,Leu^8]-bradykinin.

RESULTS

Effect of Dimerization Position on the Inhibition of Bradykinin-Induced Smooth Muscle Contraction *In Vitro*. The initial studies investigating the effects of dimerization based on position were conducted in a standard guinea pig ileum assay of bradykinin-induced smooth muscle contraction, a preparation known to contain a BK$_2$-type receptor. In addition to estimating the pA$_2$ values for these compounds, we also assessed the ability of these inhibitors to sustain their interaction with the receptor. This was measured by assessing the degree to which the preparation returned to baseline sensitivity and responsiveness after exposure to 10^{-5} M inhibitor, followed by a 40-minute recovery period wherein the tissue was washed every 10 minutes with fresh Krebs buffer. Table I is a summary of the data comparing the reference ligand (CP-0088) to the series of cysteine-substituted monomers and their corresponding bissuccinimidohexane dimers.

Table I. Effect of monomeric and dimeric cysteine-substituted analogues of CP-0088 on bradykinin-induced contractions of guinea pig ileum *in vitro*

Compound #	Structure[a]	Description Reference	pA_2[b]
CP-0088	D-Arg-Arg-Pro-Hyp-Gly-Phe-Ser-D-Phe-Leu-Arg	Monomer	6.5±0.2
CP-0140	[L-Cys^0]-CP-0088	Monomer	6.7±0.1
CP-0152	[BSH(CYS^0)-CP-0088	Dimer	<6
CP-0149	[D-CYS^0]-CP-0088	Monomer	6.7±0.5
CP-0161	[BSH(D-CYS^0)]-CP-0088	Dimer	6.5±0.1
CP-0141	[L-CYS^1]-CP-0088	Monomer	6.1±0.1
CP-0153	[BSH(L-CYS^1)-CP-0088	Dimer	7.6±0.6
CP-0142	[L-CYS^2]-CP-0088	Monomer	<6
CP-0154	[BSH(L-CYS^2)]-CP-0088	Dimer	6.9±0.3
CP-0143	[L-CYS^3]-CP-0088	Monomer	6.7±0.4
CP-0155	[BSH(L-CYS^3)]-CP-0088	Dimer	7.7±0.2
CP-0136	[L-CYS^4]-CP-0088	Monomer	Inactive
CP-0137	[BSH(L-CYS^4)]-CP-0088	Dimer	<6
CP-0173	[D-CYS^4]-CP-0088	Monomer	Inactive
CP-0203	[BSH(D-CYS^4)]-CP-0088	Dimer	Inactive
CP-0144	[L-CYS^5]-CP-0088	Monomer	6.4±0.2
CP-0156	[BSH(L-CYS^5)]-CP-0088	Dimer	7.9±0.1
CP-0126	[L-CYS^6]-CP-0088	Monomer	6.6±0.2
CP-0127	[BSH(L-CYS^6)]-CP-0088	Dimer	7.7±0.2
CP-0145	[L-CYS^7]-CP-0088	Monomer	Inactive
CP-0157	[BSH(L-CYS^7)]-CP-0088	Dimer	Inactive
CP-0146	[D-CYS^7]-CP-0088	Monomer	Inactive
CP-0158	[BSH(D-CYS^7)]-CP-0088	Dimer	Inactive
CP-0147	[L-CYS^8]-CP-0088	Monomer	Inactive
CP-0159	[BSH(L-CYS^8)]-CP-0088	Dimer	Inactive
CP-0148	[L-CYS^9]-CP-0088	Monomer	Inactive
CP-0160	[BSH(L-CYS^9)]-CP-0088	Dimer	Inactive

[a] All dimers are <u>bis</u>succinimidohexane type.   [b] pA_2 values are means ± s.e.m. of n = at least 3

Table II. Effect of monomeric and dimeric cysteine-substituted analogues of CP-0088 on bradykinin-induced contraction of rat uterus *in vitro*

Monomer	Bissuccinimidohexane dimer	pA_2[a] monomer	pA_2[a] dimer	% Recovery monomer	%Recovery dimer
CP-0088	--	7.4±0.2	--	100	--
CP-0140	CP-0152	7.1±0.4	7.9±0.1	50	50
CP-0148	CP-0153	<6	7.5±0.2	100	100
CP-0142	CP-0154	6.4±0.2	P.A.[b]	80	90
CP-0143	CP-0155	P.A.[b]	6.2±0	--	100
CP-0136	CP-0137	Inactive	Inactive	--	--
CP-0144	CP-0156	7.2±0.2	8.1±0.1	95	75
CP-0126	CP-0127	7.1±0.1	8.5±0.3	100	50
CP-0145	CP-0157	Inactive	Inactive	--	--
CP-0147	CP-0159	Inactive	Inactive	--	--
CP-0148	CP-0160	Inactive	Inactive	--	--

[a] pA2 values are means ± s.e.m. of n = at least 3   [b] P.A. = Partial Agonist

A number of points can be made from these data. First, for the majority of positions, the replacement of the reference residue with cysteine does not dramatically alter the activity of the resulting monomeric inhibitor. This is not true, however, for positions 4, 7, 8 and 9, wherein cysteine substitution completely eliminates activity. Second, except for position "0", dimers were consistently more potent than their corresponding monomer when activity remained after cysteine substitution. Maximal activity was seen with dimers formed from a monomer containing cysteine in position 3, 5, or 6 (dimers CP-0155, CP-0156, and CP-0127, respectively). Third, dimers formed from the "0" position, regardless of the chirality of the cysteine residue, are equipotent to the reference ligand, consistent with data obtained from dimers formed using the N-terminal alpha amino group (data not shown). Lastly, following a 40 minute wash-out period of all compounds which possessed antagonist activity, the dose-response curve to bradykinin was equivalent to that seen before exposure to the antagonist. This demonstrates that the effects of the antagonists in this tissue are fully reversible.

We then expanded our investigation to an assay system employing a second BK_2 receptor subtype, bradykinin-induced smooth muscle contraction in the rat uterus. Table II is a summary of the data concerning monomers and dimers formed by the introduction of L-cysteine at various positions within the ligand. Data from D-cysteine substitutions are qualitatively similar to that seen in the guinea pig ileum assay system.

As the data indicate, we again see a dramatic enhancement of activity with dimerization except for dimers formed from positions 4, 7, 8 and 9. Interestingly, dimers formed from the "0" position now show enhanced activity in this system, which is in sharp contrast to the lack of enhancement found using the guinea pig ileum assay. Finally, dimer CP-0127 (the bissuccinimidohexane dimer containing cysteine in position 6) was again found to be substantially more potent than any other dimer, including dimer CP-0156.

Another important difference between monomeric and dimeric inhibitors in rat uterine tissue is the reduced recovery seen with a number of the dimers. In particular, exposure to 10^{-5} $\underline{M}$ CP-0127 was found to reduce recovery by approximately 50%. Recovery improved another 50% (to 75% of pre-exposure responsiveness) with an additional 40-minute recovery period, and reached control levels after a third. These data suggest that reduced recovery may be a function of a sustained interaction with the receptor as opposed to a "down regulation" or inactivation of receptors in this tissue.

From these data we determined that the 6 position was optimal for enhancing the activity of these types of antagonist dimers. We recognize that dimers formed using this same type of chemistry but with cysteine residues substituted in other positions could be better suited for other bradykinin receptor types. Despite this potentially confounding variable, however, further studies concerning the effects of linker chemistry on activity utilized a monomer containing cysteine in position 6 as the "base" ligand; this compound is referred to herein as monomer CP-0126.

Effect of Alkyl Chain Length on the Inhibition of Bradykinin-Induced Uterine Smooth Muscle Contraction *In Vitro*. To assess the effects of alkyl chain length on both potency and inhibition of recovery, a series of b̲i̲s̲maleimidoalkane linkers were synthesized and then used to dimerize the cysteine-containing "base" ligand (CP-0126). The resulting compounds were then tested in the rat uterine smooth muscle assay system for inhibitory potency as well as their ability to inhibit recovery. The data from these studies are summarized in Table III.

Table III. Effect of linker length in dimeric analogues of CP-0126 on bradykinin-induced contraction of rat uterus *in vitro*

# of carbon atoms in linker	Compound #	Structure[a]	pA_2[b]	% Recovery (40 min)
n=2	CP-0162	[BSE(L-Cys⁶)]-CP-0088	8.4±0.2	90
n=3	CP-0172	[BSP(L-Cys⁶)]-CP-0088	8.6±0.2	90
n=4	CP-0209	[BSB(L-Cys⁶)]-CP-0088	8.3±0.2	50
n=6	CP-0127	[BSH(L-Cys⁶)]-CP-0088	8.5±0.3	50
n=8	CP-0211	[BSO(L-Cys⁶)]-CP-0088	8.4[c]	25
n=9	CP-0229	[BSN(L-Cys⁶)]-CP-0088	9.3±0.4	0-10
n=10	CP-0230	[BSD(L-Cys⁶)]-CP-0088	8.6±0.2	0
n=12	CP-0166	[BSDD(L-Cys⁶)]-CP-0088	8.2±0.3	0[d]

[a] BSE = b̲i̲s̲succinimidoethane, BSP = b̲i̲s̲succinimidopropane, BSB = b̲i̲s̲succinimidobutane, BSH = b̲i̲s̲succinimidohexane, BSO = b̲i̲s̲succinimidooctane, BSN = b̲i̲s̲succinimidononane, BSD = b̲i̲s̲succinimidodecane, BSDD = b̲i̲s̲succinimidododecane.
[b] pA_2 values are the means ± s.e.m. of n = at least 3
[c] n < 3
[d] Irreversible at 80 minutes

Two important points can be made from these data. First, enhanced potency can be demonstrated for the entire series of dimers, independent of the alkyl chain length. However, potency appears to decline for alkyl chains less than 6 or greater than 10 methylene groups in length. Second, inhibition of recovery appears to increase as a function of chain length, to the point where the bissuccinimidododecane dimer (CP-0166) exhibits an essentially irreversible blockade of bradykinin-induced smooth muscle contraction after exposure to 10^{-5} $\underline{M}$ inhibitor, despite an extended (120-minute) recovery or "wash-off" period. These data suggest that this sustained interaction with the tissue may be due to hydrophobic interactions of the alkyl chain with the receptor itself or with "peri-receptor" membrane components, a mechanism which has been proposed previously to explain the long acting selective $ß_2$-adrenoceptor agonist, salmeterol.[11]

DISCUSSION

The enhanced activity of these dimers may be a function of one or more of a number of different molecular mechanisms. The most obvious of these is that the dimer is interacting with two receptors simultaneously and the increase in potency and duration of action is the result of bivalent cooperativity. This explanation is unlikely as it is difficult to visualize how two macromolecular, membrane-bound receptors can be spanned by dimers formed with alkane chain linkers of such short lengths. In addition, even if receptor crosslinking were possible, it is hard to explain why there is such a difference in potency between dimers formed with alkane linkers of 9 and 12 methylene groups in length (pA_2 values of 9.3 and 8.2, respectively) with the shorter of the two being more potent.

There are other explanations for the enhanced potency observed for this series of compounds, however. As discussed above, one possibility includes the existence of secondary binding sites in the vicinity of the primary ligand binding site that can interact with various components of the linker and/or geminal ligand. Alternatively, the existence of the linker and the geminal ligand by virtue of steric and/or electrostatic interactions may impart a certain degree of "pre-organization" to the primary ligand, so as to improve binding by decreasing the entropic nature of the free peptide in solution.

Finally, exploration of the linker's contribution to the enhanced potency and duration of action is far from complete. Simple alkane chains appear to be highly desirable but the potential for further improvements in activity using more hydrophilic linkers, linkers with more constrained geometries (cis or trans double bonds, saturated or unsaturated ring systems, etc.) and linkers based on different conjugation chemistries (other than maleimido/succinimido conjugates) will also need to be incorporated into future compounds for a complete understanding of the role these elements play in the enhancement of activity to emerge. All of these possibilities are being investigating concurrently in our laboratories.

CONCLUSIONS: It appears that dimerization of peptide-based bradykinin antagonists can improve the potency of the parent ligand by as much as 100-fold, as measured in simple *in vitro* systems. Preliminary data indicate that this improvement in activity will, in fact, transfer into improved potency and duration of activity in a number of *in vivo* model systems of both bradykinin-specific and non-specific pathophysiologic conditions. These types of compounds may be useful in the treatment of a number of disease states.

REFERENCES

1. Roth, R.A.; Cassell, D.J.; Morgan, D.O.; Tatnell, M.A.; Jones, R.H.; Schüttler, A.; Brandenburg, D. Effects of Covalently Linked Insulin Dimers on Receptor Kinase Activity and Receptor Down Regulation. *FEBS Letters* **1984**, *170*, 360-364.

2. Fauchère, J.C.; Rossier, M.; Capponi, A.; Vallotton, M.B. Potentiation of the Antagonistic Effet of $ACTH_{11-24}$ on Steroidogenesis by Synthesis of Covalent Dimeric Conjugates. *FEBS Letters* **1985**, *183*, 283.

3. Chino, N.; Yoshizawa-Kumagaye, K.; Noda, Y.; Watanabe, T.X.; Kimura, T.; Sakakibara, S. Synthesis and Biological Properties of Antiparallel and Parallel Dimers of Human α-human Atrial Natriuretic Peptide. *Biochemical and Biophysical Res. Communications* **1986**, *141*, 665-672.

4. Shimohigashi, Y.; Ogasawara, T.; Koshizaki, T.; Waki, M.; Kato, T.; Izumiya, N.; Kurono, M.; Yagi, K. Interaction of Dimers of Inactive Enkephalin Fragments with μ Opiate Receptors. *Biochemical and Biophysical Res. Communications* **1987**, *146*, 1109-1115.

5. Kodama, H.; Shimohigashi, Y.; Sakagushi, K.; Waki, M.; Takono, Y.; Yamada, A.; Hatae, Y.; Kamiya, H-O. Dimerization of Neurokinin A and B COOH-terminal Heptapeptide Fragments Enhanced the Selectivity for Tachykinin Receptor Subtypes. *Eur. J. Pharmacol.* **1988**, *151*, 317-320.

6.   Sakaguchi, K.; Shimogashi, Y.; Matsumoto, H.; Komada, H.; Shimazaki, H.; Waki, M.; Takano, Y.; Higuchi, Y.; Kamiya, H-O.   Characteristic *in vitro* and *in vivo* activities of tachykinin peptide dimers. In *Peptide Chemistry*; Veki, M., ed.; Protein Research Foundation: Osaka, Japan, 1989; pp. 57-60.

7.   Higuchi, Y.; Takano, Y.; Shimazaki, H.; Shimohigashi, Y.; Kodama, H.; Matsumoto, H.; Sakaguchi, K.; Nonaka, S.; Saito, R.; Waki, M.; Kamiya, H-O. Dimeric Substance P Analogue Shows Highly Potent Activity of the *in vivo* Salivary Secretion in the Rat. *Eur. J. Pharmacol.* **1989**, *160*, 413-416.

8.   Vavrek, R.J.; Stewart, J.M.   Succinyl bis-Bradykinins: Potent Agonists with Exceptional Resistance to Enzymatic Degradation. In *Peptides: Proceedings of the Eighth American Peptide Symposium*; Hruby, V.J., Rich, D.H., Eds.; Pierce Chemical Company: Rockford, IL, 1983; pp. 381-384.

9.   Caporale, L.H.; Chorev, M.; Levy, J.J.; Goldman, M.E.; DeHaven, P.A.; Gay, C.T.; Reagan, J.E.; Rosenblatt, M.; Nutt, R.F. Characterization of Parathyroid Hormone Antagonists.   In *Peptides: Proceedings of the Tenth American Peptide Symposium*; Marshall, G.R., Ed.; Pierce Chemical Co.: Rockford, IL, 1988; pp. 449-451.

10. Regoli, D.; Rhaleb, N.E.; Dion, S.; Drapeau, G.   New Selective Bradykinin Antagonists and Bradykinin B_2 Receptor Characterization.   *Trends in Pharmacological Sciences* **1990**, *11*, 156-161.

11. Jack, D.   A Way of Looking at Agonism and Antagonism: Lessons from Salbutamol, Salmeterol and Other ß-adrenoceptor Agonists.   *Brit. J. Clin. Pharmacol.* **1991**, *31*, 501-514.

AAS 38/I
Recent Progress on Kinins
© 1992 Birkhäuser Verlag Basel

NEW AND HIGHLY POTENT BRADYKININ ANTAGONISTS

J. Knolle, G. Breipohl, S. Henke, K. Wirth and B. Schölkens
HOECHST AG, P.O.B. 80 03 20, D-6230 Frankfurt/Main 80, Germany

SUMMARY: The results obtained underline the unique properties of **HOE 140** and suggest its use in the therapy of allregic conditions, asthma and athritis (ref. 1).

INTRODUCTION

The nonapeptide bradykinin (BK) (Arg-Pro-Pro-Gly-Phe-Ser-Pro-Phe-Arg) is one of the main mediators which are released when the body responds to traumata and injury. It is produced from its precursor kininogens by the action of proteases termed kallikreins. Similar to other kinins bradykinin influences vascular tone and permeability, decreases blood pressure and initiates or enhances the release of mediators from leukocytes. BK is involved in pain, inflammation and certain allergic reactions (e.g. rhinitis, asthma etc.).

Specific and potent bradykinin antagonists therefore are considered to be a new therapeutic principle for the treatment of such diseases where pathologically elevated bradykinin levels are involved.

The fundamental work of Stewart and Vavrek (ref. 2) after almost 25 years led to the discovery that replacement of Pro^7 by $D\text{-}Phe^7$ yields antagonists of BK. The bradykinin antagonists emerging from their synthetic efforts e.g. $D\text{-}Arg[Hyp^2, Thi^{5,8}, D\text{-}Phe^7]$ BK have been used widely as pharmacological tools to evaluate the role of BK in many biological processes (ref. 3).

The compounds, however, are like BK susceptable to rapid degradation and only active in a micromolar range.

For use in therapy therefore compounds with enhanced metabolic stability and significantly increased biological activity are desirable.

RESULTS

Biological activity of BK-antagonists was measured by the effect on isolated guinea pig pulmonary arteries contracted with BK and are represented at IC_{50}-values in table 1. The structure of unnatural amino acids used is given in figure 1.

TABLE 1. Structure activity studies of BK-antagonists measured by the effect on isolated guinea pig pulmonary arteries contracted with BK (IC_{50}) and receptor binding assay on guinea pig ileum with radiolabelled BK (K_i)

PEPTIDE SEQUENCE	IC_{50} [nM]	K_i [nM]
H-D-Arg-Arg-Hyp-Pro-Gly-Thi-Ser-D-Phe-Thi-Arg-OH	6400	67.2
(Stewart et al.)		
H-D-Arg-Arg-Hyp-Pro-Gly-Thi-Ser-D-**Tic**-Thi-Arg-OH	2100	6.4
H-D-Arg-Arg-Hyp-Pro-Gly-Thi-Ser-D-**Tic**-**Pro**-Arg-OH	190	2.6
H-D-Arg-Arg-**Pro**-**Hyp**-Gly-Thi-Ser-D-**Tic**-**Tic**-Arg-OH	95	4.5
H-D-Arg-Arg-Hyp-Pro-Gly-Thi-Ser-D-**Tic**-**Aoc**-Arg-OH	56	0.3
H-D-Arg-Arg-**Pro**-**Hyp**-Gly-Thi-Ser-D-**Tic**-**Aoc**-Arg-OH	11	1.0
H-D-Arg-Arg-**Pro**-**Hyp**-Gly-Thi-Ser-D-**Tic**-**Oic**-Arg-OH	5.4	0.3

| Thi | D-Tic | Aoc | Oic |

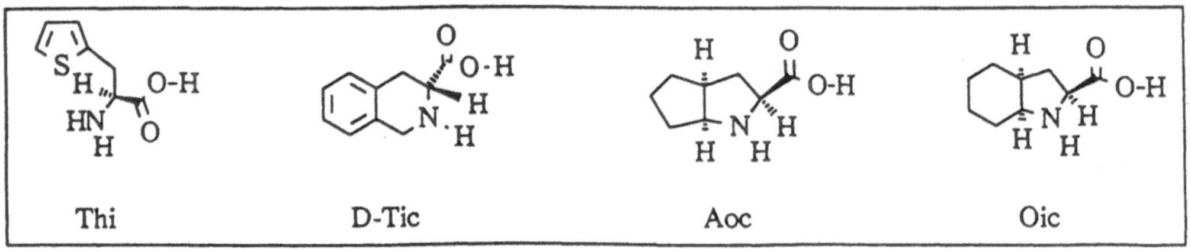

Fig. 1.   Structures of unnatural amino acids

Structure activity relationship of the peptides are discussed in the following. In an attempt to increase potency as well as metabolic stability of BK-antagonists we modified several positions in the peptide sequence by introduction of unnatural amino acids. First we replaced D-Phe[7] by the imino acid D-Tic. This exchange resulted in a slight increase in potency of over the reference substance. When we replaced the aromatic amino acid in position 8 by proline, we observed in addition an approximately 10-fold enhanced biological activity. Further we introduced in addition the imino acid L-Tic in position 8. But this replacement did not result in a very pronounced effect. However, when we used the more lipophilic bicyclic Aoc, we observed a significant increase in antagonistic potency. This effect was additionally enhanced by interchanging Hyp[2] and Pro[3], resulting in an IC_{50}-value of 11 nM.

When we used the even more lipophilic Oic in position 8, we again obtained a further increase in antagonistic potency. This antagonist has an IC_{50}-value of 5.4 nM. The activity of this compound has reached the order of magnitude like bradykinin itself. Replacement of Aoc or Oic by their D-enantiomer resulted in a significant diminution of activity indicating a highly stereo-specific structural requirement in this position. A potency in the nanomolar range like bradykinin itself was obtained by incorporation of unnatural amino acids in the peptides. In table 1 receptor binding data for some antagonists are summarized, which underline the high potency of the compounds. The structure activity studies discussed above demonstrate that we achieved a very pronounced enhancement of antagonistic activity with our new bradykinin antagonists. D Arg[0] [Hyp[3], Thi[5], D-Tic[7], Oic[8]] BK with the code name **HOE 140** was chosen for a more intensive investigation and further development. All data of this peptide obtained so far confirm the high potency of this compounds.

BIOLOGICAL RESULTS

In addition to the results in the guinea pig pulmonary artery assay listed in table 1, the potency of **HOE 140** has been confirmed in other in vitro assays (ref. 4,7).

IN VITRO

HOE 140 inhibits the BK-induced effects in a variety of organs (figure 2). **HOE 140** is a selective B_2 receptor antagonist, demonstrated by its inactivity in the rabbit aorta, a tissue only expressing B_1 receptors.

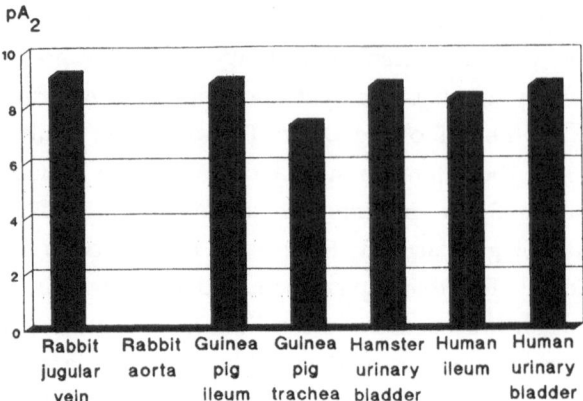

Fig.2 . Activities of HOE 140 in isolated organs

HOE 140 and its parent compounds are the **first bradykinin antagonists**, which inhibit the BK-induced effects at the guinea pig trachea (ref. 8-11). The metabolic stability of **HOE 140** in vitro was demonstrated by its stability for at least 72 hrs in synovial fluids (ref. 12). HOE 140 antagonizes the BK-induced EDRF release.

IN VIVO

In vivo experiments demonstrate that 100 pmol/kg of **HOE 140** applied as an aerosol leads to a marked and long lasting inhibition of a BK-induced bronchoconstriction (figure 3).

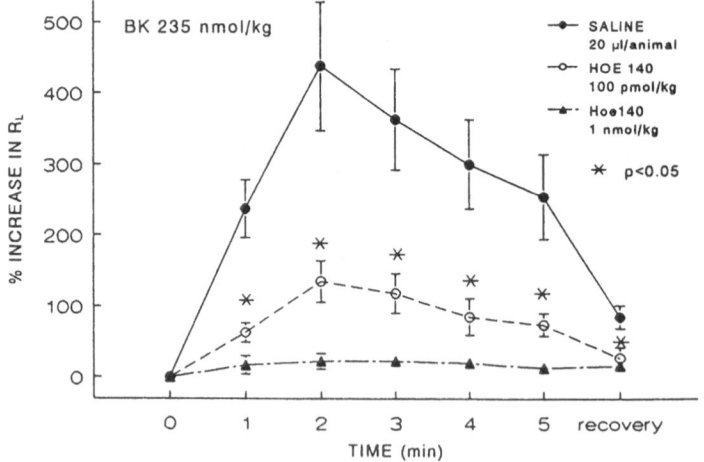

Fig. 3. Bradykinin induced bronchoconstriction in guinea pigs
         HOE 140 aerosol against Bradykinin Aerosol

Recently BK is recognized as the crucial mediator for the inflammation observed in asthmatics (ref. 13).

The antiinflammatory effect was demonstrated in the model of carrageenan induced pedal inflammation in the rat. Here a 83 % reduction in paw swelling after 2 hrs. was observed at a dose of 0,1 mg/kg.

HOE 140 exhibits also under in vitro conditions a remarkable metabolic stability.

CLINIC

HOE 140 is currently evaluated in clinical trials.

REFERENCES

1. D. Proud, C.R. Baumgarten, R.M. Naclerio, P.E. Ward, J. Immun. 138, *Kinin Metabolism in Human Nasal Secretions During Experimentally Induced Allergic Rhinitis,* 428 - 434 (1987).

2.a) R.J. Vavrek and J.M. Stewart, Peptides 6, *Competitive antagonists of bradykinin,* 161 - 164 (1985).

2.b) J.M. Stewart and R.J. Vavrek, Adv. Biosci. 65, *Bradykinin competitive antagonists: design and activities,* 73 - 80 (1987).

3. R.M. Burch, S. Farmer and L.R. Steranka, Medicinal Research Reviews 10, 237 - 269 (1990).

4. S. Henke, H. Anagnostopoulos, G. Breipohl, H. Gerhards, J. Knolle, B.A. Schölkens, F. Lembeck, Pure Appl. Chem., *Novel highly potent bradykinin antagonists and their impact on allergic diseases* (in press).

5. F.J. Hock, K. Wirth, U. Albus, W. Linz, H.J. Gerhards, G. Wiemer, S.Henke, G. Breipohl, W. König, J. Knolle and B.A. Schölkens, Brit. J. Pharmacol., *HOE 140 a new potent and long acting bradykinin-antagonist: in vitro studies,* 102, 769 - 773 (1991).

6. K. Wirth, F.J.Hock, U. Albus, W. Linz, H.G. Alpermann, H. Anagnostopoulos, S.Henke, G. Breipohl, W. König, J. Knolle and B.A. Schölkens, Brit. J. Pharmacol., *HOE 140 a new potent and long acting bradykinin-antagonist: in vivo studies,* 102, 774 - 777 (1991).

7. F. Lembeck, T. Griesbacher, S. Henke, G. Breipohl, and J. Knolle, Brit. J. Pharmacol., *New, long-acting, potent bradykinin antagonists,* 102, 297 - 304 (1991).

8. D. Proud (personal communication).

9. D. Regoli (personal communication).

10. M.N. Perkins, G.M Burgess, E.A. Campbell, A. Hallett, R.J. Murphy, S. Naeem, I.A. Patel, A. Rueff, and A. Dray (poster presented at the Winter Meeting of the British Pharmacological Society, December 1990).

11. S.G. Farmer (data presented at the meeting on "Advances in Inflammation Research", London 1990).

12. D. Bhoola, Kinin 91 (München).

13. S.G. Farmer in Bradykinin Antagonists, Marcel Dekker Inc., New York, 213 - 236 (1991).

AAS 38/I
Recent Progress on Kinins
© 1992 Birkhäuser Verlag Basel

PSEUDOPEPTIDE ANALOGS OF BRADYKININ AND BRADYKININ ANTAGONISTS

Raymond J. Vavrek, Lajos Gera and John M. Stewart

Department of Biochemistry, University of Colorado School of Medicine
4200 East 9th Avenue, Denver, CO 80262 USA

SUMMARY: Over 100 reduced-bond analogs of bradykinin and bradykinin antagonists were designed, synthesized, and assayed in the classic smooth muscle and blood pressure assays in a further study of the structure-activity relationships of bradykinin. Both potent BK-like agonists and antagonists of BK activity were found among the reduced-bond analogs.

INTRODUCTION

The search for modifications of the bradykinin sequence (BK: Arg-Pro-Pro-Gly-Phe-Ser-Pro-Phe-Arg) which can shed additional light on the physiological and pharmacological roles of the kallikrein-kinin system continues with renewed vigor in many laboratories. Much of the recent emphasis has been on developing more potent, more selective and metabolically stable analogs of [DPhe[7]]-BK, the prototype of peptide BK antagonists (1,2,3). We have synthesized a group of BK analogs containing one type of pseudopeptide bond modification, the reduced peptide bond, at various positions in BK and BK antagonist sequences. In this modification the carbonyl group of a peptide bond (-CO-NH-) is reduced to a methylene group (-CH$_2$-NH-). We report here the results of that study.

METHODS

The various reduced bond analogs were prepared by methods reported recently (4). Except for the peptide analogs containing a reduced bond at the C-terminal position (i.e., Phe[CH$_2$NH]Arg) [abbreviated Phe(R)Arg], which were made by modified Sasaki-Coy methods (5), Boc-reduced dipeptides were synthesized and introduced into the growing peptide during solid phase synthesis, using the BOP/HOBt coupling method. Otherwise, standard methods for solid phase synthesis and purification of the analogs were used, and have been described (1). Bioassays were performed on isolated rat uterus (RUT), guinea pig ileum (GPI) and rat blood pressure (RBP) as previously described (1).

RESULTS AND DISCUSSION

Table 1 lists the structures and biological actions of the reduced-bond analogs of BK. Reduction of the Pro-Pro (003-004), Gly-Phe (005-008), or Phe-Ser (009-016) bonds of BK antagonists generally destroys biological activity. A reduced peptide bond at Ser-Pro in BK agonist sequences (023-026) yields potent agonists (7) that evidently act through a BK receptor-mediated mechanism, since the agonist activity is blocked by the standard BK antagonist NPC-567 (002).

Reduction of the Ser-DPhe bond of the antagonist NPC567 converts it to an agonist in the uterus assay (034), and protects the analog from inactivation by angiotensin converting enzyme (ACE) in the pulmonary circulation. This modification eliminates activity on the ileum.

A reduced bond at Pro-Phe (035-038) in BK agonists reduces BK-like activity in all our assays. We do not confirm a report (8) that long-acting BK agonists in the blood pressure assay are produced by this modification.

Analogs with a reduced peptide bond between positions 7 and 8 of BK antagonist sequences containing the normal phenylalanine at position eight do not retain antagonist activity (042-050). We have previously found that the most potent antagonists with a DPhe residue at position 7 possess an aliphatic residue in sequence position 8 (see compounds 051, 060 and 065) instead of the usual phenylalanine. This pattern of biological activity is maintained in the DPhe(R)aliphatic (7-8) analogs (051-069 and 080-087), with the analogs having Ile, Leu and Pro at position 8 showing the best spectrum of antagonist actions. It is interesting that N-ethylisoleucine at position 8 (075-078) is not an acceptable substitute for proline.

Drapeau et al. (9) reported that certain BK analogs with a reduced peptide bond between Phe and Arg (positions 8 and 9) are stable to both ACE and the carboxypeptidase kininase-II. We found a general loss of potency in BK agonists (096-099) and complete loss of activity in antagonist sequences (100-105) upon reduction of the Phe-Arg bond. Remarkably, this reduced (8-9) modification did not reliably confer total resistance to pulmonary destruction in the rat upon analogs having agonist activity. Our blood pressure assay technique does not allow estimation of pulmonary destruction of antagonists.

Multiple reduced peptide bonds in the C-terminal portion of the BK sequence (106-120) have little positive effect on agonist or antagonist activity, except some Ser(R)Pro(6,7)-Phe(R)Arg(8,9) agonist analogs in which ileum activity is destroyed while both uterus and blood pressure activity are retained. One analog (119) has remarkably high potency on the uterus and is fully resistant to pulmonary degradation. In this analog, reduction of the (6-7) bond of peptide 098 has produced a dramatic change in potency and pattern of biological activities.

TABLE 1 - Bradykinin Analogs Containing Reduced Dipeptide Bonds[a]

Analog Number	Peptide Structure 0 1 2 3 4 5 6 7 8 9		Biological Activities RUT	GPI	IA	%D
001 BK	Arg - Pro - Pro - Gly - Phe - Ser - Pro - Phe - Arg		100%	100%	100%	99%
002-N567	DArg-Arg - Pro - Hyp - Gly - Phe - Ser -DPhe - Phe - Arg [b]		6.5*	5.9*	I	-
003-8446	Arg - Pro(R)Pro - Gly - Phe - Ser -DPhe - Phe - Arg		AG	5.5*	AG	0
004-8448	DArg-Arg - Pro(R)Pro - Gly - Phe - Ser -DPhe - Phe - Arg		AG	5.9*	AG	-
005-7058	Arg - Pro - Pro - Gly(R)Phe - Ser -DPhe - Phe - Arg		0	0	0.1%	20%
006-7060	DArg-Arg - Pro - Pro - Gly(R)Phe - Ser -DPhe - Phe - Arg		0	0	0.2%	44%
007-7062	Arg - Pro - Hyp - Gly(R)Phe - Ser -DPhe - Phe - Arg		0	0.7%	0	-
008-7064	DArg-Arg - Pro - Hyp - Gly(R)Phe - Ser -DPhe - Phe - Arg		I(P)	I(P)	I	-
009-6168	Arg - Pro - Pro - Gly - Phe(R)Ser -DPhe - Thi - Arg		0.3%	I(P)	0	-
010-6170	DArg-Arg - Pro - Pro - Gly - Phe(R)Ser -DPhe - Thi - Arg		0.1%	5.2*	I	-
011-6172	Lys-Arg - Pro - Pro - Gly - Phe(R)Ser -DPhe - Thi - Arg		0.1%	0	0	-
012-6174	K-K-Arg - Pro - Pro - Gly - Phe(R)Ser -DPhe - Thi - Arg		0.2%	0	-	-
013-6176	Arg - Pro - Hyp - Gly - Phe(R)Ser -DPhe - Thi - Arg		0.3%	0	I(P)	-
014-6178	DArg-Arg - Pro - Hyp - Gly - Phe(R)Ser -DPhe - Thi - Arg		0.3%	0	0.1%	44%
015-6180	DArg-Arg - Pro - Hyp - Gly - Phe(R)Ser -DPhe - Thi - Arg		0.5%	0	0	-
016-6182	K-K-Arg - Pro - Hyp - Gly - Phe(R)Ser -DPhe - Thi - Arg		0.4%	0	0.1%	50%
017-6052	Ac - Ser(R)Pro - Thi - Arg		0.1%	I(P)	0.2%	80%
018-6054	Ppa - Ser(R)Pro - Thi - Arg		0	0	0	-
019-6056	Ac - Thi - Ser(R)Pro - Thi - Arg		0	0	0	-
020-6058	Ppa - Thi - Ser(R)Pro - Thi - Arg		0	0	0.1%	81%
021-6060	Ac - Gly - Thi - Ser(R)Pro - Thi - Arg		0	I(P)	0	-
022-6062	Ppa - Gly - Thi - Ser(R)Pro - Thi - Arg		0	0	AG	94%
023-6014	Arg - Pro - Hyp - Gly - Thi - Ser(R)Pro - Thi - Arg [c]		140%	80%	180%	0
024-6016	DArg-Arg - Pro - Hyp - Gly - Thi - Ser(R)Pro - Thi - Arg [c]		175%	10%	140%	0
025-6018	Lys-Arg - Pro - Hyp - Gly - Thi - Ser(R)Pro - Thi - Arg [c]		225%	36%	450%	0
026-6020	K-K-Arg - Pro - Hyp - Gly - Thi - Ser(R)Pro - Thi - Arg [c]		160%	5%	480%	15%
027-8426	Arg - Pro - Pro - Gly - Phe - Ser - Leu(R)Leu - Arg		0	0	AG	8%
028-8428	DArg-Arg - Pro - Pro - Gly - Phe - Ser - Leu(R)Leu - Arg		AG	0	0	-
029-8430	Arg - Pro - Hyp - Gly - Phe - Ser - Leu(R)Leu - Arg		AG	0	0	-
030-8432	DArg-Arg - Pro - Hyp - Gly - Phe - Ser - Leu(R)Leu - Arg		AG	0	0	-
031-5876	Ppa -Ser(R)DPhe - Phe - Arg		0	0	0	-
032-5882	Ppa - Thi -Ser(R)DPhe - Phe - Arg		0	0	0	-
033-5880	Ppa -DAla - Phe -Ser(R)DPhe - Phe - Arg		0	0	0	-
034-5884	DArg-Arg - Pro - Hyp - Gly - Phe -Ser(R)DPhe - Phe - Arg [d]		13%	0	2%	0
035-6196	Arg - Pro - Pro - Gly - Phe - Ser - Pro(R)Phe - Arg [e]		31%	18%	0	-
036-6198	DArg-Arg - Pro - Pro - Gly - Phe - Ser - Pro(R)Phe - Arg		5%	7%	1%	-
037-6200	Arg - Pro - Hyp - Gly - Phe - Ser - Pro(R)Phe - Arg		13%	2%	0	-
038-6202	DArg-Arg - Pro - Hyp - Gly - Phe - Ser - Pro(R)Phe - Arg		4%	0.3%	0.1%	0

Analog Number	Peptide Structure										Biological Activities			
	0	1	2	3	4	5	6	7	8	9	RUT	GPI	IA	%D
039-5866					Ppa -	Ser -	DPhe(R)Phe -	Arg			0	0	0.1%	75%
040-5868				Paa -	Thi -	Ser -	DPhe(R)Phe -	Arg			0	0	0	-
041-5870			Paa -	DAla -	Thi -	Ser -	DPhe(R)Phe -	Arg			0	5.4*	0	-
042-5872	DArg-Arg -	Pro -	Hyp -	Gly -	Phe -	Ser -	DPhe(R)Phe -	Arg			0.1%	5.9*	I	-
043-6618	Arg -	Pro -	Pro -	Gly -	Phe -	Ser -	DPhe(R)Phe -	Phe			0	I(P)	2%	87%
044-6620	DArg-Arg -	Pro -	Pro -	Gly -	Phe -	Ser -	DPhe(R)Phe -	Phe			0	5.5*	0	-
045-6622		Pro -	Hyp -	Gly -	Phe -	Ser -	DPhe(R)Phe -	Phe			0	0	0.4%	70%
046-6624	DArg -	Pro -	Hyp -	Gly -	Phe -	Ser -	DPhe(R)Phe -	Phe			0	0	0	-
047-6226	Arg -	Pro -	Hyp -	Gly -	Thi -	Ser -	DPhe(R)Phe -	Phe			0	I(P)	1%	92%
048-6228	DArg-Arg -	Pro -	Hyp -	Gly -	Thi -	Ser -	DPhe(R)Phe -	Phe			0	5.3*	1%	92%
049-6230	DArg -	Pro -	Hyp -	Gly -	Thi -	Ser -	DPhe(R)Phe -	Phe			0	0	0	-
050-6232	DArg-Arg -	Pro -	Hyp -	Gly -	Thi -	Ser -	DPhe(R)Phe -	Phe			I(P)	0	0	-
051-7188	DArg-Arg -	Pro -	Hyp -	Gly -	Thi -	Ser -	DPhe -	Aib -	Arg		7.0*	5.8*	I	-
052-7340	Arg -	Pro -	Pro -	Gly -	Phe -	Ser -	DPhe(R)Aib -	Arg			0	0	0	-
053-7342	DArg-Arg -	Pro -	Pro -	Gly -	Phe -	Ser -	DPhe(R)Aib -	Arg			5.0*	0	0	-
054-7344	Arg -	Pro -	Hyp -	Gly -	Phe -	Ser -	DPhe(R)Aib -	Arg			0	0	I	-
055-7346	DArg-Arg -	Pro -	Hyp -	Gly -	Phe -	Ser -	DPhe(R)Aib -	Arg [d]			0	0	I	-
056-7378	Arg -	Pro -	Pro -	Gly -	Thi -	Ser -	DPhe(R)Aib -	Arg			0	0	0	-
057-7380	DArg-Arg -	Pro -	Pro -	Gly -	Thi -	Ser -	DPhe(R)Aib -	Arg			I(P)	I(P)	0	-
058-7382	Arg -	Pro -	Hyp -	Gly -	Thi -	Ser -	DPhe(R)Aib -	Arg			0	0	0	-
059-7384	DArg-Arg -	Pro -	Hyp -	Gly -	Thi -	Ser -	DPhe(R)Aib -	Arg			0	0	I	-
060-7850	DArg-Arg -	Pro -	Hyp -	Gly -	Thi -	Ser -	DPhe -	Leu -	Arg		7.0*	6.4*	I	-
061-8220	Arg -	Pro -	Hyp -	Gly -	Phe -	Ser -	DPhe(R)Leu -	Arg			0.03%	5.3*	I	-
062-8222	DArg-Arg -	Pro -	Hyp -	Gly -	Phe -	Ser -	DPhe(R)Leu -	Arg [d]			6.1*	6.1*	I	-
063-8224	Arg -	Pro -	Hyp -	Gly -	Thi -	Ser -	DPhe(R)Leu -	Arg			0.01%	5.4*	0	-
064-8226	DArg-Arg -	Pro -	Hyp -	Gly -	Thi -	Ser -	DPhe(R)Leu -	Arg			6.4*	6.3*	I	-
065-7418	DArg-Arg -	Pro -	Hyp -	Gly -	Phe -	Ser -	DPhe -	Ile -	Arg		7.7*	6.8*	I	-
066-7772	Arg -	Pro -	Hyp -	Gly -	Phe -	Ser -	DPhe(R)Ile -	Arg			6.9*	6.5*	0	-
067-7774	DArg-Arg -	Pro -	Hyp -	Gly -	Phe -	Ser -	DPhe(R)Ile -	Arg [d]			7.0*	7.0*	I	-
068-7776	Arg -	Pro -	Hyp -	Gly -	Thi -	Ser -	DPhe(R)Ile -	Arg			6.9*	7.0*	0	-
069-7778	DArg-Arg -	Pro -	Hyp -	Gly -	Thi -	Ser -	DPhe(R)Ile -	Arg			7.3*	7.0*	I	-
070-7198	DArg-Arg -	Pro -	Hyp -	Gly -	Thi -	Ser -	DPhe -	NMF -	Arg		6.0*	5.5*	0	-
071-6430	Arg -	Pro -	Pro -	Gly -	Phe -	Ser -	DPhe(R)NMF -	Arg			0.2%	I(P)	0.2%	73%
072-6432	DArg-Arg -	Pro -	Pro -	Gly -	Phe -	Ser -	DPhe(R)NMF -	Arg			0.2%	5.2*	0	-
073-6436	Arg -	Pro -	Hyp -	Gly -	Phe -	Ser -	DPhe(R)NMF -	Arg			0.3%	I(P)	0.1%	93%
074-6438	DArg-Arg -	Pro -	Hyp -	Gly -	Phe -	Ser -	DPhe(R)NMF -	Arg			0.2%	5.6	0	-
075-7930	Arg -	Pro -	Hyp -	Gly -	Phe -	Ser -	DPhe(R)NEI -	Arg			0.02%	0	0.2%	57%
076-7932	DArg-Arg -	Pro -	Hyp -	Gly -	Phe -	Ser -	DPhe(R)NEI -	Arg			0.01%	I(P)	0	-
077-7934	Arg -	Pro -	Hyp -	Gly -	Thi -	Ser -	DPhe(R)NEI -	Arg			0	0	0	-
078-7936	Arg -	Pro -	Hyp -	Gly -	Thi -	Ser -	DPhe(R)NEI -	Arg			I(P)	I(P)	I	-

Analog Number	Peptide Structure 0-9	RUT	GPI	IA	%D
079-4436	DArg-Arg - Pro - Hyp - Gly - Phe - Ser -DPhe- Pro - Arg [f]	6.3*	6.0*	I	-
080-6664	Arg - Pro - Pro - Gly - Phe - Ser -DPhe(R)Pro - Arg	0	5.9*	0.1%	76%
081-6666	DArg-Arg - Pro - Pro - Gly - Phe - Ser -DPhe(R)Pro - Arg	5.4*	6.4*	0.1%	80%
082-6668	Arg - Pro - Hyp - Gly - Phe - Ser -DPhe(R)Pro - Arg	6.0*	5.5*	I	-
083-6670	DArg-Arg - Pro - Hyp - Gly - Phe - Ser -DPhe(R)Pro - Arg [d]	5.8*	6.0*	0.1%	0
084-6674	Arg - Pro - Pro - Gly - Thi - Ser -DPhe(R)Pro - Arg	5.9*	6.1*	0.1%	34%
085-6676	DArg-Arg - Pro - Pro - Gly - Thi - Ser -DPhe(R)Pro - Arg	6.1*	6.4*	0	-
086-6678	Arg - Pro - Hyp - Gly - Thi - Ser -DPhe(R)Pro - Arg	5.9*	5.6*	I	-
087-6680	DArg-Arg - Pro - Hyp - Gly - Thi - Ser -DPhe(R)Pro - Arg	6.1*	6.3*	I	-
088-6876	Arg - Pro - Pro - Gly - Phe - Ser -DPhe(R)Pro-NH$_2$	0	I(P)	0	-
089-6878	DArg-Arg - Pro - Pro - Gly - Phe - Ser -DPhe(R)Pro-NH$_2$	0	I(P)	0	-
090-6880	Arg - Pro - Hyp - Gly - Phe - Ser -DPhe(R)Pro-NH$_2$	0	0	0	-
091-6882	DArg-Arg - Pro - Hyp - Gly - Phe - Ser -DPhe(R)Pro-NH$_2$	I(P)	0	0	-
092-7098	Arg - Pro - Pro - Gly - Thi - Ser -DPhe(R)Pro-NH$_2$	0	I(P)	0	-
093-7100	DArg-Arg - Pro - Pro - Gly - Thi - Ser -DPhe(R)Pro-NH$_2$	I(P)	I(P)	I	-
094-7102	Arg - Pro - Hyp - Gly - Thi - Ser -DPhe(R)Pro-NH$_2$	0	I(P)	0	-
095-7104	DArg-Arg - Pro - Hyp - Gly - Thi - Ser -DPhe(R)Pro-NH$_2$	0	0	0	-
096-7642	Arg - Pro - Hyp - Gly - Phe - Ser - Pro - Phe(R)Arg	0.4%	6%	23%	0
097-7644	DArg-Arg - Pro - Hyp - Gly - Phe - Ser - Pro - Phe(R)Arg	54%	1%	55%	0
098-7646	Arg - Pro - Hyp - Gly - Thi - Ser - Pro - Phe(R)Arg	41%	2%	86%	45%
099-7648	DArg-Arg - Pro - Hyp - Gly - Thi - Ser - Pro - Phe(R)Arg	55%	0.2%	174%	0
100-S438	Arg - Pro - Pro - Gly - Phe - Ser -DPhe - Phe(R)Arg	0.07%	0	0.1%	0
101-S442	DArg-Arg - Pro - Pro - Gly - Phe - Ser -DPhe - Phe(R)Arg	I(P)	0	0	-
102-7632	Arg - Pro - Hyp - Gly - Phe - Ser -DPhe - Phe(R)Arg	0.03%	0	0	-
103-7634	DArg-Arg - Pro - Hyp - Gly - Phe - Ser -DPhe - Phe(R)Arg [e]	0.01%	I(P)	2%	97%
104-7636	Arg - Pro - Hyp - Gly - Thi - Ser -DPhe - Phe(R)Arg	0.1%	0	2%	98%
105-7638	DArg-Arg - Pro - Hyp - Gly - Thi - Ser -DPhe - Phe(R)Arg	0.01%	I(P)	0.1%	37%
106-7110	DArg-Arg - Pro - Pro - Gly(R)Phe - Ser - DPhe(R)Pro - Arg	0	0	0.1%	26%
107-7112	Arg - Pro - Hyp - Gly(R)Phe - Ser - DPhe(R)Pro - Arg	0.1%	0	0	-
108-7114	DArg-Arg - Pro - Hyp - Gly(R)Phe - Ser - DPhe(R)Pro - Arg	0	0	0.3%	74%
109-6186	Arg - Pro - Pro - Gly - Phe(R)Ser - Pro(R)Phe - Arg	0.1%	0.4%	0.1%	0
110-6188	DArg-Arg - Pro - Pro - Gly - Phe(R)Ser - Pro(R)Phe - Arg	0.3%	0	0	-
111-6190	Arg - Pro - Hyp - Gly - Phe(R)Ser - Pro(R)Phe - Arg	0.4%	I(P)	0	-
112-6192	DArg-Arg - Pro - Hyp - Gly - Phe(R)Ser - Pro(R)Phe - Arg	0.3%	I(P)	0	-
113-6442	Arg - Pro - Pro - Gly - Phe(R)Ser -DPhe(R)NMF - Arg	8%	0	0	-
114-6444	DArg-Arg - Pro - Pro - Gly - Phe(R)Ser -DPhe(R)NMF - Arg	5%	0	0.4%	65%
115-6446	Arg - Pro - Hyp - Gly - Phe(R)Ser -DPhe(R)NMF - Arg	8%	0	0.3%	70%
116-6448	DArg-Arg - Pro - Hyp - Gly - Phe(R)Ser -DPhe(R)NMF - Arg	12%	0	AG	-
117-7742	Arg - Pro - Hyp - Gly - Phe - Ser(R)Pro - Phe(R)Arg	34%	0.1%	24%	71%
118-7744	DArg-Arg - Pro - Hyp - Gly - Phe - Ser(R)Pro - Phe(R)Arg	32%	0.1%	16%	0
119-7746	Arg - Pro - Hyp - Gly - Thi - Ser(R)Pro - Phe(R)Arg	245%	0.4%	5%	0
120-7748	DArg-Arg - Pro - Hyp - Gly - Thi - Ser(R)Pro - Phe(R)Arg	43%	0.1%	19%	48%

Footnotes to Table 1 are on the next page.

Footnotes to Table 1

[a] Numbering of analogs in Table 1 is sequential (001-120) for this list, followed by the four digit "B"-number used in this laboratory. Standard assays on rat uterus (**RUT**), guinea pig ileum (**GPI**), and rat blood pressure following intraaortic bolus administration (**IA**) were used (1). **%D** is the percent destruction of the analog on initial passage through the pulmonary circulation. **Agonist** activity is given as per cent (%) of BK activity. Unquantitated weak BK-like agonist activity is given as **AG**. **Antagonist** activity is given as the pA_2 value determined on 4 - 10 tissues and is followed by an asterisk (*). I indicates unquantitated antagonist activity. **I(P)** indicates weak partial antagonist action. **Abbreviations:** (R) = [CH$_2$NH], except in X-Pro analogs, which lack a proton. Ac- (acetyl-); Aib (alpha aminoisobutyryl); Hyp (trans-4-hydroxyprolyl); K-K-(Lys-Lys-); NEI (N-ethyl isoleucyl); NMF (N-methyl-phenylalanyl);Paa (phenylacetyl-); Ppa (phenylpropionyl-); Thi (beta-2-thienylalanyl). Other footnotes are to literature references: [b] Ref. 6; [c] Ref. 7; [d] Ref. 4; [e] Ref. 8; and [f] Ref. 2.

Changing the -CO-NH- moiety of a peptide - the peptide bond - to -CH$_2$-NH- causes major alteration in both the conformation and basicity of the resulting peptide. The normal peptide moiety is planar and rigid, with the large substituents in the *trans* orientation. In contrast, the carbon in the -CH$_2$-NH- group is tetrahedral, allowing greatly increased flexibility in the peptide backbone. Moreover, the normal peptide moiety is neutral, while the amino group in the reduced peptide is basic, and can be expected to exist as a salt at physiological pH, introducing a positive charge into the peptide. Both these alterations can be expected to alter the way a peptide may interact with receptors for the parent hormone. The goal of studies with pseudopeptides is to explore the peptide-receptor interaction to see if it is possible to make an analog having a conformationally much more favorable interaction with receptors. At the same time, since reduced peptide bonds are not cleaved by the usual peptidases, very potent and long-acting agonists or antagonists could be achieved. This type of modification offers great potential for drug development, and could even lead to orally active peptide drugs.

ACKNOWLEDGEMENTS

This work was supported by grant #HL-26284 from the US-NIH, and by Nova Pharmaceutical Corporation. Amino acid analyses were performed by Robert Binard. The authors thank Robin Reed, Frances Shepperdson and Steven Durrance for technical assistance.

REFERENCES

1. Vavrek RJ, Stewart JM. Competitive antagonists of bradykinin. Peptides 1985: 6: 161-5.

2. Vavrek RJ, Stewart JM. Development of bradykinin antagonists: Structure-activity relationships for new categories of antagonist sequences. In: Kinins V. Abe K, Moriya H, Fujii S, editors. New York: Plenum. 1989: 395-400 (Adv. Exp. Med. Biol. 1989: 247B).

3. Stewart JM, Vavrek RJ. Chemistry of peptide B2 bradykinin antagonists. In: Bradykinin Antagonists: Basic and Clinical Aspects. Burch RM, editor. New York: Marcel Dekker. 1991: 51-96.

4. Gera L, Vavrek RJ, Stewart JM. Facile synthesis of reduced dipeptides for bradykinin analogs. In:Peptides, Proceedings of the 12th American Peptide Symposium. Smith J, editor. Leiden: ESCOM, 1992 (in press).

5. Sasaki Y, Coy DH. Solid phase synthesis of peptides containing the CH_2NH peptide bond isostere. Peptides 1987: 8: 119-21.

6. Stewart JM, Vavrek RJ. Bradykinin competitive antagonists for classical kinin systems. In: Kinins IV. Greenbaum LM, Margolius HS, editors. New York: Plenum. 1986: 537-42 (Adv. Exp. Med. Biol. 198A).

7. Vavrek RJ, Gera L, Stewart JM. Bradykinin analogs with reduced peptide bonds at the Ser-Pro position: potent agonist analogs. In: Peptides 1990, Proceedings of the 21st European Peptide Symposium. Giralt E, Andreau D, editors. Leiden: ESCOM. 1991: 642-3.

8. Tourwe D, De Cock E, Van Marsenille M, Van Der Auwere L, Van Binst G, Viville R, Degelen J, Scarso A. Synthesis and biological activity of bradykinin analogues with reduced and ethylenic isosteric peptide bond replacements. In: Peptides 1988, Proceedings of the 20th European Peptide Symposium. Jung G, Bayer E, editors. Leiden: ESCOM. 1989: 562-4.

9. Drapeau G, Rhaleb N-E, Dion S, Jukic D, Regoli D. [Phe[8](CH_2NH)Arg[9]]bradykinin, a B_2 receptor selective agonist which is not broken down by either kininase I or kininase II. Eur. J. Pharmacol. 1988: 155: 193-5.

AAS 38/I
Recent Progress on Kinins
© 1992 Birkhäuser Verlag Basel

BRADYKININ ANTAGONISTS DO NOT REQUIRE A D-AROMATIC AMINO ACID RESIDUE AT POSITION 7

Raymond J. Vavrek, Lajos Gera and John M. Stewart

Department of Biochemistry, University of Colorado School of Medicine
4200 East 9th Avenue, Denver, Colorado 80262, USA

SUMMARY: More than 200 new analogs of bradykinin have been synthesized and assayed. Analogs containing a D-aliphatic amino acid residue at position 7 and an L-aliphatic residue at position 8 are very potent antagonists of BK action on classical systems. Thus the "conventional wisdom" that a D-aromatic amino acid residue is required at sequence position 7 of BK antagonists must be modified.

INTRODUCTION

The first description of competitive antagonists of bradykinin (BK: Arg-Pro-Pro-Gly-Phe-Ser-Pro-Phe-Arg) established the requirement for a D-aromatic amino acid residue replacing the aliphatic proline residue at sequence position 7 (1). Additional modifications at the amino terminus and positions 3,5 and 8 yielded the potent first-generation BK antagonists. Later the combination of a D-aromatic amino acid residue at position 7 with an L-proline residue replacing the aromatic phenylalanine residue at position 8 was shown to yield good antagonists (2). Recently, BK analogs with a modified D-phenylalanine residue at position 7 combined with proline derivatives at position 8 were demonstrated to be the most potent and long acting antagonists of BK yet reported (3). Also, BK analogs possessing alkyl ethers of the aliphatic D-hydroxyproline at position 7, combined with a similar L-residue at position 8, have been reported to be potent antagonists of BK (4). This last publication, which appeared as we were finishing the extensive study reported here, is the first report that the D-amino acid residue at position seven of potent BK antagonists is not necessarily aromatic.

Some years ago, as a natural extension of our work with proline at position 8 of BK antagonists (2), we began to look into the influence on antagonist activity of the side chains of residues at positions 6 and 8, which sit on either side of the then presumably obligate D-aromatic residue at position 7. From previous work (5) it was known that analogs containing a D-aromatic amino acid residue replacing serine at position 6 of the antagonist sequence (ie, a sequence with a D-aromatic amino acid at both positions 6 and 7) could show antagonist action (for instance [DPhe^6,CDF^7]-BK), but that analogs containing aliphatic residues (Ala, Pro, Hyp) other than the normal serine at position 6 of antagonist sequences generally did not. Little work had been reported on the requirements for, and limitations of, substitutions at position 8 of BK antagonists. We report a large series of BK analogs containing aliphatic amino acid residues in positions 6, 7 and 8.

METHODS

Peptides were synthesized by the solid phase method, purified and characterized as previously described (1). They were assayed in the classical BK assay systems (isolated rat uterus and guinea pig ileum, and rat blood pressure) by our standard methods (1). Antagonist activities on smooth muscles are expressed as the pA$_2$ value of Schild. Antagonist potency on rat blood pressure was not quantitated precisely, since such determinations require extended measurements. A mixture of an ED$_{25}$ dose of BK (the amount required to lower arterial blood pressure by 25mm) and the antagonist were injected as a bolus. A rough estimate of antagonist potency was obtained from the amount of antagonist needed to give 50% inhibition of the depressor response to BK, but due to potential inaccuracies of this method only the fact of antagonism is reported here. Pulmonary inactivation of agonists was estimated from the ratio of the molar dose of peptide required by the intraaortic versus intrajugular route to lower blood pressure by 25mm. This method does not allow estimation of pulmonary degradation of antagonists.

RESULTS AND DISCUSSION

Table 1 lists the structures and biological activities of these new BK analogs. Replacement of serine at position 6 of antagonists by valine generally converts them into agonists on the rat uterus, and significantly decreases antagonist potency on the guinea pig ileum (peptides 007-014). It is interesting that lysine at position 6 generally yields uterus-specific antagonists (015-017). Beta-branched residues (Ile, Val) flanking DPhe generally destroy uterus biological activity, but allow decreased antagonist activity on the ileum (018-033). Single aliphatic beta-branched residues (especially Leu and Ile) at position 8 of antagonist sequences frequently yield potent antagonists in all assays (038-077). A thienylalanine (Thi) residue at position 5, although often dramatically increasing potency of BK antagonists containing DPhe at position 7, generally decreases antagonist potency of these 8-aliphatic analogs. In this group of 8-aliphatic analogs containing a D-aromatic residue at position 7, DArg-[Hyp^3,DPhe^7,Ile^8]-BK (065) is the most potent antagonist of BK on smooth muscle reported here. Cyclic aliphatic residues at position 8 of DPhe-7 antagonists containing serine or threonine at position 6 provide good antagonists (082-129). A series of new analogs having DPhe at position 7 and aromatic

TABLE 1 - New Bradykinin Analogs

Analog	Peptide Structure										Biological Activities			
Number	0	1	2	3	4	5	6	7	8	9	RUT	GPI	IA	%D
001 BK	Arg - Pro - Pro - Gly - Phe - Ser - Pro - Phe - Arg										100%	100%	100%	99%
002-N567	DArg-Arg - Pro - Hyp - Gly - Phe - Ser -DPhe - Phe - Arg [b]										6.5*	5.9*	I	-
003-7450	Arg - Pro - Pro - Gly - Thi - Thr -DPhe - Phe - Arg										9%	5.7*	I	-
004-7452	DArg-Arg - Pro - Pro - Gly - Thi - Thr -DPhe - Phe - Arg										0.1%	5.9*	I	-
005-7454	Arg - Pro - Hyp - Gly - Thi - Thr -DPhe - Phe - Arg										0.2%	5.4*	0	-
006-7456	DArg-Arg - Pro - Hyp - Gly - Thi - Thr -DPhe - Phe - Arg										6.3*	5.7*	0	-
007-7514	Arg - Pro - Pro - Gly - Phe - Val -DPhe - Phe - Arg										39%	0	2%	59%
008-7516	DArg-Arg - Pro - Pro - Gly - Phe - Val -DPhe - Phe - Arg										15%	I(P)	I	-
009-7518	Arg - Pro - Hyp - Gly - Phe - Val -DPhe - Phe - Arg										72%	I(P)	6%	79%
010-7520	DArg-Arg - Pro - Hyp - Gly - Phe - Val -DPhe - Phe - Arg										25%	I(P)	0	-
011-7524	Arg - Pro - Pro - Gly - Thi - Val -DPhe - Phe - Arg										5%	0.1%	2%	54%
012-7526	DArg-Arg - Pro - Pro - Gly - Thi - Val -DPhe - Phe - Arg										16%	5.5*	I	-
013-7528	Arg - Pro - Hyp - Gly - Thi - Val -DPhe - Phe - Arg										127%	0	0	-
014-7530	DArg-Arg - Pro - Hyp - Gly - Thi - Val -DPhe - Phe - Arg										8%	0	0	-
015-8044	DArg-Arg - Pro - Pro - Gly - Phe - Lys -DPhe - Phe - Arg										5.5*	5.3*		-
016-8046	Arg - Pro - Hyp - Gly - Phe - Lys -DPhe - Phe - Arg										5.9*	0	0	-
017-8048	DArg-Arg - Pro - Hyp - Gly - Phe - Lys -DPhe - Phe - Arg										5.6*	0	0	-
018-7558	Arg - Pro - Pro - Gly - Phe - Ile -DPhe - Ile - Arg										0	5.2*	0.1%	0
019-7560	DArg-Arg - Pro - Pro - Gly - Phe - Ile -DPhe - Ile - Arg										0.05%	5.9*	I	-
020-7562	Arg - Pro - Hyp - Gly - Phe - Ile -DPhe - Ile - Arg										0.3%	I(P)	0.1%	79%
021-7564	DArg-Arg - Pro - Hyp - Gly - Phe - Ile -DPhe - Ile - Arg										0.01%	6.0*	0.1%	53%
022-7600	Arg - Pro - Pro - Gly - Thi - Ile -DPhe - Ile - Arg										0.08%	5.4*	I	-
023-7602	DArg-Arg - Pro - Pro - Gly - Thi - Ile -DPhe - Ile - Arg										0.08%	5.7*	AG	-
024-7604	Arg - Pro - Hyp - Gly - Thi - Ile -DPhe - Ile - Arg										0.06%	I(P)	0.3%	86%
025-7606	DArg-Arg - Pro - Hyp - Gly - Thi - Ile -DPhe - Ile - Arg										6.2*	5.9*	0.3%	81%
026-7536	Arg - Pro - Pro - Gly - Phe - Val -DPhe - Val - Arg										0.1%	I(P)	0	-
027-7538	DArg-Arg - Pro - Pro - Gly - Phe - Val -DPhe - Val - Arg										0.03%	0	0	-
028-7540	Arg - Pro - Hyp - Gly - Phe - Val -DPhe - Val - Arg										0.07%	I(P)	I	-
029-7542	DArg-Arg - Pro - Hyp - Gly - Phe - Val -DPhe - Val - Arg										5.7*	5.6*	0	-
030-7546	Arg - Pro - Pro - Gly - Thi - Val -DPhe - Val - Arg										0.04%	5.2*	0.5%	57%
031-7548	DArg-Arg - Pro - Pro - Gly - Thi - Val -DPhe - Val - Arg										0.1%	5.5*	I	-
032-7550	Arg - Pro - Hyp - Gly - Thi - Val -DPhe - Val - Arg										0.07%	I(P)	I	-
033-7552	DArg-Arg - Pro - Hyp - Gly - Thi - Val -DPhe - Val - Arg										0.02%	5.6*	I	-
034-7782	Arg - Pro - Hyp - Gly - Phe - Ser -DPhe - Gly - Arg										0.01%	0	I	-
035-7784	DArg-Arg - Pro - Hyp - Gly - Phe - Ser -DPhe - Gly - Arg										0	0	I	-
036-7820	Arg - Pro - Hyp - Gly - Thi - Ser -DPhe - Gly - Arg										0	0	0.1%	91%
037-7822	DArg-Arg - Pro - Hyp - Gly - Thi - Ser -DPhe - Gly - Arg										0	0	0	-

Analog Number	Peptide Structure 0 1 2 3 4 5 6 7 8 9	Biological Activities RUT	GPI	IA	%D
038-7610	Arg - Pro - Pro - Gly - Phe - Ser -DPhe - Aib - Arg	5.4*	5.4*	I	-
039-7612	DArg-Arg - Pro - Pro - Gly - Phe - Ser -DPhe - Aib - Arg	5.7*	6.0*	I	-
040-7614	Arg - Pro - Hyp - Gly - Phe - Ser -DPhe - Aib - Arg	5.5*	5.3*	I	-
041-7616	DArg-Arg - Pro - Hyp - Gly - Phe - Ser -DPhe - Aib - Arg	5.9*	5.8*	I	-
042-7182	Arg - Pro - Pro - Gly - Thi - Ser -DPhe - Aib - Arg	5.2*	5.4*	I	-
043-7184	DArg-Arg - Pro - Pro - Gly - Thi - Ser -DPhe - Aib - Arg	6.1*	6.1*	0	-
044-7186	Arg - Pro - Hyp - Gly - Thi - Ser -DPhe - Aib - Arg	5.7*	5.6*	0	-
045-7188	DArg-Arg - Pro - Hyp - Gly - Thi - Ser -DPhe - Aib - Arg	7.0*	5.8*	I	-
046-7826	Arg - Pro - Hyp - Gly - Phe - Ser -DPhe - Ala - Arg	5.0*	I(P)	0.1%	52%
047-7828	DArg-Arg - Pro - Hyp - Gly - Phe - Ser -DPhe - Ala - Arg	5.6*	0	0	-
048-7830	Arg - Pro - Hyp - Gly - Thi - Ser -DPhe - Ala - Arg	0	I(P)	I(P)	-
049-7832	DArg-Arg - Pro - Hyp - Gly - Thi - Ser -DPhe - Ala - Arg	5.8*	0	I	-
050-7844	Arg - Pro - Hyp - Gly - Phe - Ser -DPhe - Leu - Arg	0.5%	5.9*	0.1%	33%
051-7846	DArg-Arg - Pro - Hyp - Gly - Phe - Ser -DPhe - Leu - Arg	7.4*	6.5*	I	-
052-7848	Arg - Pro - Hyp - Gly - Thi - Ser -DPhe - Leu - Arg	0.1%	6.1*	MXD	-
053-7850	DArg-Arg - Pro - Hyp - Gly - Thi - Ser -DPhe - Leu - Arg	7.0*	6.4*	I	-
054-7392	Arg - Pro - Pro - Gly - Phe - Ser -DPhe - Val - Arg	0.03%	6.0*	I	-
055-7394	DArg-Arg - Pro - Pro - Gly - Phe - Ser -DPhe - Val - Arg	5.8*	6.2*	I	-
056-7396	Arg - Pro - Hyp - Gly - Phe - Ser -DPhe - Val - Arg	5.8*	5.4*	0.02%	50%
057-7398	DArg-Arg - Pro - Hyp - Gly - Phe - Ser -DPhe - Val - Arg	6.7*	6.3*	I	-
058-7400	Arg - Pro - Pro - Gly - Thi - Ser -DPhe - Val - Arg	0.2%	5.4*	3%	98%
059-7402	DArg-Arg - Pro - Pro - Gly - Thi - Ser -DPhe - Val - Arg	6.2*	6.3*	I	-
060-7404	Arg - Pro - Hyp - Gly - Thi - Ser -DPhe - Val - Arg	0.1%	5.3*	I	-
061-7406	DArg-Arg - Pro - Hyp - Gly - Thi - Ser -DPhe - Val - Arg	6.3*	6.5*	I	-
062-7412	Arg - Pro - Pro - Gly - Phe - Ser -DPhe - Ile - Arg	0.2%	6.0*	0	-
063-7414	DArg-Arg - Pro - Pro - Gly - Phe - Ser -DPhe - Ile - Arg	6.9*	6.2*	I	-
064-7416	Arg - Pro - Hyp - Gly - Phe - Ser -DPhe - Ile - Arg	6.6*	6.1*	0	-
065-7418	DArg-Arg - Pro - Hyp - Gly - Phe - Ser -DPhe - Ile - Arg	7.7*	6.8*	I	-
066-7422	Arg - Pro - Pro - Gly - Thi - Ser -DPhe - Ile - Arg	0.7%	6.1*	0.8%	86%
067-7424	DArg-Arg - Pro - Pro - Gly - Thi - Ser -DPhe - Ile - Arg	6.8*	6.8*	I	-
068-7426	Arg - Pro - Hyp - Gly - Thi - Ser -DPhe - Ile - Arg	6.8*	6.0*	I	-
069-7428	DArg-Arg - Pro - Hyp - Gly - Thi - Ser -DPhe - Ile - Arg	7.0*	6.7*	I	-
070-7762	Arg - Pro - Hyp - Gly - Phe - Ser -DPhe - Nle - Arg	0.1%	6.1*	I	-
071-7764	DArg-Arg - Pro - Hyp - Gly - Phe - Ser -DPhe - Nle - Arg	7.1*	6.4*	I	-
072-7766	Arg - Pro - Hyp - Gly - Thi - Ser -DPhe - Nle - Arg	0.3%	6.7*	0	-
073-7768	DArg-Arg - Pro - Hyp - Gly - Thi - Ser -DPhe - Nle - Arg	7.3*	6.7*	I	-
074-7952	Arg - Pro - Hyp - Gly - Phe - Ser -DPhe - tLeu - Arg	5.4*	5.4*	0	-
075-7954	DArg-Arg - Pro - Hyp - Gly - Phe - Ser -DPhe - tLeu - Arg	6.2*	5.9*	0	-
076-7956	Arg - Pro - Hyp - Gly - Thi - Ser -DPhe - tLeu - Arg	5.4*	5.4*	0	-
077-7958	DArg-Arg - Pro - Hyp - Gly - Thi - Ser -DPhe - tLeu - Arg	5.9*	5.9*	0	-
078-7202	Arg - Pro - Pro - Gly - Thi - Ser -DPhe - Thr - Arg	0	I(P)	0	-
079-7204	DArg-Arg - Pro - Pro - Gly - Thi - Ser -DPhe - Thr - Arg	I(P)	I(P)	I	-
080-7206	Arg - Pro - Hyp - Gly - Thi - Ser -DPhe - Thr - Arg	0	I(P)	I	-
081-7208	DArg-Arg - Pro - Hyp - Gly - Thi - Ser -DPhe - Thr - Arg	0	5.4*	I	-

Analog Number	Peptide Structure										Biological Activities			
	0	1	2	3	4	5	6	7	8	9	RUT	GPI	IA	%D
082-4432	DArg-Arg - Pro - Pro - Gly - Phe - Ser -DPhe - Pro - Arg [b]										5.9*	6.6*	I	-
083-4434	Arg - Pro - Hyp - Gly - Phe - Ser -DPhe - Pro - Arg [b]										5.7*	5.6*	I	-
084-4436	DArg-Arg - Pro - Hyp - Gly - Phe - Ser -DPhe - Pro - Arg [b]										6.3*	6.0*	I	-
085-5438	DArg-Arg - Pro - Pro - Gly - Thi - Ser -DPhe - Pro - Arg [c]										6.0*	6.6*	0	-
086-7496	Arg - Pro - Hyp - Gly - Phe - Thr -DPhe - Pro - Arg										5.3*	0	I	-
087-7498	DArg-Arg - Pro - Hyp - Gly - Phe - Thr -DPhe - Pro - Arg										6.0*	5.7*	I	-
088-7502	Arg - Pro - Pro - Gly - Thi - Thr -DPhe - Pro - Arg										0.01%	5.6*	0.1	42%
089-7504	DArg-Arg - Pro - Pro - Gly - Thi - Thr -DPhe - Pro - Arg										I	5.8*	I	-
090-7506	Arg - Pro - Hyp - Gly - Thi - Thr -DPhe - Pro - Arg										5.2*	5.3*	0	-
091-7508	DArg-Arg - Pro - Hyp - Gly - Thi - Thr -DPhe - Pro - Arg										5.9*	5.6*	0	-
092-7724	Ppa-DArg-Arg - Pro - Hyp - Gly - Phe - Ser -DPhe - Pro - Arg										6.1*	5.4*	0	-
093-7726	Pba-DArg-Arg - Pro - Hyp - Gly - Phe - Ser -DPhe - Pro - Arg										6.5*	5.9*	I	-
094-7728	Tba-DArg-Arg - Pro - Hyp - Gly - Phe - Ser -DPhe - Pro - Arg										5.7*	5.6*	0	-
095-7730	Cha-DArg-Arg - Pro - Hyp - Gly - Phe - Ser -DPhe - Pro - Arg										6.5*	6.6*	I	-
096-7732	Cpa-DArg-Arg - Pro - Hyp - Gly - Phe - Ser -DPhe - Pro - Arg										6.3*	6.1*	I	-
097-7734	Nba-DArg-Arg - Pro - Hyp - Gly - Phe - Ser -DPhe - Pro - Arg										6.5*	6.1*	I	-
098-8324	DArg-Arg - Pro - Pro - Gly - Phe - Ser - FDF - Pro - Arg										5.6*	6.7*	0	-
099-8328	DArg-Arg - Pro - Hyp - Gly - Phe - Ser - FDF - Pro - Arg										5.7*	I(P)	0	-
100-8332	Arg - Pro - Pro - Gly - Phe - Ser -DPhe - DHP - Arg										5.6*	6.5*	I	-
101-8334	DArg-Arg - Pro - Pro - Gly - Phe - Ser -DPhe - DHP - Arg										5.1*	7.1*	I	-
102-8336	Arg - Pro - Hyp - Gly - Phe - Ser -DPhe - DHP - Arg										5.7*	I/0*	0	-
103-7164	Arg - Pro - Pro - Gly - Phe - Ser -DPhe - Thz - Arg										5.9*	6.0*	I	-
104-7166	DArg-Arg - Pro - Pro - Gly - Phe - Ser -DPhe - Thz - Arg										6.1*	6.1*	0	-
105-7168	Arg - Pro - Hyp - Gly - Phe - Ser -DPhe - Thz - Arg										5.5*	5.4*	0	-
106-7170	DArg-Arg - Pro - Hyp - Gly - Phe - Ser -DPhe - Thz - Arg										6.2*	5.6*	I	-
107-7172	Arg - Pro - Pro - Gly - Thi - Ser -DPhe - Thz - Arg										5.5*	5.7*	I	-
108-7174	DArg-Arg - Pro - Pro - Gly - Thi - Ser -DPhe - Thz - Arg										5.7*	6.3*	0	-
109-7176	Arg - Pro - Hyp - Gly - Thi - Ser -DPhe - Thz - Arg										5.6*	5.8*	0	-
110-7178	DArg-Arg - Pro - Hyp - Gly - Thi - Ser -DPhe - Thz - Arg										6.8*	6.1*	I	-
111-8372	Arg - Pro - Pro - Gly - Phe - Ser -DPhe - Azt - Arg										0	0	0	-
112-8374	DArg-Arg - Pro - Pro - Gly - Phe - Ser -DPhe - Azt - Arg										0	5.6*	I	-
113-8376	Arg - Pro - Hyp - Gly - Phe - Ser -DPhe - Azt - Arg										0	0	0	-
114-8378	DArg-Arg - Pro - Hyp - Gly - Phe - Ser -DPhe - Azt - Arg										5.0*	I(P)	I	-
115-8382	Arg - Pro - Pro - Gly - Phe - Ser -DPhe - Pip - Arg										5.4*	5.8*	0	-
116-8384	DArg-Arg - Pro - Pro - Gly - Phe - Ser -DPhe - Pip - Arg										5.0*	6.6*	I	-
117-8386	Arg - Pro - Hyp - Gly - Phe - Ser -DPhe - Pip - Arg										5.6*	5.6*	I	-
118-8388	DArg-Arg - Pro - Hyp - Gly - Phe - Ser -DPhe - Pip - Arg										6.6*	6.3*	I	-
119-7942	Arg - Pro - Hyp - Gly - Phe - Ser -DPhe - cAib - Arg										I(P)	I(P)	0	-
120-7944	DArg-Arg - Pro - Hyp - Gly - Phe - Ser -DPhe - cAib - Arg										5.3*	5.4*	0	-
121-7946	Arg - Pro - Hyp - Gly - Thi - Ser -DPhe - cAib - Arg										0	0	0	-
122-7948	DArg-Arg - Pro - Hyp - Gly - Thi - Ser -DPhe - cAib - Arg										5.2*	5.7*	0	-
123-7854	Arg - Pro - Hyp - Gly - Phe - Ser -DPhe - cLeu - Arg										5.8*	5.4*	I	-
124-7856	DArg-Arg - Pro - Hyp - Gly - Phe - Ser -DPhe - cLeu - Arg										6.0*	5.7*	I	-
125-7858	Arg - Pro - Hyp - Gly - Thi - Ser -DPhe - cLeu - Arg										I/0	5.4*	I	-
126-7860	DArg-Arg - Pro - Hyp - Gly - Thi - Ser -DPhe - cLeu - Arg										6.7*	6.0*	0	-

Analog number	Peptide Structure 0 1 2 3 4 5 6 7 8 9	RUT	GPI	IA	%D
127-7886	DArg-Arg - Pro - Hyp - Gly - Phe - Ser -DPhe - Cpg - Arg	7.2*	6.2*	I	-
128-7888	Arg - Pro - Hyp - Gly - Thi - Ser -DPhe - Cpg - Arg	2%	5.9*	0	-
129-7890	DArg-Arg - Pro - Hyp - Gly - Thi - Ser -DPhe - Cpg - Arg	7.0*	6.5*	I	-
130-3852	Arg - Pro - Hyp - Gly - Phe - Ser - DPhe - Phe - Arg [b]	0.4%	5.6*	I	-
131-7304	Arg - Pro - Hyp - Gly - PFF - Ser -DPhe - PFF - Arg	0.06%	0	I	-
132-7306	DArg-Arg - Pro - Hyp - Gly - PFF - Ser -DPhe - PFF - Arg	0.01%	5.7*	I	-
133-7300	Arg - Pro - Hyp - Gly - Thi - Ser -DPhe - PFF - Arg	0.1%	0	I	-
134-7302	DArg-Arg - Pro - Hyp - Gly - Thi - Ser -DPhe - PFF - Arg	0.01%	5.8*	0	-
135-7752	Arg - Pro - Hyp - Gly - Phe - Ser -DPhe - PNF - Arg	0.3%	0	I	-
136-7754	DArg-Arg - Pro - Hyp - Gly - Phe - Ser -DPhe - PNF - Arg	6.1*	5.7*	I	-
137-7756	Arg - Pro - Hyp - Gly - Thi - Ser -DPhe - PNF - Arg	0.06%	5.3*	0	-
138-7758	DArg-Arg - Pro - Hyp - Gly - Thi - Ser -DPhe - PNF - Arg	0.06%	5.3*	I	-
139-8062	Arg - Pro - Hyp - Gly - Phe - Ser -DPhe - Trp - Arg	0.05%	0	0	-
140-8064	DArg-Arg - Pro - Hyp - Gly - Phe - Ser -DPhe - Trp - Arg	0.08%	I(P)	I	-
141-8066	Arg - Pro - Hyp - Gly - Thi - Ser -DPhe - Trp - Arg	0.1%	I(P)	0	-
142-8068	DArg-Arg - Pro - Hyp - Gly - Thi - Ser -DPhe - Trp - Arg	0.2%	5.4*	0	-
143-8082	Arg - Pro - Hyp - Gly - Phe - Ser -DPhe - Nal - Arg	1%	I(P)	0	-
144-8084	DArg-Arg - Pro - Hyp - Gly - Phe - Ser -DPhe - Nal - Arg	5.3*	5.5*	0	-
145-8086	Arg - Pro - Hyp - Gly - Thi - Ser -DPhe - Nal - Arg	0.8%	5.4*	0	-
146-8088	DArg-Arg - Pro - Hyp - Gly - Thi - Ser -DPhe - Nal - Arg	0.2%	5.7*	0	-
147-8072	Arg - Pro - Hyp - Gly - Phe - Ser -DPhe - Pal - Arg	I(P)	0	I	-
148-8074	DArg-Arg - Pro - Hyp - Gly - Phe - Ser -DPhe - Pal - Arg	5.8*	I	I	-
149-8076	Arg - Pro - Hyp - Gly - Thi - Ser -DPhe - Pal - Arg	0	I(P)	I	-
150-8078	DArg-Arg - Pro - Hyp - Gly - Thi - Ser -DPhe - Pal - Arg	5.6*	0	I	-
151-7192	Arg - Pro - Pro - Gly - Thi - Ser -DPhe -NMF - Arg	0.3%	6.2*	2	-
152-7194	DArg-Arg - Pro - Pro - Gly - Thi - Ser -DPhe -NMF - Arg	0.2%	5.4*	0.1%	0
153-7196	Arg - Pro - Hyp - Gly - Thi - Ser -DPhe -NMF - Arg	0.05%	I(P)	0	-
154-7198	DArg-Arg - Pro - Hyp - Gly - Thi - Ser -DPhe -NMF - Arg	6.0*	5.5*	0	-
155-3934	Arg - Pro - Pro - Gly - Thi - Ser -DPro - Thi - Arg [c]	0.01%	0	0	-
156-4062	Arg - Pro - Pro - Gly - Thi - Ser -DVal - Thi - Arg [c]	1%	0	-	-
157-4064	Arg - Pro - Pro - Gly - Thi - Ser - DIle - Thi - Arg [c]	AG	0	0.3%	0
158-8616	DArg-Arg - Pro - Pro - Gly - Phe - Ser - DIle - Phe - Arg	0.2%	0	0	-
159-8618	Arg - Pro - Hyp - Gly - Phe - Ser - DIle - Phe - Arg	0.1%	0	0	-
160-8620	DArg - Arg - Pro - Hyp - Gly - Phe - Ser - DIle - Phe - Arg	1%	I(P)	0	-
161-8302	Arg - Pro - Pro - Gly - Phe - Ser - DAlg - Phe - Arg	0.6%	4%	0	-
162-8304	DArg-Arg - Pro - Pro - Gly - Phe - Ser - DAlg - Phe - Arg	3%	1%	0	-
163-8306	Arg - Pro - Hyp - Gly - Phe - Ser - DAlg - Phe - Arg	4%	0.1%	0	-
164-8308	DArg-Arg - Pro - Hyp - Gly - Phe - Ser - DAlg - Phe - Arg	8%	0	0	-
165-8178	Arg - Pro - Pro - Gly - Phe - Ser -DCpg - Phe - Arg	0.9%	0	0	-
166-8180	DArg-Arg - Pro - Pro - Gly - Phe - Ser -DCpg - Phe - Arg	0.5%	0	0	-
167-8182	Arg - Pro - Hyp - Gly - Phe - Ser -DCpg - Phe - Arg	0.8%	0	0	-
168-8184	DArg-Arg - Pro - Hyp - Gly - Phe - Ser -DCpg - Phe - Arg	AG	0	I	-

Analog	Peptide Structure										Biological Activities			
Number	0	1	2	3	4	5	6	7	8	9	RUT	GPI	IA	%D
169-8276		Arg - Pro - Hyp - Gly - Phe - Ser - cLeu - Phe - Arg									4%	0.6%	0	-
170-8278	DArg-Arg - Pro - Hyp - Gly - Phe - Ser - cLeu - Phe - Arg										4%	0.2%	0.02%	0
171-8292		Arg - Pro - Pro - Gly - Thi - Ser - cLeu - Thi - Arg									0.5%	0.7%	0.8%	64%
172-8294	DArg-Arg - Pro - Pro - Gly - Thi - Ser - cLeu - Thi - Arg										0.6%	0	0.2%	18%
173-8296		Arg - Pro - Hyp - Gly - Thi - Ser - cLeu - Thi - Arg									0.9%	0	0	-
174-8298	DArg-Arg - Pro - Hyp - Gly - Thi - Ser - cLeu - Thi - Arg										2%	0	AG	0
175-7086	DArg-Arg - Pro - Hyp - Gly - Phe - Ser - DPro -Pro - Arg										I(P)	0	0	-
176-7096	DArg-Arg - Pro - Hyp - Gly - Thi - Ser - DPro -Pro - Arg										0	0	0	-
177-8516		Arg - Pro - Pro - Gly - Phe - Ser - DPro - Ile - Arg									0	0	0	-
178-8518	DArg-Arg - Pro - Pro - Gly - Phe - Ser - DPro - Ile - Arg										0	0	0	-
179-8520		Arg - Pro - Hyp - Gly - Phe - Ser - DPro - Ile - Arg									0	0	0	-
180-8522	DArg-Arg - Pro - Hyp - Gly - Phe - Ser - DPro - Ile - Arg										I(P)	0	I	-
181-8526		Arg - Pro - Pro - Gly - Thi - Ser - DPro - Ile - Arg									0.1%	0	0	-
182-8528	DArg-Arg - Pro - Pro - Gly - Thi - Ser - DPro - Ile - Arg										I(P)	0	I	-
183-8530		Arg - Pro - Hyp - Gly - Thi - Ser - DPro - Ile - Arg									I(P)	0	0	-
184-8532	DArg-Arg - Pro - Hyp - Gly - Thi - Ser - DPro - Ile - Arg										0	0	0	-
185-8594		Arg - Pro - Pro - Gly - Phe - Ser - DVal - Ile - Arg									5.4*	0	AG	-
186-8596	DArg-Arg - Pro - Pro - Gly - Phe - Ser - DVal - Ile - Arg										6.2*	6.2*	I	-
187-8598		Arg - Pro - Hyp - Gly - Phe - Ser - DVal - Ile - Arg									5.9*	5.8*	0	-
188-8600	DArg-Arg - Pro - Hyp - Gly - Phe - Ser - DVal - Ile - Arg										7.1*	6.1*	I	-
189-8644		Arg - Pro - Pro - Gly - Phe - Ser - DLeu - Ile - Arg									0.2%	5.7*	AG	-
190-8646	DArg-Arg - Pro - Pro - Gly - Phe - Ser - DLeu - Ile - Arg										5.9*	6.0*	I	-
191-8648		Arg - Pro - Hyp - Gly - Phe - Ser - DLeu - Ile - Arg									5.3*	I(P)	0	-
192-8650	DArg-Arg - Pro - Hyp - Gly - Phe - Ser - DLeu - Ile - Arg										6.3*	5.3*	I	-
193-8492		Arg - Pro - Pro - Gly - Phe - Ser - DIle - Ile - Arg									5.5*	5.6*	I	-
194-8496	DArg-Arg - Pro - Pro - Gly - Phe - Ser - DIle - Ile - Arg										6.2*	5.4*	0	-
195-8498		Arg - Pro - Hyp - Gly - Phe - Ser - DIle - Ile - Arg									5.9*	5.1*	I	-
196-8500	DArg-Arg - Pro - Hyp - Gly - Phe - Ser - DIle - Ile - Arg										5.9*	5.9*	I	-
197-8508		Arg - Pro - Hyp - Gly - Thi - Ser - DIle - Ile - Arg									5.9*	5.2*	I	-
198-8510	DArg-Arg - Pro - Hyp - Gly - Thi - Ser - DIle - Ile - Arg										6.1*	5.6*	I	-
199-8554		Arg - Pro - Pro - Gly - Phe - Ser - DNle - Ile - Arg									7.1*	6.6*	0	-
200-8556	DArg-Arg - Pro - Pro - Gly - Phe - Ser - DNle - Ile - Arg										6.2*	6.0*	I	-
201-8558		Arg - Pro - Hyp - Gly - Phe - Ser - DNle - Ile - Arg									5.9*	5.9*	I	-
202-8590	DArg-Arg - Pro - Hyp - Gly - Phe - Ser - DNle - Ile - Arg										7.0*	6.3*	I	-
203-8312		Arg - Pro - Pro - Gly - Phe - Ser - DAlg - Ile - Arg									5.0*	5.3*	0	-
204-8314	DArg-Arg - Pro - Pro - Gly - Phe - Ser - DAlg - Ile - Arg										5.8*	5.2*	0	-
205-8316		Arg - Pro - Hyp - Gly - Phe - Ser - DAlg - Ile - Arg									5.6*	5.3*	0	-
206-8318	DArg-Arg - Pro - Hyp - Gly - Phe - Ser - DAlg - Ile - Arg										5.8*	5.6*	I	-
207-8282		Arg - Pro - Hyp - Gly - Phe - Ser - cLeu - Ile - Arg									0.1%	0	0	-
208-8284	DArg-Arg - Pro - Hyp - Gly - Phe - Ser - cLeu - Ile - Arg										0.04%	0	0	-
209-8286		Arg - Pro - Hyp - Gly - Thi - Ser - cLeu - Ile - Arg									0	0	0	-
210-8288	DArg-Arg - Pro - Hyp - Gly - Thi - Ser - cLeu - Ile - Arg										0.06%	0	22%	99%

Analog Number	Peptide Structure										Biological Activities			
	0	1	2	3	4	5	6	7	8	9	RUT	GPI	IA	%D
211-8654		Arg - Pro -	Pro -	Gly -	Phe -	Ser -	DLeu -	Nle -	Arg		1.1%	I	I	-
212-8656	DArg-	Arg - Pro -	Pro -	Gly -	Phe -	Ser -	DLeu -	Nle -	Arg		0.1%	5.5*	I	-
213-8658		Arg - Pro -	Hyp -	Gly -	Phe -	Ser -	DLeu -	Nle -	Arg		0.02%	I(P)	0	-
214-8660	DArg-	Arg - Pro -	Hyp -	Gly -	Phe -	Ser -	DLeu -	Nle -	Arg		5.1*	5.6*	0	-
215-8700		Arg - Pro -	Hyp -	Gly -	Phe -	Ser -	DLeu -	Pip -	Arg		0	5.2*	0	-
216-8702	DArg-	Arg - Pro -	Hyp -	Gly -	Phe -	Ser -	DLeu -	Pip -	Arg		I(P)	I(P)	0	-
217-8706		Arg - Pro -	Pro -	Gly -	Phe -	Ser -	DIle -	DHP -	Arg		0	0	0	-
218-8708	DArg-	Arg - Pro -	Pro -	Gly -	Phe -	Ser -	DIle -	DHP -	Arg		I(P)	I(P)	AG	-
219-8710		Arg - Pro -	Hyp -	Gly -	Phe -	Ser -	DIle -	DHP -	Arg		0	0	0	-
220-8712	DArg-	Arg - Pro -	Hyp -	Gly -	Phe -	Ser -	DIle -	DHP -	Arg		0	0	I	-
221-8624		Arg - Pro -	Pro -	Gly -	Phe -	Ser -	DAlg -	Pro -	Arg		0	0	0	-
222-8626	DArg-	Arg - Pro -	Pro -	Gly -	Phe -	Ser -	DAlg -	Pro -	Arg		0	0	AG	-
223-8628		Arg - Pro -	Hyp -	Gly -	Phe -	Ser -	DAlg -	Pro -	Arg		0	I(P)	0	-
224-8630	DArg-	Arg - Pro -	Hyp -	Gly -	Phe -	Ser -	DAlg -	Pro -	Arg		I(P)	I(P)	0	-
225-8634		Arg - Pro -	Pro -	Gly -	Phe -	Ser -	DAlg -	Nle -	Arg		5.1*	5.8*	I	-
226-8636	DArg-	Arg - Pro -	Pro -	Gly -	Phe -	Ser -	DAlg -	Nle -	Arg		6.0*	5.6*	I	-
227-8638		Arg - Pro -	Hyp -	Gly -	Phe -	Ser -	DAlg -	Nle -	Arg		5.0*	0	0	-
228-8640	DArg-	Arg - Pro -	Hyp -	Gly -	Phe -	Ser -	DAlg -	Nle -	Arg		7.0*	5.1*	I	-
229-8536		Arg - Pro -	Pro -	Gly -	Phe -	Ser -	DCpg -	Ile -	Arg		15%	5.2*	AG	-
230-8538	DArg-	Arg - Pro -	Pro -	Gly -	Phe -	Ser -	DCpg -	Ile -	Arg		5.4*	6.7*	I	-
231-8540		Arg - Pro -	Hyp -	Gly -	Phe -	Ser -	DCpg -	Ile -	Arg		7.5*	6.0*	I	-
232-8542	DArg-	Arg - Pro -	Hyp -	Gly -	Phe -	Ser -	DCpg -	Ile -	Arg		7.1*	6.0*	I	-
233-8198		Arg - Pro -	Pro -	Gly -	Phe -	Ser -	DCpg -	Cpg -	Arg		0.2%	5.9*	AG	-
234-8200	DArg-	Arg - Pro -	Pro -	Gly -	Phe -	Ser -	DCpg -	Cpg -	Arg		7.1*	6.9*	-	-
235-8202		Arg - Pro -	Hyp -	Gly -	Phe -	Ser -	DCpg -	Cpg -	Arg		7.3*	7.6*	-	-
236-8204	DArg-	Arg - Pro -	Hyp -	Gly -	Phe -	Ser -	DCpg -	Cpg -	Arg		8.3*	6.6*	-	-
237-8212		Arg - Pro -	Hyp -	Gly -	Thi -	Ser -	DCpg -	Cpg -	Arg		7.1*	6.8*	-	-
238-8214	DArg-	Arg - Pro -	Hyp -	Gly -	Thi -	Ser -	DCpg -	Cpg -	Arg		7.7*	6.6*	I	-

[a] **Analog numbering** is sequential (001-238) followed by the B numbers used in our laboratory. **Agonist activity** is given relative to BK = 100% in the isolated rat uterus (RUT) and guinea pig ileum (GPI) assays. The activity on rat blood pressure is by intraaortic administration (IA). Apparent percent destruction (%D) on initial passage through the pulmonary circulation is given for agonists; it is not determined for antagonists. **Antagonist data:** 6.5* indicates BK antagonist pA_2 value of 6.5 determined on 4 - 12 tissues. (The pD_2 for BK is 8.7 in the RUT and 7.6 in the GPI assay in our laboratory.) **For all assays,** AG indicates unquantitated (usually weak) agonist activity; MXD indicates mixed agonist-antagonist activity; I indicates unquantitated BK antagonist activity; I(P) indicates partial antagonism; I/O indicates weak antagonism. **Other Abbreviations:** Aib (aminoisobutyryl); Alg (allyl-Gly); Azt (azetidinecarboxyl); cAib (1-aminocyclopropanecarboxyl); CDF (*p*-cloro-D-Phe); cLeu (1-aminocyclopentanecarboxyl); Cha (cyclohexaneacetyl-); Cpa (cyclopentaneacetyl-); Cpg (cyclopentyl-Gly); DAlg (D-allyl-Gly); DCpg (D-cyclopentyl-Gly); DHP (3,4-dehydro-Pro); FDF (*p*-fluoro-D-Phe); Nal (β-2-naphthyl-Ala); Nba (norbornaneacetyl-); Nle (norLeu); NMF (N-methyl-Phe); Pal (β-3-pyridylalanine); Pba (phenylbutyryl); Pip (pipecolyl); PNF (*p*-nitro-Phe); Ppa (phenylpropionyl-); Tba (*t*-butylacetyl-); tLeu (*tert*-Leu); Thz (thiazolidinecarboxyl). Literature references: [a] Ref. 2; [b] Ref. 5.

residues at position 8 had low antagonist potency on ileum, and for the most part had very weak agonist activity on rat uterus (130-154).

Acylation of the amino terminus of BK antagonists with a bulky acyl group has been reported to increase *in vivo* stability (6). We found that such acylated derivatives having proline in position 8 (092-097) maintained good antagonist potency, but did not show prolonged antagonism in the rat blood pressure assay.

Table 1 also presents structure-activity studies showing that D-aliphatic amino acid residues at position 7 in combination with L-aliphatic residues (175-238) [but not L-aromatic residues (155-174)] at position 8 produce BK antagonists. Bulky, beta-branched or cyclic D-aliphatic amino acid residues at position 7 combined with bulky or cyclic L-aliphatic residues at position 8 yield the best antagonists so far in this new series of analogs. A D-aliphatic or D-cyclic amino acid residue at position 7 of the BK sequence by itself (155-174) does not provide a BK antagonist. Although analogs having D-cyclopentylglycine (Cpg) at position 7 in analogs having the usual phenylalanine at position 8 are almost inactive (165-168), the combination of D-Cpg at position 7 with L-Cpg or L-Ile at position 8 (229-238) yields very potent antagonists. Analog 236 is the most potent BK antagonist described in this series. Certain of these also showed much longer activity *in vivo* in the rat than the "first generation" antagonists previously described.

The discovery of potent antagonists having aliphatic amino acid residues in positions seven and eight opens the way for development of an entirely new series of bradykinin antagonists.

ACKNOWLEDGEMENTS

This work was supported by grant #HL-26284 from the US-NIH, and by Nova Pharmaceutical Corporation. The authors thank Frances Shepperdson and Steven Durrance for the biological assays, Robert Binard for the amino acid analyses, and Robin Reed for technical assistance. We thank Dr. Floyd Dunn for gifts of thienylalanine and other unusual amino acids.

REFERENCES

1. Vavrek RJ, Stewart JM. Competitive antagonists of bradykinin. Peptides 1985: 6:161-5.

2. Vavrek RJ, Stewart JM. Development of bradykinin antagonists: Structure-activity relationships for new categories of antagonist sequences. In: Kinins V. Abe K, Moriya H, Fujii S, editors. New York: Plenum. 1989: 395-400. (Adv. Exp. Med. Biol. 1989: 247B).

3. Lembeck F, Griesbacher T, Eckhardt M, Henke S, Breipohl G, Knolle J. New, long-acting, potent bradykinin antagonists. Brit. J. Pharmacol. 1991: 102: 297-304.

4. Kyle DJ, Martin JA, Burch RM, Carter JP, Lu S, Meeker S, Prosser JC, Sullivan JP, Togo J, Noronha-Blob L, Sinsko JA, Walters RF, Whaley LW, Hiner RN. Probing the bradykinin receptor: Mapping the geometric topography using ethers of hydroxyproline in novel peptides. J. Med. Chem. 1991: 34: 2649-53.

5. Stewart JM, Vavrek RJ. In: Bradykinin Antagonists; Basic and Clinical Aspects. Burch RM, editor. New York: Marcel Dekker. 1991: 51-96.

6. Lammek B, Wang Y-X, Gavras I, Gavras H. A new highly potent antagonist of bradykinin. Peptides 1990: 11: 1041-3.

AAS 38/I
Recent Progress on Kinins
© 1992 Birkhäuser Verlag Basel

METABOLISM AND CHARACTERISATION OF KININS AND HOE 140 (KININ ANTAGONIST) IN THE SYNOVIAL FLUID OF PATIENTS WITH INFLAMMATORY JOINT DISEASES

A. P. Bond, G. Breipohl[1], K. Worthy, G. Campion[1], P.A. Dieppe[2] and K.D. Bhoola

Departments of Pharmacology and Rheumatology[2], University of Bristol, School of Medical Sciences, University Walk, Bristol BS8 1TD.[1] Hoechst AG, Pharmaceutical Division, P.O. Box 80 03 20, D-6230, Frankfurt/M.80

SUMMARY: Methods have been optimised for the collection of synovial fluid and the chromatographic separation of individual kinins (bradykinin and kallidin) in the fluid by HPLC. In addition, the stability of the kinin antagonist, Hoe 140, in synovial fluid was compared with that of synthetic bradykinin. Although bradykinin was completely degraded after incubation for only 6 h in pooled synovial fluid obtained from patients with rheumatoid arthritis, Hoe 140 was stable for as long as 2 weeks under the same conditions. These studies will provide quantitative information regarding levels of kinins in inflamed joints and an insight into the therapeutic potential of kinin antagonists.

INTRODUCTION

Inflammatory arthropathies, such as rheumatoid arthritis (RA), are conditions characterised by pain, swelling and tissue destruction in the synovial joints. Kinins have been reported in the synovial fluid (SF) of patients with RA (1-3), and it has been proposed that these vasoactive peptides may act locally, contributing to the classical symptoms of the disease (4).

In previous studies the methods used to measure kinins lacked specificity; the present study therefore aimed to develop procedures to identify and measure kinins in SF. Since BK and kallidin are produced by the action of different enzymes (plasma and tissue kallikrein respectively), the separate measurement of these two peptides will provide insights into the relative importance of each kallikrein in synovitis. The development of a chromatographic procedure to separate BK and kallidin was, therefore, essential. Techniques using two different HPLC systems were optimised and compared. The most appropriate method for collection of SF and extraction of kinins before HPLC analysis was also determined.

If kinins are involved in the pathogenesis of RA, intra-articular injection of a potent kinin antagonist should provide a new therapy for the disease. One criteria for such an antagonist is that it must be resistant to the kininases present in SF, which cause the rapid breakdown of BK

(5). The survival in SF of both BK and a new kinin antagonist, Hoe 140 (Hoechst), was, therefore, investigated.

MATERIALS AND METHODS

Sample collection: SF was taken, by artherocentesis, from the knees of patients with rheumatoid, osteo and psoriatic arthritis, attending Rheumatology Clinics at Bristol Royal Infirmary. A proportion of each sample was mixed immediately with a cocktail of inhibitors to prevent any formation (40 mg/l trasylol, 4 mg/ml SBTI; Sigma Chemicals, U.K.) or breakdown (10 μM phosphoramidon, 10 μM captopril, 6 mM 1,10–phenanthroline, Sigma Chemicals, U.K; and 60 mM EDTA, Analar grade, BDH, U.K.) of kinins. The remainder of the SF was collected into plain plastic tubes, without the addition of inhibitors, and all were stored on ice. Samples were centrifuged (5 min, 5,000 rpm, 4oC) and the supernatant stored at −20oC.

Preparation of SF: Before use, the SFs were treated with hyaluronidase (22.5 IU per ml SF; Sigma Chemicals) for 30 min at 37oC to reduce viscosity. Samples were then centrifuged (10,000 rpm, 10 min, 4oC) to remove debris and the supernatant was divided into aliquots and stored at −20oC until required.

Measurement of kinins by SMART^{TM} System: The SMART^{TM} system consisited of microprecision pumps and a micro mixer, equipped with a UV–detector measuring at fixed wavelengths (Pharmacia, Milton Keynes, U.K.). Kinin separation was carried out on a C$_{18}$ reversed phase 3.2 mm x 30 mm column. The mobile phase consisted of A: 0.025% TFA in water and B: 0.025% TFA in acetonitrile (far–UV grade; BDH, U.K.)/water (60:40) (v/v). Elution was carried out over a linear gradient from 0% to 60% B over 20 min, at a flow rate of 240 μl/min. Detection was by measurement of UV–absorbance at 214 nm.

Measurement of kinins by HPLC (Gilson): The Gilson HPLC system (Gilson Medical Electronics) consisted of two 306 pumps, 811 mixer and 621 data master, equipped with a 1000S diode array UV–detector (applied Biosystems). Kinins were separated on a reversed phase, 4.6 mm x 250 mm, column with 5 μm particle size and 300Å pore size (Rainin Instrument Company). The mobile phase consisted of A: 0.025% trifluoroacetic acid (TFA) in water/acetonitrile (95:5) (v/v) and B: 0.025% TFA in acetonitrile/water (90:10) (v/v). Elution was performed at a flow rate 1 ml/min, using a gradient from 20% to 60% B over 20 min, with a halving of the gradient between 5 and 15 min. Detection was carried out by measurement of UV–absorbance at 210 nm.

Pretreatment of SF Before Measurement by HPLC and SMART™ Systems: Before the SF could be measured using the SMART™ or Gilson HPLC techniques described, they first required treatment to remove other molecules, such as proteins, which may otherwise interfere with measurement of kinins. Studies were performed to determine the optimal method for treating the fluid. An acid–alcohol extraction was first carried out by the following procedure: the sample was added to an equal volume of acid–alcohol (0.1% 5 M HCl in absolute alcohol) and this was then vortexed and kept at –20⁰C for 40 min. Samples were centrifuged (3,000 rpm, 5 min, 4⁰C) and the supernatant decantered. Each precipitate was washed in one volume of the acid–alcohol and, after recentrifugation, the corresponding supernatants pooled. The extracts were then evaporated to dryness overnight at 50⁰C and the residue resuspended in one volume of distilled water. The extract was then filtered through membranes with a 10K nominal, molecular weight cut–off (Millipore, U.K.) and the filtrate collected.

Measurement of endogenous kinins in SF: Prior to measurement of the SF (containing a 1:1 inhibitor solution (v/v)), a proportion of each sample was spiked with 1 ng/μl synthetic BK and kallidin to allow assessment of recovery. The acid–alcohol extraction was carried out on the SF, using 0.1% 5 M HCl in absolute alcohol according to the method described above. The extract was then filtered and the filtrate stored at –20⁰C, until measurement of 50 μl on the SMART™ system.

Stability studies of kinins and Hoe 140 in SF: Synthetic kinins or Hoe 140 were added to SF (250 μg/ml). Thimerosal (0.1 mg/ml) was also added to prevent bacterial breakdown of the kinin and the antagonist during the incubation period. These samples were then incubated at 37⁰C. After the required incubation times, aliqouts of sample were removed, diluted 1:10 and internal standard added (25 ng/μl BK or Hoe 140). An acid alcohol extraction with the 0.1% 5 M HCl in absolute alcohol was then carried out on the diluted sample to extract the kinins or antagonist for measurement (method as described above). The extract was filtered through the 10K cut–off membrane filters, and the filtrate stored at –20⁰C. For measurements these samples were all diluted 1:1, and 20 μl measured, in duplicate, by the Gilson HPLC system.

Synthetic kinins: BK, kallidin and Hyp³ BK were purchased from Sigma Chemicals U.K., and Hyp³ kallidin from Protagen AG, Switzerland. Hoe 140 was a gift from Hoechst AG (Frankfurt, Germany).

RESULTS

Using the chromatographic procedures developed, a good resolution of synthetic kinins was achieved. The elution profiles for mixtures of synthetic BK, kallidin and Hoe 140 and also Hyp³ BK and Hyp³ kallidin measured by the SMART™ and Gilson HPLC systems are shown in figure 1. Mixtures of kallidin and Hyp³ BK were not resolved using these techniques. Dose-response curves for each synthetic kinin were determined by measuring the area under the relevant peak obtained on injection of varying concentrations of synthetic kinin. Figure 2 shows such curves for BK and kallidin, Hyp³ BK and Hyp³ kallidin, and for Hoe 140, measured on the SMART™ system. The sensitivity for the two HPLC techniques was high and both allowed detection of as little as 4 ng of synthetic kinin.

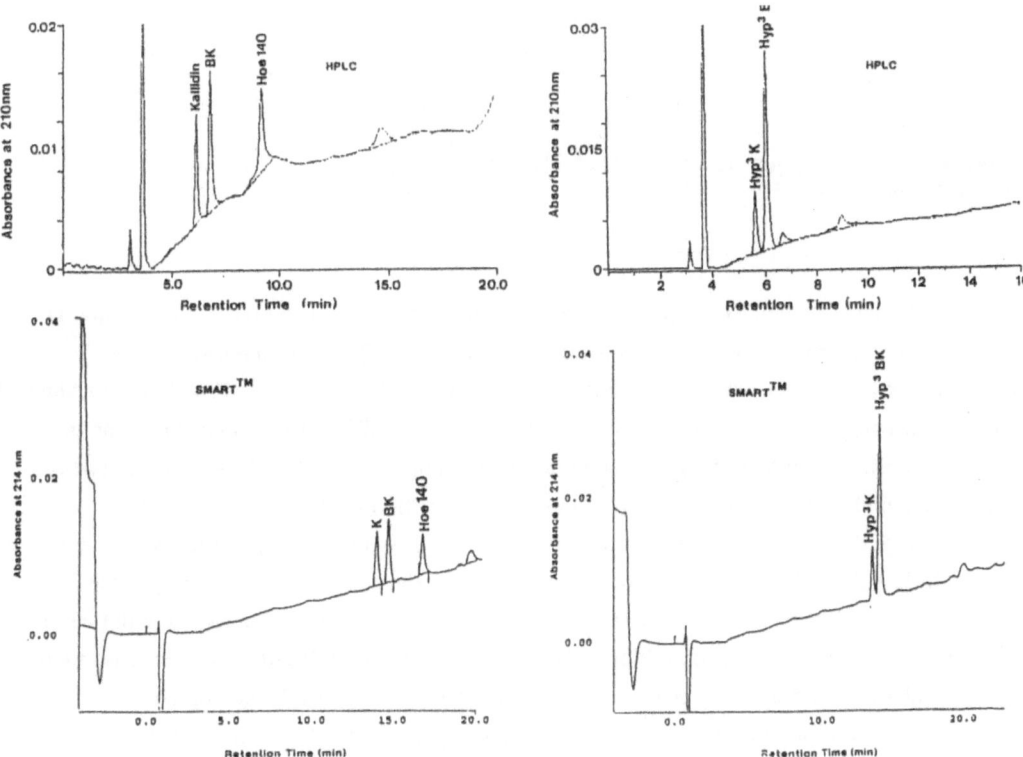

Figure 1. High performance liquid chromatography of kallidin (K), bradykinin (BK) and Hoe 140, and Hyp³ kallidin and Hyp³ BK. Peaks represent 50 ng of kinin injected.

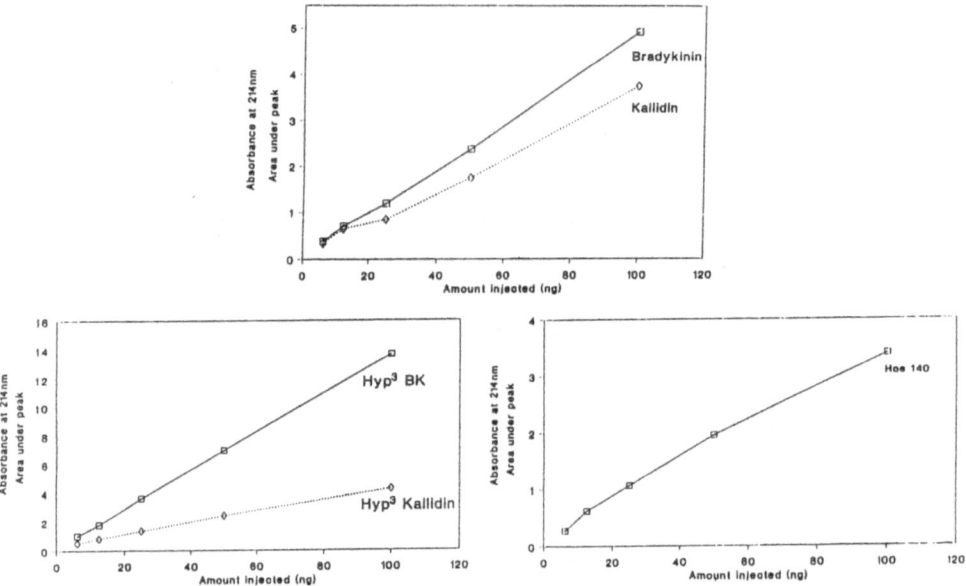

Figure 2. Dose–response relationships of BK, kallidin, Hyp³ BK, Hyp³ kallidin and Hoe 140 measured on SMART™ system. Values show mean of duplicate measurements.

The acid–alcohol extraction followed by dialysis resulted in an efficient purification of the SF, with the protein concentration being reduced from 40.2 mg/ml to 33.4 µg/ml by that treatment. Studies using SF with inhibitors spiked with 1 ng/µl synthetic BK and kallidin showed that the recovery for the synthetic kinins was approximately 80% for this procedure. The trace obtained for measurement of the RA SF with inhibitors on the SMART™ showed that peaks due to the inhibitors were also present, but none had retention times corresponding to those of the measured synthetic kinins. Spiking a proportion of each sample with standards (synthetic BK and kallidin) allowed assessment of precise recovery for the extraction procedure in each case.

The stability of Hoe 140 in pooled RA SF was investigated and compared with that of synthetic BK under the same conditions. The results are shown in figure 3 and demonstrate that after incubation for only 6 h at 37ºC, BK was completely metabolised. No degradation of a similar concentration of Hoe 140 occurred during this period, and furthermore, Hoe 140 was not degraded after 96 h in SF. In fact, Hoe 140 was still present even after a 2 week incubation. The results shown were all performed in spun, cell–free SF, but similar studies using SF to which cells had been added, and also with one fresh, un–spun SF showed no degradation of Hoe 140 in a 72 h period of incubation.

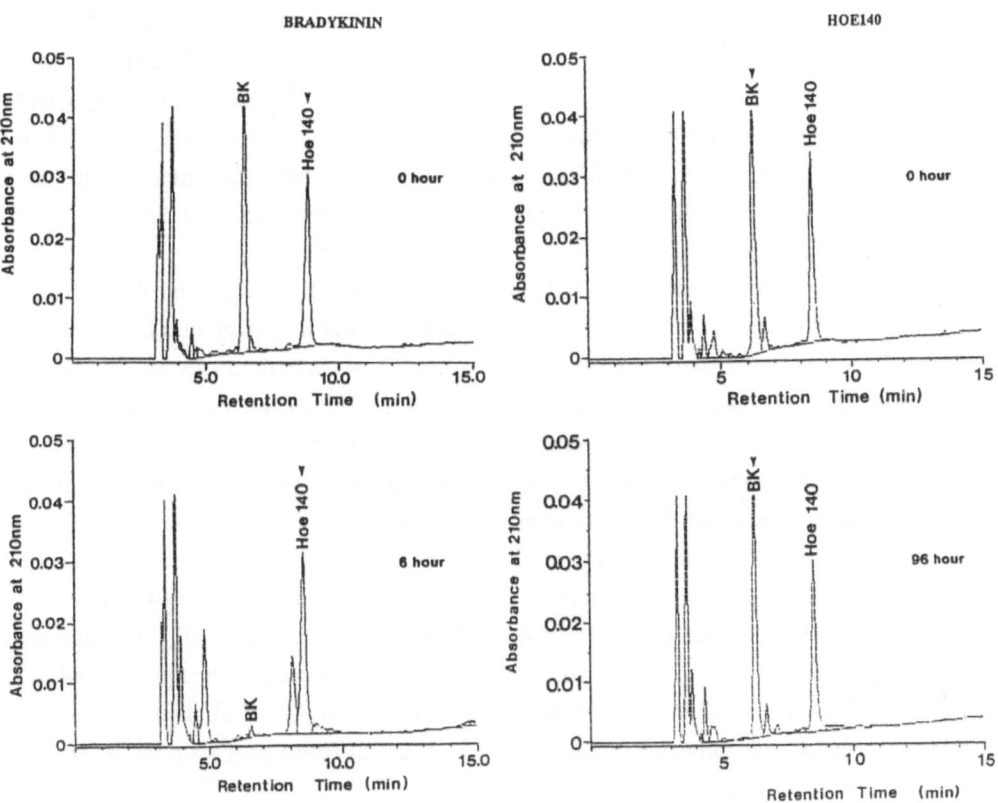

Figure 3. Metabolism of synthetic bradykinin (BK) and Hoe 140 after incubation in pooled RA SF at 37°C.   Arrows indicate internal standards.

DISCUSSION

Detection and precise values for free kinins in biological fluids is necessary in order to assess their role in inflammation. In order to achieve this objective two steps are necessary: firstly, the collection of the fluid and extraction of the endogenous kinins. This collection step must include the inactivation of kinin metabolising and forming enzymes, immediately after sample collection in order to maintain steady state kinin levels. Secondly, confirmation of kinin detection by HPLC must be carried out by radio immunoassay (RIA) or bioassay with the activity inhibited by a kinin antagonist.

This study describes methods for the collection of SF and extraction of kinins, and the subsequent separation of individual kinins (BK and kallidin) in the sample by SMART™ and Gilson HPLC systems. Future work must involve collection of the kinin HPLC fractions, and their subsequent measurement by a kinin ELISA (Enzyme–linked immunosorbant assay), which is necessary for the further characterisation and quantification of each kinin moiety in SF. Data collected for the levels of each kinin in SF from patients with different arthropathies (rheumatoid, osteo and psoriatic arthritis) will provide an insight into the role of individual kinins in inflammatory joint disease.

The first antagonists were successfully synthesised in 1985 by Stewart and Vavrek (6) by replacing proline in position 7 of BK with a D amino acid. Numerous antagonists have since been synthesised and such compounds antagonise many BK effects, both in vitro and in vivo. The usefulness of these molecules in therapy has, however, proved somewhat limited to date due to their susceptibility to fast enzymatic degradation. The new antagonist, Hoe 140, has been demonstrated to be a specific and potent BK2 receptor antagonist in vitro (7) and in vivo (8). This study clearly demonstrates that Hoe 140 has overcome the problem of enzymatic degradation in SF, by the substitution of several unnatural amino acids into its structure. The conditions used in this study were similar to those that may be encountered within the joint, except in the unlikely event of a synovial membrane kininase not occuring in SF. Therefore, the true stability of Hoe 140 in the inflamed joint will only become apparent in the light of clinical studies. The importance of kinins in the pathogenesis of RA and other inflammatory joint diseases will only become fully apparent with the clinical use of Hoe 140 or a similar potent kinin antagonist.

ACKNOWLEDGEMENTS

We thank the Arthritis and Rheumatism council for financial support. We are grateful to Dr. E. Hill, S. Cresswell and A. Davies from Pharmacia LKB.

REFERENCES

1. Armstrong D, Jepson JP, Keele KA, Stewart JW. Pain producing substance in human inflammatory exudates and plasma. J. Physiol 1957; 135: 350-370.

2. Eisen V. Plasma kinins in synovial exudates. Br J Exp Pathol 1970; 51: 322-327.

3. Melmon KL, Webster ME, Goldfinger SE, Seegmiller JE. The presece of kinins in inflammatory synovial effusions from arthritides of varying etiologies. Arth Rheum 1967; 10: 13-20.

4. Kaplan AP. Kinins and bone resorption in rheumatic disease. Arth Rheum 1987; 30: 589-592.

5. Sheikh IA, Kaplan AP. Assessment of kininases in the rheumatic diseases and the effects of therapeutic agents. Arth Rheum 1987; 30: 138-145.

6. Vavrek RJ, Stewart JM. Competitive antagonists of bradykinin. Peptides 1985; 6: 161-164.

7. Wirth K, Hock FJ, Albus U, Linz W, Alperman HG, Anagnostopoulos H, Henke S, Breipohl G, König W, Knolle J, Schölkens BA. Hoe 140 a new potent long-acting bradykinin antagonist: in vitro studies. Br J Pharmacol 1991; 102: 774-777.

8. Hock FJ, Wirth K, Albus U, Linz W, Gerhards HJ, Weimer G, Henke S, Breipohl G, König W, Knolle J, Schölkens BA. Hoe 140 is a new potent long-acting bradykinin antagonist: in vivo studies. Br J Pharmacol 1991: 769-773.

Localization of Kallikreins and Kininogens

AAS 38/I
Recent Progress on Kinins
© 1992 Birkhäuser Verlag Basel

IMMUNOVISUALISATION OF PLASMA PREKALLIKREIN AND H-KININOGEN ON HUMAN NEUTROPHILS AND IN HUMAN HEPATOCYTES

L.M. Henderson[1], C.D. Figueroa[2], W. Muller-Esterl[3], A. Stain[4], & K.D. Bhoola[5].

Departments of Biochemistry[1] and Pharmocology[5], University of Bristol, U.K.; Institute of Histology & Pharmacology[2], Austral University, Valdivia, Chile; Department of Pathobiochemistry[3], Institute of Physiological Chemistry, University of Mainz, Germany; Liver Unit[4], Queen Elizabeth Horpital and School of Biochemistry, University of Birmingham, U.K.

SUMMARY: Both plasma prekallikrein and H-kininogen were immunolocalised in human hepatocytes by the use of immunocytochemical techniques in conjunction with the confocal optical scanning microscopy, In contrast, both proteins were demonstrated on the external surface of human blood neutrophils. However, detection of H-kininogen on non-fixed but not on fixed neutrophils with the anti-domain 6 antibody (directed at the prekallikrein binding site on H-kininogen), suggested that access to the epitope was blocked by the presence of the bound plasma prekallikrein. Therefore, we prepose that H-kininogen provides the binding site for plasma prekallikrein on circulating neutrophils.

INTRODUCTION

The occurrence of tissue kallikrein in human neutrophils, and both H- and L- kininogens on their exterior surface has been demonstrated previously through the use of immunocytochemical techniques (1, 2). The localization of tissue kallikrein was restricted to neutrophils, being undetectable in eosinophils, lymphocytes, macrophages, megakaryocytes and platelets (1). Plasma prekallikrein is synthesized in hepatocytes, and released into the circulation where it forms a 1:1 complex with H-kininogen.

The confocal optical scanning microscope is cabable of taking optical sections through whole cells or tissues in a non-invasive manner, as it collects the emitted fluorescence light from only within the plane of focus of the objective lens (3). This property of the microscope permits not only the immunological detection of antigens but also the determination of their location within a cell and on the external surface of the cell membrane. With the use of confocal microscopy, we have identified plasma prekallkrein (prePK) on H-kininogen (HK) attached to the plasma membrane of the neutrophil. In addition, we immunolocalised both H-kininogen and plasma prekallikrein in human hepatocytes.

MATERIALS AND METHODS

Isolation of human neutrophils: The neutrophils were isolated from human buffy coats obtained from the South West Regional Blood Transfusion Service, Southmead Hospital, Bristol. The red blood cells were removed by a 1 x g sedimentation in 1%(w/v) dextran in PBS (NaCl 137 mM, KCl 3 mM, Na2HPO4, 1.5 mM KH2PO4; pH 7.4). They were separated from other whole blood cells by spinning the resulting supernatant through Lymphoprep at 800 x g for 20 min. Any remaining red blood cells were removed by hypotonic lysis.

Preparation of cytoplasts from neutrophils: Cytoplasts are enucleated cells which lack the internal organelles of their parent neutrophils. They are right side out and retain most of the membrane characteristics of their parent cells (4, 5). They can be prepared from neutrophils on a Ficoll 70 step–gradient. The neutrophils were resuspended in 12.5% Ficoll 70 containing 5 μgml^{-1} cytochalasin B , 5 mM glucose and preincubated for 10 min at 37°C before being layered on top of a step–gradient consisting of 25% and 16% Ficoll 70, each containing 5 μgml^{-1} cytochalasin B and 5 mM glucose. The cytoplasts are harvested, by aspiration, from the 16– 12.5% interface after centrifugation at 81000 x g at 37°C for 1 h.

Isolation of hepatocytes: Hepaocytes were prepared from liver tissue, removed from adult human donors, but surgically trimmed prior to graft transplantation in paediatric patients (6). The trimmed segments were maintained aseptically at 4° C in a preservation fluid for about 12 to 24 h. The hepatocytes were isolated by sequential perfusion with HEPES (pH 7.4) and an enzyme solution (0.05% collagenase, 0.05% hyaluronidase, 0.1% dipase, 0.005% DNAase with 5 mM Ca Cl2) through catheters inserted into the blood vessels. The cell suspension containing dissociated cells was first filtered through a 60 μM nylon mesh and then the cells were harvested by centrifugation at 50 x g. All proceedures were performed aseptically.

Immunocytochemistry: The neutrophils were attached to round coverslips by a 1 x g sedimentation for 10 min. The hepatocytes were cytospun on to microscope slides. The cells were washed 3 times with PBS. The cells, if required, were fixed by treating them with 4% formaldehyde for 10 min. Non–fixed cells were treated with PBS. The cells were washed 3 x 5 min with PBS 1% (v/v) human IgG to block nonspecific binding to the Fc receptor. The cells were incubated with the primary antibody diluted in PBS containing 1% (v/v) human IgG for 2– 16 h; the anti plasma prekallikrein antibody (AS176) was used in a dilution of 1:500, and that for H–kininogen (HKL16, directed against residues 569–595) was used in a dilution of 1:100. Next the cells were washed again 3 x 5 min in PBS–1% (v/v) human IgG, before incubating them with the FITC labelled second antibody. The second antibodies used were all F(ab) fragments to prevent binding to the Fc receptors on the neutrophils. The cells were finally washed 2 x 5 min with PBS before being imaged on the confocal microscope. Controls slides with both no primary and no secondary antibody were included.

Reagents: Ficoll 70, cytochalasin B, FITC–labelled second antibody were purchased from Sigma Chemicals, U.K., Lymophoprep from Nycomed, U.K. and HEPES buffer from BDH, U.K.

RESULTS AND DISCUSSION

Antibodies have access to only the antigens/epitopes exposed on the exterior of a non–fixed cell. Internal antigens and epitopes are only accessible following permeabilisation of the plasma membrane. The polyclonal rabbit anti–plasma prekallikrein antibody AS176 gave an annular pattern of staining on non–fixed neutrophils (Plate 1 a, b). The pattern of staining was more extensive on formaldehyde fixed neutrophils. This result demonstrates the presence of plasma prekallikrein on the exterior of the neutrophil plasma membrane. Using AS176 antibody, plasma prekallikrein was also detected on non–fixed and fixed cytoplasts, which have only a plasma membrane, thereby confirming their location on the external surface of the neutrophil. The monoclonal anti H–kininogen antibody HKL16 was raised to residues 569–595 of domain 6. This is the region reported to be involved in the binding to plasma prekallikrein. Using this antibody we failed to detect H–kininogen on non–fixed neutrophils (Plate 1 c). However, H–kininogen has previously been detected on neutrophils using other antibodies and was detected with HKL16 on formaldehyde fixed neutrophils (Plate 1 d).and fixed cytoplasts (Plate 1 e). The failure to detect H–kininogen using HKL16 suggests that the access to the epitope is blocked on non–fixed neutrophils. Therefore, we propose that HKL16 epitope is blocked due to the binding of plasma prekallikrein to domain 6 of H–kininogen.

Both plasma kallikrein and its endogenous substrate H–kininogen were immunolocalised in isolated hepatocytes (Plate 1 f, g) by confocal microscopy, and in sections of human liver by light microscopy.

CONCLUSION

We have demonstrated the presence of plasma prekallikrein complexed to domain 6 of H–kininogen on blood neutrophils. The plasma prekallikrein binding site on H–kininogen is not accessible on non–fixed neutrophils. Therefore, we propose that H–kininogen acts as the plasma kallikrein carrier on the circulating human neutrophil. These molecules, present on the surface of the neutrophil, may be involved in the local release of kinins and the diapedesis of neutrophils between endothelial cells.

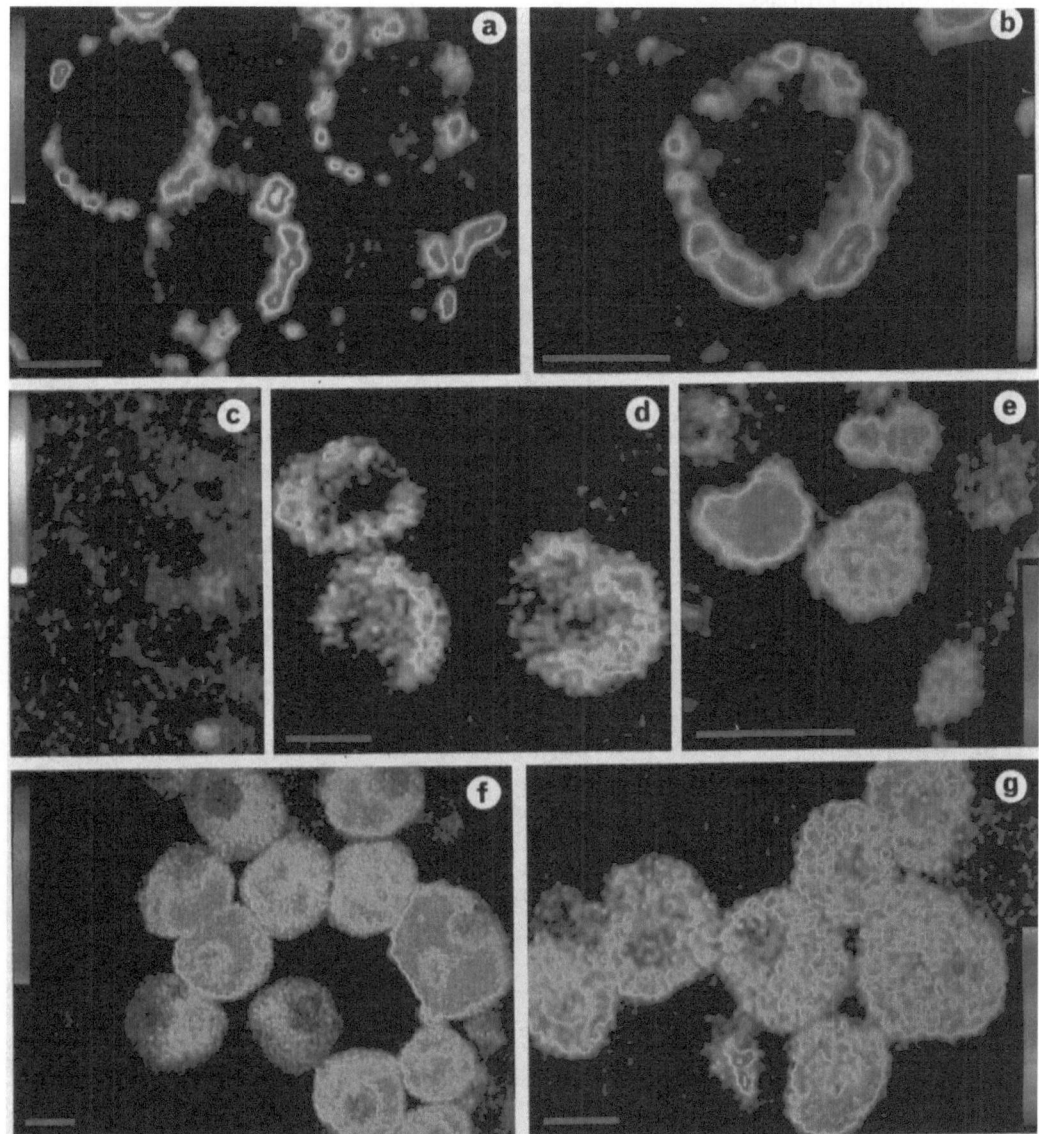

Plate 1. Images taken with the confocal laser scanning microscope showing immunological reactivity to prePK and HK.

a and b) plasma prekallikrein (AS176) on the membrane of non–fixed neutrophils; H–kininogen (HKL16, anti HK–domain 6 antibody) c) on non–fixed neutrophils and d) on fixed neutrophils and e) on fixed cytoplasts; f) plasma prekallikrein (AS176) in human hepatocytes; g) H–kininogen (HKL16) in human hepatocytes.

The fluorescent colour intensity ranged from blue (nil), green (minimal), yellow (moderate) and red/white (maximal). Bar indicates 5 μM.

ACKNOWLEDGMENTS

The confocal microscope and Dr. L.M. Henderson were funded by a Wellcome Trust grant to Profs J.B. Chappell and O.T.G. Jones, Department of Biochemistry, University of Bristol. KDB thanks the Medical Research Council (U.K.) for research grant support.

REFERENCES

1. Figueroa CD, MacIver AG, Bhoola KD. Identification of   immunoreactive tissue kallikrein in human polymorphonuclear leucocytes. Brit J Haemat 1989; 72:321–328.

2. Figueroa CD, Henderson LM, Kaufmann J, De la Cadena RA, Colman RW, Muller–Esterl W, Bhoola KD. Immunovisualisation of high (HK) and low (LK) molecular weight kininogens on isolated human neutrophils. Blood 1992; 79:754–759.

3. Shotton DM. Confocal scanning optical microscopy and its applications for biological specimens. J Cell Sci 1989; 94:175–206.

4. Roos D, Voetman AA, Meerhof LJ. Functional activity of enucleated human polymorphonuclear leukocytes J Cell Biol 1983; 97:368–377.

5. Henderson LM, Chappell JB, Jones OTG. The superoxide–generating NADPH oxidase of human neutrophils is electrogenic and associated with an H^+ channel. Biochem J 1988; 246:325–329.

6. Ismail I, Howl J, Wheatly M, McMaster P, Neuberger JM, Strain AJ. Hepatology 1991; 14:1076–1082.

AAS 38/I
Recent Progress on Kinins
© 1992 Birkhäuser Verlag Basel

LOCALIZATION OF KALLIKREIN GENE FAMILY
PROTEASES IN RAT TISSUES

J.A.V. Simson, J. Chao and L. Chao

Departments: Anatomy and Cell Biology, and Biochemistry and Molecular Biology,
Medical University of South Carolina, Charleston, S.C., USA

SUMMARY: Monoclonal antibodies specific for three kallikrein gene family enzymes (tissue kallikrein, esterase A and tonin) have been used to determine the tissue and cellular distributions of these proteases as well as their association with other relevant molecules (kininogen, kallikrein-binding protein, and Na,K-ATPase α-subunit). Secretion of these enzymes from salivary glands was also analyzed. The results of these localization studies provide important clues to the functions of different members of this closely related family of serine proteases.

INTRODUCTION

Tissue kallikrein, isolated from rodent salivary glands and kidney, is one of a sizeable group of genetically related serine proteases (1-4). The existence of kallikrein-like enzymes in salivary glands, pancreas and kidney has been known for several decades (5-8); their functional role in these glands continues to be a subject of intense investigation. Tissue kallikrein was initially believed to function in the production of vasoactive peptides in the stroma of secreting glands (9). As studies on the cellular localization of these enzymes have supplemented physiological and pharmacological studies, the proposed roles of tissue kallikrein, and members of its multigene family, have expanded. Mounting evidence suggests that, in addition to the production of vasoactive peptides, kallikreins are involved in a wide range of physiological processes including prohormone cleavage (1,10,11) and epithelial ion transport (probably via kinins) (12). The function of the enormous concentration and diversity of kallikrein gene family proteases within salivary glands, where these enzymes are found in greatest abundance, remains a biological enigma.

The questions posed in this overview of the tissue and cellular localization of tissue kallikrein gene family members are as follows. 1) Where are kallikreins expressed and localized in tissues and cells? 2) What does the localization and molecular associations of a kallikrein gene family member suggest about its function? The basic premise of cytochemistry, i.e., that cellular localization reflects function, has been highly productive in kallikrein investigations. Thus, the presence of kallikrein in transporting epithelium such as salivary gland ducts (7,13), kidney tubules (14,15), and gut epithelium (16) is consistent with an ion transporting role for either the enzyme itself or a peptide product. Likewise, the localization of kallikrein-like enzymes in peptide hormone producing cells, such as pituitary (17), hypothalamic nuclei (neouronal cell aggregates) (18), and atrial myocytes (19, 20) is strong support for a role of these enzymes in proteolytic processing of hormone precursors. These observations expand the prohormone processing roles of kallikrein suggested initially by genetic studies (1).

We have examined the tissue and cellular localization of three proteases of the rat kallikrein gene family (2,3) for which we have highly specific monoclonal antibodies (21,22). Kallikrein, tonin and esterase A have been localized in two transporting epithelia, salivary glands and kidney. The tissue and cellular distribution of kallikrein has been compared to the distribution of other proteins relevant to kallikrein function: kininogen and kallikrein-binding protein (KBP), as well as to Na,KATPase. In addition, we have investigated secretion of kallikrein gene family enzymes from salivary glands in response to α- and β-adrenergic, and cholinergic agonists.

MATERIALS AND METHODS

Specific monoclonal antibodies have been generated that do not cross-react with other kallikrein gene family members in Western blots of salivary glands (21,22). These were used in an indirect immunoperoxidase method, as described previously (18-21, 23, 24) for localizing three kallikrein gene family members: tissue kallikrein, tonin, and esterase A. Buffered formaldehyde-fixed tissues were sectioned (5u) and incubated in primary antisera at dilutions of 1:50 or 1:100, for 2 hr at 25°C or overnight at 4°C, followed by peroxidase-conjugated goat or rabbit anti-mouse immunoglobulin antisera. Peroxidase was demonstrated by standard peroxidase cytochemistry with 3,3' diaminobenzidine and H_2O_2 as substrates. Polyclonal antisera were used for localizing kininogen (25), KBP (26) and Na,K-ATPase (27). Immunocytochemistry was performed as described previously for polyclonal antibodies (7,27), using either the immunoglobulin-enzyme bridge technique or an indirect immunoperoxidase method with peroxidase-conjugated goat anti-rabbit antiserum as the secondary antibody. In all cases, both positive and negative controls were run in every immunostaining experiment; several experiments were performed to confirm each observation. In saliva collection experiments, in anesthetized animals, the submandibular duct was cannulated, followed by arterial cannulation and perfusion with ringer's bicarbonate containing the secretagogue at appropriate concentration. Saliva and venous effluent were collected and analyzed for kallikrein-like TAME esterase activity.

RESULTS AND DISCUSSION

This paper summarizes results of previous studies performed on kallikreins in salivary glands and kidney (23,24) and includes new information on localization of rat kallikrein message, kininogen and KBP, and on secretion of kallikrein-like proteases from salivary glands.

Kallikreins in Salivary Glands and Kidney. Kallikrein, tonin, and esterase A are not identically distributed in salivary glands or kidney. In salivary glands, tissue kallikrein appears to be present in granules of essentially all submandibular gland granular convoluted tubule (GCT) cells, whereas tonin and esterase A are present in only a subpopulation of these cells (Figure 1a-c). Moreover, kallikrein is found in small, apical granules of striated duct cells in all three major salivary glands (7,13), whereas esterase A (23) and tonin are not (Table I). *In situ* hybridization, using a tissue kallikrein cDNA probe (3), revealed that kallikrein message is present in GCT cells and in a short segment of intralobular striated duct cells (Figure 1d) consistent with data obtained in mouse submandibular glands (28), but is not present further downstream in interlobular ducts. Since apical kallikrein is often present in the epithelium of interlobular striated ducts, this must represents secondary uptake of kallikrein from upstream sources. When the distribution of tissue kallikrein and Na,K-ATPase are compared in parotid striated ductal cells, kallikrein is in apical granules (13), whereas Na,K-ATPase is associated with basal membranes (24). Electron microscopic immunogold studies indicate that the two enzymes do not overlap intracellularly (29).

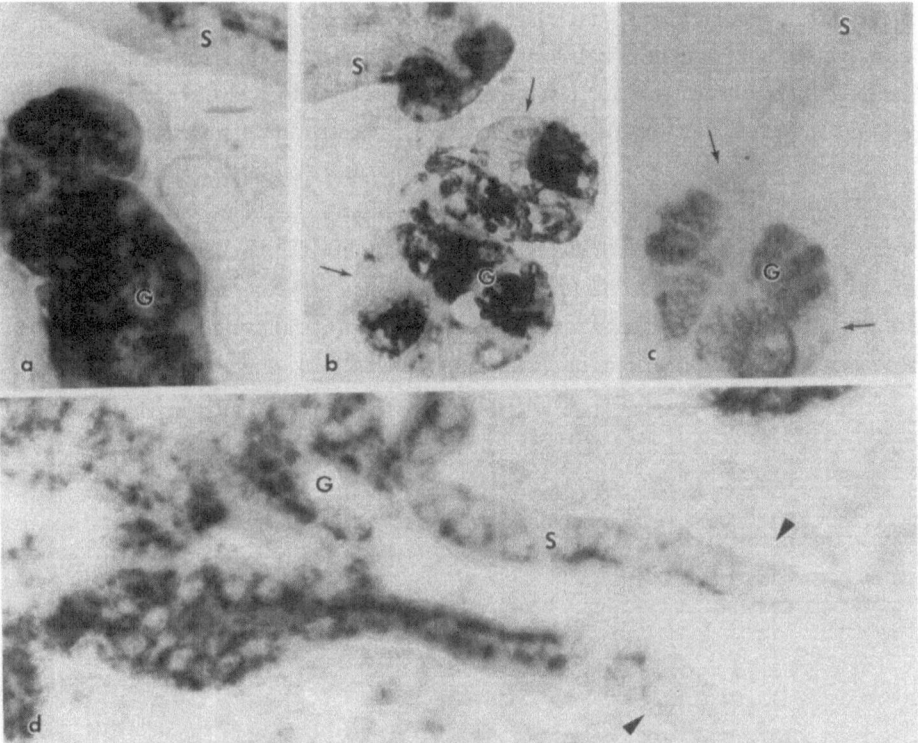

Figure 1. Rat submandibular gland with GCT (G) and striated duct (S) segments: immunostaining with monoclonal antibodies for: **a**) kallikrein **b**) tonin and **c**) esterase A; and **d**) *in situ* hybridization with kallikrein cDNA. Note in **b** & **c** the presence of unstained GCT cells (arrows), and in **d**, the transition between striated duct cells with and without message (arrowheads). (**a-c** X600; **d** X800).

Table 1. Monoclonal antibody staining of rat salivary glands for kallikrein gene family proteases*

| | Submandibular | | Parotid | Sublingual |
	GCT	SD	SD	SD
Anti-kallikrein V_4D_{11} & V_4G_6	++++	++ς	++ς	++ς
Anti-tonin $1F_{11}$	+++	-	-	-
Anti-esterase.A $6C_{11}$ & $5A_{10}$	++	+/-ς	+/-ς	+/-ς

* Scoring of stain from "not above control background" (-) to "very high" (++++) includes both intensity and distribution of staining. GCT= granular convoluged tubules; SD= striated ducts ⸗apical staining; ς basal staining.

In epithelia of kidney, kallikrein is present primarily in the apical region of distal/connecting tubules (Figure 2a). Its apical location in kidney (7,14,24) suggests a role for kallikrein or kinins in apical transport or permeability, rather than in basal transport. Esterase A (24) by contrast, is present primarily in straight tubules of medullary rays and outer medulla (Figure 2b), overlapping the Na,K-ATPase (27) distribution (Figure 2c). No staining in kidney has been seen with our monoclonal antibodies for tonin. Thus, in kidney, kallikrein is strategically placed to modify permeability of the apical membrane of connecting tubules and/or cortical collecting ducts, an important site of mineralocorticoid action, whereas esterase A overlaps vasopressin-dependent sites in thick straight tubules (30).

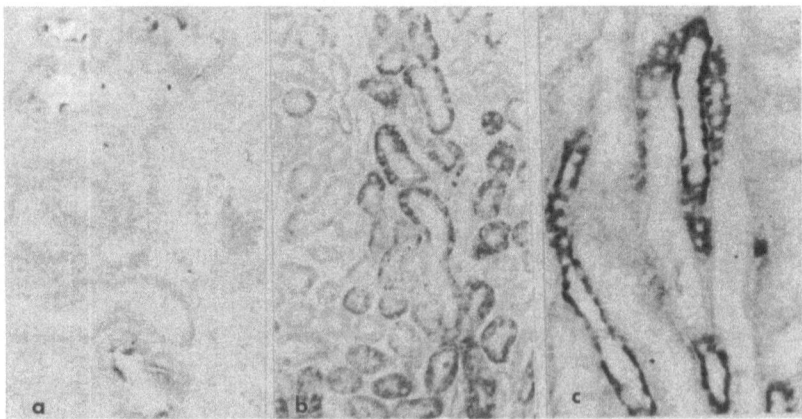

Figure 2. Kidney, a) interlobular zone, b,c) outer medulla/medullary rays. Immunostaining for: a) kallikrein, b) esterase A, and c) Na,K-ATPase. (a,c X300; b X160)

Distribution of Kininogen and Kallikrein-Binding Protein (KBP). Other components of the
tissue kallikrein system have also been studied. Using polyclonal antibodies for kininogen (25)
and KBP (26), both have been found primarily extracellularly in the stroma of submandibular
glands, around interlobular ducts and at the base of GCT cells (figure 3a,b). Some kininogen
staining is in endothelium, although some apparently represents substrate bound to connective
tissue. Kininogen is also present in kidney, in both vasculature and cortical collecting tubules
(Figure 3c), whereas KBP is found exclusively in stroma and the lumen of blood-vessels, but not
in epithelia (not shown). Since both kininogen and KBP appear extracellular in those tissues in
which kallikrein gene family proteases are intracellular, we also suspect endocrine/paracrine (i.e.,
stromal) release of these enzymes, as suggested in other studies (15).

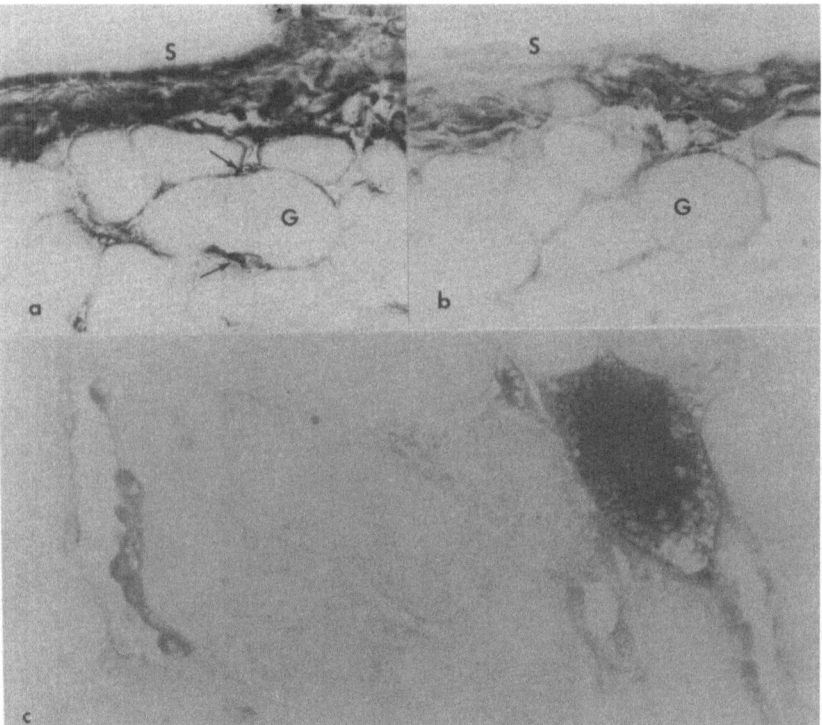

Figure 3. Immunostaining with polyclonal antibodies in submandibular gland for: a) kininogen
and b) KBP; and c) in kidney for kininogen. Note the stromal immunoreactivity for both
kininogen and KBP around interlobular striated duct (S) and GCT (G). In a, capillary
endothelium (arrows) around GCT is intensely stained for kininogen. In c) the stained collecting
tubule on the right abuts on a vein near the cortico-medullary junction. a, b (X300); c (X400).

Salivary Kallikrein Secretion. Preliminary studies on secretion of salivary kallikreins reveal several interesting differences in the pattern of release of these enzymes from their storage sites. Both biochemical and histochemical evidence strongly suggest that, although most secretion is apical, at least some of the enzymes are secreted basolaterally in submandibular glands (Table 2; Figure 4), which would bring the enzyme into contact with kininogen substrate. Of interest are several observations: phenylephrine (α-adrenergic) stimulated maximum release of kallikrein from GCT cells, but not from striated duct cells, whereas isoproterenol (β-adrenergic) elicited loss of kallikrein from the apex of striated duct cells, but was much less potent than phenylephrine in eliciting secretion from GCT cells. Pilocarpine resulted in demonstrable loss of immunoreactivity for kallikrein and esterase A, but not for tonin in GCT cells (Figure 4). Taken together, these results suggest that, although all rat kallikrein gene family members so far characterized may be found in GCT cells of submandibular salivary glands, they are apparently individually regulated in terms both of synthesis and secretion.

Table 2. TAME esterase released from secretagogue-stimulated submandibular glands*

Secretagogue	time interval	Venous effluent EU/min	Saliva EU/ml	Total EU/interval
Phenylephrine	0-30 min	5.1	13.4	555
	30-60 min	3.9	2.3	186
Acetylcholine	0-25 minutes	0.4	5.1	138
	25-60 min	0.3	1.1	49
Isoproterenol	0-65 min	#	1.9	#

*Esterase was measured using tosyl arginine methyl ester (TAME) as substrate. One esterase unit (EU) is equivalent to the cleavage of 1 umole TAME/min. # Venous effluent was not collected

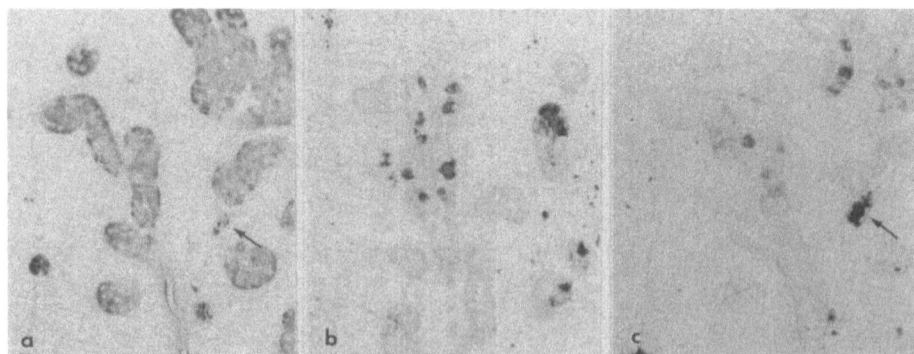

Figure 4. Pilocarpine stimulated (1 hr) submandibular gland: sequential sections stained with monoclonal antibodies to a) kallikrein, b) tonin and c) esterase A. Kallikrein and esterase A staining intensity is decreased in GCT cells (a,c), whereas tonin immunoreactivity remains strong (b). Note also immunoreactivity in vascular channels (a, c, arrows). (X160).

CONCLUSION

Immunocytochemical localization provides an important added dimension to biochemical and physiological data concerning the distribution and function of kallikrein gene family members. We have found that, in salivary glands and kidney, the distribution of three kallikrein gene family members differ at the cellular level. Kallikrein is positioned to act apically in transporting epithelia, whereas esterase A is generally basolateral. In salivary glands, some kallikreins are secreted into the stromal/vascular compartment during stimulated secretion. Kallikrein, tonin and esterase A exhibit a differential response to secretagues. The ability to combine the powerful reagents and tools of biochemistry and molecular biology with the visual and integrating power of morphology allows a more complete understanding of the tissue kallikrein system as a whole.

ACKNOWLEDGEMENTS: Several individuals in addition to the authors have contributed importantly to these studies: J. Condon, R. Williams, J. King, L.-M. Chen, M. Tillman, and Drs. C. Woodley-Miller, S. Murray, J. R. Martinez, and K. Geering. Supported in part by NIH grant #RO1 DE09731, HL 29737 and Fogarty International Fellowship #F06 TW01292.

REFERENCES

1. Shine J, Mason AJ, Evans BA and Richards RI. The kallikrein multigene family: specific processing of biologically active peptides. Cold Spring Harbor Symp Quant Biol 1983; 48:419-426.
2. Gerald WL, Chao J, Chao L. Immunological identification of rat tissue kallikrein cDNA and characterization of the kallikrein gene family. Biochim Biophys Acta 1986; 866:1-14.
3. Murray, SR, Chao J, Lin F-K, Chao L. Kallikrein multigene families and the regulation of their expression. J Cardiovasc Pharmacol 1990; 15 (suppl 6):S7-S16.
4. Clements JA. The glandular kallikrein family of enzymes: tissue specific expression and hormonal regulation. Endocr Rev 1989; 10:393-419.
5. Werle E. Kallikrein, kallidin and related substances. In: Polypeptides Which Affect Smooth Muscle and Blood Vessels. M. Schacter, Ed. Pergamon Press, Oxford 1960; pp 199-209.
6. Orstavik TB, Brandtzaeg P, Nustad K, Halvorsen KM. Cellular localization of kallikreins in rat submandibular and sublingual salivary glands. Acta Histochem 1975: 54:183-192.
7. Simson JAV, Spicer SS, Chao J, Grimm L, Margolius HS. Kallikrein localization in rodent salivary glands and kidney with the immunoglobulin-enzyme enzyme bridge technique. J Histochem Cytochem 1979; 27:1567-1576.
8. Schachter M. Kallikreins (kininogenases) - a group of serine proteases with bioregulatory actions. Pharmacol Rev 1979; 31:1-17.
9. Hilton SM, Lewis GP. The relationship between glandular activity, bradykinin formation and functional vasodilatation in the submandibular salivary gland. J. Physiol 1956; 134:471-483.
10. Bothwell MA, Wilson WH, and Shooter EM. The relationship between glandular kallikrein and growth factor-processing proteases of mouse submaxillary gland. J Biol Chem 1979; 254:7287-7294.
11. Currie MG, Geller DM, Chao J, Margolius HS, Needleman P. Kallikrein activation of a high molecular weight atrial peptide. Biochem Biophys Res Commun 1984 120:461-466.
12. Cuthbert AW, Margolius HS. Kinins stimulate net chloride secretion by the rat colon. Br J Pharmac 1982; 75:587-598.
13 Simson JAV, Fenters R, and Chao J. Electron microscopic immunostaining of kallikrein in rat submandibular glands. J Histochem Cytochem 1983; 31:301-306.

14. Orstavik TB, Inagami T Localization of kallikrein in the rat kidney and its anatomical relationship to renin. J Histochem Cytochem 1982; 30:385-390.
15. Vio CP, Figueroa CD Subcellular localization of renal kallikrein by ultrastructural immunocytochemistry. Kidney Int 1985; 28:36-42
16. Schachter M, Peret MW, Billing AG, and Wheeler GD. Immunolocalization of the protease kallikrein in the colon. J Histochem Cytochem 1983; 31:1255-1260.
17. Powers CA, Nasjletti A. A kininogenase resembling glandular kallikrein in the rat pituitary pars intermedia. Endocrinology 1983; 112:1194-1200.
18. Simson JAV, Dom R, Chao J, Woodley C, Chao L, Margolius HS. Immunocytochemical localization of tissue kallikrein in brain ventricular epithelium and hypothalamic cell bodies. J Histochem Cytochem 1985; 33:951-953.
19. Simson JAV, Currie MG, Chao L and Chao J. Co-localization of a kallikrein-like serine protease (arginine esterase A) and atrial natriuretic peptide in rat atrium. J Histochem Cytochem 1989; 37:1913-1917.
20. Xiong W, Chen L-M, Woodley-Miller C, Simson JAV, Chao J. Identification, purification and localization of tissue kallikrein in rat heart. Biochem J 1990; 267:639-646.
21. Woodley CM, Chao J, Simson JA, Margolius HS, Chao L. A monoclonal antibody to rat tissue kallikrein: use in biochemical and immunohistochemical studies. Kinins IV: Adv Exper Biol Med 1986; 198B:503-513.
22. Chao J, Chao L. Identification and expression of kallikrein gene family in rat submandibular and prostate glands using monoclonal antibodies as specific probes. Biochim Biophys Acta 1987; 910:233-239.
23. Simson JAV, Condon J, Fenters R, Chao L, and Chao J. Immunocytochemical localization of a kallikrein-like serine protease (esterase A) in rat salivary glands. Anat Rec 1988; 221:475-481.
24. Simson JAV, Condon Jl, Chao L, and Chao J. Comparison of the distribution of tissue kallikrein and esterase A, a kallikrein-like enzyme, in rat kidney using specific monoclonal antibodies. J Histochem Cytochem 1988; 36:1251-1254.
25. Chao S, Chao L, Chao J. Sex dimorphism and inflammatory regulation of T-kininogen and T-kininogenase. Biochim Biophys Acta 1989; 991:477-483.
26. Chao J, Chai KX, Chen L-M, Xiong W, Chao S, Woodley-Miller C, Wang L, Lu HS, Chao L. Tissue kallikrein-binding protein is a serpin. 1. Purification, characterization, and distribution in normotensive and spontaneously hypertensive rats. J Biol Chem 1990; 265:16394-16401.
27. Graves JS, Inabnett T, Geering K and Simson JAV. Cross-reactivity of an antiserum to the a-subunit of the Na+,K+-ATPase of toad (Bufo marinus) kidney with basal and apical membranes of transporting epithelia of the rat. Cell Tiss Res 1989; 258:137-145.
28. Penschow JD, Haralambidis J and Coghlan JP. Locaton of glandular kallikrein mRNAs in mouse submandibular gland at the cellular and ultrastructural level by hybridization histochemistry using 32P- and 3H-labeled oligodeoxyribonucleotide probes. J Histochem Cytochem 1991; 39:835-842.
29. Simson JAV, Chao J. Subcellular distribution of a regulated secretory protein (tissue kallikrein) and a basal membrane protein (Na$^+$,K$^+$-ATPase α-subunit in rat parotid striated duct cells. (submitted for publication).
30. Madsen KM, Verlander JW, Tisher CC. Relationship between structure and function in distal tubule and collecting duct. J Electron Mic Tech 1988; 9:187-208.

AAS 38/I
Recent Progress on Kinins
© 1992 Birkhäuser Verlag Basel

HORMONAL REGULATION OF PITUITARY GLANDULAR KALLIKREIN: A MORPHOMETRIC STUDY

Jorge P. Roa, C. Andrew Powers and Carlos P. Vio

Laboratory of Cell Physiology and Pathology, Department of Physiology, Pontificia Universidad Católica de Chile, Santiago, Chile. Department of Pharmacology, New York Medical College, New York, USA

SUMMARY: We have previously identified the lactotrophs as the Glandular Kallikrein (GK) containing cells in the rat anterior pituitary using immunocytochemistry, this localization has been independently confirmed with similar methods by other groups. The purpose of the present work was to evaluate the estrogen and dopaminergic control of the GK-containing cells using a morphometric analysis.

Female (200-250 g) ovariectomized rats (n=40) were treated with estradiol (5, 10, 50 µg/rat) in the presence or absence of haloperidol (2.5 mg/Kg). The pituitaries were fixed by perfusion with Bouin's and immunostained for prolactin (PRL) or GK. The number of cells and the intensity of the staining were determined by morphometric analysis.

Little GK staining was observed in pituitaries from ovariectomized rats, whereas estradiol treatment produced a marked increase in GK staining; GK-positive lactotrophs increased from 4% in control to 75% with 5 µg of estradiol, higher doses produced little further increase. However, GK staining intensity in lactotrophs was markedly dependent upon estradiol dose increasing 4-fold between 5 µg and 50 µg. Haloperidol (2.5 mg/Kg) elicited weak GK staining in 46% of the lactotrophs in the absence of estradiol, and potentiated GK staining intensity elicited with low doses of estradiol.

Estradiol also produced a dose-dependent increase in pituitary mass and % lactotrophs indicating lactotroph proliferation. Estradiol produced a dose dependent increase in pituitary wet weight, % PRL-positive cells and % GK-positive cells. Pituitary weight was correlated with % lactotrophs (r=0.992), and % GK cells (r=0.874), and % lactotrophs was correlated with % GK cells (r=0.978). Haloperidol slightly increased pituitary weight, % PRL or % GK cells at all estrogen doses.

The results show that estrogen induction of rat anterior pituitary GK appears likely to involve a primary action to increase GK synthesis and intracellular levels in most lactotrophs, and that the dopamine receptor blockade with haloperidol has a modulator effect.

INTRODUCTION

Glandular Kallikrein (GK) (EC 3.4.21.35) is a serine proteinase which hydrolyses, by limited proteolisis, the plasmatic low molecular weight kininogen to release the vasoactive peptide, kallidin (1). It is well known that GK is widely distributed in the body (eg. pancreas, kidney, submandibular gland, etc.), therefore it is presume that GK may play other important physiological role besides the production of kinins.

It has been demonstrated that GK-like enzymatic activity is present in the rat anterior pituitary. This enzyme possesses properties identical to GK from rat urine or renal cortex and predominantly exists as a latent zymogen that can be activated in vitro, by trypsin (2). The anterior pituitary GK is 20 times higher in females than males owing to powerful induction by ovarian estrogen. GK mRNA has also been demonstrated in the anterior pituitary and its levels are sex-dependent and estrogen-induced (3). Chronic dopamine receptor blockade with haloperidol has been demonstrated to more than double GK enzyme activity, mRNA and gene transcription in the anterior pituitary. The dual estrogen and dopaminergic regulation of anterior pituitary GK parallels that of prolactin (PRL) suggesting a localization in PRL-producing cells. By using an immunocytochemical method, we and other independent studies (4-6), have identified lactotrophs as the GK-containing cells in the rat anterior pituitary. The coregulation and colocalization of GK with PRL in lactotrophs has suggested a functional interrelationship of some kind. Recent studies have documented that GK can process PRL in vitro to novel forms which appear to correspond to novel estrogen-dependent PRL variants present in vivo (7).

Although the estrogen and dopaminergic regulation of lactotroph GK is now well documented, the cellular mechanisms involved in this regulation has not been established. Examination of the estrogen induction and dopaminergic repression of anterior pituitary GK at a cellular level is one approach to address this issue. Thus, we report here a morphometric, immunocytochemical study of pituitaries from rats treated with various doses of estrogen in the presence or absence of haloperidol.

MATERIALS AND METHODS

3-5 month old virgin female Sprague-Dawley rats (200-250 g) (n=40) were ovariectomized under ether anesthesia and were housed in groups of five (8 groups) in a constant temperature (22 $^\circ$C), light controlled (lights on daily from 08:00 h-20:00 h) room with free access to food and water. Two weeks later they were treated for 10 days with estradiol (5, 10 and 50 µg, 48 h, s.c.) with or without haloperidol (2.5 mg/kg/day, i.m.). The anterior pituitaries were removed, weighted, split and fixed in Bouin's fluid (24-48 h), dehydrated in alcohol, embedded in paraplast and methacrylate (6 µm and 1 µm sections). The sections were immunostained for GK or PRL by the unlabeled method as previously described (4). The antibodies and PAP complexes were diluted in buffer (Tris 0.05 M, pH 7.6, 0.7% lambda carrageenan, 0.25% Triton X-100). The tissue was incubated for 24-48 h with primary antisera GK (1: 2.000) or PRL (1:10.000), second antibody (1:20) for 30 min, PAP complex (1:150) for 30 min, DAB-H_2O_2 for 14 min and counterstained with hematoxylin.

The population of GK and PRL-immunoreactive cells were counted in paraplast sections, using a light microscope at a magnification of x 200 in sample areas delineated by an ocular squared grid (0.16 mm^2) and expressed as cells per mm^2 of area. Their percentages were calculated in relation to the whole cell population. The cells were counted in five sections from each rat of each experimental group, and only cells with nuclear profile and clearly defined borders were counted. The intensity of GK immunostaining within the cells was estimated by a "blind observer" with a single ordinal ranking (1 to 5), being 1 a faint staining and 5 the strongest staining. Results were analyzed by one-way analysis of variance, with differences between means determined by using Newman-Keuls' test.

RESULTS

Estradiol produced a dose-dependent increase in pituitary wet weight, % lactotrophs and % GK positive cells. Increase in pituitary weight was correlated with increase in % lactotrophs (r=0.992), and % GK positive cells (r=0.874). Similarly, the increase in % lactotrophs was correlated with increase in GK positive cells (r=0.978). Haloperidol slightly increased pituitary weight and % PRL positive and % GK positive cells in all treatment groups. The haloperidol effect on pituitary wet weight was similar at all estrogen levels. The greatest effect of haloperidol on % lactotrophs was observed at 0 and 5 µg estradiol doses, and on % GK positive was on the 0 µg control group. Only 4% of the lactotrophs stained for GK in the absence of estradiol or haloperidol. 5 µg estradiol increased this percentage to 75% and further increase in estradiol doses produced little further increase in this %. In the absence of estradiol, haloperidol increased the % GK positive lactotrophs from 4% to 46%, but it had little effect on the % of GK positive lactotrophs in the presence of estradiol (Table 1).

TABLE 1: Effects of differents doses of estradiol with and without haloperidol on Glandular Kallikrein (GK) and Prolactin (PRL) immunoreactive cells, and pituitary wet weight in female rats.

Treatment	%GK	%PRL	%GK /%PRL	weight(mg)
E_0	1.2	28.6	0.04	8.7±0.3
E_0H	16.0	35.0	0.45	12.8±0.3
E_5	36.8	49.1	0.75	13.7±0.5
E_5H	41.2	56.1	0.73	17.2±1.6
E_{10}	42.3	61.3	0.69	16.9±0.7
$E_{10}H$	51.0	64.9	0.79	20.2±0.6
E_{50}	55.4	66.1	0.84	19.5±1.6
$E_{50}H$	63.9	68.2	0.94	25.4±0.8

E= 17 ß-Estradiol (5, 10, 50 µg)   H= Haloperidol (2.5 mg/Kg)

Estradiol produced a dose-dependent increase in GK-staining intensity in individual pituitary cells. In the absence of estradiol stimulation, GK immunoreactivity was virtually undetectable; weak brown staining was seen with the 5 μg estradiol dose, and this staining deepened to dark brown and black, and included a larger cellular area as the estradiol dose increased further. Each estrogen dose produced a significant increase in GK-staining intensity above the previous dose, and the staining intensity achieved with 50 μg estradiol was 4-fold greater than that achieved with 5 μg. In the absence of estradiol, haloperidol elicited weak GK-staining below that achieved with the lowest dose of estradiol. Haloperidol enhanced GK-staining intensity achieved with the two lower doses of estradiol, but had no effect on GK-staining intensity at the highest estradiol dose (Table 2).

Table 2: Intensity of kallikrein immunostaining (I_{GK}).

Treatment	E_0	E_0H	E_5	E_5H	E_{10}	$E_{10}H$	E_{50}	$E_{50}H$
I_{GK}	1.2±0.26	1.8±0.26	2.4±0.32	3.6±0.32	3.2±0.26	3.8±0.27	4.4±0.30	4.8±0.27

Values are means ± SEM

DISCUSSION

In a previous publication, we reported that kallikrein-positive cells in the anterior pituitary corresponded to prolactin-producing cells using an immunocytochemical technique. The present work was done to evaluate the estrogen and dopaminergic control by a morphometric, immunocytochemical analysis. The present results confirm that GK-positive cells in the anterior pituitary are invariably lactotrophs. Very few lactotrophs exhibit GK-immunostaining in the absence of estrogen, and estradiol produced a dose-dependent increase, in the number of GK-positive cells and in the GK staining intensity. The initial rise in the % GK-positive cells (increased from 4% in control to 75% with 5 μg of estradiol) probably reflects increase in GK levels above the detection limit rather than an estrogen-induced phenotype transition. On the other hand, estradiol produced a dose-dependent increase in pituitary mass closely correlated with increase in the percent of cells containing PRL. This increase in lactotroph proportion was paralleled by increase in the proportion of GK-positive cells. Haloperidol alone elicited weak but detectable GK immunostaining and increased the number of cells expressing kallikrein in response to estradiol and produced a marked enhancement of GK-staining intensity elicited by lower doses of estradiol. Thus, estrogen induction of lactotroph GK appears to be accomplish by two complimentary mechanisms. First, estrogen induces GK gene expression and protein synthesis in most lactotrophs, resulting in large increases in cellular GK levels. This is consistent with the present finding showing marked increases in GK staining intensity in individual lactotrophs, as well as previous reports of large increases in GK enzyme activity, immunoreactivity, and mRNA after estrogen treatment (2,3,8). Second, estradiol selectively stimulates lactotrophs proliferation - resulting in an increased number of cells in which GK can be induced. It is well known that estrogen can produce marked increases in lactotroph proliferation (9) and multiple lactotroph populations exist which vary in their secretory products (10). The effects of haloperidol support the concept that dopamine is primarily modulating estrogen effects on lactotroph kallikrein levels. The dopaminergic neuroendocrine input acts to inhibit GK induction by low to moderate estrogen levels - decreasing intracellular GK levels but producing little change in the percentage of GK-positive lactotrophs. This dopaminergic modulation may shift estrogen regulation of GK to physiological events associated with either large surges in estradiol levels, or sharp decreases in dopaminergic input.

The function of glandular kallikrein in the normal lactotrophs is not fully understood. Of the major pituitary hormones, only PRL shows an analogous pattern of regulation and the colocalization of GK with PRL in lactotrophs would be of particular interest in view of the reports that kallikrein may function to process PRL to novel forms in rat lactotrophs (7) and that proteolytic processing is essential before the growth-promoting or mitogenic actions of PRL can be expressed (11).

CONCLUSION

Estrogen induction of rat anterior pituitary GK appears likely to involve primary actions to increase GK synthesis and intracellular levels in most lactotrophs, effects which are modulated by dopaminergic neuroendocrine input. GK is the only member of its gene family known to be estrogen-induced. The tissue-specificity of the induction, together with the colocalization of GK with PRL, points to a role in lactotrophs - perhaps as a PRL processing protease.

ACKNOWLEDGEMENTS

This work was supported by grants Fondecyt 346/89, 32/90, NIH DK32783 and DIUC. We thank Maria Alcoholado and Nora Loyarte for their technical assistance.

REFERENCES

1.   MacDonald RJ, Margolius HS, Erdös EG: Molecular biology of tissue kallikrein. Biochem. J. 1988; 253: 313-321.

2.   Powers CA: Anterior pituitary glandular kallikrein: trypsin activation and estrogen regulation. Mol. Cell. Endocrinol. 1986; 46: 163-174.

3.   Clements JA, Fuller P, McNally M, Nikolaidis J, Funder J: Estrogen regulation of kallikrein gene expression in the rat anterior pituitary. Endocrinol. 1986; 119: 268-273.

4.   Vio CP, Roa JP, Silva R, Powers CA: Localization of immunoreactive glandular kallikrein in lactotrophs of the rat anterior pituitary. Neuroendocrinol. 1990; 51: 10-14.

5.   Jones TH, Figueroa CD, Smith C, Cullen DR, Bhoola KD: Characterization of a tissue kallikrein in human prolactin- secreting adenomas. J Endocrinol. 1990; 124:327-331.

6.   Kitagawa A, Kizuki K, Moriya H, Kudo M, Noguchi T: Kallikrein- and prolactin-producing cells in the rat anterior pituitary are the same. J Biochem. 1990; 108:971-975.

7.   Powers CA Hatala MH: Prolactin proteolysis by glandular kallikrein: In vitro reaction requirements and cleavage sites, and detection of processed prolactin in Vivo. Endocrinol. 1990; 127: 1916-1927.

8.   Chao J, Chao L Swain Ch Tsai J Margolius H: Tissue Kallikrein in rat brain and pituitary: Regional distribution and estrogen induction in the anterior pituitary. Endocrinol. 1987; 120: 475-482.

9.   Dannies PS: Control of prolactin production by estrogens. In: Litwack G (ed). Biochemical Actions of Hormones. Vol XII. Academic Press, New York, 1987: pp. 289-310.

10.   Frawley LS: Mammosomatotropes: currents status and possible functions. Trends Endocrinol Metabol 1989; 1: 31-34.

11.   Mittra J: Somatomedins and proteolytic bioactivation of prolactin and growth hormone. Cell 1984; 38: 347-348.

AAS 38/I
Recent Progress on Kinins
© 1992 Birkhäuser Verlag Basel

KALLIKREIN-PRODUCING CELLS IN THE RAT PITUITARY AND PINEAL GLAND

K. Kizuki, A. Kitagawa, K. Aoki, H. Moriya, T. Noguchi* and M. Kudo**

Department of Biochemistry, Science University of Tokyo, Tokyo 162, Japan. *Department of Physiology and **Department of Pathology, Toho University School of Medicine, Tokyo 143, Japan

SUMMARY: By using an immunohistochemical technique, kallikrein-producing cells in the anterior pituitary of rats were identified to be the same as prolactin-producing cells. Kallikrein was localized at the Golgi apparatus, the rough endoplasmic reticulum and secretory granules. Kallikrein was also located in the perivascular cells of the pineal gland.

INTRODUCTION

Kallikrein-like activity or immunoreactive tissue kallikrein has been reported in the pituitaries of rats(1-3) and pigs(4) and other various regions of the rat brain(5,6). On the other hand, although tissue kallikrein has extremely high substrate specificity for kininogens, others, such as proinsulin, apolipoprotein B100, atrial natriuretic peptide, Met-enkephalin containing peptide BAM22P, are hydrolyzed by tissue kallikrein in vitro(7). These observations indicate that tissue kallikrein may play an important role in pituitary and brain physiology besides the liberation of kinin. However, in order to elucidate the physiological function(s) of tissue kallikrein, more detailed information on the localization of kallikrein would appear to be essential.

The localization of tissue kallikrein in rat pituitaries and pineal gland was therefore studied by an immunohistochemical technique, using antiserum against rat urinary kallikrein (RUK).

MATERIALS AND METHODS

Antibodies

The RUK used for the preparation of rabbit anti-RUK serum was
purified from the urine of Wistar rats(7) and rabbit antibody
for RUK was produced by the immunization procedures previously
described for human urinary kallikrein(8).

Antisera raised in rabbits against rat luteinizing hormone
(LH), against adrenocorticotrophic hormone(ACTH) were purchased
from Cosmo Bio Co., Ltd(Tokyo, Japan). Antisera raised in
rabbits against rat growth hormone(GH) and against prolactin
were kindly supplied by Dr. A.F.Parlow through the NIADDK
(Bethesda, MD,U.S.A.).

Immunohistochemistry

Wistar rats(7-8 weeks old) were used. Rats were sacrificed by
a transcardiac perfusion technique with a solution of 4%(w/v)
paraformaldehyde in 0.1 M phosphate buffer, pH 7.4, and the
pituitaries and pineal glands were removed and enbedded in
paraffin by standard procedures. Immunostaining for kallikrein
was carried out using an avidin-biotin-horseradish peroxidase
complex(ABC-HRP Vectastain kit, Vector laboratories Inc., Burl-
ingame, CA,U.S.A.). Double immunostaining for kallikrein and
prolactin was carried out using an ABC-HRP and an avidin-biotin
-alkaline phosphatase complex(ABC-AP Vectastain kit), respectively.

Immunoelectron microscopic study

This was carried out by the methods previously reported using
17β-estradiol(ES)-treated rat(9). Namely, in our preliminary
experiments, we observed that the immunostaining intensities of
the kallikrein-positive cells in the anterior pituitaries of
rats at proestrus, postestrus, and diestrus were extremely weak,
while strong immunostaining was noted at estrus on immunohistochemical analysis under a light microscope. We also observed
that the immunostaining intensity of the kallikrein-positive
cells in rats treated with ES was even stronger than that of
rats at estrus. Therefore, ES was subcutaneously injected 5

times into female rats (7 weeks old) at 48 h intervals (1mg/kg
body weight/injection) to facilitate the examination of the
kallikrein-positive cells in the anterior pituitary. Namely,
1.5 mg of ES was dissolved in 100 µl of benzyl alchol, then
900 µl of sesame oil was added. This solution was injected into
the rats (100 µl/150 g body weight). For the control rats, a
mixture of 100 µl of benzyl alchol and 900 µl of sesame oil was
used. Following the last injection, the control rats at estrus
were killed after checking their estrus cycle and the pituitary
glands were dissected out using the method described above.
The ES-treated rats were also killed on the same day as the
control rats.

Animals for immunostaining of pineal gland kallikrein
Rats (7 weeks) were fed *ad libitum* and exposed to a 12-hour
light-dark cycle (light on daily from 8 a.m.- 8 p.m.). After
one week, the rats were sacrificed by the transcardiac perfusion
technique described above.

RESULTS

Identification of kallikrein-positive cells in the anterior
pituitary
Kallikrein-positive cells were detected in the anterior and the
intermediate lobes of the pituitary of both male and female rats
but were not observed in the posterior lobe of the pituitary in
either sex.

Many kallikrein-positive cells were scattered through the
anterior lobe of the pituitary of female rats in estrus. The
positive reaction was restricted to the cytoplasm of the cells,
the nuclei remaining unstained. Next, we tried to identify the
kallikrein-positive cells in the anterior pituitary and the
kallikrein-positive cells in the anterior pituitary of female
rats in estrus were found to correspond to the prolactin-
producing cells by the double immunostaining for both kallikrein

and prolactin, whereas the cells producing GH, LH and ACTH were negative for kallikrein (see color photos in Ref. 7).

The kallikrein-positive cells in the anterior pituitary were further confirmed to be the same as prolactin-producing cells by using an immunoelectron microscopic method. As shown in Fig. 1-a, kallikrein positivity was specifically observed within organelles of certain cells. The immunoreactivity was observed at the Golgi apparatus, the rough endoplasmic reticulum and secretory granules, and the intensity of immunoreactivity varied from granule to glanule (Fig. 1-a and -b). No immuno-reactivity was observed in the nucleus. The secretory granules varied considerably in size and shape (up to 150-620 nm), as is characteristic of prolactin-producing cells. Dilatations of cisternae of rough endoplasmic reticulum and Golgi apparatus were also observed, which are typical untrastructural characte-ristics of prolactin-producing cells(10). No immunoreaction was observed in any of the cells when normal control rabbit serum or preabsorbed anti-RUK serum was used.

Localization of kallikrein in the pineal gland

Kallikrein-immunoreactive substance was observed in the pineal glands in both male and female rats. Figure 2-a shows the result for a female rat. The kallikrein-immunoreactive cells were seen among the cell bodies of the pinealocytes and frequently localized in the perivascular area, although most of the pinealocytes appeared to be negative. A considerable number of immunoreactive cells with a large nucleus similar to those of the pinealocytes were detected. The immunoreactive cytoplasm of these cells extended from their polymorphic cell bodies in the form of processes. Marked immunoreactivity in the perivascular area could be due to these thick immunoreactive processes terminating within or close to the perivascular space. As shown in Fig. 2-b, no immunoreactivity was observed in the control specimens.

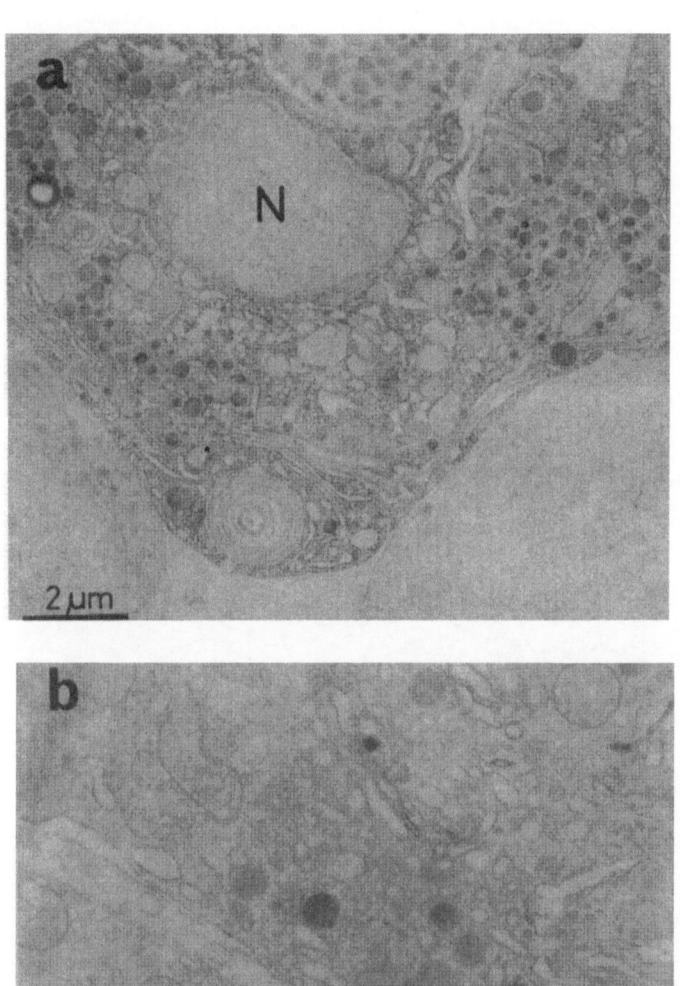

Figure 1.   Immunoelectron microscopic analyses of the kallikrein-positive cells in the anterior pituitary of 17β-estradiol-treated rat.
   N, nucleus.   Magnifications are X8,400 (a) and 17,000 (b).

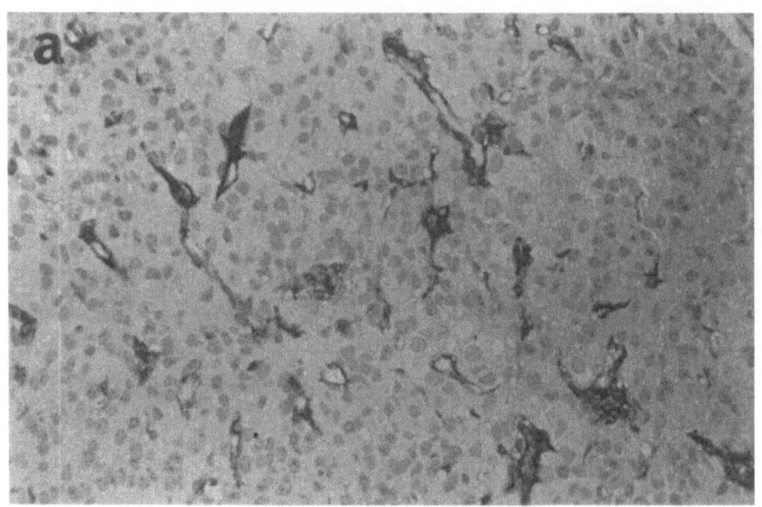

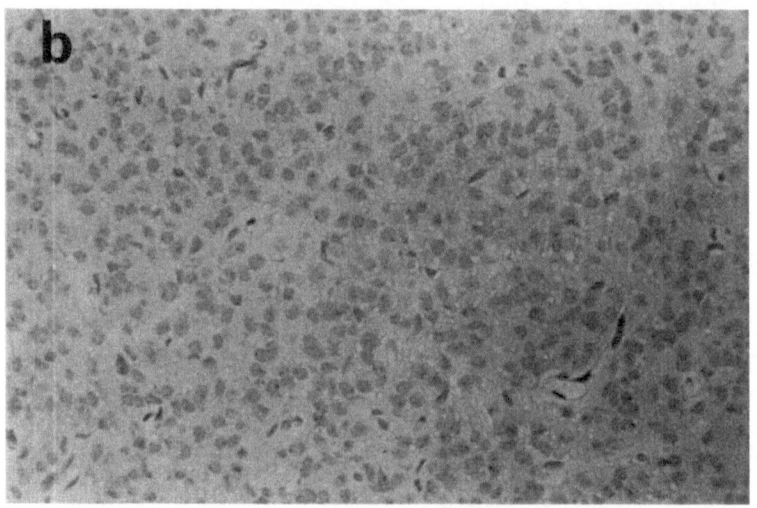

Figure 2. Immunostaining for kallikrein in female rat pineal
gland (a). Control was negative (b).
   Original magnification is X100.

DISCUSSION

We demonstrated by using an immunohistochemical analysis under a light microscopy and an immunoelectron microscopic analysis that the kallikrein-producing cells and the prolactin-producing cells in the anterior pituitary are the same. In the present work, we observed that kallikrein exists in the secretory granules in the prolactin-producing cells in the anterior pituitary and the perivascular area in the pineal glands. Thus, it seems likely that the anterior pituitary and pineal gland secrete kallikrein into the blood vessels, and it is possible to consider that a part of the tissue kallikrein in the plasma originates from the anterior pituitary and pineal gland.

Kallikrein was located in the secretory granules and the Golgi apparatus in the prolactin-producing cells of the anterior pituitary. At present, we have no information of subcellular localization of kallikrein in the pineal gland but if this subcellular localization of kallikrein holds true within the pineal glands, one can speculate that tissue kallikrein may be involved in the processing of some proteins or peptides in both the prolactin-producing cells of the anterior pituitary and the pineal gland because these organelles appear to be sites of the processing of proteins or peptides. However, further detailed biochemical and physiological studies on the function of tissue kallikrein in these glands are necessary. For example, investigations on prokallikrein activator and substrate(s) of kallikrein besides kininogens in these tissues are essential.

ACKNOWLEDGEMENT

We gratefully thank Dr. A.F.Parlow for the gift of antisera for rat prolactin and GH.

REFERENCES

1. Powers CA, Anterior pituitary glandular kallikrein: trypsin activation and estrogen regulation. Mol Cell Endocrinol 1986; 46:163-174.

2. Powers CA, Trypsin activation, partial characterization, and distribution of kallikrein-like and thrombin-like proteases in the neurointermediate lobe of rat pituitary. J Neurochem 1986; 47:145-153.

3. Chao J, Chao L, Christopher C, Swain CC, Tsai J, Margolius HS, Tissue kallikrein in the rat brain and pituitary: Regeonal distribution and estrogen induction in the anterior pituitary. Endocrinology 1987; 120:475-482.

4. Powers CA, Nasjletti A, A novel kinin-generating protease (kininogenase) in the porcine anterior pituitary. J Biol Chem 1982; 257:5594-5600.

5. Scicli AG, Forbes G, Nolly H, Dujovny M, Carretero OA, Kallikrein-kinins in the central nervous system. Clinical and Experimental Hypertension Part A - Theory and Practice 1984; 6(10&11):1731-1738.

6. Shisheva AC, Printz MP, Herman K, Ganten D, Kinin-forming activity in rat brain. Neurochem Int 1985; 7:621-629.

7. Kizuki K, Kitagawa A, Takahashi M, Moriya H, Kudo M, Noguchi T, Immunohistochemical localization of kallikrein within the prolactin-producing cells of the rat anterior pituitary gland. J Endocrinol 1990; 127:317-323.

8. Kizuki K, Kamada M, Ikekita M, Moriya H, Porcine pancreatic prokallikrein. II. Purification and some properties of prokallikrein A. 1982; 30:3354-3361.

9. Kitagawa A, Kizuki K, Moriya H, Kudo M, Noguchi T, Kallikrein- and prolactin-producing cells in the rat anterior pituitary are the same. 1990; 108:971-975.

10. Hymer WC, McShan WH, Christiansen RG, Electron microscopic studies of anterior pituitary glands from lactating and estrogen-treated rats. 1961; 69:81-90.

AAS 38/I
Recent Progress on Kinins
© 1992 Birkhäuser Verlag Basel

CELLULAR LOCALIZATION OF HUMAN KININOGENS

C.D. Figueroa[1], C.B. Gonzalez[2], W. Müller-Esterl[3] and K.D. Bhoola[4]

Institutes of Histology & Pathology[1] and Physiology[2], Austral University Valdivia, Chile; Department of Pathobiochemistry[3], Institute of Physiological Chemistry and Pathobiochemistry, University of Mainz, Germany; Department of Pharmacology[4], University of Bristol, England U.K.

SUMMARY: An immunocytochemical screening using polyclonal and monoclonal anti-kininogen antibodies was performed in various human tissues including blood cells. By comparing the spatial relationship between the cellular localizations of tissue kallikrein and kininogens it was evident that in some tissues both enzyme and substrate were present establishing a close anatomical relationship whereas in others only one of the components could be detected. This pattern of distribution suggests that within various tissues (cells) the major function of either tissue kallikrein (kininogenase, processing enzyme) or kininogen (kinin precursor, cysteine protease inhibitor, kallikrein acceptor molecule) could be different and probably specific to each cell type.

INTRODUCTION

Human kininogens, the endogenous substrates for the kallikreins, are multifunctional molecules which are synthesized by the liver and secreted into the circulation (1,2). Both, high (HK) and low (LK) molecular weight kininogens act as cysteine protease inhibitors (3) and serve as kinin precursor molecules. In addition, HK is involved in the intrinsic blood coagulation cascade (2,4). By activating specific cell receptors, kinins mediate a variety of effects such as increase in vascular permeability, contraction or relaxation of isolated smooth muscle preparations, hypotension, bone resorption and pain (5-8).

It has recently been suggested that kinins may act as paracrine hormones (9). The criteria for a paracrine function of an hormonal system in any tissue are: (i) the presence of the necessary components (enzyme and substrate) for the local generation of hormones, (ii) mechanisms involved in the release of enzyme and substrate, (iii) the presence of receptors (or binding sites) for the hormone, (iv) the functional events related to the hormones, and (v) the metabolizing enzymes for the degradation of the hormones. Many studies have been concerned with the localization of the enzyme, tissue kallikrein in various human and rat tissues however, there is little information concerning the expression of the corresponding substrate, kininogen in those tissues. This study was designed to investigate whether human tissues, in addition to the liver and the kidney contain cells which express immunoreactive kininogen.

MATERIALS AND METHODS

Immunocytochemical methods offer one of the most adventageous approaches to investigate the presence of kininogens in different organs and cells. Moreover, polyclonal or monoclonal antibodies raised against specific regions of the kininogen molecule can be used to elucidate which particular kininogen is present in each of the cell types.

Tissue processing. The human tissues used in this study were kindly provided by the Department of Pathology, National Health Service, Valdivia, Chile. All tissue samples selected for immunocytochemistry corresponded to conserved areas of tissues surgically removed due to inflammation and the presence of adenomas or carcinomas. Tissue fragments were fixed in 10% formaldehyde for 24 h, dehydrated in ethanol and embedded in paraffin wax as previously described (10).

Isolation of human neutrophils. Neutrophils were isolated from whole anticoagulated human blood using dextran sedimentation and Ficoll-Hypaque centrifugacion (11). Briefly, 20 ml of blood were mixed with 20 ml of 6% dextran-0.9% NaCl (M_r 266,000, Sigma Chemicals, U.S.A.) and 60 ml of PBS-0.4% sodium citrate. After 15 min the upper leucocyte-enriched plasma was gently layered over Ficoll-Hypaque (Pharmacia-LKB Biotechnology, Sweden) and centrifuged at 400 g for 20 min at 20°C. The cell pellet was resuspended in an erythrocyte lysis buffer composed of 155 mM NH_4Cl, 2.7 mM $KHCO_3$ and 3.7 mM EDTA. The suspension was centrifuged at 400 g for 10 min and the cell pellet was washed three times in excess of PBS-0.4% sodium citrate pH 7.4. Finally, the cells were resuspended in PBS containing 2% normal human or goat serum to block Fc receptors present on the leucocyte surface and then were immunostained in suspension or on cell smears (11). Smears containing all blood cellular components were prepared after dextran sedimentation.

Antibodies to human kinonogens. Six different antibodies which recognize HK (I-108, HKL-16 and HKL-10), LK (LKL-3 and R7) or HK and LK (III-279) were used to localize kininogens in various human tissues and isolated blood cells (Table 1).

Table 1.   **Characteristics of kininogen antibodies**

III-279	PoAb against LK (rabbit). It cross-react with HK
I-108	PoAb against HK (sheep) < 5% cross-reactivity with LK
HKL-16	MoAb directed against residues 569-595 of the HK light chain (prekallikrein binding site)
HKL-10	MoAb directed against residues 402-420 of the HK light chain (NH$_2$-terminal portion of the His-rich region)
LKL-3	MoAb raised against the synthetic peptide: NH$_2$-Cys-Gly-Try-Lys-Gly-Arg-Pro-Pro-Lys-Ala-Gly-Ala-Gln-Pro-Ala-Ser-Glu-Arg-Glu-Val-Ser-COOH, corresponding to residues 389-409 of the LK light chain
R7	PoAb directed to the same LK portion as LKL-3

PoAb = Polyclonal antibody; MoAb = Monoclonal antibody

Immunocytochemistry.   Tissue sections (5 μm thick) were dewaxed, rehydrated and incubated with polyclonal anti-kininogen sera (1:300 to 1:2000) followed by a sandwich peroxidase-anti-peroxidase method as previously described (10). Visualization of bound antibody was achieved by incubation in a diaminobenzidine (0.1%)-hydrogen peroxide (0.03%) solution. Monoclonal antibodies recognized HK or LK only when frozen sections were used. Smears prepared using isolated blood leucocytes were immunostained according with the immunogold-silver staining method to avoid interference with neutrophil myeloperoxidase. Both tissue sections and cell smears were lightly counterstained with haematoxylin, dehydrated and mounted in Canada balsam.

Aliquots of non-fixed neutrophils were immunostained in the presence of 0.2% sodium azide, to prevent internalization of the antibody by the cells. Goat anti-rabbit or anti-mouse IgG labelled with 30 nm and 10 nm gold particles respectively were used to visualize the bound antibodies. After immunostaining was completed, the neutrophils were fixed with 5% glutaraldehyde, post-fixed with 1% osmium tetroxide and embedded in epon-araldite as described elsewhere (11).

Immunocytochemical controls.   Controls included omission of the first antibody or replacement of the kininogen antibodies by non-immune sera or unrelated IgG of the same species.

C. D. Figueroa et al.

RESULTS

A list of the human tissues included in this study and their reactivity to the various kininogen antibodies is shown in Table 2. It can be observed that some tissues contain both kininogen and the enzyme tissue kallikrein (kidney, submaxillary gland, sweat glands and neutrophils; Figs. 1-11) while others display immunoreactivity only to tissue kallikrein (tracheo-bronchial glands, pancreas, pituitary, stomach and gallbladder) or kininogen (liver, platelets, endometrial glands, large blood vessels and arterioles; see Table 2 and Figs. 1-11).

Table 2.   **Cellular localization of human kininogens**

Organ (cell)	PoAb		MoAb	
	LK/HK	HK	HK[a]	LK[a]
Liver (hepatocytes)	+	+	+	+
Nasopharynx[b]	-	-	-	-
Trachea[b]	-	-	-	-
Lung	-	-		
Pancreas[b]	-	-		
Kidney[b] (principal cells)	+	±		
Sweat glands[b] (dark cells)	+	+	+	+
SMG[b] (acinar cells)	±	+		
Pituitary[b]	-	-		
Stomach[b]	-	-		
Gallbladder[b]	-	-		
Blood (neutrophils)[b]	+	+		+
(platelets)	+	+		
Breast	-	-		
Ovary	-	-		
Fallopian tube	-	-		
Uterus				
endometrium (glands)	+	+		
myometrium (arterioles)	+	+		
Prostate	-	-		
Blood vessels				
large vessels (EC)	+	+		
arterioles (SMC)	+	+		

[a] Immunocytochemistry performed on frozen sections. EC= endothelial cells; SMC= smooth muscle cells; SMG= submaxillary gland.   [b] Tissues in which glandular kallikrein was also detected.   + = presence; − = Absence; ± = weak immunoreactivity. PoAb= Polyclonal antibody; MoAb= Monoclonal antibody.

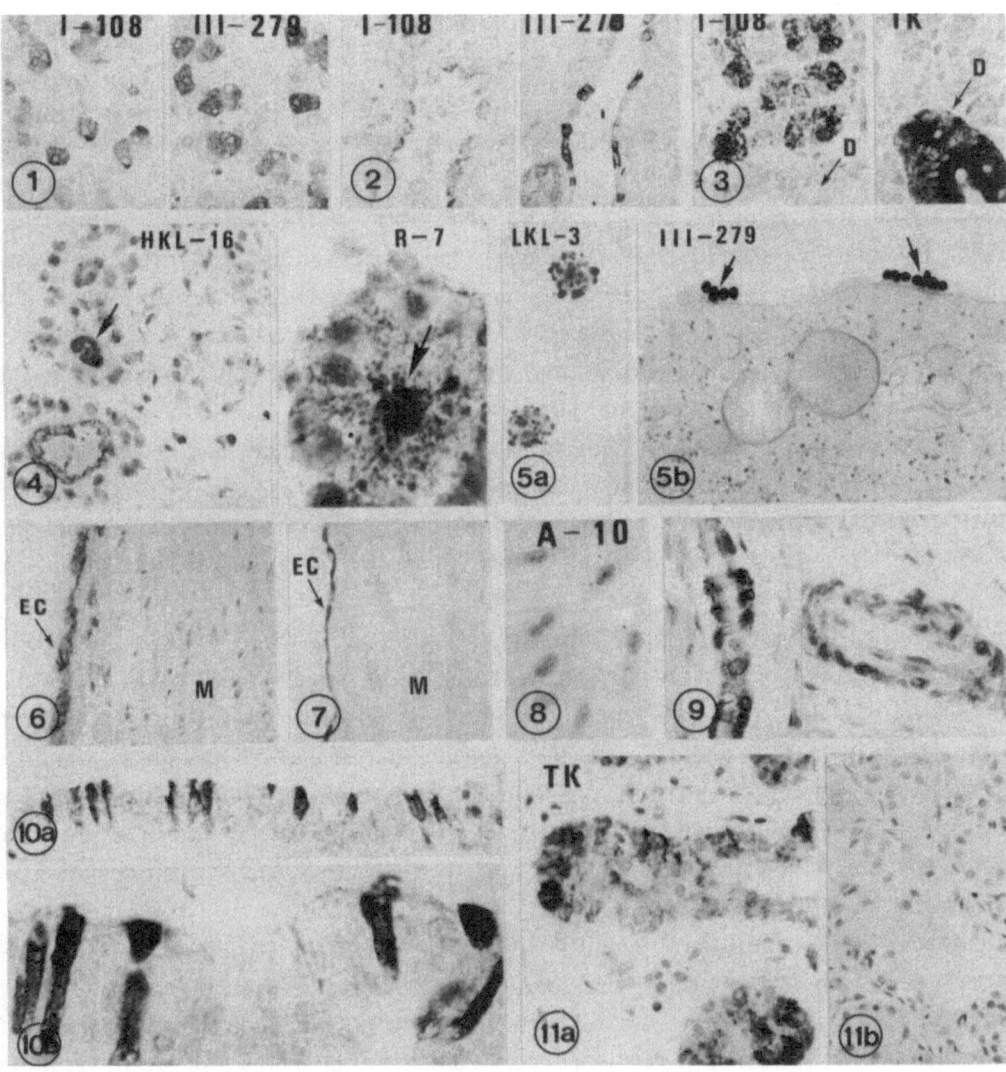

Figs. 1-3 Immunoreactive kininogen in human liver (**Fig. 1**), in renal collecting ducts (**Fig. 2**) and in submaxillary gland acini (**Fig. 3**). Submaxillary gland ducts (D) are devoid of HK but contain tissue kallikrein (TK); **Fig. 4** Sweat glands; **Fig. 5** Human neutrophils at light (a) and electron (b) microscopy. Immunogold particles (arrows) localize on the plasma membrane; Human (**Fig. 6**) and rat (**Fig. 7**) aorta show kininogen only in endothelial cells (EC) whereas the media layer (M) and A-10 cells in culture (**Fig. 8**) remain unstained; **Fig. 9** Uterine arterioles; **Fig. 10** Endometrial glandular epithelium at low (a) and high (b) power; **Fig. 11** Respiratory mucosa. Only TK (a) is present in the serous glands (arrows), (b) kininogen.

DISCUSSION

For many years the presence of kininogens was thought to be restricted to liver and plasma however, more recent studies have shown that these molecules are expressed by several other cell types such as, collecting duct cells of the human kidney (10,12), dark cells of sweat glands (13), platelets (14,15), endothelial cells (16,17) and human neutrophils (11,18,19). Our study confirmed the existence of kininogens in these cells and describes for the first time the presence of the kinin precursors in acinar cells of human submaxillary gland, in smooth muscle cells of arterioles and in some epithelial cells of the human endometrial glands during the early secretory phase. Immunoreactivity to kininogen in the human submaxillary gland seems to be similar to that reported by Chao et al. (20) in the rat after acute-phase inflammation. With the exception of liver, kidney and endothelial cells (1,16,21), kininogen biosynthesis (e.i. specific [^{35}S] incorporation) or mRNA expression has not been demonstrated in other human tissues leaving the question open whether the kininogens are synthesized by these cells or are taken up from plasma or other biological fluids.

An interesting observation became apparent after comparing the cellular localization of kininogens with that of the enzyme tissue kallikrein in the human kidney, sweat glands and submaxillary gland. At these sites the cells that contain the enzyme and its substrate are in close proximity one to another. Given a concomitant release of the enzyme and its substrate(s), this morphological relationship would support the idea that the major function of kininogens in these tissues would be to serve as kinin precursor molecules (Fig. 12). Kinins formed in this paracrine manner may in turn participate in the regulation of electrolyte and/or local blood flow.

Unexpectedly, immunoreactive kininogen was also found in smooth muscle cells of arterioles in various human tissues and specially in the uterus. This localization contrasted with that seen in large blood vessels like the human aorta and umbilical blood vessels where the substrate was restricted to endothelial cells. Similarly, the media layer of the rat aorta (the only non-human tissue included in this study) and a cell line derived from aortic smooth muscle cells (A-10 cells) were both devoid of staining. These results therefore differ from those of Oza et al. (22) who detected release of kinins by trypsin in homogenates prepared from rat aorta denuded of endothelium and from rat aortic smooth muscle cells in culture. At present we cannot exclude the possibility that the higher sensitivity of the methods used by Oza et al. (22) results in the observed discrepancies.

This study describes for the first time the presence of kininogen in human uterus. In the rat, however, the isolated estrogenized uterus has been reported to contain kininogen (23-

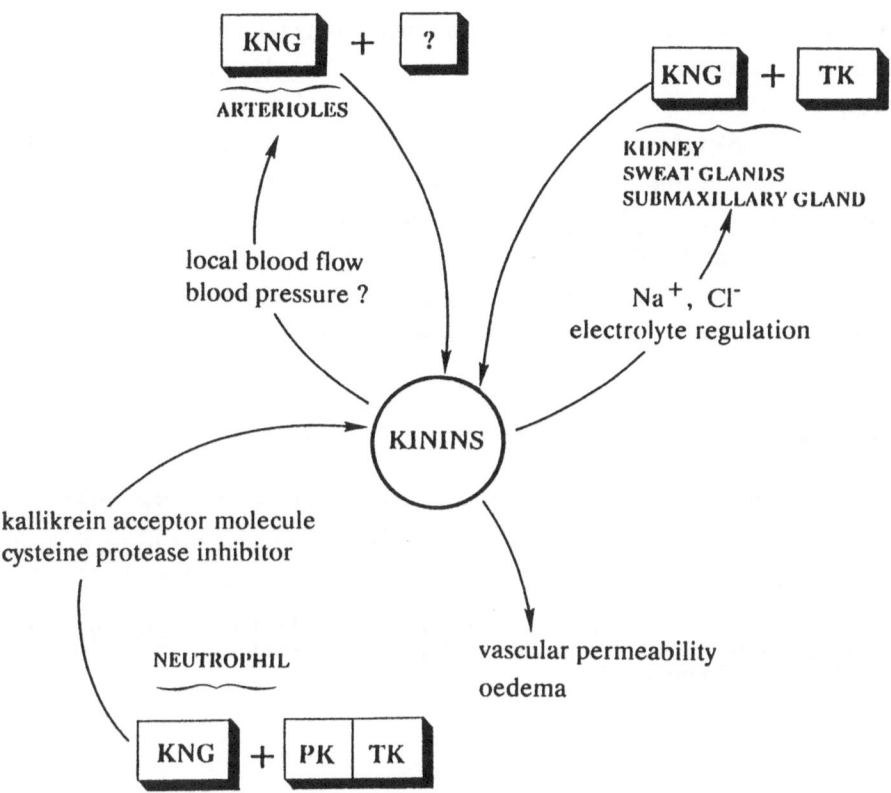

Fig. 12 Schematic representation of the possible roles of kininogen (KNG) in various tissues and in neutrophils. PK = plasma kallikrein; TK = tissue kallikrein.

26) thereby providing a rational basis for the well known contractile response of this tissue to glandular kallikrein. Recent studies show that kininogen is present in the uterine tissue in a concentration of 1.5 $\pm$ 0.3 ng of bradykinin equivalents per mg wet wt and that no more than 15% of this amount would be due to plasma contamination (26). On the other hand, approximately 80% of this kininogen was resistant to tissue kallikrein but, sensitive to trypsin suggesting that in the rat, some of the uterine kininogen would correspond to T-kininogen.

Isolated human neutrophils have been reported to contain HK and possess receptors for this molecule on its surface (18). We found that both HK and LK localized as clusters of immunogold particles on the cell membrane. Similar high affinity binding sites are present on endothelial cells and platelets (27,28). It could be suggested that kininogens anchored to specific cell receptors may serve two functions: (i) in the case of platelets and endothelial cells HK may act as an acceptor protein for plasma kallikrein and factor XI which could locally initiate and propagate the intrinsic coagulation cascade and the kinin-generating pathway. (ii) In the case of neutrophils, proteolytic cleavage of surface bound LK and HK by tissue (29,30) and plasma kallikrein respectively (or another leucocyte kininogenase) could produce a discrete and circumscribed formation of kinins that may in turn facilitate the local diapedesis of neutrophils and oedema formation during acute inflammation.

ACKNOWLEDGMENTS

We would like to thank Dr M.T. Poblete and Mr J. Delannoy of the Department of Pathology, National Health Service, Valdivia, Chile for their valuable help in collecting the specimens used in this study. We also wish to thank Mrs G. Garces for her technical assistance.

This work was supported by FONDECYT, (91/0961) and DID-UACH (S/91/32), Chile; the Deutsche Forschungsgemeinschaft and the Fonds der Chemischen Industrie, Germany; and the Medical Research Council, U.K.

REFERENCES

1. Nakanishi S.   Substance P precursor and kininogen: their structures, gene organizations, and regulation. Physiol Rev 1987; **67**:1117-1142.

2. Müller-Esterl W.   Kininogens, kinins and kinships. Thromb Haemostas 1989; **61**:2-6.

3. Müller-Esterl W.   Novel functions of kininogens. Semin Thromb Hemostas 1987; **13**:115-126.

4. Kaplan AP, Silverberg M.   The coagulation-kinin pathway of human plasma. Blood 1987; **70**:1-15.

5. Bhoola KD, Calle JD, Schachter M.   The effect of bradykinin, serum kallikrein and other endogenous substances on capillary permeability in the guinea pig. J Physiol (Lond) 1960; **152**:75-86.

6. Frey EK, Kraut H, Werle E. Kallikrein (Padutin). Enke, Stuttgart, 1950.

7. Lerner UH, Jones IJ, Gustafson GT.   Bradykinin, a new potential mediator of inflammation-induced bone resorption. Arth Rheum 1987; **30**:530-540.

8. Whalley ET, Clegg S, Stewart JM, Vavrek RJ. The effect of kinin agonists and antagonists on the pain response of the human blister base. Naunyn-Schmiedeberg's Arch Pharmacol 1987; 336:652-655.

9. Carretero OA, Scicli AG. Kinins, paracrine hormones, in the regulation of blood flow, renal function, and blood pressure. In: Endocrine Mechanisms in Hypertension. Laragh JH, Brenner BM, Kaplan NM, editors. New York: Raven Press, 1989: 219-239.

10 Figueroa CD, MacIver AG, Mackenzie JC, Bhoola KD. Localisation of immunoreactive kininogen and tissue kallikrein in the human nephron. Histochemistry 1988; 89:437-442.

11. Figueroa CD, Henderson LM, Kaufmann J, De la Cadena RA, Colman RW, Muller-Esterl W, Bhoola KD. Immunovisualisation of high (HK) and low (LK) molecular weight kininogens on isolated human neutrophils. Blood 1992; (in press).

12. Proud D, Perkins M, Pierce JV, Yates K, Highet P, Herrig P, Mark MM, Bahu R, Carone F, Pisano JJ. Characterization and localization of human renal kininogen. J Biol Chem 1981; 256:10634-10639.

13. Poblete MT, Reynolds NJ, Figueroa CD, Burton JL, Müller-Esterl W, Bhoola KD. Tissue kallikrein and kininogen in human sweat glands and psoriatic skin. Br J Dermatol 1991; 124:236-241.

14. Schmaier AH, Zuckerberg A, Silverman C, Kuchibhotla J, Tuszynski GP, Colman RW. High molecular weight kininogen. A secreted platelet protein. J Clin Invest 1983; 71:1477-1489.

15. Schmaier AH, Smith PM, Purdon AD, White JG, Colman RW. High molecular weight kininogen: localization in the unstimulated and activated platelet and activation by platelet calpain(s). Blood 1986; 67:119-130.

16. Schmaier AH, Kuo A, Lundberg D, Murray S, Cines DB. The expression of high molecular weight kininogen on umbilical vein endothelial cells. J Biol Chem 1988; 263:16327-16333.

17. van Iwaarden F, de Groot PG, Sixma JJ, Berrittini M, Bouma BN. High molecular weight kininogen is present in cultured human endothelial cells: Localization, isolation and characterization. Blood 1988; 71:1268-1276.

18. Gustafson EJ, Schmaier AH, Wachtfogel YT, Kaufman N, Kucich U, Colman RW. Human neutrophils contain and bind high molecular weight kininogen. J Clin Invest 1989; 84:28-35.

19. Figueroa CD, Henderson LM, Colman RW, De la Cadena RA, Müller-Esterl W, Bhoola KD. Immunoreactive H- and L-kininogens in human neutrophils. J Physiol (Lond) 1990; 425:65P.

20. Chao J, Swain C, Chao S, Xiong W, Chao L. Tissue distribution and kininogen gene expression after acute-phase inflammation. Biochim Biophys Acta 1988; 964:329-339.

21. Iwai N, Matsunaga M, Kita T, Tei M, Kawai C. Detection of low molecular weight kininogen messenger RNA in human kidney. J Hypertens 1988; **6 (Suppl)**:399-400.

22. Oza NB, Schwartz JH, Goud HD, Levinsky NG. Rat aortic smooth muscle cells in culture express kallikrein, kininogen, and bradykininase activity. J Clin Invest 1990; **85**:597-600.

23. Nustad K, Pierce JV. Purification of rat urinary kallikreins and their specific antibody. Biochemistry 1974; **13**:2312-2319.

24. Beraldo WT, Lauar NS, Siqueira GRT, Heneine IF, Catanzaro OL. Pecularities of the oxytocic action of rat urinary kallikrein. In: Chemistry and Biology of the Kallikrein-Kinin System in Health and Disease. Pisano JJ, Austen KF, editors. DHEW Publication (NIH). Bethesda, MD. 1976: 375-378.

25. Figueiredo AFS, Salgado AHI, Siqueira GRT, Velloso CR, Beraldo WT. Rat uterine contraction by kallikrein and its dependence on uterine kininogen. Biochem Pharmacol 1990; **39**:763-767.

26. Orce GG, Carretero OA, Scicli G, Scicli AG. Kinins contribute to the contractile effects of rat glandular kallikrein on the isolated rat uterus. J Pharmacol Exp Ther 1989; **249**:470-475.

27. van Iwaarden F, de Groot PG, Bouma BN. The binding of high molecular weight kininogen to cultured human endothelial cells. J Biol Chem 1988; **263**:4698-4703.

28. Greengard JS, Griffin JH. Receptors for high molecular weight kininogen on stimulated washed human platelets. Biochemistry 1984; **23**:6863-6869.

29. Figueroa CD, MacIver AG, Bhoola KD. Identification of a tissue kallikrein in human polymorphonuclear leucocytes. Br J Haematol 1989; **72**:321-328.

30. Cohen WM, Wu H, Featherstone GL, Jenzano JW, Lundblad RL. Linkage between blood coagulation and inflammation: Stimulation of neutrophil tissue kallikrein by thrombin. Biochem Biophys Res Comm 1991; **176**:315-320.

AAS 38/I
Recent Progress on Kinins
© 1992 Birkhäuser Verlag Basel

IMMUNOLOCALIZATION OF HIGH MOLECULAR WEIGHT KININOGEN (HKg) AND T KININOGEN (TKg) IN THE RAT HYPOTHALAMUS

J.P. Richoux, J. Bouhnik*, G. Grignon and F. Alhenc-Gelas*

Laboratoire d'Histologie-Embryologie, Faculté de Médecine, BP 184, F 54505
Vandoeuvre-les-Nancy Cedex. *INSERM U-36, 17, rue du Fer à Moulin, F 75005
Paris

SUMMARY: Specific HKg immunostaining detected with antiserum against the
light chain (LC) of HKg was restricted to SRIF neurons of the hypothalamic
periventricular area projecting to median eminence (ME). Heavy chain (HC) immunoreactivity related to HKg and/or low molecular weight kininogen (LKg) was
found in some other hypothalamic territories. Specific TKg was mainly associated with vasopressin in neurons of suprachiasmatic (SCN), supraoptic (SON)
and paraventricular (PVN) nuclei. By direct RIA, hypothalamus was found to
contain the highest level of TKg (10ng/mg protein) and after trypsin hydrolysis and HPLC separation of kinins, 10,3 pg BK and 7,3 pg T-kinin/mg protein.

INTRODUCTION

Recently, some components of the kallikrein-kinin system have been demonstrated in the brain. Kinin releasing enzymes (kallikreins) have been identified
by direct RIA, in vitro biosynthesis (1) and mRNA hybridization (2). Bradykinin (BK) was detected in rat hypothalamus by immunocytochemistry in first (3)
and combined HPLC and RIA (4,5).

BK receptors have been characterized using biochemistry (6,7,8) and autoradiography (9). Kinin destroying enzyme (converting enzyme) has been found in
some brain area by immunocytochemistry (10), captopril autoradiography
(11,12) and biochemistry (13,14). Presence of kininogens (kinin precursors)
has been documented only indirectly after trypsin hydrolysis and RIA of re-

leased kinins from brain extracts (4) or CSF (15). In the rat three kininogens have been identified in the plasma (16): HKg and LKg susceptible to kallikreins (BK release) and produced from the same gene; TKg which is kallikrein resistant and releases T-kinin under trypsin hydrolysis. HKg, LKg and TKg mRNA are very homologous but are differentially regulated. In addition, the three kininogens are cysteine proteinase inhibitors through their highly homologous HC. In this report, we identify specifically two kinin precursors in the rat hypothalamus using both immunocytochemistry and biochemistry.

MATERIALS AND METHODS

Antisera. Rabbit anti-rat TKg and HKg, mouse monoclonal anti-TKg have been described previously (17,18,19); LC of HKg was obtained (20) and specific LC antiserum raised in rabbit.

Kininogen biochemistry in cerebellum and hypothalamus. TKg and HKg RIAs have been reported elsewhere (17,18,21). Kinin contents of brain homogenates were measured by RIA (22) after trypsin hydrolysis before and after HPLC kinin separation.

Immunocytochemistry. Wistar control and dehydrated rats by drinking water deprivation, homozygous and heterozygous Brattleboro rats were used in this study. Half receives intracisternal colchicine injection (100ug/50ul saline) before sacrifice. Brains were fixed by perfusion (Bouin-Hollande + glutaraldehyde) and embedded in paraplast.

Immunocytochemistry and controls were performed as follow : diluted primary antiserum 24h at 4°C; biotinylated IgG anti-rabbit 1/250th for 45 min; Streptavidine-peroxidase conjugate 1/600th for 30 min. Peroxidase activity was detected using DAB 0.01%, H2O2 0.003%. HKg-gel, HC(HKg)-gel, TKg-gel were used for specificity tests and cross reactivity study.

RESULTS

Biochemistry. TKg RIA gives mean values of 10ng TKg/mg protein of hypothalamus and 5,3ng TKg/mg protein of cerebellum. Unfortunately, dilution curves of brain homogenates are not parallel to standard curve of HKg. Trypsin releases high level of immunoreactive BK in hypothalamus, and HPLC separation allows to detect 10,3 pg BK and 7,3pg T kinin per mg protein in the hypothalamus.

HKg specific immunostaining. Antiserum directed against the specific LC of HKg or HKg antiserum exhausted with HC (HKg)-gel allows to stain bipolar neurons of the periventricular area of the hypothalamus (fig.1) and their projections and terminals in external zone of ME (fig.2). Colchicine enhances greatly the number of positive neurons and the intensity of the staining which is specifically abolished by preadsorption with HKg-gel. These neurons are SRIF neurons.

HC immunostaining. The diluted unadsorbed HKg antiserum stains magnocellular mostly oxytocinergic neurons in PVN (fig.3), SCN and parvocellular SRIF neurons in SCN. In addition, HC positive cell bodies only stain after colchicine in arcuate nucleus, lateral and dorso median hypothalamus. LC antiserum does not stain these neurons whereas preadsorption of HKg antiserum with HC-gel inhibits the detection. Thus, HC immunoreactivity may be due to LKg and/or HKg.

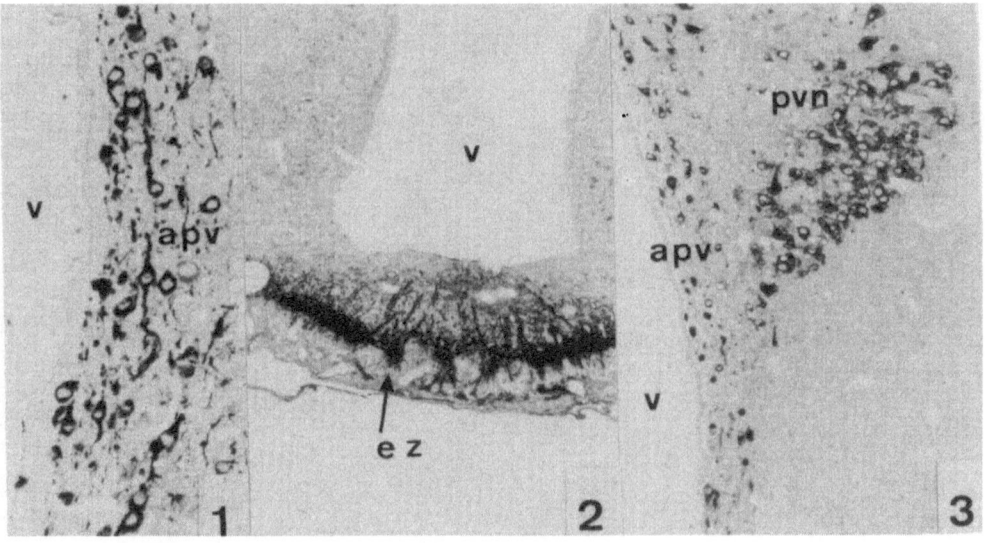

Fig. 1: Demonstration of specific HKg using LC (HKg) antiserum in cell bodies of pva (X 320). **Fig. 2:** These LC (HKg) specific positive neurons project to the external zone (ez) of median eminence (X 130). **Fig. 3:** HKg staining using unadsorbed HKg antiserum; note the presence of positive HKg bipolar neurons (LC specific) in the periventricular area (pva) and magnocellular neurons (related to HC) in paraventricular nucleus. (pvn) (X 130).

TKg immunostaining. In absence of colchicine treatment, no cell body stains. Colchicine allows to detect positive TKg neurons in all rat strains studied, except homozygous Brattleboro. The specific staining occurs only in PVN-SON magnocellular vasopressinergic neurons of the hypothalamo-neurohypohysial system (fig.4). Fibers are easily detectable throughout the hypothalamus and in the internal zone of ME (fig.5) but rarely in the neural lobe. TKg is undetectable in homozygous Brattleboro but reappears in the heterozygous. In dehydrated Wistar rat, TKg staining disappears at the level of cell bodies, even after colchicine. Monoclonal and polyclonal antibodies reveal the same neurons and fibers. Adsorption of TKg with TKg-gel abolishes specifically the staining whereas HKg-gel has no effect.

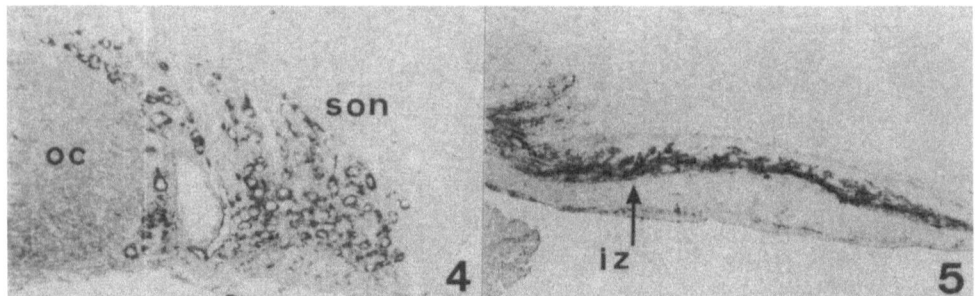

Fig. 4: Specific TKg immunostaining in magnocellular neurons of the supraoptic nucleus (son). **Fig. 5:** TKg containing neurons project towards the internal zone (iz) of median eminence (X 130). v: third ventricle; oc: optic chiasma.

DISCUSSION

The present study is the first specific immunocytochemical localization of two kinin precursors, HKg and TKg in rat hypothalamus. In parallel, we have identified TKg by direct RIA and BK and T-kinin after HPLC separation of released kinin by trypsin hydrolysis.

Immunocytochemical identification of HKg in neurons requires the use of antibodies directed against the specific LC, since HKg and LKg have a identical
HC. In this way, specific LC (HKg) antiserum and HC antibody free HKg antiserum allowed us to define a specific HKg system related to the SRIF periventricular hypothalamic system. However, few positive BK neurons and fibers have been reported in this area (3). HC immunoreactivity related to HKg and LKg
colocate mostly with other known major peptides (SRIF, oxytocin) in various
neuron systems.

Presence of BK precursor in magnocellular neurons of the hypothalamo-neurohy-
pophyseal system agrees with the highest concentration of BK measured in
hypothalamus and neurohypophysis (5). Presence of a wide HC neuron system
scattered throughout the dorsomedian and lateral hypothalamus parallels with
BK staining previously reported (3). But full identification of HC immunoreactivity requires isolation of pure LC of LKg and production of specific
antisera. Finally, biochemical measurement of true BK parallels with K kininogen immunostaining. Our data are in good agreement with earliest biochemical BK determinations (4,24).

TKg appears closely associated with vasopressin. Tkg immunostaining and RIA
agree with the recent demonstration of TKg mRNA in the brain (23). Moreover,
high molecular weight TKg protein (24) and mRNA (23) have been detected in
the brain. Our TKg antibodies could cross-react with this compound of which
the gene is unidentified as yet. TKg immunostaining parallels with vasopressin during stimulation of the vasopressinergic system, since both TKg and vasopressin staining disappears at the perikarya level during drinking deprivation. In the same way, altered vasopressin biosynthesis in homozygous Brattleboro rat is accompanied by the complete loss of TKg staining.

K kininogens could act as BK precursors in neurons. Endogenous BK could be
coreleased together with the major hormones SRIF, oxytocin and vasopressin to
modulate the release of these peptides at the terminal level. BK might have
also a releasing factor activity on secretion of some antehypophyseal hormones (25). In interneurons (SCN, dorsomedian and lateral hypothalamus), BK
could play the role of neuromodulator-neurotransmitter.

The role of TKg is unknown, since no T kinin releasing enzyme has been reported in the brain as yet. Because HKg, LKg and TKg are powerfull cysteine proteinase inhibitors, it can be proposed that these compounds are implicated in
peptidic hormone maturation and inactivation processes.

REFERENCES

1. Chao J, Woodley C, Chao L, Margolius HS. Identification of tissue kallikrein in brain and in the cell free translation product encoded by brain
   mRNA. J Biol Chem 1983; 258:15173-15178.

2. Chao J, Chao L, Swain CC, Tsai JJ, Margolius HS. Tissue kallikrein in rat
   brain and pituitary: regional distribution and estrogen induction in the
   anterior pituitary. Endocrinology 1987; 120:465-482.

3. Corrêa FMA, Innis RB, Uhl GR, Snyder SH. Bradykinin like immunoreactive
   neuronal systems localized histochemically in rat brain. Proc Natl Acad
   Sci USA 1979; 76:1489-1493.

4. Perry DC, Snyder SH. Identification of bradykinin in mammalian brain. J
   Neurochem 1984; 43:1072-1080.

5. Kariya K, Yamauchi A, Sasaki T. Regional distribution and characterization of kinin in the CNS of the rat. J Neurochem 1985; 44:1892-1897.

6. Lewis RE, Childers SR, Philipps MI.[^{125}I] Tyr-Bradykinin binding in pri
   mary rat brain cultures. Brain Res 1985; 346:263-272.

7. Fujiwara Y, Mantique CR, Yamamura HI. Identification of ß bradykinin bin
   ding sites in guinea-pig brain. Eur J Pharmacol 1988; 147:487-488.

8. Lee RTW, Lolait SJ, Muller JM. Molecular characteristics and peptide specificity of bradykinin binding sites in intact neuroblastoma glioma cells
   inculture (NG 108-15). Neuropeptides 1989; 14:51-57.

9. Steranka LR, Manning DC, Dehaas CJ, Ferkany JW, Borosky SA, Connor JR,
   Vavrek RJ, Stewar JM, Snyder SH. Bradykinin as a pain mediator: receptor
   are localized to sensory neurons, and antagonists have analgesic actions.
   Proc Natl Acad Sci USA 1988; 85:3245-3249.

10. Defendini R, Zimmerman EA, Weare JA, Alhenc-Gelas F, Erdös Eg. Angioten-
    sin-converting enzyme in epithelial and neuroepithelial cells. Neuroendo-
    crinology 1983; 37:32-40.

11. Strittmatter SM, De Souza EB, Lynch DR, Snyder SH. Angiotensin-converting
    enzyme localized in the rat pituitary and adrenal glands by [^{3}H] capto-
    pril autoradiography. Endocrinology 1986; 118:1690-1699.

12. Corrêa FMA, Plunkett LM, Saavedra JM. Quantitative distribution of angio-
    tensin-converting enzyme (kininase II) in discrete areas of the rat brain
    by autoradiography with computerized microdensitometry. Brain Res 1986;
    375:259-266.

13. Saavedra JM, Fernandez Pardal J, Chevillard C. Angiotensin-converting en-
    zyme in discrete areas of the rat forebrain and pituitary gland. Brain
    Res. 1982; 245:317-326.

14. Chevillard C, Niwa M, Saavedra JM. Angiotensin-converting enzyme in discrete forebrain areas of spontaneously hypertensive rats. Brain Res 1984; 309:389-392.

15. Scicli AG, Forbes G, Nolly H, Dujovny M, Carretero OA. Kallikrein-kinins in the central nervous system. Clin Exp Hypertens 1984; A6:1731-1738.

16. Nakanishi S. Substance P precursor and kininogen: their structures, gene organizations and regulation. Physiol Rev 1987; 67:1117-1142.

17. Baussant T, Michaud A, Bouhnik J, Savoie F, Alhenc-Gelas F, Corvol P. Effect of dexamethasone on kininogen production by a rat hepatoma cell line. Biochem Biophys Res Commun 1988; 154:1160-1165.

18. Suzuki H, Alhenc-Gelas F, Bouhnik J, Corvol P, Menard J. Differential effects of nephrectomy and surgery on plasma kininogens and angiotensinogen in the rat. Endocrinology 1988; 122:2809-2815.

19. Lesage S, Bouhnik J, Richoux JP, Baussant T, Gauthier F, Eager K, Corvol P, Alhenc-Gelas F. Immunological characterization of rat kininogens with monoclonal antibodies to T-kininogen. Distinction between the different domains of T-kininogen and the multiple rat kininogens. Eur J Biochem 1992; in press.

20. Kerbiriou DM, Griffin JH. Human high molecular weight kininogen: studies of structure-function relationships and of proteolysis of the molecule oc curing during contact activation of plasma. J Biol Chem 1979; 254:12020-12027.

21. Bouhnik J, Baussant T, Savoie F, Alhenc-Gelas F, Gauthier F, Esnard F. Di rect radioimmunoassay for rat T-kininogen. Biochem Biophys Res Commun 1987; 144:1090-1097.

22. Alhenc-Gelas F, Marchetti J, Allegrini J, Corvol P, Menard J. Measurement of urinary kallikrein activity. Species differences in kinin production. Biochem Biophys Acta 1981; 677:477-488.

23. Mann EA, Lingrel JB. Developmental and tissue specific expression of rat T-Kininogen. Biochem Biophys Res Commun 1991; 174:417-423.

24. Marks N, Stern F, Chi LM, Berg MJ. Diversity of rat brain cysteine protei nase inhibitors: isolation of low molecular weight cystatins and a higher molecular weight T-Kininogen like glycoprotein. Arch Biochem Biophys 1988; 267:448-458.

25. Drouhault R, Abrous N, David JP, Dufy B. Bradykinin parallels thyrotropin-releasing hormone actions on prolactin release from rat anterior pituitary cells. Neuroendocrinology 1987; 46:360-364.